D1432717

STRESS A-Z

STRESS A-Z

A SOURCEBOOK FOR FACING EVERYDAY CHALLENGES

ADA P. KAHN, PH.D.

Facts On File, Inc.

Stress A–Z: A Sourcebook for Facing Everyday Challenges

Copyright © 1998 by Ada P. Kahn, Ph.D.

Facts On File, Inc.
11 Penn Plaza
New York NY 10001

Library of Congress Cataloging-in-Publication Data

98-99

Kahn, Ada P.
Stress A–Z / Ada P. Kahn.
390 p.   cm.
Includes bibliographical references and index.
ISBN 0-8160-3295-5
1. Stress, Physiology—Encyclopedias. 2. Stress, Psychology—Encyclopedias. I. Title.
QP82.2.S8K34   1998
616.9'8—dc21   97-51580

Cover design by Cathy Rincon

Printed in the United States of America

MP Hermitage 10 9 8 7 6 5 4 3 2 1

This book is printed on acid-free paper.

CONTENTS

ACKNOWLEDGMENTS

ADVISORY BOARD:

J. Sean Callan, M.D.   Dr. Callan has more than 30 years of clinical and administrative experience in medicine. He is a surveyor for the Joint Commission on Accreditation of Health Care Organizations (JCAHO). Dr. Callan is certified by the American Board of Psychiatry and Neurology and has served as medical editor of the American Medical Association's *AMA/Medicine Today,* a weekly nationwide television program. He was also a contributing editor of the *Journal of the American Medical Association* and at one time published *Good Health,* a medical newspaper for the general public. He has written *Your Guide to Mental Health,* a consumer's guide to psychiatry, and edited *The Physician* and *The Family Medical Guide.*

Delbert H. Meyer, M.D.   Dr. Meyer, a native of Oklahoma with more than 30 years' experience in medicine, performed his graduate studies at the Kansas University School of Medicine and served his internship and residency at Wayne County General Hospital at the University of Michigan. He is a member of the American Thoracic Society, the American College of Chest Physicians, the California Medical Association and the American Medical Association. He is a clinical instructor at the University of California at Davis, California, and a medical adviser for the School of Respiratory Therapy at American River College in Sacramento, California. He is on staff at Mercy San Juan Hospital in Carmichael, California, and affiliated with several other California hospitals. Dr. Meyer has also written extensively for a number of medical journals.

Pam Peeke, M.D., M.P.H.   A native of San Francisco, California, Dr. Peeke received both the baccalaureate in science and a master's degree in public health policy from the University of California at Berkeley. After receiving her M.D. from Michigan, Dr. Peeke completed her clinical training at the George Washington University Medical Center in Washington, D.C., and was later awarded the Pew Foundation Postdoctoral Scholarship in clinical nutrition and metabolism at the University of California at Davis. She was then appointed to the National Institutes of Health (NIH), where she has conducted her research for the past three years. Presently Dr. Peeke is a clinical research fellow holding a joint appointment with the National Institute of Child Health and Human Development and the NIH Office of Alternative Medicine (OAM).

EDITORIAL RESEARCH ASSISTANT: Henrie Moise

FOREWORD

Stress is a contemporary and pervasive public health issue in the United States as evidenced in individuals, families, workplaces, homes, and communities.

Stress, in medicine and psychology, is any strain or interference that disturbs a person's normal functioning. Stress can be caused by external physical stress, e.g., noise or heat; internal physiologic stress of an ailment, e.g., heart or lung disease; external psychologic stress, e.g., job frustrations or spousal abuse; or internal psychologic stresses, e.g., chronic anxieties or depression. These all interact and interrelate with each other in various complex physiologic and psychologic [defense] mechanisms. Physical and physiologic stress can produce psychologic diseases and psychologic stress can cause medical diseases. Because of this, it is important to take a broad view of the causes, effects and treatments of stress.

Ada Kahn has made an excellent selection of many contemporary issues in *Stress A–Z*, covering a variety of stress-related areas such as diet, environment, occupational illness and sick building syndrome, coping in today's work environment, downsizing, aging, and end-of-life issues. She treats child and spouse abuse as well as the larger topic of domestic violence, a much greater public health problem than is generally realized. She looks at information anxiety, a product of our current information explosion and a form of stress that has not been generally appreciated. She examines culture shock, which may become an increasing problem in this era of world-wide travel, and highlights anniversary reaction, holiday stress, and weekend depression.

Kahn has taken a holistic approach to dealing with stress. Just as the field of holistic health focuses on the whole person, not just the headache or backache, similarly stress must focus on the whole mind-body interaction. The author, although mentioning mind-altering medications and the pharmacologic approach, emphasizes what patients can do for themselves in mind-altering alternative techniques, self-help, and self-healing. She has, however, included an entire section on use of medications for some conditions.

Many patients are acquiring new insight and learning about health matters in response to HMOs and managed care. Others are checking up on their own diagnoses and treatment plans on the Internet; as patients learn how their medications interact with each other, they also become aware of the side effects and complications of every drug prescribed. For many, this has not only heightened awareness, but also markedly increased anxieties and overall stress. Physicians are now seeing patients who have discontinued important medications because of anxiety occurring after reading about relatively mild or rare side effects.

In this era of medical cost cutting and managed care, the problem of stress will become even more important. It has been estimated that at least two-thirds of the visits to physicians' offices are for stress-related problems. Patients may experience more stress as consultations and special tests are discouraged. Physicians may also experience anxieties and increased stress as they implement the HMO and managed care restrictions.

As stress becomes a greater factor in our everyday lives, it is fortuitous to be presented with this very readable, user-friendly compendium. *Stress A–Z* includes more than 500 entries adding up to 225,000 words. It contains many entries on the types of conditions that physicians see every day—physical disorders with emotional components. The book is not intended to provide complete information on any one topic. Instead, this reference is designed for individuals who want a comprehensive overview of stress-related topics, suggestions for self-help, and information about medical treatment.

Kahn's prior compendium, *The Encyclopedia of Mental Health*, was written for the lay reader, but became a desk reference for many professionals. *Stress A–Z* will also be an important volume for the professional, one to have next to the *Physicians' Desk Reference* so that a topic can quickly and easily be referred to by doctor and patient alike. It gives the appropriate information rapidly—the type that clinicians, and their patients, frequently need.

—Delbert H. Meyer, M.D.

abortion The interruption or loss of any pregnancy before the fetus is capable of living outside the womb. However, the term usually refers to induced or intentional termination of pregnancy, while *spontaneous* abortion, the natural loss of pregnancy, is usually referred to as "miscarriage."

The subject of abortion is stressful to society as well as to individuals. In the late 1990s, there are issues of social pressure as well as differing religious, moral, and political points of view. Some viewpoints hold that life begins at conception and regard abortion as a criminal act. Other viewpoints hold that life begins when the baby is capable of sustaining itself beyond the womb.

In 1973, the United States Supreme Court declared that under the Constitution a woman was entitled to undergo an abortion at any time during the first trimester (three months) of pregnancy; the individual states retained the right to regulate for health reasons where and by whom abortions could be performed during the second trimester. Since then, those who oppose abortion on moral and religious grounds (known as Pro-lifers) have fought to reverse and limit this decision, and the issues themselves have become incorporated into political party platforms during presidential and congressional campaigns.

Throughout history, many women have coped with the stress surrounding the decision to abort, and the method to use. Until the Supreme Court decision, society at large condemned women who had intercourse outside of marriage and ignored the dilemma arising from an unwanted pregnancy. Making the choice to abort was made secretly and often without the knowledge and support of family or the man involved. Today, however, there is a large group (known as Pro-choicers) who,

whether they are for or against abortion, campaign for the right of a woman to make that choice.

Before the legalization of abortion, the choice of method was largely limited to "abortifacients"—oral remedies such as castor oil, quinine pills, or other strong laxatives, or an injection of concentrated soap solutions, hot baths, or physical exertions such as climbing stairs. If women had the money, they would seek the services of illegal, "backstairs" abortionists who were doctors (usually unlicensed) or other unscrupulous people ready to take advantage of them, but who assumed no responsibility for the success or failure of the procedures. As a result, many women died or incurred permanent injury, often affecting their future ability to bear children.

In the United States, procedures used for elective termination depend on the length of the pregnancy. In the early stages, procedures are relatively simple, involve minimal pain and discomfort, and rarely require an overnight hospital stay. For later stages, procedures are more complicated, but all of these procedures, when performed in a sterile environment by competent physicians, are safe.

The key to relieving the stress of an abortion is knowing where to turn for information and counseling. If at all possible, the support of family and friends should be sought as early as possible. Organizations, such as Planned Parenthood, with offices in many large cities, local health departments, women's and other health clinics, family doctors, or local hospital gynecology staff are resources for help. While the lasting effects of an unwanted pregnancy cannot be completely eliminated, making a decision that is based on knowledge of all the options is more likely to reduce the stress. In many cases, the subject of abortion also causes stress for the fathers-to-be who may share in the decision-making process regarding continuation of the pregnancy.

See also PREGNANCY.

FOR FURTHER INFORMATION:
Planned Parenthood Federation of America
810 Seventh Avenue
New York, N Y 10019
Phone: (212) 541-7800

SOURCES:
Kahn, Ada P., and Linda Hughey Holt. *The A To Z of Women's Sexuality.* Alameda, Calif.: Hunter House, 1992.
Holt, Linda Hughey, and Melva Weber. *AMA Book of Womancare.* New York: Random House, 1982.

absenteeism   Absenteeism or frequent absence from work may be related to employees' stress on the job and/or in their personal lives. According to a survey conducted by Northwestern National Life of Minneapolis, 17% of the 600 employees interviewed missed one or more days of work in 1990 due to stress, almost half (46%) felt highly stressed, and three-quarters (75%) experienced three or more stress-related illnesses somewhat or very often.

STRESSFUL FACTORS AT WORK THAT MAY CAUSE ABSENTEEISM

- Lack of recognition by superiors
- Role conflict (particularly with peers)
- Deadlines
- Job unsuitability or unpreparedness
- Concerns about job security and career paths
- Environmental discomforts ("sick building syndrome")
- Sexual concerns
- Marital difficulties
- Concerns about children/grandchildren
- Concerns about elderly parents
- Financial problems
- Health problems (self or family members)
- Other family pressures

Another source of stress for employees is the need to balance time for work, family, and self. This stressor can lead to health problems, decreased productivity, and employee turnover. It can be expected to remain a major factor since the hours spent by men and women in the workplace are increasing.

Employees experiencing stressors may exhibit persistent physical symptoms such as irregular sleep patterns, fatigue, anxiety, and weight change. There is also evidence that these employees may be more subject to colds, flu, headaches, gastric upsets, and other illnesses, all of which lead to an increase in absenteeism.

The high rate of absenteeism among the nation's workers results in high losses for business and industry. A study in the early 1980s by the Bureau of National Affairs indicated that approximately 50% of worker absences could be avoided by attending to employee needs—both physical and emotional. As a result, many corporations have undertaken preventive efforts, such as health examinations, health risk appraisals and employee assistance (EAPs) and wellness programs for weight control, smoking cessation, exercise, and stress reduction. Because the bureau study also showed a positive correlation between absences and the attitudes of employees to their superiors, some employers have introduced programs aimed at job enrichment, career ladders, and worker participation.

See also EMPLOYEE ASSISTANCE PROGRAMS; MARITAL THERAPY; SCHOOL; WORKING MOTHERS; WORKPLACE.

FOR FURTHER INFORMATION:
American Industrial Hygiene Association
345 White Pond Drive
Akron, OH 44321
Phone: (216) 873-2442

abuse   See ADDICTION; DOMESTIC VIOLENCE.

access to care   The financial, geographic, or physical accessibility of health care to those in need. Access to care causes many individuals a great deal of stress because they are uninsured or underinsured and cannot pay the costs of health care themselves. Many people are denied such care because they are ineligible for health insurance or government aid. Such individuals worry that an illness might devastate any family savings.

Access to care can also refer to geographic accessibility of physicians and facilities. In general, people in rural and isolated areas in the United States have less access to health care than those in metropolitan areas in which major teaching institutions are located. They have serious worries about obtaining appropriate care should an emergency arise. For this reason, many of them choose to move near a metropolitan area during their later years.

Access to care also implies physical ability to enter the building where care is provided. Individuals who have disabilities are often stressed by consideration of whether entranceways, elevators, etc., are accessible in health care facilities. The availability of appropriate transportation services to the health care facility is another concern.

See also DISABILITIES.

acculturation The process of adjusting to a new culture. In situations where there are linguistic or cultural communication barriers or an individual's expectations are not congruent with what takes place, stress can be heightened.

The stress of adjusting to an unfamiliar culture may lead to behavior changes, such as increased alcohol and tobacco consumption. Furthermore, when various family members become accustomed to the new culture at different rates, conflicts can arise between the generations, contributing to tensions within the family.

There are many community service programs available in cities in the United States designed to help acquaint newcomers to the country with customs, costs, and ways to locate needed services. Many are geared to helping newcomers learn the language, while others emphasize the sociocultural aspects of relocating. Local public libraries are a good source of such programs. Frequently, ethnic groups welcoming newcomers in their communities will help them learn how to shop in local markets, find good merchandise at a discount, and obtain legal services and medical care.

Health care needs of immigrants
Many immigrant patients in the United States do not use the Western medical model. Some of these patients see Western medicine as one of many healing systems. Cultural expectations can cause stress for these individuals as well as the physicians who treat them. For example, some East Indian women will not allow pelvic examination by male physicians, even those from their own culture. Because such procedures can be construed as grounds for divorce, a relatively simple physical examination becomes both a cultural and a medical issue.

Health care professionals should address the clinical issues surrounding folk beliefs and behaviors in a culturally sensitive manner, according to an article in *The Journal of the American Medical Association* (March 1, 1994). Lee M. Pachter, D.O., St. Francis Hospital and Medical Center, Hartford, Connecticut, wrote: "A culturally sensitive health care system is one that is not only accessible, but also respects the beliefs, attitudes and cultural lifestyles of its patients. It is a system that is flexible and acknowledges that health and illness are in large part molded by variables such as ethnic values, cultural orientation, religious beliefs, and linguistic considerations."

Dr. Pachter explained that most medical folk beliefs and practices are not harmful and do not interfere with biomedical therapy. Under these circumstances the clinician should not attempt to dissuade the patient from these beliefs, but instead educate him or her as to the importance of the biomedical therapy in addition to the patient-held belief. Any ethnomedical practice that has the potential for serious negative outcome needs to be discouraged, but this must be done in a sensitive and respectful way. Replacing dangerous practices with alternatives that fit into the patient's ethnocultural belief system is often met with acceptance.

As reported in an editorial in *Canadian Family Physician* (October 1995), the stress of the acculturation experience is especially severe for individuals whose future residency status is in question, such as those entering a new country as a student, or those hoping to find work and remain on a permanent basis. Local community agencies can help relieve some of the stresses these individuals encounter.

See also ALTERNATIVE THERAPIES; MIGRATION, PERSONAL SPACE.

SOURCES:
Cave, Andrew, et al. "Physicians and Immigrant Patients." *Canadian Family Physician* 41 (October 1995): 1685–90.
Pachter, Lee M. "Culture and Clinical Care: Folk Illness Beliefs and Behavior and Their Implications for Health Care Delivery." *Journal of the American Medical Association* 271, no. 9 (March 1, 1994): 690–94.

TIPS TO REDUCE STRESS OF MEDICAL ENCOUNTERS WITH IMMIGRANT PATIENTS

- Become aware of the commonly held folk medical beliefs and behaviors of the patient's community.
- Assess the likelihood of a particular patient or family acting on these beliefs during a specific illness episode.
- Arrive at a way to successfully negotiate between the two belief systems.
- Be aware of your own cultural biases.
- Determine whether language will be an issue during office visits.
- Develop an office guide for immigrant patients, including typical questions asked during an examination, needs for disrobing, and types of examinations and testing procedures and their importance.
- Prepare a list of local agencies that are available to help with multicultural issues.
- Encourage patients to share their culture and life-style with you so that you have information for accurate diagnoses and appropriate therapy.
- Ask before going ahead with any procedures. By seeking permission and explaining the procedures you remove the mystery and patients become partners in the activity rather than objects of scrutiny. Compliance improves with understanding.
- Take advantage of opportunities for cross-cultural learning in group discussions with other professionals from different cultural backgrounds.

acne Very common skin condition; occurs on the face but can also occur on the back, chest, shoulders, and neck. It consists of blackheads, whiteheads, pimples and deeper, boil-like lesions called nodules and can be a source of extreme stress for the sufferer.

It has been estimated that 80% to 90% of teenagers suffer from acne at one time or another, and about one in every five young people visit a dermatologist because of acne. The prevalence of the problem is no comfort to the high school student who feels that the blemishes will keep him or her from being socially accepted. Although primarily a disease of adolescence, acne occurs among older persons as well. In many cases untreated acne clears up after several years; however, it can leave lifelong scars that affect the person's self-image.

Coping with acne

In addition to seeking help from a dermatologist, a person who has acne might relieve some of his or her stress by joining a peer support group at school or at a local community center, or visiting a psychotherapist who counsels adolescents. Parents can be particularly helpful to their son or daughter who has acne by being supportive, offering encouragement for treatment, and contributing to the young person's self-esteem. In cases of extreme scarring a plastic and reconstructive surgeon's opinion on treatment might be sought.

Causes of acne

Acne is activated by male-type hormones, which occur in both males and females and cause the sebaceous glands of the skin to enlarge. The sebaceous glands make sebum, an oily substance that reaches the surface by emptying through the opening of a follicle or hair-containing canal on the surface of the skin. The material in the oil stimulates the lining of the follicle wall and the cells shed more rapidly and stick together, plugging the openings at the surface of the skin. Additionally, the mixture of oil and cells helps bacteria in the follicles grow and produce chemicals that cause the wall of the follicle to break, allowing sebum, bacteria, and shed skin cells to escape, and lead to production of pimples. Thus, the blackness of a blackhead is not dirt; it is caused by dried oil and shed skin cells in the opening of the hair follicles.

Self-care to relieve acne

There is no instant or permanent cure for acne, but it can be controlled and sufferers should be encouraged to follow appropriate care and treatment to prevent permanent scars. Washing the face with soap and warm water no more than twice a day is a good routine to follow. Men with acne who shave and prefer using a safety rather than an electric razor have particular concerns. They should soften the beard thoroughly with soap and warm water. To avoid nicking pimples, they should shave as lightly as possible, and shave only when necessary, always using a sharp blade. Dermatologists have differing opinions on the importance of diet in managing acne. Some people however, find that their acne becomes worse when they eat certain foods, such as chocolate, milk products, or nuts. Individuals can often determine what foods cause their acne and learn to avoid them.

Diagnosis and treatment

Dermatologists recommend that sufferers not pick, scratch, pop, or squeeze pimples, which may lead to additional inflammation and scarring. However, when treating acne, the dermatologists may open pimples or remove blackheads and whiteheads.

Depending on the type of acne, a dermatologist will recommend different therapies. In some cases, an acne-like rash is due to another cause, such as make-up, lotions, or medications. When visiting a dermatologist, it is important to provide a history of relevant habits.

For milder cases of acne, many non-prescription lotions and creams may be helpful. If used too often, however, many of them lead to excessively dry skin. Dermatologists advise that when buying makeup, people should choose "noncomedogenic" or "nonacnegenic" products. "Noncomedogenic" means that using the cosmetic should not result in the formation of whiteheads and blackheads. Topical preparations in cream or lotion form are sometimes prescribed by dermatologists to help unblock the pores and reduce the bacteria.

In more severe cases, female-type hormones and other medications that decrease the male-type hormones are used. Another oral medication, isotretinoin (Accutane), is sometimes used to treat acne that has not responded to other treatments. However, frequent visits with the dermatologist are necessary to monitor and control the side effects; the drug can cause severe birth defects if taken during pregnancy.

See also BODY IMAGE; PUBERTY; SELF-ESTEEM.

FOR FURTHER INFORMATION:
American Academy of Dermatology
930 N. Meacham Road
Schaumburg, IL 60168
Phone: (708) 330-0230

Society for Investigative Dermatology, Inc.
1001 Potrero Street (Bldg. 100, Room 269)

San Francisco, CA 94110
Phone: (415) 647-3992

SOURCE:
Acne, Schaumburg, Ill.: American Academy of
Dermatology, 1993.

acquired immunodeficiency syndrome (AIDS)

AIDS is a deficiency of the IMMUNE SYSTEM due
to infection with HIV (HUMAN IMMUNODEFI-
CIENCY VIRUS). As yet, there is no curative
treatment and no vaccine for AIDS; however,
in many individuals, symptoms and complications respond in varying degrees to antiviral agents, antibiotics, radiation therapy, and
anti-cancer drugs.

Considered by many the "plague" of the
20th century, no other disease in modern
times has had such an impact on the civilized
world. It is a source of stress for those who are
infected, for all who fear acquiring it, and for
family and friends of AIDS patients.

At the end of 1995, reported cases of AIDS
had reached 476,899 in the United States, with
at least between one and two million more
believed to be infected with the HIV virus.
AIDS occurs throughout the world, but those
in Africa suffer disproportionately. The following statistics for the United States were
reported by the Centers for Disease Control in
mid-1995:

CUMULATIVE REPORTED AIDS CASES IN THE UNITED STATES

Group	Total
Cases	476,899
Male	408,874
Female	68,021
Adult/Adolescent	470,288
Pediatric	6,611
White, not Hispanic	228,644
Black, not Hispanic	160,148
Hispanic	82,910
Asian/Pacific Is	3,265
Am. Indian/Alaska	1,202
Unknown	730

The virus is transmitted through body fluids—usually semen or blood, but also through
saliva and tears. AIDS is also transmitted from
mother to infant *in utero* or via passage
through the birth canal or via infected breast
milk. More rarely, doctors and nurses exposed
to infected patients have caught the virus.
There have also been isolated case reports of
infection through organ donations, artificial
inseminations, and exposure to infected dentists. In the early 1980s, when AIDS was first
recognized as a syndrome and the full extent
of the disease acknowledged, most of the
patients were homosexual males and intravenous drug users or their partners. Within a
few years, there was recognition that the disease was also spreading into the heterosexual
population, and that women and children
were dying of AIDS.

In many developed countries, public
health measures have helped to level off the
rate of AIDS. For example, donated blood
and semen samples are screened for AIDS.
Also, guidelines have been developed for
"safe sex" between partners in risk groups.
"Safe sex" eliminates the exchange of body
fluids through such means as using condoms,
avoiding oral intercourse, and limiting to a
single, steady partner. Western medical centers advise "universal precautions," which
mean carefully covering any body surfaces
that might be exposed to an infected person's
body fluids.

Stresses of HIV on mental health

Individuals at high risk for developing the
disease live in fear and have concerns about
acquiring the disease through casual contact.
Death from AIDS has touched many families
in the United States. For most, it has meant
recognizing their children's homosexual
behavior as well as facing their illness and
death in their 20s, 30s, and 40s.

Mark Etkin, M.D., University of Manitoba,
Canada, described mental health needs of
patients as well as caregivers during a semi-

nar in 1991. According to Dr. Etkin, to properly coordinate the care of HIV patients, family physicians must be prepared to deal with an array of psychiatric and neurological syndromes, including depression and dementia.

There is a high suicide rate among HIV patients as reported by Dr. Etkin. People with HIV are much more likely to commit suicide than cancer patients as a result of the stress of their affliction. Most are at an age when they are not nearly ready to accept death. Psychosocial changes in an HIV patient involve changes in life-style and sexuality, work, financial status, SELF-ESTEEM, BODY IMAGE, and uncertainty about the future.

The period of time after learning that a person is infected with the HIV virus is characterized by anxiety and stress stemming from his or her own DENIAL, family reactions, the homophobia of both family and friends, and employment and insurance concerns. HIV patients need nonjudgmental, forward-looking sources of support, people skilled in LISTENING carefully, letting them ventilate their fears, and dealing with their physical symptoms. SUPPORT GROUPS, helping the person maintain as much CONTROL as possible, counseling them in legal decisions before dementia sets in, and identifying referral programs, are extremely helpful.

Choosing a physician

Choosing a physician experienced in treating AIDS may be the AIDS patient's most important decision. A study showed those patients whose physicians rarely treat the disease die a year sooner than those with experienced doctors. The research, presented at a conference in Washington, D.C., in January 1996, indicated that being a physician's first AIDS patient, or even the second or third, is risky. These patients appear more likely to miss important treatment to forestall life-threatening problems.

"Results support the hypothesis that practice makes perfect," said Dr. Mari Kitahata of the University of Washington, who conducted the study. She based her results on 403 men with AIDS who were treated at the Group Health Cooperative of Puget Sound, a health maintenance organization in Washington State, between 1984 and 1994. She found the risk of dying on any particular day was a third lower for AIDS patients with experienced doctors, compared with those whose doctors are seeing AIDS for the first time.

Stresses on health care professionals

There is enormous personal stress among many health care professionals who work with AIDS patients. There is the medical complexity of the disease, as well as the stigma of AIDS and AIDS risk behaviors. Some health care workers fear contracting the disease from the patients, while some inwardly rebel against caring for people whose concepts of behavior differ so radically from theirs.

Pediatric AIDS

Pediatric AIDS causes special stresses for the infected child and his or her family. Many infected children require foster care because of parental inability to provide the needed care. Unfortunately, many AIDS-infected children do not live long, and parents must face grief after watching the child suffer. Although it is controversial, most communities have accepted the opinion of the Centers for Disease Control that infected children in a normal classroom would not pose a hazard to their classmates. However, the reality is that few infants or young children with AIDS live long enough to be in school for very long. Meanwhile, schoolchildren with AIDS live with the stresses of being different and have difficulties maintaining the grade level because of frequent treatment. In many cases, they are cut off from teachers and other students, which leads to FRUSTRATION, despair and DEPRESSION.

Runaway adolescents, many of whom subsist through prostitution, are especially vulnerable to HIV infection. These teenagers have few support systems, are usually school dropouts, and have severed family connections.

Women and AIDS

Women accounted for an increasing percentage of AIDS cases in the United States, according to a 1991 report from the Centers for Disease Control. The numbers nearly doubled between 1985 and 1990, from 6.6% to 11.5%.

At an AIDS conference at Stanford University in 1991, then U.S. surgeon general Dr. Antonia Novello emphasized that women are increasingly victims of AIDS, not just caretakers of men suffering from the deadly disease. "Women have almost been forgotten in the AIDS questions . . . if there ever was a day when we thought women would serve only as caretakers for AIDS patients, that day has long passed," she said. "Previously, attention has been given to the social and economic impact of this pandemic [AIDS] on women, particularly mothers and children. Now women should be seen as victims of the disease itself."

Novello predicted that over the next decade, the heterosexual mode of transmission of HIV will become the primary means of spreading HIV infection in most industrialized countries, and by the year 2000, the number of worldwide AIDS cases of women will begin to equal those of men. "The fight against AIDS requires coordinated action among a wide spectrum of private and public sector groups, including women who must in many cultures have the courage to stand up to a society, and perhaps a family, that may condemn them for assuming a non-traditional role," Novello said.

Novello said that men and women are unequal in terms of abilities to protect themselves against AIDS. She believes that it is easier for the man to protect himself from AIDS than for the woman, and probably this is because the women's protection is much more problematic. Although the condom is seen as the most effective method of preventing the spread of AIDS from an infected partner, to many women this safeguard is denied because of cultural restraints. In some societies, suggesting to a husband or partner that he use a condom may be a social taboo, because it is perceived as a COMMUNICATION of insolence or defiance against the man. In many societies, the price of challenging authority to protect herself against AIDS is too high a price.

AIDS and pregnancy

Recommendations by the Centers for Disease Control in the late 1990s included testing of pregnant women for the HIV virus who acknowledge having engaged in high-risk behavior. More recently, researchers have suggested that HIV screening be routinely offered to all pregnant women so that those testing positive can make decisions about continuing their pregnancies, about future pregnancies, and about early medical treatment for their newborns.

See also CHRONIC ILLNESS.

FOR FURTHER INFORMATION:
AIDS-Hotlines National
AZT Hotline
Phone: (800) 843-9388

CAIN (Computerized AIDS Information Network)
San Francisco AIDS Foundation
54 Tenth St.
San Francisco, CA 94103
Phone: (415) 864-4368

Centers for Disease Control and Prevention/American Social Health Association
Phone: (800) 341-AIDS

National AIDS Information Clearinghouse
Centers for Disease Control
Box 6003
Rockville, MD 20850
Phone: (800) 458-5231

Physician Link (List of MDs with expertise in AIDS treatment and research)
Phone: (800) 344-5500

SOURCES:

Andre, Pierre. *People, Sex, HIV & AIDS: Social, Political, Philosophical and Moral Implications.* Huntington, W.Va.: University Press, 1995.

Donovan, Catherine A., and Elizabeth Stratton. "Changing Epidemiology of AIDS," *Canadian Family Physician* 40 (August 1994).

Epstein, Steven. *Impure Science: AIDS, Activism and the Politics of Knowledge.* Berkeley: University of California Press, 1996.

Gifford, Allen, *Living Well With HIV & AIDS.* Palo Alto, Calif.: Bull Publishers, 1997.

Goldfinger, Stephen E. ed. "AIDS: A Glimmer of Hope." *Harvard Health Letter* 20, no. 9 (July 1995).

"Panel Backs New AIDS Drug." *Chicago Tribune,* November 7, 1995.

acrophobia   A fear of heights. It is one of the most common PHOBIAS and is a source of stress to phobic individuals. The fear, which may include being on top of mountains, on high floors of skyscrapers, or even of riding to a high floor in an elevator is usually out of proportion to the real danger. There is a high level of stress and anxiety even when these individuals approach overlooks or bridges. Some individuals who experience acrophobia may also fear being injured or falling, which are related phobias.

See also ANXIETY DISORDERS.

ACTH (adrenocorticotrophic hormone)   A secretion by the pituitary gland that controls release of steroid hormones from the adrenal cortex. ACTH is also known as corticotrophin. Under conditions of STRESS, both ACTH and beta-endorphins are released into the bloodstream.

See also ENDORPHINS.

acupressure   Sometimes referred to as ACUPUNCTURE without needles, acupressure embraces the same concepts of energy flow and point stimulation as the original science but uses the pressure of the therapist's fingers for point stimulation. Acupressure is used by many people for relief of physical and psy-

chological stresses. It is thought to combine the science of acupuncture with the power of the healing touch and has been most widely used for pain control.

In Oriental medicine, acupressure is helpful in conditions where the body's energy balance has been upset by a variety of physical and/or emotional stresses. Because it is an extremely gentle technique, acupressure is sometimes used by the therapist with individuals who are fearful of needles.

See also ALTERNATIVE THERAPIES; SHIATSU.

acupuncture   A technique used to relieve stress for many people. It has been used for thousands of years as a component of Chinese medicine, and is based on the theory that the body's "vital energy" (Chi) circulates through "meridians" along the surfaces of the body. The ancient theory holds that illness and disease result from imbalances in vital energy, which can be remedied when therapy is applied to "acupuncture points" located along the meridians. The goal of acupuncture is to rebalance the flow of energy, promoting health and preventing future imbalance. The points are believed to have certain electrical properties, which when stimulated can alter chemical neurotransmitters in the body and bring about a healing response. Practitioners of acupuncture insert hair-thin stainless steel needles into the patient's body surfaces at acupuncture points.

In addition to stress reduction and relaxation, many people have used acupuncture for a variety of conditions, including stress reduction and relaxation, osteoporosis, asthma, back pain, painful menstrual cycles, and migraine headaches.

Research with acupuncture

Over the last two decades in the 20th century, acupuncture has become one of the most intensively studied of medical procedures, says Dr. Bruce Pomeranz, professor of medicine, University of Toronto Medical School.

He reported to the *Toronto Star* (September 10, 1995) that scores of scientifically rigorous animal experiments and clinical studies have allowed researchers to uncover a mechanism to explain how acupuncture controls chronic pain. Evidence points to a similar mechanism accounting for acupuncture's success in treating addictions to alcohol, cocaine, and opiate, he said. The acupuncture points on the body and ear correlate to sites where there are unusually large concentrations of nerves. The needles stimulate the nerves, which send an electrical message to the brain. Dr. Pomeranz explains that the brain releases endorphins (morphine-like brain chemicals), which block pain messages from getting through and take away the emotional components of pain.

Further, the endorphin system is linked to a system that releases cortisone, a chemical that alleviates inflammation in the body. Heroin and cocaine addicts suffer from depressed endorphin levels. Their bodies compensate for the high levels of narcotics in their blood by producing less of the naturally-occurring substance. The agonies of withdrawal result from low levels of the painblocking endorphins. Stimulation of the endorphin system through acupuncture gets it going in a natural way, says Dr. Pomeranz. He also points out that acupuncture has been successful in treating alcoholism.

Increasing acceptance of acupuncturists
In the mid-1990s, acupuncture is permitted in all 50 states. In some states, only physicians are permitted to practice acupuncture, while other states allow the procedure to be performed by lay acupuncturists under medical supervision or by unsupervised lay persons. In the United States, an estimated 3,000 medical doctors and osteopaths have studied acupuncture and use it in practice, up from 500 a decade before. Additionally, some 7,000 nonphysicians use acupuncture for a wide array of problems, sometimes in conjunction with massage, herbal therapies, and other tra-

ditional Eastern techniques. In 1990, the U.S. secretary of education recognized the National Accreditation Commission for Schools and Colleges of Acupuncture and Oriental Medicine as an accrediting agency. However, the Food and Drug Administration considers acupuncture needles to be "investigational" devices and has not approved the use of acupuncture for any disease treatment. In the early 1990s, the U.S. Food and Drug Administration estimated that nine to 12 million acupuncture treatments are performed annually in the United States. In the mid-1990s, nearly 100 private insurers and Medicaid programs in some states cover acupuncture for some conditions.

Choosing an acupuncturist
Individuals choosing a therapist to perform acupuncture should be examined by their physician first. Some conditions are beyond the scope of acupuncture treatment and demand immediate medical attention. However, many physicians may agree to have their patients undergo acupuncture along with traditional treatment. In some cases they will agree that a patient try acupuncture first, if postponing traditional treatment will not be injurious. When arranging to meet with an acupuncturist, follow the suggestions below.

See also ACUPRESSURE; ADDICTION; ALTERNATIVE THERAPIES.

TIPS TO AVOID STRESS WHEN USING ACUPUNCTURE

- Discuss your expectations with the acupuncturist. Ask how long until you can expect to see a change in your condition. Be suspicious of promises of a quick cure, especially if you have had your problem for some time. If you don't see progress after six to eight treatments, reevaluate your choice of treatment and the practitioner.

(Continues)

TIPS TO AVOID STRESS WHEN USING ACUPUNCTURE (continued)

- Check the credentials of the acupuncturist you are considering. Ask whether he or she is certified by the National Commission for the Certification of Acupuncturists. To become certified, an acupuncturist must pass both a written and practical exam. To be eligible to take the exam, he or she must be licensed, have at least two years of training at an acupuncture school, or must have worked as an apprentice acupuncturist for at least four years.
- If your prospective acupuncturist is a physician, ask whether he or she belongs to the American Academy of Medical Acupuncture, which requires at least 200 hours of acupuncture training for membership. Approximately 500 of the 3,000 physicians practicing acupuncture in the United States belong to the AAMA.
- Discuss the costs of the procedure. Depending on the area of the country, and whether or not the acupuncturist is a physician, fees vary. Usually the first visit is considerably higher than subsequent visits.
- Weigh the risks of acupuncture. There have been reports of serious complications attributed to acupuncture needles. However, most acupuncturists use sterile, disposable needles that come in a sealed package.

SOURCES:

Martyn, Peter. "Acupuncture Successful in Treating Addictions." *The Toronto Star,* Sept. 10, 1995.

Weiss, Rick. "Medicine's Latest Miracle." *Health,* January/February 1995.

addiction Usually refers to psychological or physical dependence on a chemical substance or behavior. Some individuals develop addiction to alcohol, tobacco, drugs, food, and sedatives prescribed by physicians. Others are addicted to activities such as dieting, exercising, GAMBLING, and sex. An addiction is often the result of stressful situations and the inability of the individual to cope with them. Once addicted, he or she suffers from new stresses, including the physical or mental symptoms of the addiction or obtaining the money for his or her habit. In the meantime, family, friends and employers also suffer from stress, which can lead to situations such as DIVORCE, low job productivity or loss of job.

Criteria for addiction are a compulsive or obsessive craving leading to persistent substance use or repeated actions; a need to increase the substance dose or level of activity as the addict's tolerance increases; and, with certain drugs (alcohol, narcotics, barbiturates, etc.), possibly acute withdrawal symptoms if the drug is reduced or withdrawn abruptly. Withdrawal symptoms alone do not necessarily imply addiction. However, physical dependence can develop with prolonged use of a drug (e.g., morphine for pain). Psychological dependence can involve a loss of control of the substance use, and a tendency to orient behavior or life priorities toward obtaining the drug or pursuing the addictive behavior.

Recognizing an addiction

Warning signs of drug or alcohol addiction include withdrawal from responsibilities; deterioration of family relationships, school or work performance; negative personality changes, such as depression; changes in sleep patterns, such as insomnia or sleeping too much; and legal problems, such as shoplifting or stealing money.

Overcoming addictions

To overcome an addiction the addict must recognize that it exists and acknowledge his or her responsibility for the situation. Once the addict has confronted his/her problem, relief from addictions is usually best accomplished with a multidimensional approach. This may include psychological, medical, and spiritual therapies. Additionally, ALTERNATIVE THERAPIES, such as MEDITATION and GUIDED IMAGERY, may be of use.

The addict also needs help from family members and an outside support group. Many self-help organizations exist to help recovering addicts and can be located through local public health departments or libraries. Groups are available to help the addicts themselves as well as spouses and children, who will also experience anxiety and stress because of the addict's behaviors. In many cases, relief from certain stressors, such as work pressure and family problems, can help an addict recover from his or her dependency.

Addiction Severity Index
The addiction severity index is a tool that mental health professionals generate from a questionnaire that gathers information about an individual's stressors leading to or resulting from the addiction, as well as social, legal, employment, drug and alcohol use, and other habits. Using the index, the mental health professional can assess the individual's function and level of stress in each dimension independently at the beginning of treatment and later, after treatment interventions.

See also AGING; ALCOHOLISM AND ALCOHOL DEPENDENCE; ANXIETY; BEHAVIOR THERAPY; PSYCHOTHERAPIES.

FOR FURTHER INFORMATION:
American Society on Addiction Medicine
5225 Wisconsin Avenue NW (Suite 409)
Washington, DC 20015
Phone: (202) 244-8948

SOURCE:
E'Archangelo, E. "Substance Abuse in Later Life." *Canadian Family Physician* 39 (September 1993): 1986–93

adolescence See PUBERTY.

adoption When individuals take by choice a child of other parents as their own child. Couples or singles choose to adopt for various personal reasons; some are unable to have children and may have undergone a variety of tests and treatments to no avail. Adopting a child is a stressful process and with each step new anxieties appear to replace previous ones.

Planning for adoption puts stress on personal relationships. Referring to emotional highs and lows, the book *Adopting Your Child* suggests, "Most adoptions are roller coaster rides. There are long straight stretches, sudden lurches upward, and swooping plunges to the ground. There are people for whom adoption seems to go like clockwork, but they are in the minority. Because there are so many areas over which you have no control, you cannot plan your way to a certain result."

Next, the avenue of adoption must be chosen and the many players involved in aiding and approving adoptive parents identified. Adoptive parents in the late 1990s have many choices to make: private channels versus public agencies versus adoption through intermediaries, adoption directly from birth mother, or domestic versus international. Furthermore, far more adoption litigation is taking place today, in courtrooms in the United States, and far more stories of birth parents changing their minds permeate our media than in earlier times. Other issues that could arise include disqualification after a study of the adoptive home by a social worker, refusal of a child that is referred, and court denial of the adoption.

Finally, once adoption occurs, there will be the many stresses that are the norms of parenthood. However, for adoptive parents other stressful events may lie ahead: deciding how and when to tell children they are adopted, dealing with the anxiety this information may bring to them at various stages of their lives, and recognizing the possibility that when they are older they may want to find their birth parents.

See also COMMUNICATION; INFERTILITY; PARENTING.

FOR FURTHER INFORMATION:
National Adoption Center
1218 Chestnut Street
Philadelphia, PA 19107
Phone: (215) 925-0200

SOURCE:
Reynolds, Nancy Thalia. *Adopting Your Child: Options, Answers, & Actions.* Bellingham, Wash.: Self-Counsel Press, 1993.

adrenaline   A catecholamine (also known as epinephrine) produced and released by the adrenal medulla in response to stimulation from the nervous system, such as stressful events. Regulated by the sympathetic nervous system, it is a potent stimulator of the organs and may play a role in controlling certain aspects of immune functions. Adrenaline produces an increase in heart rate, rise in blood pressure, and contraction of abdominal blood vessels. These sympathetic changes can be reversed by activation of the parasympathetic system.

See also IMMUNE SYSTEM; NEUROTRANSMITTERS; STRESS.

adultery   Voluntary   sexual   intercourse between a married man or woman and a person of the opposite sex who is not the legal spouse; it is also known as extramarital sex. Historically, in many countries, adultery has been considered a TABOO and a major (and sometimes the only) ground for divorce. In the United States, adultery is a source of stress within marriages, and in many cases contributes to DEPRESSION in one or both partners in the MARRIAGE.

Since the early 1980s, when AIDS was discovered, adultery and extramarital affairs carry the strong threat of acquiring the deadly virus or another SEXUALLY TRANSMITTED DISEASE.

See also LIVE-IN.

SOURCE:
Kahn, Ada P., and Linda Hughey Holt. *The A–Z of Women's Sexuality.* Alameda, Calif.: Hunter House, 1992.

advance directives   See DEATH; END OF LIFE CARE.

advertising   Propaganda for commercial purposes; designed to influence the consumer in making decisions to buy by emphasizing advantages of one particular product over its competitors. Choosing from the wide array of products and services available in the marketplace today can be an extremely stressful experience.

Advertising is just one part of a complicated process of marketing that includes determining what goods and services should be created for a specific segment of customers, finding suitable pricing structures and methods of distribution, and influencing prospective purchasers.

In an ideal world, consumers would be educated and use technical guidelines and consumer guides to help in making purchasing decisions. Unfortunately, there are few educated consumers and most live their lives prey to the pressures and stresses of advertising. Children, particularly, can be victims since they are unable to discriminate between what is real and what is unreal, what is good and what is bad. In turn, children may place demands on parents for products that can be unhealthy or poorly made, and which the parents cannot afford.

Two of the 20th century's newer advertising tools, direct mail and telemarketing, are playing an increasingly important role in the advertising process. Both tend to apply greater pressure in their selling messages and often produce a great deal of stress for potential customers in the form of unwelcome mail and telephone calls both at the office and at home.

Advertising campaigns are usually a combination of print ads and radio and TV commercials. They nudge, tease, scold, amuse, prod, and provoke potential customers in order to get them to try and then buy. Often, the campaign is centered not on the product itself, but on surrounding issues—how or where it is being used or who is using it. Techniques used to accomplish this include testimonials by well-known spokespersons, often athletes or movie stars who are paid to lend their names or faces as an endorsement for products. In many cases, products are merely repackaged and promoted as new and improved.

Advertising campaigns are usually directed to women, who have, since the turn of the century, accounted for more than 80% of all consumer spending. Until recently, Madison Avenue was dominated by males and the images of women in the advertising they created reflected their fantasies and fears. Advertisers have told consumers what they should and should not be and/or do, and advertising has spun pictures of perfection that often reminded consumers of their many shortcomings. Advertising, at its best, reflects styles and values. But it also can be overbearing when it takes the lead, sets the agenda, and attempts to dictate consumer behavior.

See also MONEY; SHOPAHOLISM.

FOR FURTHER INFORMATION (INQUIRIES AND COMPLAINTS):
Federal Trade Commission
Pennsylvania Avenue at Sixth St. NW
Washington, DC 20580
Phone: (202) 326-2222

aerobic activities   See EXERCISE.

affective disorders   An individual who has an affective disorder (also known as mood disorder) may have feelings of extreme sadness or intense, unrealistic elation with corresponding disturbances in mood that are not due to any other physical or mental disorder. It is stressful enough for the individual as well as those around him or her at work or at home to warrant professional attention.

Affective disorders differ from thought disorders; schizophrenic and paranoid disorders are primarily disturbances of thought, although individuals who have those disorders may also have some distortion of mood or affect.

The death rate for individuals with chronically depressed moods is about 30 times as high as that for the general population because of the higher incidence of SUICIDE. Manic (to be defined) individuals also have a high risk of death, which can be attributed to their tendencies to exhaust themselves physically, to neglect their health, and to have accidents (often alcohol related).

Types of affective disorders
Affective disorders can be subcategorized as major depression and bipolar disorders. These disorders can be acute or chronic; both show symptoms by changes in the biological, psychological and sociological functioning of the individual. In some individuals, bipolar disorders and DEPRESSION occur according to a seasonal pattern, with a regular cyclic relationship between the onset of the mood episodes and particular seasons.

A *mood syndrome* (depressive or manic) is a group of associated symptoms that occur together over a short duration. For example, Major Depressive Syndrome is defined as a depressed mood or loss of interest, of at least two weeks' duration, along with several associated symptoms, such as difficulty in concentrating and sleeping, fatigue, hopelessness, loss of pleasure, and weight loss or gain, with suicidal thoughts sometimes present.

A *mood episode* (major depressive, manic, or hypomanic) is a mood syndrome not due to a known organic factor and not part of a non-mood psychotic disorder such as schizophrenia, schizoaffective disorder, or delusional disorder. Psychiatrists diagnose a mood disorder by the pattern of mood episodes. For example, the diagnosis of major depression, recurrent type, is made when an individual has had one or more major depressive episodes without a history of a manic or hypomanic episode.

Manic episodes are distinct periods during which the individual experiences a predominant mood that is either elevated, expansive, or irritable. Such individuals may have inflated self-esteem, increased energy, accelerated and loud speech, flight of ideas, distractibility, grandiose delusions, and decreased need for sleep. The disturbance may cause marked impairment in working, social activities, or relationships; an episode may require that the affected person be hospitalized to prevent his harming himself or others. There may be rapid shifts of mood, with sudden changes to depression or anger. The mean age for the onset of manic episodes is in the early 20s, but many new cases appear after age 50.

Hypomanic episodes are mood disturbances less severe than mania, but they may be severe enough to cause several symptoms: marked impairment in judgment; financial, social or work activities associated with increased energy and busyness; exaggerated self-confidence; hypertalkativeness; euphoria or increased sense of humor. Often not recognized as illness by others, these behaviors are nevertheless associated with what are known as hypomanic episodes. Hypomanic episodes may be followed by depressions of moderate to great severity.

Major depressive episodes

Major depression affects approximately 10% of the adult population. A major depressive episode includes either depressed mood (in children or adolescents, irritable mood) or loss of interest or pleasure in all, or almost all, activities for at least two weeks. Associated symptoms may include feelings of worthlessness or excessive or inappropriate guilt, difficulty in concentrating, restlessness, appetite disturbance, change in weight, sleep disturbance, decreased energy, an inability to sit still, pacing, hand-wringing, and recurrent thoughts of death or of attempting suicide.

Depressive episodes are more common among females than among males. The average age of onset of depressive episodes is the late 20s, but a major depressive episode may begin at any age.

Bipolar disorders (episodes of mania and depression) are equally common in males and females. Bipolar disorder seems to occur at much higher rates in first-degree biologic relatives of people with bipolar disorder than in the general population.

Cyclothymia involves numerous periods of hypomanic episodes and numerous periods of depressed mood or loss of interest or pleasure that are not severe enough to meet the criteria for bipolar disorder or major depressive episode.

Dysthymia involves a history of a depressed mood for at least two years that is not severe enough to meet the criteria for a major depressive episode. This is a common form of depression, and the person who has this condition may have periods of major depressive episodes as well.

Causes of affective disorders

There are many explanations for affective disorders, including the psychoanalytic, interpersonal, cognitive, behavioral, learned helplessness, biologic, and genetic theories.

All these theories have common points of focus that can be roughly categorized as biological, psychosocial, and sociocultural. Personality characteristics of some individuals, such as lack of self-esteem and negative views of themselves and their future, predispose them to affective disorders. A stressful life event can also activate previously dormant negative thoughts.

Individuals who become manic generally are ambitious, outgoing, energetic, care what others think about them, and are sociable before their episodes and after remission. However, depressive individuals appear to be more anxious, obsessive, and self-deprecatory. They often are prone to feelings of self-blame and guilt. Depressed individuals tend to interact with others differently from the way manics do. For example, some manic individuals dislike relying on others and try to establish social roles in which they can dominate others. On the other hand, depressed individuals take on a role of dependency and look to others to provide support and care. Feelings of a loss of hope and helplessness are central to most depressive reactions. In severe depression, "learned helplessness" may occur in which the individual sees no hope and gives up trying to cope with his or her situation.

Incidence of affective disorders is higher among relatives of individuals with clinically diagnosed affective disorders than among the general population, indicating a hereditary predisposition.

Biologic factors also play an important role. There was considerable research during the 1970s and 1980s to explore the view that depression and manic episodes both may arise from disruptions in the balance of the levels of brain chemicals called biogenic amines. Biogenic amines serve as neutral transmitters or modulators to regulate the movement of nerve impulses across the synapses from one neuron to the next. Two such amines involved in affective disorders are NOREPINEPHRINE and 5-hydroxytryptamine (SEROTONIN). Some drugs are known to have antidepressant properties and to biochemically increase concentrations of one or the other (or both) of these transmitters.

In many individuals, psychosocial and biochemical factors work together to cause affective disorders. For example, stress has been considered as a possible causative factor in many cases. Stress may also affect the biochemical balance in the brain, at least in some predisposed individuals. Some individuals experience mild depression following significant life stresses, such as the death of a family member. Other major life events, especially those involving reduced self-esteem, physical disease or abnormality, or deteriorating physical condition, may precipitate changes in mood.

Treatment of affective disorders
A variety of treatments including pharmaceutical medications and BEHAVIOR THERAPY are used to treat affective disorders. Some behavioral approaches, known as cognitive and cognitive-behavioral therapies, include efforts to improve the thoughts and beliefs (implicit and explicit) that underlie the depressed state. Therapy includes attention to unusual stressors and unfavorable life situations, and observing recurrence of depression.

Prescription medications used to treat affective disorders include antidepressants, tranquilizers, and antianxiety drugs. Lithium carbonate, a simple mineral salt, is used to control manic episodes and is also used in some cases of depression where the underlying disorder is basically bipolar. For many individuals, lithium therapy is often effective in preventing cycling from depressive to manic episodes.

Support groups for the affected individuals as well as their families are available in many areas.

See also AGORAPHOBIA; ALCOHOLISM; MANIC-DEPRESSIVE DISORDER; PHARMACOLOGICAL APPROACH; PSYCHOTHERAPIES; SEASONAL AFFECTIVE DISORDERS.

FOR FURTHER INFORMATION:
National Depressive and Manic Depressive Association
222 S. Riverside Plaza (Suite 2812)
Chicago, IL 60606
Phone: (312) 993-0066

National Institute of Mental Health
Office of Scientific Information
Public Inquiries Section
5600 Fishers Lane (Room 15C-17)
Rockville, MD 20857
Phone: (301) 443-4513

National Mental Health Association
1021 Prince Street
Alexandria, VA 22314
Phone: (703) 684-7722

SOURCES:
Kahn, Ada P., and Jan Fawcett. *The Encyclopedia of Mental Health.* New York: Facts On File, 1993.
McFarland, Gertrude K., and Mary Durand Thomas. *Psychiatric Mental Health Nursing.* Philadelphia: J.B. Lippincott, 1991.

age-associated memory impairment   See FORGETTING; MEMORY.

age discrimination Usually refers to adults ages 55 to 65 and older who are often the first workers to be let go in company downsizings and MERGERS and are overlooked as potential employees when applying for new jobs. Both of these factors of age discrimination are a source of stress. However, with the slumping economy of the '90s, age discrimination, which is usually defined by negative stereotypes depicting older adults as less productive than younger workers and unable to be trained in new technology, has taken on new meaning. According to Patricia O'Toole in the May 1992 issue of *Lear's* magazine, during 1990 and 1991 the ranks of unemployed men and women between the ages of 45 and 54 swelled by more than 50% to almost one million. Much too young to retire, they are finding that employers consider them too old and too expensive to hire.

Hard as a recession can be on employees and job-hunters over age 40, age discrimination cannot be blamed on the economy alone. Although Congress banned age discrimination with the Age Discrimination in Employment Act of 1967, discrimination has continued and there have been increasing numbers of unemployed adults. Polls conducted by the Commonwealth Fund, a New York-based foundation, showed that there are six million unemployed Americans older than 55, half of whom are women who want to continue working. Traditionally, women have been subjects of both age and sex discrimination. Those with jobs were slow in getting the recognition their male counterparts received. Women were often the first to be forced out of work because of LAYOFFS or cutbacks, but employers used the excuse that they did not really have to work and did not really need the money. Although women were often essential to the organizations in which they worked, they were frequently made to feel incompetent and forced out or "encouraged" to take early retirement.

Despite the fact that there has been much research to disprove the stereotypes attributed to aging, they continue to influence judgments made concerning employment. Statistics have shown that workers age 40 and older take less time off than any other age group and are less accident-prone than younger workers. Members of this age group have also experienced more massive changes in technology over their lifetime than any past generation and are no less—if no more—adept at learning and using technology than those who are younger.

Middle-aged, mid-career adults in the age 40 to 55 range who lose their jobs are experiencing loss of income and benefits at a time when their families are still young and in need of their support and protection. They are often the most rooted in their communities and unwilling to move. Even when they are willing to leave, they can have difficulty in breaking even on heavily mortgaged homes. Older workers, on the other hand, may be more mobile because their families are grown and have realized equity in their home investments.

For those older adults in the age 55 to 65 and older range, loss of work may also mean loss of health insurance and/or pension benefits at a time when they need them most. These losses and the efforts older adults make to seek new employment are sources of great stress. Corporations who have ignored the stereotypes and made a point of hiring older workers have said it pays. For a decade, Travelers Corporation, an insurance company, has operated an in-house temporary service staffed mainly by its retirees who need little training and are highly productive because of their knowledge of the company.

See also AGING; JOB SECURITY.

FOR FURTHER INFORMATION:
National Institute on Aging
National Institutes of Health
Department of Health and Human Services
9000 Rockville Pike, MD 20892
Phone: (301) 496-1752

Administration on Aging
330 Independence Ave. SW (Room 4640)

Washington, DC 20201
Phone: (202) 619-0641

ageism   See AGE DISCRIMINATION.

aggression   A general term for a variety of behaviors that appear outside the range of what is socially and culturally acceptable. It includes extreme self-assertiveness, social dominance to the point of producing resentment in others, and a tendency toward hostility. Individuals who show aggression may do so for many reasons including stress, frustration, as a compensatory mechanism for low SELF-ESTEEM, lack of affection, hormonal changes, or illness. Aggression may be motivated by ANGER, overcompetitiveness or a need to harm or defeat others. Aggression is stressful for the victim of the aggressor as well as for the aggressor him or herself.

An individual with an aggressive personality may behave unpredictably at times, causing stress for those around him or her. For example, such an individual may start arguments inappropriately with friends or members of the family and may harangue them. The individual may write letters of an angry nature to government officials or others with whom he or she has some quarrel. In addition to stressful circumstances, hormonal imbalances may account for some aggression. Excessive androgens, the male sex hormones, seem to promote aggression (e.g., the use of androgenic steroids to promote development of muscle mass in athletes has been known to make the user more aggressive). Individuals who are continuously aggressive may show changes in brain wave patterns in electroencephalograms (EEG).

The term *passive aggression* relates to behavior that seems to be compliant, but in which "errors, mistakes, or accidents" for which no direct responsibility is assumed result in difficulties or harm to others. Patterns of behavior such as making "mistakes" that harm others are considered "passive aggressive." ("Gee, I'm sorry, I didn't mean to ruin all your work.")

SOURCE:
Kahn, Ada P., and Sheila Kimmel, *Empower Yourself: Every Woman's Guide to Self-Esteem.* New York: Avon Books, 1997.

aging   The aging process begins the day one is born, but for many individuals, stress related to aging increases as the years go by. Anxieties about health status, financial capabilities, standard of living, and surviving loved ones mount as one grows older. Additionally, the aging process often brings with it a decrease in the body's ability to adapt to stress. Consequently, there is an increase in the body's vulnerability, often resulting in more susceptibility to colds, headaches, and minor gastrointestinal upsets. Stress also affects a person's likelihood of developing more serious diseases in older age, including high blood pressure, heart disease, arthritis, ulcers, and possibly cancer. Stress has also been shown to worsen diseases such as diabetes in people who already have them.

Achieving successful aging
There have been three major theories for achieving old age. One is the biblical theory, which holds that the righteous are granted long life. Second is the theory that there are special places in the world where people live long. Third is the modern theory of lifestyle, diet, exercise, and moderation. This theory states that to some extent people have an influence on the length as well as the quality of their lives. Genetic makeup is also an influence, but that is a situation over which there is no control. The object of successful aging should be making the best use of what one has.

During the first half of the century, life expectancy was increased by reducing neonatal, infant, and maternal deaths. Since the 1980s, there has been an increase in life expectancy even after the age of 60 that is probably due in part to the decreasing incidence of cardiovascular risk factors. Now, there seems to be a consensus by geriatricians that certain lifestyle components can help people age successfully.

(See chart below.)

Some characteristics associated with aging can be slowed down by regular exercise programs. Exercise strengthens the body while improving one's mental outlook and widening one's social contacts. Older adults are now jogging, walking, bicycling, and swimming. These exercises improve the condition of the heart and lungs, aid in weight control, and decrease many stress factors.

Many older adults skip meals or seem to have a reduced appetite. Eating well is important in keeping up vitality in old age. Even people who come from families with a history of heart disease can lower their own risk of becoming ill by following a low-fat diet, eliminating smoking, controlling their weight, and exercising regularly.

One of the sad effects of aging is the loss of loved ones and treasured relationships. A nine-year study of 7,000 Alameda County (California) residents indicated that people with few relationships died at rates two to five times higher than those with more friendships. Another study, in England, of females who had suffered severe DEPRESSION, revealed that women who experienced severe stress and did not have a confidante were approximately 10 times more likely to be depressed than women who had companionship of some sort. Even caring for pets has a beneficial effect on aging; being responsible for something other than oneself is a morale booster.

Planning for retirement helps one stay active. In a study by the American Association of Retired Persons, members ranked BOREDOM as one of the most serious problems of retirement.

Many healthy people move into RETIREMENT communities or buildings during their later years so that they will have companionship as well as available health care nearby. Among the concerns of the aging population are the ability to continue managing one's own affairs, the desire to remain independent and not be a burden to children or society, and the dread of living out one's last years in a nursing home.

See also AGE DISCRIMINATION; ELDERLY PARENTS; INTERGENERATIONAL CONFLICTS.

FOR FURTHER INFORMATION:
American Association of Retired Persons
601 E Street NW
Washington, DC 20049
Phone: (202) 434-2277

SOURCES:
Beer, Ralph. "Hello Mother, Hello Father: Here We Are at . . . Middle Age." *Modern Maturity*, January-February 1996.
Kahn, Ada P., and Jan Fawcett. *The Encyclopedia of Mental Health*. New York: Facts On File, 1993.

aging parents   See ELDERLY PARENTS.

agoraphobia   An ANXIETY DISORDER; it is a complex syndrome characterized by extreme ANXIETY about being in situations from which escape may be difficult or embarrassing or in which help may not be available in the event

---

**COPING WITH THE STRESSES
OF AGING**

- Maintain friendships and relationships with others.
- Keep physically and intellectually active.
- Make constructive use of time.
- Eat a proper diet with a reasonable amount of fiber.
- Reduce intake of salt and cholesterol.
- Avoid smoking and excessive alcohol intake.
- Do a reasonable amount of exercise.
- Protect skin from the sun.
- Undergo periodic health examinations.
- Examine risk factors; determine necessary life-style changes.

of having a PANIC ATTACK. Agoraphobia includes fears of losing control of oneself and of developing embarrassing or incapacitating symptoms, such as dizziness, fainting, or sudden illness.

Typically, the anxiety leads to a pervasive avoidance of situations that may include being alone outside or in the home; being in a crowd of people; traveling in an automobile, bus, or airplane; or being on a bridge or in an elevator. According to *Diagnostic and Statistical Manual of Mental Disorders, Fourth Edition,* some individuals are able to expose themselves to the feared situations but endure these experiences with considerable dread. Often an individual is better able to confront a feared situation when accompanied by a companion.

Agoraphobia causes stress for the sufferer as well as for family members and friends. Individuals' avoidance of situations may impair their ability to travel to work or to carry out homemaking responsibilities, such as grocery shopping and taking children to the doctor. Agoraphobia can be socially disabling. Many agoraphobics refuse invitations or make excuses for not going out. Thus, adjustments are necessary to compensate for the agoraphobic's lack of participation in family life and activities outside the home.

Prevalence

Agoraphobia usually occurs in adults; the ratio of agoraphobia in woman vs. men is three to one. Shy, anxious women form the group of individuals most prone to agoraphobia. Many agoraphobics are indecisive, lack initiative, feel guilty because they are unable to get out of situations themselves, and may gradually withdraw into a restricted lifestyle.

The majority of agoraphobics are married at the time they come for treatment. In most cases involving agoraphobics, spouses seem well-adjusted and integrated individuals. Agoraphobia may strain a marriage because the agoraphobic person may ask the spouse to take over chores that require going out, such as

shopping or picking up children; spouses often must fulfill social obligations without the companionship of their mates. Spouses are additionally stressed by having to be "on call" in case anxiety attacks occur that require an emergency trip home to soothe the agoraphobic. Thus, a couple that may have been happy may be driven apart by the disorder, with each blaming the other for a lack of understanding. The husband may think that the wife is not trying to overcome her phobic feelings, and the agoraphobic wife may think that her husband does not understand her suffering. The wife may become so preoccupied with fighting her daily terrors that she focuses little attention on their marital relationship and her husband's needs. However, in cases where the agoraphobic has an understanding, patient, and loving spouse, this support can be an asset in overcoming the agoraphobic condition. The spouse can attend training sessions with the therapist, attend group therapy sessions, and act as the "understanding companion" when the agoraphobic is ready to venture out.

Symptoms

Many agoraphobics were formerly active, sociable, outgoing persons; however, when they seek treatment, they are often in a constant state of extreme stress. Typically, the agoraphobic admits to being generally anxious and expresses feelings of helplessness and discouragement. In some cases, agoraphobics abuse alcohol and drugs.

Characteristic symptoms in addition to general anxiety include an intense fear of dizziness or falling, loss of bladder or bowel control, vomiting, palpitations, and chest pain. There may be a fear of having a heart attack because of the rapid heart action, of fainting if the anxiety becomes too intense, and of being surrounded by unsympathetic onlookers. The individual then develops a fear of the fear, which brings about anxiety in anticipation of a panic reaction, resulting in avoidance of the feared situation.

Occasionally, depersonalization occurs; depersonalization is a change in the perception or experience of the self so that the feeling of one's own reality is temporarily lost. Often in agoraphobia there is a history of panic attacks; however, agoraphobia may occur with or without a history of panic attacks.

Many agoraphobics have episodes of DEPRESSION. The first episode may occur within weeks or months of the first panic attack. Individuals complain of feeling "blue," having crying spells, feeling hopeless and irritable, lacking interest in work, and having difficulty in sleeping. Agoraphobia is often aggravated during a depressive episode. The increased anxiety may make individuals less motivated to work hard at tasks (such as going out) that they previously did with difficulty.

Some agoraphobics are also claustrophobic. Usually CLAUSTROPHOBIA is present before the agoraphobia develops. The common factor between the two phobias is that escape is blocked, at least temporarily. Symptoms of the phobic anxiety in agoraphobia may include many physical sensations that accompany other anxiety states, such as dry mouth, sweating, rapid heart beat, hyperventilation, faintness, and dizziness. Many women report that generalized anxiety and panic in agoraphobia tends to be worse just prior to and during MENSTRUATION.

Some agoraphobics experience obsessions, which are persistent and recurrent ideas, thoughts, impulses, or images that occur involuntarily and invade the consciousness. Obsessional behavior is usually present before an individual develops agoraphobia. Individuals may develop obsessional thinking about certain places, situations, or objects that might stimulate their fear reaction. Obsessional thinking is difficult to control, often distorts or exaggerates reality, and causes much anticipatory anxiety. Individuals may develop compulsive behavior in an attempt to reduce obsessional thoughts and resultant stress and anxiety.

Causes of agoraphobia

Agoraphobia frequently results from panic attacks, which are attacks of overwhelming anxiety, leading the victim to fear a fatal heart attack or loss of mental control. After repeated panic attacks, sufferers avoid crowds, enclosed places (tunnels, airplanes, large groups of people, even leaving home) for fear that a repeat panic attack might occur.

Some individuals regard the world as a dangerous place because of learned experiences. Many agoraphobics had at least one agoraphobic parent and many have had at least one parent who is somewhat fearful. In some cases, they received mixed messages from their parents. While they were encouraged to achieve, they were not well prepared to deal with the world, either because they were overprotected and taught that home is the only safe place, or underprotected, having to take on too much responsibility at an early age.

Additionally, there may be a genetic predisposition to panic disorder; it may be as much as 10 times more frequent in the biological relatives of those with panic disorder as among those without such a family history.

The biological basis for panic attacks and resultant agoraphobia is being researched, and there are many theories. For example, symptoms of panic attacks, such as palpitations, sweating, and tremulousness, have lead to a theory that they are the result of massive discharges from the adrenergic nervous system (part of the autonomic nervous system, which controls activities of organs, blood vessels, glands and many other tissues in the body).

Treatments for agoraphobia

Treatment for agoraphobia is usually directed toward several aspects of the agoraphobic syndrome: agoraphobia, panic attacks and anticipatory anxiety. A variety of treatments are often used for the same individual, sometimes in sequence or combination.

BEHAVIOR THERAPY includes educating individuals about their reactions to anxiety-producing situations, and teaching BREATHING exercises to help overcome HYPERVENTILATION. In many cases, three to six months of behavior therapy is effective, and subsequent supportive and behavioral techniques reduce the anxiety level and help individuals master fears of recurrent attacks in specific situations.

Many treatments for agoraphobia are based on varieties of techniques known as exposure therapy. Typically, treatment involves exposing the agoraphobic to situations that are commonly avoided and frightening in order to demonstrate that there is no actual danger. Treatment may include direct exposure, such as having the individual move away from a safe place or person, or enter a crowded shopping center in a structured way. Indirect exposure is also used; this may involve use of films with fear-arousing cues. Systematic desensitization is a procedure characterized by exposure (either in imagination or *in vivo*) to the least reactive elements of a situation or object until the anxiety response no longer occurs. Another imaginal procedure for anxiety treatment includes flooding, or continuous presentation of the most reactive elements of a situation until anxiety reduction occurs.

Facing the fearful situation with appropriate reinforcement may help an individual undo the learned fear. For example, some therapists set progressive goals for the patient for each week, such as walking one block from home, then two and three, and taking a bus. In the early stages of treatment, many therapists accompany their patients as they venture into public places, and in some cases spouses or family members are trained to accompany them. Other therapists recommend structured group therapy with defined goals and social skill training for agoraphobics and their families.

Involvement of spouses and family members usually produces better results than treatment involving the agoraphobic alone.

Home-based treatment, where individuals proceed at their own pace within a structured treatment program, produces fewer dropouts than the more intensive, prolonged exposure or pharmacological treatments.

Some agoraphobics develop ways to live more comfortably with their disorder. For example, those who go to church or a movie theater may prefer aisle seats so that they can make a fast exit if they experience a panic attack. Having a telephone nearby is another comfort.

Pharmacological approach
The treatment of choice today for agoraphobia involves use of both behavior therapy and pharmaceutical medication, with the latter withdrawn as progress is made. Particularly for those who have panic attacks, drug therapy initially seems to enhance results of exposure-based treatments. In many cases, drugs are used for three to six months and then discontinued once the individual has some control over bodily sensations. Some individuals never experience recurrence of attacks, while others experience a return months or years later. When attacks recur, a second course of drug therapy is often successful.

A variety of drugs are used to treat panic attacks associated with agoraphobia. These include the tricyclic antidepressant medications, the monoamine oxidase inhibitors (MAOIs, which are also used to treat severe depression), and ALPRAZOLAM, an antianxiety drug. For many individuals, panic attacks are successfully controlled with use of particular tricyclic antidepressants (imipramine, desipramine, or clomipramine). Monoamine oxidase inhibitors (MAOIs) are often used as second-line medications when patients do not respond to a tricyclic.

Free-floating or anticipatory anxiety is often treated with selective use of a benzodiazepine (for example, oxazepam) or alprazolam (Xanax) alone, because such agents reduce anticipatory anxiety and block panic attacks. Xanax has been approved by the Food and Drug Administration to treat symptoms of panic attacks. Clonazepam (trade name, Klonopin) is a newer benzodiazepine that is also thought to have antipanic properties. Buspirone (trade name, Buspar), a nonbenzo-diazepine antianxiety agent, is less sedating and less prone to being abused than are the benzodiazepines, but its efficacy in panic disorder is still under study.

Agoraphobia and alcoholism
Some agoraphobics use alcohol in an unsuccessful attempt to avoid anticipatory anxiety and panic attacks. However, alcohol may exacerbate panic by bringing about a feeling of loss of control both mentally and physically. Also, use of alcohol may interfere with effective treatment of the agoraphobia, as central nervous system depressants in alcohol reduce the efficacy of exposure treatment. However, some agoraphobic people believe that alcohol helps to calm them before they venture out into public.

There is some evidence that both agoraphobics who abuse alcohol and agoraphobics who don't may have histories of disturbed childhoods that include familial ALCOHOLISM and depression. Also, children whose early attachments to caretakers were non-supportive as well as frightening or dangerous may fail to develop a sense of trust and security. Such individuals may be particularly vulnerable to later psychopathology, including panic attacks and agoraphobia; alcoholism may be one mode of coping for such individuals.

The clinical picture of both agoraphobia and alcoholism often involves depression. Agoraphobics who are alcohol abusers may also be more socially anxious than their non-alcoholic peers. High rates of SOCIAL PHOBIA have been noted among inpatient alcoholics, and major depression has been found to increase both the likelihood and intensity of agoraphobia and social anxieties.

Self-help groups for agoraphobics
As recovery from agoraphobia is a long-term process, self-help groups can provide valuable support. Participating individuals share common experiences and coping tips, and have an additional social outlet. Some agoraphobic SUPPORT GROUPS get together for outings, help take each other's children to and from school, arrange programs, and retrain themselves out of their fears and anxieties.

See also PHARMACOLOGICAL APPROACH; PSYCHOTHERAPIES.

FOR FURTHER INFORMATION:
American Psychiatric Association
Division of Public Affairs
1400 K Street NW
Washington, DC 20005
Phone: (212) 682-6000

Anxiety Disorders Association of America
11900 Parklawn Drive (Suite 100)
Rockville, MD 20852
Phone: (301) 231-9350

SOURCES:
American Psychiatric Association. *Diagnostic and Statistical Manual of Mental Disorders, Fourth Edition.* Washington, D.C.: American Psychiatric Association, 1994.
Frampton, Muriel. *Agoraphobia: Coping with the World Outside.* Wellingstorough, Northamptonshire, England: Turnstone Press, Ltd., 1984.
Kahn, Ada P., "Panic attacks." *Chicago Tribune,* June 23, 1991.
Kahn, Ada P., and Jan Fawcett. *The Encyclopedia of Mental Health.* New York: Facts On File, 1993.

AIDS See ACQUIRED IMMUNODEFICIENCY SYNDROME; HUMAN IMMUNODEFICIENCY VIRUS.

airplanes Many individuals are phobic about flying. Estimates indicate that one of every six adults is afraid to fly. Some people choose to spend days traveling by train or experience the stresses of highway travel in place of flying.

Anticipation of taking an airplane flight is a major source of stress for many people. Some are fearful of being in an enclosed place (CLAUSTROPHOBIA), while others fear being out of CONTROL or becoming ill, and are just generally anxious about all the safety and weather factors associated with traveling by air.

Many common phrases related to flying in airplanes, such as "terminal," "final boarding," "final approach," and "departure lounge," have a morbid connotation and produce stress. These terms are augmented by oxygen masks, life jackets, emergency exits, crash procedures, and other reminders of adverse consequences of flying. In addition, news reports of air crashes and television and movie productions centering on trouble on airplanes can contribute to the ANXIETY.

Reasons for stress
There are two major areas of stress relating to flying. One is anticipating the situation and the other is the flying situation itself. Anticipatory anxiety occurs when one makes a commitment to fly by making the reservation, purchasing the ticket, and telling people about the trip. People experiencing anticipatory anxiety usually feel dread, rapid pulse, body sensations such as tension and warmth, and have fear-producing images and thoughts.

The anticipatory fear is usually not of the airplane itself but of uncontrollable outcomes such as fear of losing control of oneself in the plane, embarrassing oneself in public, fear of separation from loved ones, fears of relinquishing control to the pilot, or thoughts of falling from the sky and dying in a crash.

People who fear flying can learn to become less fearful. Flying can be viewed as an opportunity to begin overcoming this fear. Skills can be acquired to visualize flying comfortably, and relaxation techniques can be learned to help cope with the fears. One can practice desensitization; this involves going to the airport, watching planes take off and land and imagining feeling comfortable in the planes being watched. Finally, one can make a tape to relax with reminders and ideas to help cope while flying. With preparation, practice, and more flying, this fear can be diminished.

Treating stresses and fears surrounding airplanes
Treatments for the stresses involved in airplane travel includes behavior therapies, particularly exposure therapy, HYPNOSIS, RELAXATION techniques, and use of some pharmacological approaches. Propranolol and ALPRAZOLAM are two drugs commonly used for fear of flying. They are both fast-acting and produce relatively few side effects.

Many people turn to alcohol to relieve their stresses and fears related to flying. While alcohol reduces autonomic arousal, it tends to produce anxiety-like sensations including dizziness, loss of balance, mental confusion, and lack of control of perceptual-motor functions, which in turn can trigger more stress and an anxiety response.

There may also be stress related to feelings about a place or person the individual associated with either at the point of departure or of arrival.

See also ALCOHOLISM AND ALCOHOL DEPENDENCE; ANXIETY; BEHAVIOR THERAPY; PHOBIAS; PHARMACOLOGICAL APPROACH; POST-TRAUMATIC STRESS DISORDER.

SOURCE:
Kahn, Ada P. and Ronald M. Doctor. *Encyclopedia of Phobias, Fears and Anxieties.* New York: Facts On File, 1989.

airports See AIRPLANES; RANDOM NUISANCES; VACATIONS.

Alcoholics Anonymous See ALCOHOLISM AND ALCOHOL DEPENDENCE.

alcoholism and alcohol dependence Alcoholism (alcohol dependence) is characterized by compulsive, habitual, long-term and heavy consumption of alcohol and with withdrawal symptoms when intake of alcohol suddenly ceases.

Many factors interact to lead to alcohol dependence. People who abuse alcohol often begin to drink to relieve personal, social, or business stresses. When they find temporary relief, even at the cost of occasional hangovers, they may gradually begin to drink whenever they feel tense or anxious. The more they need alcohol to fight their ANXIETY, the less they can do without it. Some individuals may start out as moderate drinkers and then begin to depend on alcohol during times of extreme STRESS, such as bereavement, loneliness, job difficulties, DIVORCE, or their illness or an illness of a close family member.

Some agoraphobics become alcoholic as a way of coping with their fears. Because some agoraphobic individuals do not go out, it is fairly easy for them to conceal their alcoholic habit. Some depressed individuals turn to alcohol to temporarily improve their mood; instead of mood elevation, it results in sedation.

Genetic factors as well as personality and environmental factors play a role in causing dependence in some cases, but it is widely understood that anyone can become addicted to alcohol if she or he drinks heavily and regularly for a prolonged period of time.

Stress on family members

When an individual drinks to excess, it can cause stress on family members as well as employers. For example, abusers may neglect home or child care responsibilities and may often be absent from their jobs. They may be difficult to live with because they are often irritable and sometimes violent. Abusers may be drunk under physically hazardous circumstances, such as operating machinery. There may be legal difficulties, such as an arrest for driving while under the influence of alcohol. Alcohol is an important factor in deaths and injuries from industrial and motor vehicle accidents, suicides, domestic violence, marriage breakdown, child abuse, and other types of crime.

Physical tolerance for alcohol varies between individuals. The shift from social drinking to alcoholism can happen almost imperceptibly over a long period of time, or may occur rapidly. Drinking habits vary, too. Some individuals are "binge" drinkers who go on drinking sprees, while others drink constantly and are never quite sober. Spouses, friends, and employers of binge drinkers must cope with the stresses of unpredictable variations in the mood behavior of the drinker, making everyday life a challenge.

Alcoholism: public health problem and disease

Alcoholism is considered a major public health problem in the United States. Estimates indicate that there are approximately five million alcohol-dependent persons in the United States. According to the American Psychiatric Association's *Diagnostic and Statistical Manual of Mental Disorders, Fourth Edition,* as many as 90% of adults in the United States have had some experience with alcohol, and a substantial number (60% of males and 30% of females) have had one or more alcohol-related adverse life events, such as driving after consuming too much alcohol or missing school or work due to a hangover.

Most authorities including the American Medical Association and the American Bar Association recognize alcoholism as a disease; others say that it is a self-inflicted condition and cannot properly be designated a disease. However, as a physiological and psychological dependence on alcohol, alcoholism must be considered an ADDICTION.

Contrary to popular belief, alcohol is a depressant, not a stimulant. The effects of alcohol are felt most noticeably in the central nervous system. As sensitivity is reduced in the nervous system, the higher functions of the brain are dulled, leading to impulsive actions, loud speech, and lack of physical control. The drinker's face may turn red or pale. While drinking, the alcoholic loses any sense of guilt or embarrassment, gains more self-confidence, and sheds inhibitions as the alcohol deadens restraining influences of the brain. Large quantities of alcohol impair physical reflexes, coordination, and mental acuteness.

Symptoms and stages of alcoholism

There are four stages of alcoholism. In the first phase, the heavy social drinker may feel no effects from alcohol. In the second phase, the drinker experiences lapses of memory relating to drinking episodes. In the third phase, there is lack of CONTROL over alcohol and the drinker cannot be certain of discontinuing drinking by choice. The final phase begins with long binges of intoxication and observable mental or physical complications.

Behavior symptoms may include aggressive or grandiose actions, irritability, jealousy or uncontrolled anger, frequent changing of jobs, repeated promises to give up drinking, hiding of bottles, and neglect of proper eating habits and personal appearance. Physical symptoms may include unsteadiness, confusion, poor memory, nausea, vomiting, shaking, weakness in the legs and hands, irregular pulse, and redness and enlarged capillaries in the face. In general, alcohol-dependent persons are more susceptible than others to a variety of physical and mental disorders.

Diagnosis of alcoholism by physicians

In a study published in the *Journal of the American Medical Association* (February 4, 1992), Diana Chapman Walsh, Ph.D., Harvard School of Public Health, underscored the need for physicians to advise patients of potential hazards associated with heavy or problem drinking,

Dr. Walsh and colleagues reported on 200 problem drinkers at a large New England manufacturing plant. Participants' drinking problems were identified by the company's EMPLOYEE ASSISTANCE PROGRAM (EAP) between February 1, 1982 and June 20, 1987. Each sub-

ject was followed for two years. Mean age of the subjects was 32 years. Subjects were overwhelmingly male (96%) and white (90%). About half (51%) graduated from high school, but not college; 47% had annual family incomes under $25,000. The report stated: "Of the 200 seriously impaired workers in the sample, only 15 percent recalled warning that their abuse of alcohol might be compromising their health during the year before being identified on the job. Fully 74 percent (148) of the workers identified on the job had seen physicians in that year, but only 22 percent of them recalled health warnings. That the manifestations of alcohol abuse are overt enough to bring these heavy drinkers to the attention of intervention programs at work during the course of the year in which they have visited physicians lends further weight to the argument that many physicians are not sufficiently alert to their patients' alcohol use and abuse."

In an editorial accompanying the study, Thomas L. Delbanco, M.D., Division of General Medicine and Primary Care, Beth Israel Hospital, Boston, wrote: "Walsh and colleagues bring us both good and bad news. Welcome is their suggestion that when doctors address alcoholism with their patients, the outcome may improve. Confirming earlier reports, however, the bad news is the continuing inference that doctors are often loathe to intervene with patients who abuse alcohol."

Delbanco noted that physicians' reticence may result from a desire not to stigmatize or insult their patients, from confusion over what to do once a diagnosis of alcoholism is made, from concern about the time demands treating an alcoholic requires, or discomfort addressing the issue if the physician himself drinks. Delbanco pointed to an increase in the number of teaching institutions with programs focusing on the diagnosis and treatment of alcoholism and a "growing public consciousness" of the toll alcoholism takes on individuals and society. He concluded by saying: "As we grapple increasingly with chronic diseases, we encounter few where our intervention can be pivotal in turning patients away from a progressive, debilitating, and often tragic illness toward a fully healthy life. Alcoholism provides both patient and doctor with that opportunity."

Professional treatment and self-help groups

Medical help for alcohol dependence includes detoxification, which is assistance in overcoming withdrawal symptoms, and psychological, social and physical treatments. Psychotherapy is usually done in groups and uses a variety of techniques. Therapists for alcoholic dependent persons may be psychiatrists, psychologists, or social workers. Family members are involved in the treatment process.

Many alcohol dependent persons benefit from involvement in SELF-HELP GROUPS. These groups are also available for other family members.

Alcoholics Anonymous (AA) is an international organization, founded in 1935, devoted to maintaining the sobriety of its members and helping them control the compulsive urge to drink through self-help, mutual support, fellowship, and understanding. Medical treatment is not used. The program includes the individual's admission that he (or she) cannot control his (her) drinking, the sharing of experiences, problems, and concerns at meetings, and helping others who are in need of support.

At the core of the AA program is the "desire to stop drinking." Members follow a 12-step program, which stresses faith, disavowal of personal responsibility, passivity in the hands of God or a higher power, confession of wrongdoing, and response to spiritual awakening by sharing with others.

The first step involves the idea of despair and a breakdown of denial concerning alcohol. Second is the idea of hope, or seeing the light. Third is the shifting of responsibility from one-self to a higher authority figure. The next steps involve confessing, making amends, continuing confirmation of a new image of oneself, and redirecting energy to help others.

Life expectancy may increase with abstinence

Alcoholics who go dry may increase their life expectancy, according to results of a study published in the *Journal of the American Medical Association* (January 4, 1992). Results supported the notion that achievement of stable abstinence reduces the risk of premature death among alcoholics. Kim D. Bullock, Psychiatry and Research Services, Veterans Affairs Medical Center, San Diego, and colleagues reported on 199 men who had histories of at least five years of drinking at alcoholic levels. All were current or former patients of the V.A. Alcoholism Treatment Program and/or members of Alcoholics Anonymous. Follow-up on relapse and mortality was obtained; 101 men had relapsed and 98 were abstinent. A control group of 92 nonalcoholics equated for age, education, and sex was also studied for mortality. There were 19 deaths among the relapsed alcoholics compared with the expected number of 3.83. Among abstinent alcoholics there were four deaths. Alcoholic men who achieved stable abstinence did not differ from nonalcoholic men in mortality experience. However, alcoholics who relapsed died at a rate 4.96 times that of an age-, sex-, and race-matched representative sample.

See also AGORAPHOBIA; CODEPENDENCY; DEPRESSION; SUPPORT GROUPS.

FOR FURTHER INFORMATION:
AL-ANON Family Group Headquarters
1372 Broadway (7th floor)
New York, NY 10018
Phone: (212) 302-7240

Alcoholics Anonymous World Services
486 Park Avenue South
New York, NY 10016
Phone: (212) 686-1100

Children of Alcoholics Foundation
200 Park Avenue (31st Floor)
New York, NY 10166
Phone: (212) 949-1404

Mothers Against Drunk Driving
P.O. Box 541688
Dallas, TX 75354-1688
Phone: (214) 744-6233

National Institute of Alcohol Abuse and
   Alcoholism
National Clearinghouse for Alcohol Information
9000 Rockville Pike
Bethesda, MD 20892
Phone: (301) 443-3860

SOURCES:

American Psychiatric Association. *Diagnostic and Statistical Manual of Mental Disorders, Fourth Edition.* Washington, D.C.: American Psychiatric Association, 1994.

Clayman, Charles B., ed. *Encyclopedia of Medicine.* New York: Random House, 1989.

O'Brien, Robert, and Morris Chafetz. *The Encyclopedia of Alcoholism.* New York: Facts On File, Inc., 1982.

Tarini, Paul. American Medical Association news releases, Oct. 1, 1991, January 4, 1992 and February 4, 1992.

Alexander technique Method of realigning body posture for relief of stress, chronic pain, or muscle tension, and to increase well-being and health. With verbal and gentle physical instruction from trained teachers, individuals learn how to eliminate common habits such as hunching, slouching, and tensing the spine that often accompany periods of stress.

The technique was developed by F. Matthias Alexander (1869–1955), an Australian Shakespearean actor who moved to England and established his first school for the technique in England in 1924. It has drawn many actors, dancers, and musicians who experience the stresses of tightness, injuries, or physical ailments related to the practice of their arts. The technique also appeals to people suffering from orthopedic or neurological problems, joint pain, headaches, and fatigue.

With Alexander exercises, individuals become aware of their bodies and learn to make conscious changes. They are taught that when they are able to release muscles, the muscles will work efficiently and without strain for the task at hand. Additionally, some of them find it helpful to lie down for 15 to 20 minutes each day and visualize the Alexander instructions.

See also ALTERNATIVE THERAPIES; BODY THERAPIES; MEDITATION.

alopecia See HAIR LOSS.

allergies A collection of disease symptoms caused by exposure of the skin to a chemical, or the respiratory system to particles of dust or pollen, or of the stomach or intestines to food. Allergies are sources of stress for many people because symptoms of allergies are unpredictable and may make people uncomfortable.

Allergies are often exacerbated by emotional stress. Though apparently not a direct cause, stress can trigger allergic attacks. If individuals are prone to allergies, it is likely that they will have less trouble with them if they can reduce the stress and tension in their lives. While they cannot eliminate an allergy, they can usually learn how to live with it, sometimes with the aid of RELAXATION techniques and GUIDED IMAGERY, or with prescription medications.

Allergy reactions

Some allergic reactions limit the sufferer's participation in certain activities, such as hiking in forests or partaking of certain foods. Such seemingly harmless, everyday encounters as with a vase of flowers, a glass of milk, or the neighbor's cat can bring on misery for the sufferer. Depending on the allergy, the reactions can vary greatly, from coughing, sneezing and a runny nose to skin irritations such as HIVES and rashes, to vomiting and diarrhea. Some people must curtail their social activities during periods when their allergy symptoms are severe.

According to the American Academy of Allergy and Immunology, 41 million American people (1 in 6) have ASTHMA and allergies. Of these, 22.4 million have hay fever and 10 million are affected with eczema, urticaria (hives) and angioedema (swelling); and by allergic reactions to food, medications, and insect stings. These last are dangerous as well as uncomfortable, accounting for at least 50 deaths a year.

The most common type of allergy, known as allergic rhinitis, affects the upper respiratory tract. Sufferers of this type of allergy often complain of cold-like symptoms such as runny eyes, drippy noses, coughing, and congestion. Since allergic rhinitis is often caused by pollen, molds, and spores, it is primarily a seasonal affliction, striking in spring and fall.

Asthma is an allergic reaction that affects the lungs and afflicts some 10 million Americans. Sufferers complain of "attacks," in which the chest tightens and breathing becomes extremely difficult. Some people gasp and feel that they might die at any moment. Asthma is also stressful for those around the sufferer. An asthma attack may be brought on by a wide variety of allergens, including house dust, certain foods, and feathers. Exercise as well as stress can also induce attacks. Effective prescription medications are available for asthma. Other common allergies include those that affect the skin, which are caused by a number of allergens, and those that affect the digestive system, most often caused by foods such as dairy and wheat-based products.

Pets, especially cats, can provide severe reactions, usually within the allergic rhinitis and skin allergy range of symptoms.

Foods can set off reactions. For example, eggs, even in tiny quantities, make many people ill. If you have an allergy and suspect that food is responsible, you can leave one item at a time out of your diet for periods of several weeks, then reintroduce it until you discover the allergen or allergens.

Allergic contact dermatitis is a skin condition produced by substances that touch the skin directly, in contrast to eruptions that occur on the skin from an internal or systemic reactions. Fabrics and dyes may do this. POISON IVY is another example of allergic contact dermatitis. Knowing that one is allergic to poison ivy makes for a stressful situation while walking in a wooded or forested area.

Diagnosis and treatment

Most allergies begin during childhood, some 80% before the age of 15 years. The first step is to identify the allergen and then to remove it from the person's environment if possible, or else to take the person away from the allergen. Sometimes a change of climate works but may result in other allergies. Some hay fever sufferers have moved to the opposite end of the country, only to find a new allergen there.

Air conditioners and filters help persons allergic to pollen. In other cases, more radical measures may be called for; for example, work-related allergens may require a change in occupation or, at the least, a face mask on the job. Hypoallergenic cosmetics (preparations that are compounded without the most common allergens) help many people who are allergic to makeup and perfume.

Many people mistake allergies for other problems and only after recurring episodes seek medical help. An allergist, or a physician who specializes in allergies, is a wise move for people who think they have an allergy but do not know its cause. In many cases, the allergist conducts skin tests in which the skin is exposed to minute amounts of various materials to see which one causes a reaction. Efforts are then made, wherever possible, to eliminate or reduce contact with that allergen. Prescription medications are available to relieve allergies.

See also ALTERNATIVE THERAPIES.

FOR FURTHER INFORMATION:

American Academy of Allergy and Immunology
611 E. Wells Street
Milwaukee, WI 53202
Phone: (414) 272-6071

American College of Allergy and Immunology
800 E. Northwest Highway (Suite 1080)
Palatine, IL 60067
Phone: (708) 359-2800

National Institute of Allergy and Infectious
  Diseases
Public Response
9000 Rockville Pike
Bethesda, MD 20892
Phone: (301) 496-5717

alprazolam   Anti-anxiety drug (also referred to as an anxiolytic or sedative) marketed under the trade name Xanax. A member of the drug group known as the benzodiazepines, it has been useful in treating some individuals who suffer from effects of extreme stress, anticipatory ANXIETY or PANIC ATTACKS AND PANIC DISORDER, and DEPRESSION, particularly in mixed states of depression and anxiety. The clinical reasons for its antidepressant effects are still unknown. Studies have shown that it has no effect on nerve cell receptors that are targets of some antidepressive drugs.

Alprazolam is comparable to tricyclic antidepressant medications and is used as an antidepressant for individuals who have an extremely high degree of anxiety and agitation; alprazolam causes sedation and lethargy. Because it has no apparent cardiac side effects, it is applicable in treatment of anxious or depressed cardiac patients. As with other drugs of this class, dependency develops with prolonged use and withdrawal effects can occur when treatment ends. These can be prevented by gradually tapering off the dosage of the drug.

See also BENZODIAZEPINE DRUGS; PHARMACOLOGICAL APPROACH.

SOURCES:
Fawcett, Jan A., and Howard M. Kravitz. "Alprazolam: Pharmacokinetics, Clinical Efficacy and Mechanism of Action." *Pharmacotherapy* no. 5 (September-October 1982).
Freeman, Arthur M., III, et al. *Journal of Clinical Psychopharmacology* 6, no. 1 (February 1986).
Kahn, Ada P., and Jan A. Fawcett. *Encyclopedia of Mental Health.* New York: Facts On File, 1993.

alternative therapies   A set of practices that, depending on the viewpoint, either complement or compete with conventional medicine in the prevention and treatment of stress-related disorders as well as other diseases.

According to David Edelberg, M.D., writing in *The Internist* (September 1994), alternative medicine commonly refers to anything that is not conventionally practiced or taught in medical school. In 1994, there were more than 200 fields of alternative medicine. Alternative fields can be divided into four broad categories: traditional medicine, such as Chinese or Native American; hands-on body-work; psychological or psychospiritual medicine; and many holdovers from the 19th century, such as chiropractic and homeopathy.

Alternative therapies for dealing with stress and healing mind as well as body, include emotional release therapies with or without body manipulation, emotional control or self-regulating therapies, religious or inspirational therapies, cognitive-emotional therapies, and emotional expression through creative therapies. Some of these have been known by such names as encounter groups, gestalt therapy, primal therapy, EST, bioenergetic psychotherapy, ROLFING, TRANSCENDENTAL MEDITATION, and BIOFEEDBACK. It is important to note that alternative therapies are not subject to scientific scrutiny through controlled efficacy studies with placebo or comparisons of treatments. They are accepted and promoted as helping on the basis of "anecdotal evidence" stemming from individual reports of success. Some may be truly helpful while others may be useless or ineffectual.

Many individuals find relief for stress-induced conditions from one or from a combination of alternative therapies either along with or after seeking traditional care. For example, MENTAL IMAGERY is rated one of the six most commonly used alternative treatments among cancer patients and is believed by physicians as well as patients to reduce both the pain and distress of symptoms. However, as with other medical conditions, individuals should not overlook traditional psychiatric or medical treatments in favor of alternative therapies because they may be robbing themselves of valuable time as their condition progresses.

Alternative vs. conventional care

Conventional medical practitioners adhere to scientific models and methodologies that many alternative medical practitioners believe focus too exclusively on reductionist and physiochemical explanations of biological phenomena. Proponents of alternative medicine suggest that this approach shows limited understanding of health and disease and, in particular, of interactions among mind-body connections, psychological, social, and biological factors that influence coping with stress and disease processes.

Advocates of alternative approaches, in recent decades known also as "holistic" (or "wholistic") medicine or complementary medicine, regard the influence of psychological factors and cognitive processes as equal to, if not more powerful than, the insights and methods of conventional medicine in coping with stress and disease and improving clinical outcomes.

For most of the 20th century, the generally accepted model for understanding biological phenomena and intervening therapeutically was the allopathic method. It achieved scientific, economic, and political primacy over the competing models such as osteopathic medicine, homeopathy, and chiropractic as well as

other alternative approaches. However, the public's interest in alternative therapies has grown tremendously during the last two decades of the 20th century.

In a survey by Harvard Medical School researchers reported that more than a quarter of the people they interviewed saw a physician regularly but were also employing another treatment, usually with their doctor's knowledge. One in ten respondents were relying on nontraditional treatments exclusively. The study emphasized the widespread acceptance of "alternative medicine," a variety of unrelated practices from acupuncture to yoga that are promoted as having healing benefits. The common factor between them is that they have not yet been subjected to scientific review, the process most of the Western world uses to determine whether a treatment is safe and effective.

A landmark study published in 1993 in the *New England Journal of Medicine* showed that far more people visited providers of alternative therapies—an estimated 425 million in 1990—than visited primary care physicians (388 million) during the same time period. The study, conducted by David Eisenberg and colleagues, found that one-third of Americans used alternative medical treatments. In addition, most of the expense for these visits, $10.3 billion, was out-of-pocket.

Herbal and "folk" therapies

In many cultures, herbs and other natural and botanical products are used to relieve stress-induced health conditions instead of modern diagnostic techniques and pharmacological treatments. Herbs are used both to cure specific illnesses, improve health, lengthen life, and increase sexual vigor and fertility.

Herbal medicine may have begun with the Greeks and spread across Europe with the Roman conquests. However, the development of an organized approach to using herbs took place in central Europe and the British Isles. Practices and beliefs in folk medicine are preserved in isolated, traditional cultures such as in Appalachia and among Native American tribes. Folk medical treatments have developed by trial and error and serendipity without benefit of the scientific method. Since folk cultures generally mix religious or spiritual beliefs with concepts of health and illness, they attribute disease to causes other than the natural causes recognized by conventional medicine. In folk beliefs, mental or physical illness may be caused by divine retribution for transgression or by the will of spirits or other magical beings. Folk healers pass down techniques from one generation to the next and may jealously guard their secrets.

Because of immigration to the Western world at the end of the 20th century, many practitioners of Western medicine are learning about folk medicine, so that they may better communicate with patients from other cultures.

Increasing interest by government and insurers

In 1991 the OFFICE OF ALTERNATIVE MEDICINE (OAM) was created within the National Institutes of Health. The goal of the OAM is to research and evaluate the many alternative or unconventional medical treatments.

Increasingly, some health insurers are paying for alternative therapies, removing some of the financial stress involved in seeking these treatments. A study reported in the *Journal of Health Care Marketing* (Spring 1995) included insurers from government, third-party insurance companies, and HMOs; results indicated the mechanisms through which each of three alternative therapies (chiropractic, ACUPUNCTURE, and biofeedback) gained some credibility and acceptance by insurers. Results indicated that these therapies have each achieved at least moderate success in obtaining third-party reimbursement.

Choosing alternative therapies

Individuals who decide to take an unproven therapy should let their physician know what they are doing. He or she will need to take the effects of that treatment into account when evaluating their care. Be wary when encountering claims that a treatment works miracles, such as rejuvenating skin or curing cancer with no pain or side effects. Watch out for contentions from proponents of a treatment that the medical community is trying to keep their "cure" a secret from the public. Also, be wary of any demands by the practitioner that an alternative treatment be substituted for a currently accepted practice. According to *Harvard Women's Health Watch* (June 1994), while there may be little harm in adding an alternative practice such as MEDITATION or massage therapy to a therapeutic regimen, replacing a valid treatment with one that has no proven efficacy may have serious consequences.

Watch out for claims that the treatment is better than approved remedies just because it is "natural." Natural products are not necessarily more benign than agents synthesized in a laboratory. A drug is any substance that alters the structure or function of the body, regardless of its source. It is important to remember that many plants contain toxic substances that can be harmful when taken in uncontrolled doses.

See also ACCULTURATION; AYURDEVA; CHIROPRACTIC MEDICINE; GUIDED IMAGERY; HOLISTIC MEDICINE; MIND-BODY CONNECTIONS; RELAXATION.

FOR FURTHER INFORMATION:
Ayurvedic Institute
P.O. Box 23445
Albuquerque, NM 97192-1445
Phone: (505) 291-9698

Office of Alternative Medicine
National Institutes of Health
6120 Executive Blvd. (Suite 450)
Rockville, MD 20892-9904
Phone: (301) 402-4741

Sharp Institute for Human Potential and
    Mind/Body Medicine
8010 Frost Street (Suite 300)

San Diego, CA 92123
Phone: (800) 82-SHARP

SOURCES:

Burton Goldberg Group, eds. *Alternative Medicine: The Definitive Guide.* Puyallup, Wash.: Future Medicine Publishing, 1993.

Eisenberg, D., et al. "Unconventional Medicine in the United States: Prevalence, Costs, and Patterns of Use. *New England Journal of Medicine* 328 (1993): 246–252.

Facklam, Howard. *Alternative Medicine: Cures or Myths?* New York: Twenty-First Century Books, 1996.

Gellert, George. "Global Explanations and the Credibility Problem of Alternative Medicine," *ADVANCES: The Journal of Mind-Body Health* 10, no. 4 (Fall 1994).

Goldfinger, Stephen, ed. "Alternative Medicine: Insurers Cover New Ground." *Harvard Health Letter* 22, no. 2 (December 1996).

Goleman, Daniel, and Joel Gurin, eds. *Mind Body Medicine: How to Use Your Mind for Better Health.* Yonkers, N.Y.: Consumer Reports Books, 1993.

Gordon, James S. *Manifesto For a New Medicine: Your Guide to Healing Partnerships and Wise Use of Alternative Therapies.* Reading, Mass: Addison-Wesley, 1996.

Morton, Mary and Michael. *5 Steps to Selecting the Best Alternative Medicine.* Novato, Calif.; New World Library, 1996.

Roach, Mary. "My Quest for Qi." *Health,* March 1997.

Weil, Andrew. *Eight Weeks to Optimum Health: Proven Program for Taking Full Advantage of Your Body's Healing Power.* New York: Alfred A. Knopf, 1997.

Alzheimer's disease At least 50% of all dementia cases are due to Alzheimer's disease, a progressive, irreversible disorder that attacks the brain and has sometimes been called "death of the mind." Families of Alzheimer's disease sufferers cope with stresses of care giving that are physical, emotional, social, and financial. These stresses become worse as the disease advances. The sufferers themselves experience stress, particularly during the onset of the illness when they are still able to recognize some of the symptoms of the disease.

The disease was named in 1906 by Dr. Alois Alzheimer (1864–1915), after diagnosing a 51-year-old patient. Although it may occur as early as age 40, Alzheimer's more commonly strikes people 65 years and older. It is the fourth leading cause of death for people between the ages of 75 and 84 (after heart disease, cancer, and stroke). Once diagnosed, many individuals live an average of three to 20 years.

An estimated four million Americans have Alzheimer's disease and a reported 100,000 deaths are due to the disease each year. As the population of older Americans increases, so will the number of people at risk for this disease.

Symptoms

Symptoms of Alzheimer's should not be confused with age-associated memory impairment (AAMI), a term health care professionals use to describe minor memory difficulties that come with age.

Although Alzheimer's symptoms vary in rate of change from person to person, there are three progressive stages of the disease. In Stage One, which can last two to four years, mild symptoms begin to be noticeable. There may be memory loss, but often this is associated with the AGING process. Recent memory is affected and the ability to learn and retain new information is impaired. Individuals may resort to writing themselves notes and labeling drawers and cabinets to remind themselves of items used in everyday living. There may be difficulty in concentrating or engaging in conversation without losing train of thought. Individuals exhibit tiredness and an unkempt appearance, and often blame others for what is happening to them. They feel out of CONTROL and many become depressed. Personality changes include being quick to anger, particularly at the inability to communicate thoughts clearly.

In Stage Two, symptoms become more severe, memory losses increase, and there are more marked changes in behavior. There is less ability to comprehend what is being said. Words are used wrong and in senseless combinations (paraphasia), and there is an inability to recognize objects (visual agnosia). Supervision of daily activities may become necessary. There is increasing disorientation regarding time and place. Some sufferers do not recognize themselves in the mirror and others do not recognize their spouses or children. Confusion often increases in the late evening (sundown syndrome). Bladder or bowel incontinence may develop; the individual may forget where the bathroom is or how to undress and use the facilities. Impaired gait develops and the body weakens.

In Stage Three, signs and symptoms continue to progress until deterioration causes the person to become bedridden.

Diagnosis

Before diagnosis of Alzheimer's disease is made, the physician will want to rule out other conditions, such as potentially reversible DEPRESSION, adverse drug reactions, metabolic changes, nutritional deficiencies, head injuries and stroke. Until the last decade, when more technologically sophisticated testing procedures became available, many sufferers were misdiagnosed and consequently treated incorrectly. For example, screen star Rita Hayworth was misdiagnosed with alcoholic dementia in the 1970s and only later was diagnosed as suffering from Alzheimer's disease, from which she died in 1987. Her film career ended when she could not remember her lines.

Diagnosis usually begins with a search for treatable causes for memory loss and mental changes. Evaluation includes screening for depression, previous history of mental illness, and an assessment of the overall mental state. Many diagnostic procedures may be used,

including blood studies, computerized axial tomography (CT scan), or electroencephalogram (EEG). In some cases a lumbar puncture is done to rule out neurosyphilis, which can cause inability to carry out purposeful movements (aproxia), inability to express thoughts (aphasia) and an inability to recognize items (agnosia). The CT scan for an individual who has Alzheimer's disease typically shows brain shrinkage. The EEG is typically slow in a person with Alzheimer's disease.

Research and treatment

Until the latter decades of the 20th century, there was little interest and research into its causes and treatment. Today, although there is no cure for Alzheimer's disease, research efforts have contributed significantly to the quality of life for patients.

In late 1991, Congress voted to increase the government's investment in battling Alzheimer's disease to $284 million, about twice the amount in the previous two years. Most of the funds were directed toward finding a cure or effective treatment, testing promising new drugs, and helping to reduce the burden of the disease on families of Alzheimer's sufferers. A portion of the funds was earmarked to launch a $4 million program to help states coordinate services available to families, such as respite care, adult day care and counseling.

Stresses facing caregivers of Alzheimer's patients

Jerome H. Stone, president, National Alzheimer's Disease and Related Disorders Association, has characterized Alzheimer's as "the disease that robs the mind of the victim and breaks the heart of the family." For caregivers of Alzheimer's sufferers, it is a very frustrating and dehumanizing condition to witness. Alzheimer's disease can be an extraordinarily demanding and frustrating experience, both for those afflicted with the disease and for their families. Caring for a parent, grandparent, or spouse whose mind is deteriorating requires stamina and patience. Confronted with a disease that afflicts the mind of a loved one, care-giving family members often feel alone and helpless. However, SUPPORT GROUPS and friends can be helpful, as can senior day-care centers.

In addition to the emotional strain on the CAREGIVER, there may be financial expenses, such as reconstructing living arrangements for the safety and convenience of the patient, giving up a job to devote full time to care, hiring people to provide part-time care or do household chores, and possibly providing nursing home care, which may or may not be covered by health insurance.

Information line and support groups

The Alzheimer's Association has a national, toll-free information and referral service telephone number. The 800 line offers callers the most current information available on Alzheimer's disease and support services through the association. The number is: (800) 272-3900.

The Alzheimer's Disease and Related Disorders Association (ARDRA) is a privately-funded national voluntary health organization, founded in 1980 and headquartered in Chicago. ARDRA has over 1,000 support groups and 160 chapters and affiliates nationwide. ARDRA's board of directors comprises business leaders, health professionals, and family members. A medical and scientific advisory board consults on and monitors related issues.

Goals of ARDRA include supporting research on causes, treatments, cures, and prevention; stimulating education and public awareness of both lay people and professionals; encouraging chapter formation for nationwide family support networks; implementing programs at the local level; advocating improved public policy and legislation at federal, state, and local levels; and patient and family services to aid present and future sufferers and caregivers.

Alzheimer's Disease International was formed in 1984 to share program and research developments on Alzheimer's disease worldwide. The nationwide Hot-Line number is: (800) 621-0379.

FOR FURTHER INFORMATION:
Alzheimer's Association
919 N. Michigan Avenue Chicago, IL 60611
Phone: (800) 272-3900

ADEAR Center Alzheimer's Disease Education
  and Referral
P.O. Box 8250
Silver Spring, MD 20907-8250
Phone: (800) 438-4380

SOURCE:
Kahn, Ada P., and Jan Fawcett. *The Encyclopedia of Mental Health.* New York: Facts On File, 1993.

GUIDELINES FOR CAREGIVERS OF ALZHEIMER'S PATIENTS

- Take one day at a time, tackling each problem as it arises. One cannot know how an Alzheimer's patient will behave the next day.
- Try to put yourself in the patient's shoes. You will feel less annoyed the tenth time you are asked what day it is if you imagine how unsettling it must be not to be oriented in time and space.
- Maintain a sense of humor. This is especially valuable in getting through potentially embarrassing situations.
- Arrange for time for yourself. Get another family member or friend to relieve you for an hour or two each day. Hire a part-time caretaker. Arrange for the patient to spend time at a senior day-care facility.
- Pay attention to your own needs. Be sure to maintain good nutrition and get regular exercise; develop hobbies and outside interests. Find people you can talk to, such as family members, friends or, if needed, professional counselors.

---

ambivalence Refers to the simultaneous existence of two, sometimes contradictory, feelings, attitudes, values, or goals. Feelings of ambivalence are stressful for many people. For example, some individuals have feelings of "ambivalence" toward a mate whom they love but who abuses them. Other individuals may be ambivalent about work and other major life issues.

The term "ambivalence" was introduced by Eugen Bleuler, a Swiss psychiatrist (1857–1939), to refer to the simultaneous feeling of antagonistic emotions, such as approach or avoidance of the same activity or goal.

See also EMOTIONS; PHOBIAS.

amnesia See FORGETTING; MEMORY.

anger For most individuals, anger is an intense emotional state in which there is a high level of displeasure and FRUSTRATION. It can be caused by STRESS or can be a reaction to stress and is indicated by feelings ranging from slight irritation to explosive HOSTILITY that are directed to other people, objects, or oneself.

Physiological changes occur when one feels angry. For example, anger increases heart rate, blood pressure, and flow of ADRENALINE. Suppressed anger may result in HEADACHES, HIGH BLOOD PRESSURE, and skin rashes. More clearly visible signs include frowning, gritting the teeth, pacing and clenching the hands. There may be changes in vocal tone; one may yell or shout, or, on the other extreme, speak in short, clipped sentences. Through such displays, an angry person attempts to gain CONTROL of a situation but at the same time clearly demonstrates that he or she has lost control.

Negative anger

There are two attitudes—positive and negative—with regard to anger. On the negative side, anger can be destructive, leading to inappropriate or illegal behavior. Negative anger seems to be directly related to frustration and feelings of inferiority. Sigmund Freud observed in his book, *Mourning and Melancholia,* that DEPRESSION is actually anger turned inward, directed at the self. Bigotry, for instance, appears to be anger turned against specific groups or humanity as a whole. Adults who express anger directly with physical violence or verbal abuse usually do so because they model their behavior on others in their environment or because there seems to be a reward for violent behavior. Since in most situations it is unacceptable to express anger directly, many people react by becoming sulky or indifferent, or by adopting a superior, patronizing attitude toward the person or situation that angered them.

The first cries of a baby may be an expression of anger or simply a less focused reaction to the birth experience. Small children react directly to situations that make them angry, sometimes by simply screaming, pulling, or striking the object or person who has angered them. As children mature, angry behavior becomes focused on retaliation. By the early teens, sulking and impertinence replace retaliation.

Many people who have a chronic illness react with anger. For example, some rheumatoid arthritis sufferers also have a situation of long-time, repressed anger. These people, particularly women who have been brought up to think anger is "unladylike," tend to say that everything is okay even when the opposite is true. Repressed anger and other personality and behavior patterns are the subjects of continued study, as researchers try to identify the role of psychological forces that exist in autoimmune diseases.

Positive anger

Anger may be helpful and constructive. There are psychological and medical opinions indicating that suppressing anger is physically and psychologically damaging. Further, limiting the expression of anger may bring regrets later. If an individual chooses to work off anger in an exercise program, it may do him good in other ways. For example, releasing an angry feeling sometimes brings with it a sense of pleasure. Some mental health professionals equate ambition and attempts to improve society with a healthy expression of anger.

Among athletes, anger can have both a harmful and positive effect on athletic performance. Anger at the opposition can drain energy and divert attention from winning the game. However, professional athletes such as members of the Chicago Bulls and other championship teams are competitive and able to turn their anger into playing more forcefully.

How to overcome anger

An individual in psychotherapy who expresses extremely stressful and angry feelings might be given three goals: first, to identify the feelings of anger; second, to use constructive release of the energy of anger; and third, to identify thought processes that lead to anger. For example, to identify thought processes that lead to anger and the resulting feelings of anger, one might keep a diary of what led to the angry feelings and how they were handled. By doing this, the individual will learn to recognize anger before losing control, take responsibility for his or her own emotions and stop blaming others. Also, with validation from a therapist, the individual will learn to accept that some anger is justified in certain situations. In learning to use constructive release of the energy of anger, the individual may benefit from ASSERTIVENESS TRAINING, and learn to express anger verbally to the appropriate source. Assertive techniques may help the individual increase feelings of self-esteem, demonstrate internal control over behavior, and harness energy generated by the anger in a nondestructive manner.

Also, individuals can learn to use energy through physical activity that involves the large muscles, such as running, walking, or playing tennis or racquetball. Other techniques that are helpful in controlling stress and anger are ALTERNATIVE THERAPIES such as BIOFEEDBACK, GUIDED IMAGERY, and MEDITATION.

Relationship of anger to grief

It is common to feel angry and stressed after the death of a loved one. The anger may be directed toward the deceased person for leaving the mourner alone, the medical care system for not being able to cure a disease or mend a body, God, or the fatal disease itself. In cases of accidents, there is often anger at the perpetrator of the loved one's death, whether a drunk driver, a drug-induced criminal, or the person who sold them drugs or alcohol. Anger is a normal part of the cycle of GRIEF reaction. However, prolonged anger that leads to depression may indicate a need to consult a mental health professional.

See also AGGRESSION; ANXIETY.

SOURCE:
Lee, John H. *Facing the Fire. Experiencing and Expressing Anger.* New York: Bantam Books, 1993.

angina pectoris   A chest pain usually caused by a low supply of oxygen to the heart muscle resulting from hardening and narrowing of the coronary arteries. It is stressful and disturbing to the sufferer as well as family or friends who are there when it occurs.

The term "unstable angina" refers to an accelerating pattern of chest pain where previously stable angina now occurs with less exertion, lasts longer, and is less responsive to medication. It can be a sign of an impending HEART ATTACK and immediate treatment by a physician should be sought.

See also HIGH BLOOD PRESSURE; TYPE A PERSONALITY.

anniversary reaction   The feeling of DEPRESSION that arises around the anniversary of a significant event such as a divorce or the death of a family member or close friend. The reaction brings stress because it may involve the recall and reliving of the events. Some individuals experience dreams or minor illness at the same time each year as part of this reaction.

See also GRIEF.

anorexia See EATING DISORDERS.

anorgasmia Old term meaning an inability to achieve an orgasm. This term has been replaced with psychosexual dysfunction, and refers to lack of orgasm in men or women, which may result from stress, sociocultural attitudes of the partners, anatomical or neurophysiological problems, or fear of painful intercourse. SEX THERAPY is helpful in many such cases.

See also FRIGIDITY; SEXUAL DIFFICULTIES.

antidepressant medications See DEPRESSION; PHARMACOLOGICAL APPROACH.

anxiety Feeling of tension and/or apprehension that comes from anticipating a situation, which may be known or unknown. Anxiety is different from fear: Fear is a response to a consciously recognized and usually external threat or danger, whereas anxiety is typically caused by an "internal" threat not apparent to any but the anxious individual.

Most people experience the stresses of anxiety in everyday life. For example, they may experience anxiety about getting to a job interview on time, going on a first date, or wearing the right clothes at an important social event. Others become anxious about being held up in traffic or when they hear reports of incoming bad weather.

Possible causes of anxiety
Individuals who face a threat or change in their health status often become anxious and feel stressed. These stresses may relate to the possibility of unpleasant treatment, pain, and possible disability. Many abused and psychologically traumatized individuals, such as victims of DOMESTIC VIOLENCE or RAPE, have

lifelong anxiety symptoms. Anxieties also occur for socioeconomic reasons. For example, threats of job layoffs cause many people stress and anxieties, while others become anxious over changes in stock market prices and develop constant fears that their fortunes will diminish.

Coping with the stress of anxiety
Most people learn to relieve some stress by COPING with transient anxieties; this includes taking more time, doing additional preparations, and facing the fact that most situations are temporary and/or really non-threatening. Unfortunately, some people turn to smoking and alcohol or drug use to cope with the stress caused by their anxieties. These habits are not considered healthy coping mechanisms, as they can lead to health hazards and addictions. Physicians may prescribe anti-anxiety drugs or anxiolytic drugs for some individuals who, at certain times, are experiencing severe anxieties.

See also GENERAL ADAPTATION SYNDROME.

anxiety disorders These are disorders that are characterized by anxiety and, at times, avoidance behaviors. According to the American Psychiatric Association's *Diagnostic and Statistical Manual of Mental Disorders, Fourth Edition,* they include generalized anxiety disorder (GAD), PHOBIAS, PANIC DISORDER, OBSESSIVE-COMPULSIVE DISORDER, and POST-TRAUMATIC STRESS DISORDER (PTSD). Anxiety disorders may result from extreme STRESS. They also produce ongoing stress for sufferers and those around them. An individual can have one or more anxiety disorders at the same time.

Generalized Anxiety Disorders (GAD). Excessive levels of anxiety and apprehension often are the main characteristics of GAD suffered by both men and women. Symptoms generally appear when individuals are 20 to 40 years old. GADs are caused by the fear of life circumstances such as the possible death of a loved one or losing one's job, even though there is no evidence these stress-producing events will actually happen.

Phobias. People who suffer from phobias feel terror, dread or panic when confronted with an object, situation or activity that they fear. Some people have such an overwhelming desire to avoid the source of their fear that it causes stress on the jobs and in family and social relationships.

SOCIAL PHOBIAS, such as fear of public speaking, meeting new people or eating in public, are very common. Simple phobias involve fear of one activity, such as flying, or of an object, such as snakes. AGORAPHOBIA is fear of going into public places, riding on public transportation, and entering shops and restaurants where one feels far from safety. Sufferers fabricate any number of excuses to remain at home. People seek help for agoraphobia more than for any other phobia and are usually successfully treated by psychotherapy and pharmaceutical medications.

Panic Disorder. Sufferers from panic disorders experience intense but brief acute anxiety dominated by a fear of dying or being out of control. Because many of the symptoms of panic disorder are also symptomatic of a heart attack, many people rush to emergency rooms. Treatment of panic disorder is important; untreated panic sufferers can become suicidal.

Obsessive-Compulsive Disorder. People with this disorder usually suffer from obsessions or from persistent ideas such as fear of infection by germs or dirt, which make them carry out compulsive, repetitive, ritualized acts such as hand washing, counting, and checking. These involuntary responses to their obsessions cause stress for sufferers and, particularly, the people with whom they live.

Post-traumatic Stress Disorder (PTSD). This anxiety disorder comes after a stressful or frightening event that causes an unusual, severe physical or mental trauma. This may result from such events as military combat, natural disasters, violence, rape, or serious injury. Most people recover when given counseling and support; however, some post-traumatic stress disorders last a lifetime.

Causes of anxiety disorders

There are several theories about the causes of anxiety disorders. No single condition or situation causes them; a person may even inherit or develop a biological susceptibility to anxiety disorders.

Psychoanalytic theory suggests that anxiety stems from unconscious conflicts from infancy or childhood. For example, a person may carry the unconscious conflict of sexual feelings toward the parent of the opposite sex, or may have developed problems from experiencing illness or fright as a child. According to this theory, anxiety can be resolved by identifying and resolving the unconscious conflict.

SYMPTOMS ASSOCIATED WITH GENERALIZED ANXIETY DISORDER

Motor tension
- Trembling, twitching, feeling shaky
- Muscle tension, aches, soreness
- Restlessness
- Easily tired

Autonomic hyperactivity
- Shortness of breath or smothering sensations
- Palpitations or accelerated heart rate
- Sweating, cold, clammy hands
- Dry mouth
- Dizziness, light-headedness
- Nausea, diarrhea, other abdominal distress
- Flushes (hot flashes) or chills
- Frequent urination
- Trouble swallowing or "lump in the throat"

Hypervigilance
- Feeling keyed up or on edge
- Exaggerated startle response
- Difficulty concentrating or "mind going blank"
- Trouble falling asleep or staying asleep
- Irritability

The learning theory suggests that anxiety is a learned behavior that can be unlearned. People who feel very stressed in a given situation or near a certain object will begin to avoid it. However, such avoidance can limit a person's ability to live normally. In many cases, sufferers learn that their anxiety diminishes by persistently facing the feared object or situation.

Another theory is that biochemical imbalances may lead to anxiety disorders. There may be complex electrochemical interactions in the central nervous system. Some studies indicate that infusions of certain biochemicals can bring on a panic attack in some people. According to this theory, treatment of anxiety should correct these biochemical imbalances. Biochemical changes can occur as a result of emotional, psychological or behavioral changes.

Diagnosing and treating anxiety disorders

A good diagnostic approach for anxiety disorders follows the same guidelines as for any other medical illness: a complete history, physical examination, and laboratory tests and mental status assessment.

In most cases, anxiety disorders are treated with a combination of therapies that are individualized for each person. There is no cure-all for everyone. Treatment focuses on teaching the individual how to identify feelings, counteract negative thinking, and apply what they have learned to real-life situations. Also, treatment enables the sufferer to gain skills to control the behavior that brings about the anxiety through a gradual process of identifying and controlling the anxiety-provoking situations.

Phobias and obsessive-compulsive disorders often are treated by BEHAVIOR THERAPY. This may involve exposing the sufferer to the feared object or situation under controlled circumstances until the fear is significantly reduced or cured. With this method, many phobic individuals have long-term recoveries.

Prescription medications can help reduce extreme symptoms so that an individual can make the best use of behavior therapy and other psychotherapeutic techniques. In addition to behavior modification techniques and medications, talking with a therapist during psychotherapy can be important for relief and improvement.

Research reported by the American Psychiatric Association indicates that 90% of phobic and obsessive-compulsive individuals who cooperate with their therapists and comply with instructions recover with behavior therapy. Studies have shown that while they are on medications, 70% of individuals who suffer from panic attacks improve. Medication is effective for about half of those suffering from obsessive-compulsive disorder. RELAXATION training, self-hypnosis, BIOFEEDBACK and GUIDED IMAGERY are also effective therapies for many individuals.

If one has a friend or a loved one who won't go for treatment, it is important to find out why he or she will not go. Often people think that going for treatment means that they are mentally ill, and they find that stressful to accept. Such people should be assured that seeking treatment for an anxiety disorder is the same as seeking treatment for any medical concern.

Role of support groups

Support groups are very helpful in the treatment of anxiety disorders because many people develop a secondary feeling of reduced morale, which results in lower levels of functioning. Support groups are effective in raising that morale as well as the self-esteem of their participants. Also, in learning about other people's problems, an individual's own feelings of unique inadequacy and inferiority often can be dispelled.

Social costs of anxiety disorders

The social costs of anxiety disorders far outweigh the expenses incurred for direct treatment, concluded a study reported in 1995 by

Andrew C. Leon, Ph.D., Cornell University Medical College, and Myrna M. Weissman, M.D., of Columbia University. An estimated 30 million adult Americans have had an anxiety disorder at some point in their lives. In the six months prior to the study, those who suffered from an anxiety disorder were more likely to have higher rates of drug and alcohol abuse, as well as higher rates of financial dependence and unemployment, than those who had not experienced an anxiety disorder. In particular, the researchers found that those with panic disorder or obsessive-compulsive disorder were more likely to be chronically unemployed or to receive disability or welfare payments than those without. "One problem," said Dr. Leon, "is the current lack of implementation of recently developed screening procedures. Sufferers of anxiety disorders often use the general medical system and emergency rooms for treatment; unless primary care and emergency care settings employ the screening procedures for these disorders, the burden on the health care system will remain substantial."

See also AFFECTIVE DISORDERS; COPING; PANIC ATTACKS AND PANIC DISORDER.

FOR FURTHER INFORMATION:
American Psychiatric Association
Division of Public Affairs
1400 K Street NW
Washington, DC 20005
Phone:(800)368-5777

Anxiety Disorders Association of America
11900 Parklawn Drive (Suite 100)
Rockville, MD 20852
Phone: (301) 231-9350

National Alliance for the Mentally Ill
1901 N. Fort Myer Drive (Suite 500)
Arlington, VA 22209-1604
Phone: (703) 524-7600

National Institute of Mental Health
Division of Communications
5600 Fishers Lane
Rockville, MD 20857
Phone: (301) 443-4536

SOURCES:
Kahn, Ada P., and Jan Fawcett. *The Encyclopedia of Mental Health.* New York: Facts On File, 1993.
Margolis, Simeon, ed. "Living Without Anxiety." *Health After 50,* August 1997.
Ross, Jerilyn. *Triumph Over Fear: A Book of Help and Hope for People with Anxiety, Panic Attacks, and Phobias.* New York: Bantam Books, 1994.
Warneke, Lorne. "Anxiety Disorders: Focus on Obsessive-compulsive Disorder." *Canadian Family Physician* 39 (July 1993).

arithmetic   See MATHEMATICS ANXIETY.

aromatherapy   The art and science of using essential oils from plants and flowers to reduce stress and enhance health. Essential oils are essences extracted from flowers and plants, as well as herbs, roots, leaves, bark, and wood, by distillation; they deeply penetrate the skin and have powerful medicinal and psychological effects. Practitioners of aromatherapy assess the patient's current physical, emotional, and bioenergetic condition. Then they blend essential oils from around the world and apply them with a specialized massage technique focusing on the nervous and lymphatic system. Aromatherapy massage has been used to treat conditions ranging from job stress to muscle soreness to varicose veins and allergies.

The art of aromatherapy is fairly new in the United States, but has been used for centuries elsewhere in the world, particularly in Egypt and Greece. During World War I, Dr. Jean Valnet, a Parisian physician, used essential oils to treat injured soldiers. He also influenced Marguerite Maury, a biochemist who developed a special way to apply the penetrating oils with massage.

Finding a practitioner of aromatherapy
There is no national organization overseeing training standards in this field. Techniques vary from practitioner to practitioner. Many therapists are employed in spas in larger cities or resort areas. If you are seeking this therapy, look for someone who is a licensed, certified

massage practitioner and who can show proof of training in the use of essential oils.

See also ALTERNATIVE THERAPIES.

SOURCES:
Cooksley, Valerie Gennari. *Aromatherapy. A Lifetime Guide to Healing With Essential Oils.* Englewood Cliffs, N.J.: Prentice-Hall, 1996.
Griffin, Katherine. "A Whiff of Things to Come." *Health,* November/December 1992.

arrhythmia   An abnormal heart rhythm, usually detected by an electrocardiogram. When some individuals hear this diagnosis, they became anxious and find the diagnosis stressful. An arrhythmia may or may not be of potential significance, and can be caused by several factors, such as coronary artery disease, heart valve problems, or hyperthyroidism. Individuals with this diagnosis should question their physician carefully about what it means, about possible lifestyle changes, ways to eliminate stress and the need for medication.

See also BIOFEEDBACK; BREATHING; HEART ATTACK; HIGH BLOOD PRESSURE; RELAXATION; TYPE A PERSONALITY.

arthritis   A painful, debilitating chronic condition that afflicts more than 40 million Americans, most of them women. When doctors diagnose "arthritis," they are identifying painful inflammation in a joint, which in some forms brings with it swelling and redness. The most common of these forms are osteoarthritis and rheumatoid arthritis. Osteoarthritis typically affects older adults and is caused by wear and tear on the joints, particularly hands, knees, feet, hips, and back. Rheumatoid arthritis is the most severe form and is caused by the body's IMMUNE SYSTEM attacking the joints and surrounding tissues, often leading to severe deformity of the shoulders, elbows, hands, wrists, feet, and ankles. Unlike osteoarthritis, rheumatoid arthritis strikes children as well as adults, and it is estimated that more than

250,000 children have juvenile rheumatoid arthritis.

Since the early 1900s, doctors have recognized that rheumatoid arthritis can be provoked or exacerbated by stress, continuous worry, or anxiety. Results of studies since then have agreed that emotional stress can trigger rheumatoid arthritis in a susceptible child or adult and, once the disease has established itself, can make it worse. The stress involved is usually acute, often resulting from such crises as the death of a family member, loss of a job, or a divorce.

According to Chad Helmick, M.D., chief, Epidemiology Section, Centers for Disease Control and Prevention, Atlanta, Georgia, arthritis and other rheumatic conditions will increase in prevalence by 50% by the year 2020, with the number affected growing from 40 million to 60 million people. Helmick says the number of people affected will grow because of the aging population. "Most people probably think that arthritis is part of normal aging and there is nothing you can do about it," says Helmick. "But there are things that can be done to reduce its impact, such as losing weight and limiting the risk of joint injuries from sports and occupation."

Pharmacological approaches and alternative therapies
Many pharmacological approaches are available for treating individuals who have arthritis. New prescription medications are being developed and many over-the-counter remedies are available. Increasingly, researchers are trying ALTERNATIVE THERAPIES, either in conjunction with prescription medications or as sole therapies.

As a result of early research in PSYCHONEUROIMMUNOLOGY, a few behavioral, stress-reducing programs to treat arthritis have been developed. One activity is exercise; the chief benefit is to move the blood flow to the affected joints and keep them flexible. Arthritic individuals may be advised to do stretching exercises to keep their joints moving smoothly and do strengthening exercises to maintain muscle tone. Walking and non-weightbearing exercises such as swimming are also helpful.

At the Stanford University Arthritis Center, physicians suggest relaxation tapes that also reduce PAIN for patients with arthritis. The logic behind these tapes is that if the mind is distracted by mental exercise, it will not feel the arthritis pain. Additionally, some researchers believe that the relaxation response increases the body's production of endorphins, which are natural painkillers.

Other researchers have used BIOFEEDBACK as a technique to help people deal with stress and to train people with arthritis to relax. In one study, one group of arthritics had biofeedback training; the other had a standard physical therapy program. Those in the group using biofeedback and relaxation felt better; additionally, their erythrocyte sedimentation rate (ESR), a blood test measuring the activity of the disease, showed that their immune systems held stable against the disease or that the disease had somewhat abated.

Two Chicago-area researchers, Elizabeth M. Jacobi, Ph.D., and Gerald M. Eisenberg, M.D., used GUIDED IMAGERY and MUSIC with arthritis patients. They found that as a psychological treatment approach, integrating health, mental imagery, and music with emotional expression and guided imagery appeared to be effective in reducing pain and psychological symptomatology and, ultimately, in improving the quality of life for those with rheumatoid arthritis.

Many psychological forces seem to have a role in autoimmune diseases. Psychotherapy can help arthritis patients understand the possible emotional factors associated with their symptoms. In conjunction with psychotherapy, or by themselves, techniques including RELAXATION exercises, MEDITATION, and biofeedback can be helpful.

See also ANGER; AUTOIMMUNE DISORDERS; CHRONIC ILLNESS.

FOR FURTHER INFORMATION:
Arthritis Foundation
1314 Spring St. NW
Atlanta, GA 30309
Phone: (404) 872-7100

National Institute of Arthritis and Musculoskeletal and Skin Diseases
9000 Rockville Pike
Bethesda, MD 20892
Phone: (201) 468-3235

SOURCES:
Kahn, Ada P. *Arthritis.* Chicago: Contemporary Books, 1983.
Locke, Steven, and Douglas Colligan. *The Healer Within.* New York: New American Library, 1986.

artificial insemination   See INFERTILITY.

assertiveness training   A process through which individuals can change unwanted behaviors that cause an individual stress. It teaches individuals to see themselves as equal human beings, with rights regardless of other roles and titles. It raises SELF-ESTEEM and clarifies the choices that are available to individuals when responding to others. Many people who are too inhibited or anxious to express themselves honestly in social situations can benefit from assertiveness training.

By teaching individuals to act upon their real feelings, assertiveness training helps them improve specific situations. Such situations might involve an over-demanding boss; a friend who takes advantage of one's generosity; the wife who resents that her husband does not do his share of housework, but is too meek to confront him with her true feelings; or the employee who wants to ask for a raise but lacks the courage to do so. Training sessions, conducted either with a therapist or through self-help techniques, include rehearsing how to act and what to say in common situations.

Assertiveness training can help people act more effectively in their own best interests, to make life decisions, take the initiative, trust their self-judgment, set goals and work to achieve them, and ask for help from others when necessary. It can empower them to stand up for themselves without undue anxiety, set limits on time and energy, respond to others' put-downs or anger, and express or defend personal opinions. It allows them to be comfortable and honest when expressing agreement or disagreement; when showing anger, affection, or friendship; and when admitting fear or anxiety.

Assertive behavior is self-expressive, honest, direct and firm, and respectful of the rights of others without unfair criticism or hurtful behavior, manipulation or undue CONTROL. Non-assertiveness behavior, on the other hand, involves suppression, frustration, and thinking of a proper response too late. As a result, non-assertive individuals feel uneasy and guilty and become stressed because they are not able to express their real feelings.

See also AGGRESSION.

SOURCE:
Kahn, Ada P., and Sheila Kimmel. *Empower Yourself: Every Woman's Guide to Self-Esteem.* New York: Avon Books, 1997.

assisted reproduction techniques   See INFERTILITY.

asthma   A chronic, allergic, inflammatory lung disease characterized by recurrent breathing problems. It is a source of STRESS to the sufferers, many of whom become depressed due to the chronically recurring condition and the ANXIETY experienced during asthma attacks. Families, too, become stressed and anxious as they learn to deal with the symptoms of the disease.

People with asthma typically have recurrent attacks or flareups of breathlessness, accompanied by wheezing. Some people have mild to moderate symptoms while others have severe symptoms that can be life threatening. Even in the same individual, asthma attacks vary in severity from day to day. In many individuals, attacks begin in childhood and tend to become less severe in adulthood; however, asthma attacks can begin at any age. Often attacks are brought on by stress or anxiety. Asthma is a major cause of lost time from school and work and of sleep disturbances.

During a severe attack, as breathing becomes increasingly difficult, there is wheezing, sweating, rapid heartbeat, and an increasingly high anxiety level. The individual cannot lie down or sleep, breathes rapidly, wheezes loudly, and may be unable to speak. He/she may fear dying, and those watching and trying to help the sufferer may add to the overall stress level by showing their own anxieties. Asthma may get worse at night because at that time chemical changes in the body narrow airways, the airways become cooled, and there may be delayed allergic reactions.

Contrary to a popular notion, asthma is not a psychosomatic illness. It is a disease and not a sign of emotional disturbance. Understanding the physiology involved in asthma can help one manage the disease, reduce the stress it brings about, and improve the quality of life. During an asthma attack, several things occur to inhibit the flow of air in and out of the airways. Inflammation causes a swelling in airways that blocks the passage of oxygen to the lungs, and this in turn is exacerbated by the contraction of pulmonary muscles and the production of thick mucus.

Asthma may be *extrinsic,* in which an allergy (usually to something inhaled) triggers an attack, or *intrinsic,* in which there seems to be no apparent external cause. Intrinsic asthma tends to develop later in life than extrinsic asthma.

About 10 million Americans have asthma; of these, about three million are children under the age of 18. Asthma affects women and men equally. In the United States, the reported number of cases of asthma is increasing but the death rate for asthma is still one of the lowest in the world.

What triggers an asthma attack

Many people get warning signs hours or days before an attack. Signs may include tiredness, a change in breathing, coughing, change in mucus color, trouble sleeping, itching of the chin or throat, sneezing, headache, dark circles under the eyes, and moodiness. Triggers vary from person to person, and many people with asthma have more than one. Common triggers include:

Excitement or stressful situations. Emotional factors themselves do not cause asthma. However, laughing, crying, or yelling may bring on symptoms.

Airborne allergens. An allergen is a substance that causes an allergic response. Common airborne allergens include pollen, dust mites, mold, and animal dander.

Common irritants. These include cigarette smoke (as well as secondhand smoke); smoke from other sources, such as candles, burning leaves, or wood-burning stoves; aerosol sprays and other chemicals; and strong odors.

Exercise. Exercise is a trigger for many people; however, most people with asthma can lead active lives, including playing sports. There are steps one can take to reduce the risk of problems.

Respiratory infections. Respiratory infections can be particularly troublesome for children who tend to get more colds than adults.

Cold air. Cold air is a trigger for many people. Covering the nose and mouth when outdoors can help.

Reduce stress by managing asthma triggers

A physician can help the asthma sufferer identify triggers and learn to reduce them. For example, one can reduce exposure to mold by ventilating the kitchen, bathroom, and other damp areas, running a dehumidifier in the basement, and frequently cleaning areas where mold is likely to grow. Airborne allergens can be shut out by keeping doors and windows closed or they can be reduced by an air filtration system. To deal with dust mites, the asthma sufferer should clean up clutter, remove carpets, cover fabric upholstery with plastic or replace it with leather or vinyl, use synthetic bedding instead of cotton, and have someone else do the vacuuming. The asthmatic should live in a home that is smoke-free, and avoid public places where smoking is permitted.

Diagnosis, treatment, and self-help

Asthma is sometimes difficult to diagnose because many of its symptoms resemble EMPHYSEMA, bronchitis, and lower respiratory infections. For some individuals, the only symptom is a chronic cough, especially at night, or coughing or wheezing occurring only with exercise. Diagnosis is made by consideration of medical history, thorough physical examination and certain laboratory tests.

Asthma cannot be cured, but it can be controlled with proper treatment. With current drug therapies, people who suffer repeated attacks can learn to manage episodes. Quality of life need not be impaired, as demonstrated by the successes of athletes who have had asthma. There are two main groups of medications. One is anti-inflammatory medications; these can help prevent asthma attacks by reducing swelling. Anti-inflammatory medications include corticosteroids (usually inhaled), cromolyn and nedocromil. Inhaled steroids are absorbed primarily by the lungs. That means little gets into the bloodstream, lowering the risk of side effects. The second group is the bronchodilators. These medications can open airways during asthma attacks. They include beta^2 agonists and theophylline. Asthma sufferers should have a bronchodilator handy.

Asthma sufferers should follow their health care provider's instructions for when to take the medication and how much to take. If they have an anti-inflammatory medication, it should be taken regularly, even when they feel fine.

Exercise can improve lung power and wellness. However, before embarking on an exercise program, asthmatics should talk with their health care providers who may provide extra medication. A warm-up before exercising in cold air is necessary as well as a scarf or mask over the nose and mouth.

Hospitals and local health departments offer breathing improvement programs and support groups for asthma sufferers and members of their families. Topics for discussion typically include coping with the stresses asthma produces on the sufferer as well as family members, avoiding asthma triggers, and new developments in medications. Groups can be helpful for parents of asthmatic children; family counseling is also useful for all concerned.

Research under way

Research on asthma is under way at the National Institutes of Health. Projects focus on identifying basic abnormalities that cause asthma, developing better drug treatments and emergency measures, educating people with asthma to help themselves more effectively, and training patients in asthma self-management techniques while under medical supervision.

See also ALLERGIES; CHRONIC ILLNESS; DEPRESSION; GUIDED IMAGERY; MEDITATION.

FOR FURTHER INFORMATION:
American Lung Association
1740 Broadway
New York, NY 10019
Phone: (212) 315-8700

Asthma and Allergy Foundation of America
1717 Massachusetts Avenue NW (#305)
Washington, DC 20036
Phone: (202) 265-0265

SOURCES:
Adams, Francis V. *The Asthma Sourcebook: Everything You Need to Know.* Los Angeles: Lowell House, 1995.
Garnett, Leah R., ed. "Chronic Conditions: Asthma Increases, but So Do Treatments." *Harvard Health Letter,* June 1997.

Hyde, Margaret O., and Elizabeth H. Forsyth. *Living with Asthma.* New York: Walker, 1995.
Litin, Scott C., ed. "Management of Adult Asthma." *Mayo Clinical Update* 13, no. 2 (1997).

atherosclerosis Common disease in which deposits of plaque containing fatty substances, such as CHOLESTEROL, are formed within the inner layers of the arteries. Commonly known as "hardening of the arteries," it produces anxieties and stress because potential complications may include coronary artery disease and strokes. The disease progresses over decades, chiefly affecting the arteries of the heart, brain, and extremities.

See also CHRONIC ILLNESS; HEART ATTACK; HIGH BLOOD PRESSURE.

attention-deficit/hyperactivity disorder (ADHD)
A persistent pattern of inattention and/or hyperactivity-impulsivity, occurring mostly in school-age children and occasionally in young adults. It is a source of stress to the children, their parents, and teachers because it interferes with the child's learning in school, causes disruptions in the classroom, and brings about anxieties for the parents.

ADHD sufferers are often overactive, impulsive, and easily distractible. Estimates are that ADHD affects 3% to 5% of the school-age population, and is more common in boys. Data on prevalence in adolescence and adulthood are limited.

According to the *Diagnostic and Statistical Manual of Mental Disorders, Fourth Edition,* attention deficit is the central feature of the disorder and the other symptoms are variable; the book also recognizes that ADHD exists as a separate entity from conduct disorder. The essential feature of conduct disorder is a persistent conduct pattern in which rights of others and age-appropriate societal norms or rules are violated. While the two conditions often occur in the same individual, it is not assumed that one is a necessary concomitant of the other. Making the distinction has important implications for outcome.

Diagnosing ADHD

To warrant the diagnosis of ADHD, according to the *DSM*, some of the hyperactive-impulsive or inattentive symptoms must have been present in the child before age seven, although many children are diagnosed only after symptoms have been present for a number of years. Additionally, there must be clear evidence of interference with developmentally appropriate social, academic, or occupational functioning, and the disorder cannot be better accounted for by another mental disorder, such as ANXIETY DISORDER, dissociative disorder, or personality disorder. Diagnosis is usually made by a pediatrician, psychologist, or neurologist. Often other health and education professionals, such as special education teachers or social workers, become involved in the diagnosis and treatment plan. Diagnosis is usually based on description of the child's behavior from parents and teachers, as well as observation of the child's behavior in the health professional's office. Often the children are restless while the physician talks with parents. Many parents look back and report that their child was hyperactive from a very early age, even from one to two years of age. However, many parents do not seek medical attention until the child is in first or second grade, and this presents difficulties. In children with a later onset, the disorder is more likely to be associated with social disruption or specific behavior at school.

To determine whether the child has an associated disorder, such as a learning disorder or mild mental retardation, psychological tests are useful.

Treating ADHD

Individualized management, on a case by case method, is most effective. No one approach to treatment is universally accepted. Successful treatment depends on multimodal therapy involving parents, teachers, and mental health professionals.

In an effort to reduce stress levels of both the child and the family, the physician usually explains the nature of ADHD, with the objective of reducing the family's feelings of guilt and blame while at the same time improving the child's self-esteem. When there are disorders of family dynamics or learning disorders underlying the symptoms, these must be addressed.

Physicians counseling families with an ADHD child usually address behavior management and how to avoid confrontation with the active, restless child. Such a child should be encouraged to channel energy into productive activities, such as doing errands, taking out the garbage or walking the dog. Support groups can be helpful to the child, parents, and siblings.

Behavior modification and COGNITIVE THERAPY are used in some cases of ADHD. Other approaches include dietary restrictions of food additives or refined sugar (Feingold diet) or supplementation of diet with megavitamins, trace elements, or amino acids. However, best results have been noted with multimodal therapy, including behavior management, special educational intervention, and, in some cases, use of stimulant drugs. Symptomatic treatment with stimulant medication in selected patients is effective and safe, but not curative.

A widely used but controversial stimulant medication is methylphenidate hydrochloride (trade name, Ritalin). The drug is effective for three to four hours and is often prescribed for use in the morning and at noon. Individualizing dosage is important because high doses may help hyperactivity but have also been found to impair learning. When the dose is too high, some children become excessively quiet, indecisive, and cry easily. When symptoms occur only in school, the medication may be given only on school days. A child on stimulant medication should be evaluated by the prescribing physician with some regularity.

When young people are untreated in childhood, they may develop very negative attitudes toward school and patterns of failure. Even with treatment, some develop behavioral problems in later life, including substance abuse.

FOR FURTHER INFORMATION:
Attention Deficit Information Network
475 Hillside Avenue
Needham, MA 02194
Phone: (617) 455-9895

National Attention Deficit Disorders Association
P.O. Box 972
Mentor, OH 44061
Phone: (800) 487-2282

SOURCES:
American Medical Association. *Archives of General Psychiatry* 52, no. 66 (June 1, 1995).
American Medical Association. *The Journal of the American Medical Association* 273, no. 23 (June 21, 1995).
American Psychiatric Association. *Diagnostic and Statistical Manual of Mental Disorders,* 4th ed. Washington, D.C.: American Psychiatric Association, 1994.

autogenic training RELAXATION and STRESS management technique developed in 1932 by Johannes Heinrich Schultz (1884–1970), a German neurologist. Dr. Schultz used it successfully for the treatment of high blood pressure, digestive disorders, and musculoskeletal problems. Since then, its therapeutic applications have expanded to include a wide variety of cardiovascular, respiratory, endocrine, gastrointestinal, metabolic, and sleep disorders.

In autogenic training, the individual self induces a hypnotic-like state and achieves relaxation through breathing and muscular decontraction exercises. The technique is often accompanied by MEDITATION and affirmative statements regarding feelings of relaxation, warmth, inner quietness, and calm.

A basic assumption behind autogenic training is that people are innately equipped with "self-regulatory brain mechanisms" that maintain a dynamic balance in all bodily functions. When this balance is disrupted, the body's self-regulating mechanisms have the capability of restoring a healthy equilibrium, whether by calming an escalated heart rate, lowering elevated blood pressure, or healing an ulcer.

See also ALTERNATIVE THERAPIES; BEHAVIOR THERAPY; BIOFEEDBACK; PROGRESSIVE MUSCLE RELAXATION.

SOURCES:
Kerman, D. Ariel (with Richard Trubo). *The H.A.R.T. Program: Lower Your Blood Pressure Without Drugs.* New York: HarperCollins, 1992.
Lehrer, Paul M., and Robert L. Woolfolk, eds. *Principles and Practice of Stress Management.* New York: Guilford Press, 1993.

autoimmune disorders Diseases caused by a reaction of the individuals' immune system against tissues or organs of that person's own body. Such disorders include rheumatoid ARTHRITIS, systemic lupus erythematosus, and insulin-dependent diabetes mellitus. Autoimmunity refers to the condition in which the body's immune system fails to recognize its own tissues and attempts to reject its own cells as if they were foreign matter. Autoimmunity increases with age as the immune system deteriorates.

Treatment of autoimmune disorders may include correcting major deficiencies; replacement of hormones such as thyroxin or insulin that are not being produced by a gland may be necessary. At times treatment may involve replacing components of blood by transfusion. Treatment may also include reducing the activity of the immune system, controlling the disorder while maintaining the body's ability to fight disease. Corticosteroid drugs are commonly used; in more severe cases, immunosuppressant drugs are prescribed.

Autoimmune disorders are sources of stress for the sufferer as well as family members because some of the disorders are difficult to diagnose and some drugs may cause serious side effects, such as damaging bone marrow.

automation in the workplace Automated production and service systems where machines do the repetitive elements of the work process that used to be handled by people. As a result of automation, workers may be displaced or left with mainly supervisory functions.

The introduction of automation is generally considered a positive step, if the worker is assisted by the machine but maintains some CONTROL over its services. However, if operator skills and knowledge are taken over by the machine, the resulting monotony, lack of control, and social isolation may result in stress for the worker.

Even when automation requires high skill from process operators, the monitoring of machines can become monotonous. Skills are used only during a small percentage of the work hours, and mechanical breakdowns can mean loss of work already completed. All of these elements constitute sources of stress at both the psychological and physiological level.

Many industries, particularly manufacturing, have experienced displacement of workers since the advent of computerization and as a result of automation in their production lines; offices have been automated as well. It is estimated that office workers spend as much as 90% of their time at computers. Use of computers has also meant automation of delivery of services. A good example is the automatic bank teller, which not only cashes checks and deposits money, but can also provide these services 24 hours a day.

See also AUTONOMY; BOREDOM; JOB CHANGE; JOB SECURITY.

automobiles Americans spend an increasing amount of time in their automobiles—commuting to work, running errands, chauffeuring children, shopping, banking, and seeking recreation. It has been estimated that the typical American driver covers 12,000 miles each year; stress begins when drivers realize that they are handling a machine that is potentially deadly to themselves and others.

Even the purchase of the automobile may be a stress-filled situation. The buyer is faced with decisions whether to buy or lease; purchase new or used. Next comes a multitude of choices relating to dealer, brand, model, and optional features. Finally, before the purchase is consummated, the buyer worries whether he/she has used the best buying strategy and obtained lowest possible price. Car ownership carries with it the stresses of coping with repair scams, gas-pump ripoffs, and car thefts.

Stresses of driving include unending traffic, stop lights, poor road conditions, road repairs, detours, competition for parking spaces, and ANGER at the driving mistakes of others. Driving also involves constant decisions. Steering, passing, turning, braking, and looking out for other drivers puts one in a highly reactive state. Thus many drivers, when given sufficient reason, are ready to release their pent-up frustrations, let their tempers soar, and exhibit aggressive behaviors. Some vent their stress by using the horn, shouting out their windows, or making gestures to other drivers. These techniques do little to reduce the stress inherent in the situation. Better alternatives include patience, self-control, and keeping a sense of humor.

Continued exposure to traffic jams and long-distance commuting can have many adverse effects such as higher blood pressure and greater incidence of colds and flu. Driver tensions can lead to what researchers call "inter-domain transfer." That means that drivers who are stressed going to and from work are likely to carry a negative mood into the office or back to their families when they get home.

With today's new car equipment and gadgets, drivers are encouraged to add to existing

---

TIPS FOR REDUCING DRIVING STRESS

- Allow more time than you think you need.
- Avoid the peak morning and evening commutes.
- Keep your mind on the task at hand.
- Practice patience and self-control.
- Listen to music or audiotapes.
- Keep your sense of humor.
- Relax before or after driving by using MEDITATION or another form of BREATHING exercise.

---

stressors by talking on car phones, dictating memos, eating "one-handed" food, and sipping hot and cold drinks. Others who have overslept and are already under stress because they are late to work may be seen in their cars combing hair, flossing teeth, applying makeup, or tying ties. Keeping attention focused on the task at hand is probably the best antidote to the stresses involved in driving an automobile.

See also GUIDED IMAGERY; RELAXATION.

autonomy A feeling of being in CONTROL along with feelings of independence and freedom. When people lose their sense of autonomy, they may lose SELF-ESTEEM, become frustrated, and feel very stressed.

Many stressful situations throughout life can contribute to loss of autonomy. Individuals may experience automation on the job, job loss, co-dependent relationships, sickness and disabilities, and old age. In most cases, autonomy can be regained, at least to some degree, by taking assertive steps, such as learning a new skill or forming new relationships or finding a new job.

In developing a sense of autonomy, peer groups play an important role. Children with peer group relationships in which all group members play an equal role in leadership generally acquire good feelings about themselves and develop confidence that others will like them. They will also develop the ability to

realize what others expect of them and to make choices about meeting those expectations in a flexible way and without stress.

For some individuals, particularly teenagers, peer groups may be destructive to autonomy. They are individuals whose experiences with their peers have not enabled them to develop self-confidence. Under these circumstances, their desire for approval or acceptance may lead to taking drugs, smoking cigarettes, or other unhealthy behaviors that seem to make them feel part of the group.

See also AGING; ANGER; ASSERTIVENESS TRAINING; CODEPENDENCY; ELDERLY PARENTS; FRUSTRATION.

SOURCES:

Johnson, D.S., and R.T. Johnson. "Peer Influences" in Corsini, Raymond J., *Encyclopedia of Psychology*, vol. 2. New York, Wiley, 1984.

Kahn, Ada P., and Sheila Kimmel. *Empower Yourself: Every Woman's Guide to Self-Esteem.* New York: Avon Books, 1997.

May, Rollo. *Freedom and Destiny.* New York, W.W. Norton, 1981.

Vinack, W.E. "Independent Personalities," in Corsini, *Encyclopedia of Psychology,* vol. 2.

aversion Dislike for certain situations or things. When individuals face something they extremely dislike—whether food, loud music, or a certain person or animal—it can be stressful. Aversion therapy helps them overcome habits and unwanted behaviors that cause stress by associating those habits or behaviors with painful experiences or unpleasant feelings.

Aversion therapy has been used to treat many stressful situations, including ALCOHOLISM, BEDWETTING, SMOKING, sex addiction, and NAIL BITING. The most widely used form is chemical therapy, in which the individual receives a drug to induce nausea and is then exposed to smoking, nail biting, or other stressful habits that he or she is trying to overcome. The chemical method has been used most widely in the treatment of alcoholism.

A more modern form of aversion therapy is known as covert sensitization. Based on modification of behavior, this therapy requires the individual to imagine the unwanted stressful habit and then to imagine some extremely undesirable consequence, such as pain or nausea.

The word "aversion" is commonly misused in place of PHOBIA, which is a more severe reaction.

See also BEHAVIOR THERAPY; PSYCHO-THERAPIES.

SOURCES:

Cautela, J. "Covert sensitization." *Psychological Reports,* 20, (1967), 459–68.

Kahn, Ada P., and Jan Fawcett. *The Encyclopedia of Mental Health.* New York, Facts On File, 1993.

Ayurveda Ayurveda ("the science of life," as it translates literally) originated at least 3,000 years ago in India and is considered to be the oldest system of natural medicine. Ayurveda employs the healing powers of breathing exercises, natural foods, massage, herbs and aromas to reduce stress and promote health and long life.

While Western medicine works on illness, Ayurvedic medicine focuses on the person as a complex, multi-leveled being, and treatment is highly individualized. For a person who feels well, Ayurvedic activities make the most of mental, physical, and spiritual well-being, enabling better COPING skills against the stresses of daily life. When a person is fighting illness or coping with stress, Ayurvedic therapy works by enhancing the healing potential within him- or herself. Ayurvedic beliefs hold that life is a relationship between body and mind. In the United States, Ayurvedic health care is considered a form of ALTERNATIVE THERAPY (or complementary medicine), meant to complement, not replace, modern medicine. Ayurveda is an art of insight that brings harmony to daily life and relationships and to such stressful EMOTIONS as pain, grief, and sadness.

A characteristic element of Ayurveda is the determination of an individual's mind/body type. It is a combination of three fundamental principles, known as *doshas,* which govern thousands of mental and physical processes. These three principles—*Vata* (movement), *Pitta* (metabolism) and *Kapha* (structure)—are the controlling agents of nature. Permutations of the *doshas* determine an individual's subtype; through careful history taking and pulse diagnosis, a practitioner can determine imbalances of energy. Disease is diagnosed through questioning, observation, palpation, percussion, and listening to the heart, lungs, and intestines. Another diagnostic technique associated with Ayurveda reveals the status of internal organs merely by observing the surface of the tongue. It is considered the mirror of the viscera and can reflect many pathological conditions.

Ayurveda classifies seven major causative factors in disease: heredity, congenital factors, internal factors, external trauma, seasonal influences, natural tendencies or habits, and supernatural factors. Disease can also result from misuse, overuse, and underuse of the senses: hearing, touch, sight, taste, and smell. It also can result from imbalanced emotions, such as unresolved anger, fear, anxiety, grief, or sadness.

Prana, the Ayurvedic term for energy, has counterparts in Oriental medicine (*Qi*) and homeopathy (Vital Force). Pranic energy is mental and physical and can be changed by diet exercise, herbs, or spiritual practices such as MEDITATION. Pranic energy flows along specific paths, called *nadis,* which converge and cross in energy centers called *chakras* located along the length of the body. During an Ayurvedic examination, *chakras* are studied and *doshas* may be determined to be out of balance, leading to ill health.

In the United States, physician training in Ayurveda is under the direction of the Maharishi Training Program in Fairfield, Iowa, and directed by Dr. Deepak CHOPRA, who is also a contemporary writer about Ayurvedic medicine.

See also ALTERNATIVE THERAPIES; IMMUNE SYSTEM; MIND-BODY CONNECTIONS; PSYCHONEU-ROIMMUNOLOGY.

FOR FURTHER INFORMATION:

Ayurvedic Institute
P.O. Box 23445
Albuquerque, NM 97192–1445
Phone: (505) 291–9698

Sharp Institute for Human Potential and Mind/Body Medicine

8010 Frost Street (Suite 300)
San Diego, CA 92123
Phone: (800) 82-SHARP

SOURCES:

Anselmo, Peter. *Ayurvedic Secrets to Longevity and Total Health.* New York: Prentice Hall, 1996.

Chopra, Deepak. *Perfect Health.* New York: Harmony Books, 1990.

Lad, Vasant. *Ayurveda: The Science of Self-Healing.* Santa Fe: Lotus Press, 1984.

Morrison, Judith M. *The Book of Ayurveda.* New York: Fireside, 1995.

baby boomers The 76 million Americans born between 1946 and 1964. They are products of the population explosion that began during World War II, peaked following the war, and lasted until the mid-1960s.

The baby boom has been attributed to several causes, including the wartime prosperity that followed the Great Depression, increased births as servicemen husbands returned after the war, a lower MARRIAGE age than for previous generations, and a tendency to have children in quick succession early in marriage rather than spacing child-bearing over a period of years.

This generation has experienced many stresses, both individual as well as societal. These stresses have not been static but have been influenced by the changing times in which baby boomers have lived. As young adults, their protest against the Vietnam War labeled them as hedonistic, rebellious, and undisciplined. When they reached college age, they were fighting for civil rights and were active in the women's movement. Improved birth control, more permissive sexual standards, and an emphasis on education for both sexes plunged young women of the baby boomer generation into a world of choices. The resulting questions about pursuing careers, entering marriage, and having children are issues of stress that continue to haunt women into the 21st century.

The concept of family has not been totally attractive to baby boomers, who frequently have substituted networks of FRIENDS and LIVE-IN or communal arrangements for the traditional marriage and family. When marriages occur, they are often at a later age than in previous generations. For many couples, this has meant stress that is brought about by INFERTIL-ITY problems because of the later age or, for single women, stress brought about by the ticking of their BIOLOGICAL CLOCK.

A good job market and a rapidly expanding economy greeted baby boomers upon graduation from college, and they were soon described as having tendencies toward materialism that included acquiring possessions at an early stage and "HAVING IT ALL." In reaction, baby boomers tended to become entrepreneurial and viewed a job as something that should be fulfilling and stimulating rather than simply a means to the end of supporting themselves and their families. However, the sheer numbers of the baby boom generation created a population bulge that increased competition for the remaining corporate and government positions. A changing economy, DOWNSIZING, the future of Social Security, rising health care costs, and the need for RETIRE-MENT savings, has led to frustrations and additional stress.

Today, as baby boomers approach middle age, the "generation gap" between them and their parents has narrowed and they have become increasingly accepting of the values they had rejected early on.

See also COMMUNICATION; INTERGENERA-TIONAL CONFLICTS; SEXUAL REVOLUTION; WOMEN'S MOVEMENT; WORKING MOTHERS.

SOURCES:
Light, Paul Charles. *Baby Boomers.* New York: Norton, 1988.
Mills, D. Quinn. *Not Like Our Parents: How the Baby Boom Generation Is Changing America.* New York: William Morrow, 1987.
Silver, Don. *Baby Boomer Retirement: 65 Simple Ways to Protect Your Future.* Los Angeles: Adams-Hall Publishers, 1994.

back pain Discomforts in the spinal column and supporting structures. Estimates are that

50% to 80% of the population have back problems significant enough to cause them to be out of work at some point during their lifetime. Of these, only a handful of backache sufferers, perhaps 10% to 20%, ever discover a reason for their pain. Diagnosis often remains an unsolved mystery because the causes of back injury vary widely and the pain usually goes away on its own.

The STRESS that occurs because of back pain can affect the individual and his or her family and WORKPLACE. Often appearing at a particularly stressful time in a person's life, back pains can be the result of a one-time injury, or they can occur after years of poor posture, OBESITY, emotional stress, or simple wear and tear. Back pain can lead to the loss of work days. People who do heavy lifting, carrying or sitting in one place, or are overweight, often develop backaches. Understanding how work habits can lead to back pain and making appropriate changes is a step toward alleviating chronic discomfort and the accompanying stress.

Stress, muscle strain, ligament injuries and disk damage

The most common one-time injury is muscle strain caused by falling, twisting, or improper lifting of heavy objects. When muscles are pulled and do not have strength to support the trunk of the body, they can contract into painful spasms.

Ligament injuries can also trigger back problems. Years of poor body mechanics can permanently stretch the ligaments, bands of fibrous tissue that connect bone and muscle to strengthen the joints of the back. When they are sprained, the muscles have to work harder to support the back.

Disk damage affects only a small percentage of backache sufferers. Disks are located between each vertebra. They are composed of a strong, fibrous ring of tissue. When enough pressure is placed on a disk, the ring can be torn. If the ring has become weakened through long and strenuous use, the tear can

---

TIPS FOR PREVENTING STRESS DUE TO BACK PAIN

- Stay in good physical condition and exercise regularly to keep muscles strong, particularly abdominal muscles, as they are important in back support.
- Stand tall, with your chin and abdomen tucked in and the curve of your lower back as straight as possible. When standing in one place for any length of time, put one foot up on the rung of a stool, box, or some other object to adjust your weight.
- When sitting, sit well back in your seat with your back straight. Do not slouch. Change your position from time to time.
- Sleep on your side with your knees bent, or on your back with only a small pillow under your knees to release stress on your lower back. Avoid sleeping on your stomach.
- When lifting objects, squat down with your knees and hips bent. Use your leg muscles to rise, keeping your back straight and elbows bent. Hold the object as close to your body as possible to avoid strain on other muscles.

---

occur with only a slight pressure or strain. A slipped, or ruptured, disk occurs when the spongy interior of the disk seeps out and puts pressure on the nerves coming from the spine, causing severe pain in the back and often down the leg. As people age, ruptured disks are more likely because the disks lose some of their fluid and become less elastic.

In rare cases, back pain may indicate more serious health problems, such as disease or injury to the spine itself, pelvic or abdominal disorders, and kidney disease.

When simple self-help techniques do not work, one should consult a physician about back pain.

When back pain persists over time, many individuals experience sufficient stress to lead to mild DEPRESSION and withdrawal. Persistent pain without relief makes one feel out of CONTROL of one's body. Taking a positive attitude and pursuing avenues of relief can give the individual more control over the situation.

See also ALEXANDER TECHNIQUE; ALTERNATIVE THERAPIES; BODY THERAPIES; MASSAGE THERAPY; RELAXATION.

SOURCES:
Goodfriend, Judy, ed. "Getting a Grip on Back Pain." *Vital Signs* 9 (March 1995).

Jetter, Alexis. "Fighting Back Pain." *Health,* September 1996.

Reed, Sara. "Oh, My Aching Back!" *The Quill,* Pennsylvania Hospital, Spring 1993.

Sinel, Michael S. *Win the Battle Against Back Pain: An Integrated Mind-Body Approach.* New York: Dell, 1996.

barbiturate drugs Medications that provide sedation and induce sleep. They have been prescribed by physicians for stress, tension, and anxiety; they act as depressants to the CENTRAL NERVOUS SYSTEM. These drugs slow down the activity of nerves that control many mental and physical functions, such as EMOTIONS, heart rate and BREATHING.

Some sleeping pills are "short-acting" barbiturates; their effects last only five or six hours and, if properly used, produce little or no aftereffects. When abused, barbiturates can cause addiction and exacerbate the sleeping difficulties.

There are many serious disadvantages to barbiturates, which have led to a sharp decline in their use by physicians. They are very toxic. Death through overdose, accidental or intended, is a significant danger, particularly when they are combined with alcohol. Physical and psychological dependency and mood changes can result from too much use.

In recent years, physicians are prescribing drugs in a newer class known as benzodiazepines for many stress and anxiety conditions. Benzodiazepines can produce dependency but not to the degree of dependency, toxicity, or cell death that occurs with the barbiturates.

See also BENZODIAZEPINE DRUGS; PHARMACOLOGICAL APPROACH.

SOURCE:
Kahn, Ada P., and Jan Fawcett. *The Encyclopedia of Mental Health.* New York: Facts On File, 1993.

battered child syndrome See DOMESTIC VIOLENCE.

battered women See DOMESTIC VIOLENCE.

bed-wetting Medically known as enuresis; means unconscious or unintentional urinating by a child over the age of three while asleep. This problem is a major source of stress for the child, who may be embarrassed or feel guilty, as well as for the parent, who may feel confused about how to handle the situation. About 10% of children still wet the bed at age five; many more continue to do so until the age of eight or nine. The situation seems more prevalent among boys than among girls.

Bed-wetting in young children may also be a symptom of other stresses, ranging from the arrival of a new sibling to moving to a new house, from starting nursery school to the absence of a parent. Punishing or shaming a child for bed-wetting is not advisable. Parents should not focus undue attention on the situation, as doing so may make the child feel more stressed and anxious, worsening the problem. Instead, parents should try to reassure the child and relieve his or her fears.

Understanding the causes of bed-wetting
In coping with the attendant stresses on child and parent, an understanding of some possible causes for the problem may be helpful. For example, if the cause of bedwetting seems to be emotional, the parent can begin to identify contributing factors and start taking positive steps to correct the situation. In some cases, a skilled counselor may be able to help locate and explain the habits and reactions of the child, parents, and/or other caretakers. All concerned should try to reinforce a child's successes and reward good behavior by compliments and encouragement.

Some little children fear bed-wetting, or may have reacted severely to embarrassment from a previous accident. As a result, they may have bad DREAMS about the accident and during such dreams may urinate in the bed. In other cases, children sleep very deeply and cannot awaken to normal urinary impulses. A new schedule can be another cause of bed-wetting, particularly when a child who is accustomed to napping has just begun nursery school or kindergarten.

Making a diagnosis and beginning treatment

In cases of repeated bed-wetting, a physician will try to determine whether or not the cause is emotional or physical. Physical causes such as infection or illness can be detected by assessing bladder function. There may be a structural abnormality of the urinary tract present from birth, diabetes mellitus, or an infection in the urinary tract. In these cases, the child may also have difficulty controlling urine during the day.

Because bed-wetting may lead to further shame and stressful situations, other symptomatic treatments have been used. For example, medications such as imipramine, a

---

TIPS FOR HELPING A CHILD OVERCOME THE STRESS OF BED-WETTING

- Estimate the approximate times when bed-wetting occurs and consider contributing factors before bedtime.
- Give the child less liquid in the few hours before bedtime.
- Plan on awakening the child a few hours after he has gone to sleep and have him go to the bathroom.
- Help him train reflexes during waking hours by having him visit the bathroom immediately on feeling the first impulse.
- Reward the child with a gold star on a chart for each dry night.
- For an older child, consider use of an alarm pad in the bed.

---

tricyclic antidepressant, have helped some children. The decision to medicate should be made by a pediatrician.

A nighttime alarm system is available, which consists of a moisture-sensitive pad to be placed in the child's bed between the mattress and the lower sheet. This triggers an alarm when urine is passed, and awakens the child, who can then use the toilet. After a while, the child awakens whenever the urge to pass urine is felt. This is more useful to children over seven years old than to younger children.

Whether the causes are physical or emotional, a child can be retrained regarding toilet habits to help restore coordination of mental, neurological, and physical impulses.

The National Enuresis Society is a self-help organization to help parents cope with the stresses of children's bed-wetting.

See also TOILET TRAINING; URINARY INCONTINENCE.

FOR FURTHER INFORMATION:
National Enuresis Society
7777 Forest Lane (Suite C-737)
Dallas, TX 75230-2518
Phone: (800) NEW-8080

SOURCES:
Brownstone, David, and Irene M. Franck. *The Parent's Desk Reference.* New York: Prentice-Hall, 1991.
Glenzer, Milton W. *How to End Bedwetting: Facts Not Fancy.* Des Plaines, Ill.: Habit Publications, 1980.

behavior therapy Behavior modification; includes several techniques intended to change the way an individual responds to stressful situations by influencing actions, thoughts, and feelings that result from such situations. Maladaptive (negative or self-defeating) behaviors often can be reduced or eliminated through behavior modification techniques. This therapy form became a widely used alternative to psychodynamic theory during the 1950s. It developed because mental health professionals recognized a lack of specificity and verifiability in the treatment outcomes of other approaches to stress and anxiety problems.

Behavior therapy focuses on behaviors and responses rather than on underlying causes. Therapists in this area believe that behaviors are not inherited but learned in response to environment. They help individuals learn to relax, to overcome stress, and to avert ANGER, panic, and undesirable behaviors such as avoidance and anxiety.

Instead of trying to alter the "personality" by probing into "unconscious" reasons that may motivate a person's behavior, behavior therapy is often used in conjunction with therapies such as PSYCHOTHERAPY and medication. It has proven effective in treating anxieties, DEPRESSION, PHOBIAS, obsessions, compulsions, ALCOHOLISM and sexual problems as well as other stress-related disorders.

The goal of behavior therapy is to help the individual develop self-control and an increased number of revised, adaptive behaviors. The therapist and patient together define treatment goals, often in conjunction with the family of the patient. The therapist acts as a coach or instructor and encourages the patient to make choices about how and when to learn new behaviors. Behavior therapists tailor specific treatment techniques to the needs of their patients, focusing on measurable aspects of observable behaviors such as frequency or intensity (for example, of ritualistic hand washing), physiological responses (such as sweating) and self-rating scales and verbal reports by the patient. Therapists may utilize any one or more of many techniques, including classical CONDITIONING, exposure therapy or desensitization, flooding, HYPNOSIS and BIOFEEDBACK.

Exposure therapy (desensitization)

Exposure therapy employs several techniques to reshape an individual's responses to stress-producing situations. A therapist may choose systematic desensitization, exposure at full intensity (flooding and implosive therapy) or exposure with modification of thought processes (contextual therapy). Systematic desensitization gradually exposes the individual to stress or anxiety-producing situations. Such exposure may take place in the individual's imagination or in real life. To retrain the thought processes, this technique is often combined with relaxation training.

In contextual therapy, developed by American psychiatrist Manuel Zane (1913–), the therapist tries to keep the patient anchored in the present situation and works with individual internal cues, which present stresses and anxieties.

Systematic desensitization

In 1958, John Wolpe (1915–97), an American psychiatrist with a background in learning theory, reported successful results in treating adults with a variety of stress and anxiety concerns, including phobic anxiety, reactive depression, and obsessive-compulsive disorder, with a process he called "systematic desensitization." He adapted his process from a technique developed in the 1920s for helping children overcome animal phobias. This process trains the individual to relax muscles, imagine increasing degrees of anxiety-producing stimuli, and then face these stimuli *in vivo* (in real life) until the maximum stimulus no longer causes great anxiety. Thus, an individual who fears sexual intercourse might place coitus at the top of the list of anxiety-producing stimuli; thinking about sitting with a date in a bar might rank at the bottom of the list. After going through a series of relaxation training exercises, the patient is asked to imagine, with as much detail as possible, the least anxiety-producing item from the list. While relaxing and imagining the situation, the patient tries to weaken the association between it and his or her anxieties. After becoming comfortable with imagining the least threatening situation, the patient gradually moves up the hierarchy of stress-producing situations.

While many therapists believe that facing a stress-producing situation in the imagination may be just as effective as facing it in reality, others believe that it is not. Once the patient has completed desensitization treatment and goes on to face the real stress-producing situation, he or she may regress slightly down the hierarchy of stress-producing events. For example, a socially phobic individual who has learned to remain calm while walking into a party and meeting new people, may be comfortable in small groups but not at large cocktail parties. However, eventually that individual will be able to move from non-threatening small group social events to a larger setting and progress to a desired level of social behavior.

Flooding

Like desensitization, the technique known as "flooding" involves the patient imagining or experiencing stress-producing situations in real life (*in vivo*). The technique was developed in the 1960s by Thomas Stampfl, an American psychologist at the University of Wisconsin. The patient is exposed directly to a maximum level of stress-producing stimulus without a graduated approach. The therapist, rather than the patient, controls when and which stressful scenarios are to be imagined. The therapist describes vivid scenes in a purposeful effort to make them as disturbing as possible to the patient, with no instructions for the patient to relax. Such prolonged and repeated exposure to feared situations helps eliminate the individual's stress-filled response and replace it with another that is more acceptable.

Implosive therapy, or implosion, is a variation and extension of the flooding technique. The patient is repeatedly encouraged to imagine a stress-producing situation at maximum intensity in order to experience as intense a stress response as possible. Assuming that there is no actual danger in the situation, the stress response is not reinforced and thus becomes gradually reduced.

While flooding and implosive techniques help reduce stress-filled responses in some individuals who have simple anxieties, for others, desensitization appears to be more effective and more permanent.

Modeling and covert modeling

Modeling therapy is also known as social learning or observational learning. The anxious individual watches another person, often of the same sex and age, successfully carry out a particular stress-producing action, such as speaking in front of a group of people or being introduced to members of the opposite sex. In some cases, the therapist "models" the action. The "cure" occurs when the patient experiences vicarious extinction of the previously stress-filled and anxiety-producing responses.

With COVERT MODELING the patient simply imagines another person facing the stress-producing situation without experiencing undue stress.

Biofeedback

Biofeedback is a technique that enables the individual undergoing therapy to monitor psychophysiological changes through an electrical feedback device. It offers an individual a way to self-regulate certain processes, such as reactions to stress-producing situations. The technique is useful with some individuals who get headaches in response to stress or become extremely nervous when thinking about potentially stressful situations such as public speaking.

By noting physiological reactions to stressful events, biofeedback techniques help establish a diagnostic baseline that enables therapists to relate this information to an individual's verbal reports, fill gaps in the individual's history, and encourage relaxation of the body part to which the biofeedback equipment is applied. In many cases, relaxation training is used in conjunction with biofeedback to give the patient a better sense of control and to break the cycle that elicits unwanted responses to stress-filled situations.

Aversion therapy

This form of therapy helps the individual focus on the negative consequences of self-defeating behavior. For example, when alcoholics are treated with mild electrical shocks or given a nausea-inducing medicinal substance every time they taste alcohol, they develop an aversive reaction to the smell and taste of the alcoholic beverage.

Hypnosis

Hypnosis is considered a behavioral technique because the role of the therapist is active. When successful, hypnosis produces a trance-like state in which the patient becomes very receptive to suggestions for behavior changes. With use of posthypnotic suggestion, an individual may learn to change a response to a stressful situation, such as meeting new people. Hypnosis is usually considered an adjunctive therapy, because it is used in conjunction with other therapies. It is also considered an alternative therapy because it makes use of processes outside of the mainstream of medicine and psychiatry.

See also AGORAPHOBIA; ALTERNATIVE THERAPIES; AVERSION; COVERT REHEARSAL; COVERT REINFORCEMENT; MIND-BODY CONNECTIONS; PANIC ATTACKS AND PANIC DISORDER; PSYCHOTHERAPIES.

SOURCES:
Hollandsworth, James G. *Physiology and Behavior Therapy: Conceptual Guidelines for the Clinician.* New York: Plenum Press, 1986.
Kahn, Ada P., and Jan Fawcett. *The Encyclopedia of Mental Health.* New York: Facts On File, 1993.
Kaplan, Sheldon J. *The Private Practice of Behavior Therapy: A Guide for Behavioral Practitioners.* New York: Plenum Press, 1986.

belching   See INDIGESTION.

Benson, Herbert, M.D. (1935–) Founding president of the Mind/Body Medical Institute; associate chief, Division of Behavioral Medicine, Harvard Medical School; and chief, Division of Behavioral Medicine, New England Deaconess Hospital.

He is a cardiologist who discovered and described how the RELAXATION response is a protective mechanism against overreaction to stress. He is the author or coauthor of several books relating to relaxation and stress, including *The Relaxation Response* and *The Mind/Body Effect;* hundreds of his articles have appeared in medical journals and popular magazines.

Dr. Benson discovered the relaxation response while studying people who practiced TRANSCENDENTAL MEDITATION. As a specialist in HIGH BLOOD PRESSURE, Dr. Benson's particular interests have included how the relaxation response can help people with high blood pressure and other health concerns. He warns that people with high blood pressure should not just give up their medication. What MEDITATION and the relaxation response do, he maintains, is improve upon the benefit of the medication.

See also ALTERNATIVE THERAPIES.

FOR FURTHER INFORMATION:
Mind-Body Medical Institute
New Deaconess Hospital
Harvard Medical School
185 Pilgrim Road
Cambridge, MA 02215
Phone: (617) 632-9530

SOURCES:
Benson, Herbert. *Beyond the Relaxation Response.* New York: Berkeley Press, 1985.
———. *The Mind/Body Effect: How Behavioral Medicine Can Show You the Way to Better Health.* New York: Simon and Schuster, 1979.
———. *The Relaxation Response.* New York: Avon Books, 1975.

benzodiazepine drugs   A class of prescription medications widely used to help relieve symptoms of stress and anxiety. They act as sedatives, muscle relaxants, and anticonvulsants. Different drugs in this class are approved for different conditions. For example, ALPRAZOLAM (trade name, Xanax) is approved for use in panic disorder.

Benzodiazepine drugs have less toxicity and fewer drug interaction problems than barbiturates and non-barbiturate sedative-hypnotic drugs. Also, benzodiazepines have a lower risk of cardiovascular and respiratory depression compared with barbiturates and are often used before general anesthesia.

Persons taking benzodiazepine drugs should avoid alcohol because interaction may result in depression of the central nervous system.

See also PANIC ATTACKS AND PANIC DISORDER; PHARMACOLOGICAL APPROACH.

bereavement   See GRIEF.

bibliotherapy   A form of supportive or alternative therapy in which carefully chosen readings are recommended for helping the individual gain insight into personal sources of stress. Bibliotherapy also includes learning through reading about the MIND-BODY CONNECTION in stress management. It is used in conjunction with many other therapies, such as BIOFEEDBACK, GUIDED IMAGERY, and RELAXATION training.

See also ALTERNATIVE THERAPIES; GUIDED IMAGERY.

binge eating   See EATING DISORDERS.

binge-purge syndrome   See EATING DISORDERS.

biofeedback   Technique that enables a person to use information about a normally unconscious physical function, such as blood pressure, to develop conscious control over that function. This technique is often used as a STRESS MANAGEMENT tool in conjunction with other stress reduction therapies, such as MEDITATION and GUIDED IMAGERY.

Biofeedback operates by detecting physiological changes in the individual and, by means of auditory or visual signals, informing him/her of these changes. The individual, using the information, then endeavors to make the signals change in the desired direction. With the biofeedback tool as a guide, the individual learns fairly quickly how to control the biological response system generating the biofeedback signals. For example, he or she might learn to control heart rate or body temperature. Biofeedback can be effective in treating certain types of hypertension, anxiety and migraine.

Training for biofeedback involves three basic stages. The first is acquiring awareness of the maladaptive response. The person learns that certain thoughts as well as certain physical events influence the response. In the second stage, guided by the biofeedback signal, the person learns to control the response. In the third stage, the person learns to transfer the control into everyday life and to manage stress without the biofeedback instrument.

In addition to helping individuals improve their physiological activities into better ranges of function, biofeedback also helps them realize that it is possible to control events that affect their well-being and their capacity to cope with stressful circumstances.

Early work with biofeedback helped people relax before a BEHAVIOR THERAPY procedure known as "systemic desensitization," which involves counterconditioning of anxiety with relaxation.

See also ALTERNATIVE THERAPIES; HEADACHES; HIGH BLOOD PRESSURE.

FOR FURTHER INFORMATION:
Association of Applied Psychology and
   Biofeedback
10200 W. 44th Avenue (#304)
Wheat Ridge, CO 80303
Phone: (303) 422-8436

SOURCES:

Basmajian, John V., ed. *Biofeedback: Principles and Practice for Clinicians.* Baltimore: Williams & Wilkins, 1983.

Lehrer, Paul M., and Robert L. Woolfolk, eds. *Principles and Practice of Stress Management.* New York: Guilford Press, 1993.

biological clock   For the many women in their mid- to late thirties who hope to become mothers, the words "biological clock" refer to the limited period of time in which they are biologically able to produce children. As their "biological clock runs out," unmarried women as well as wives who are in their late thirties or early forties and who are having difficulty in becoming pregnant experience a great deal of stress and anxiety. Statistics show that a woman's fertility is reduced and her ability to conceive becomes more difficult with age, and birth defects occur more frequently in infants born to older mothers.

See also BABY BOOMERS; INFERTILITY; PARENTING.

SOURCE:

McKaughan, Molly. *The Biological Clock.* New York: Penguin Books, 1989.

biorhythms   Physiological functions, such as menstrual cycles, that follow a regular temporal pattern. These biological rhythms regulate psychological as well as physiological functions in the individual: energy level, hunger, sleep, and elimination can all be affected. These rhythms vary considerably from person to person and within a single individual at different times. Such external factors as changing travel and time zones or changing routines in unpredictable and unfamiliar ways, can disrupt biorhythms and lead to stress.

To deal with the stress caused by disruptions in biorhythms, individuals develop their own techniques. For example, some traveling through time zones may prepare by waking earlier for several days before the trip, or getting more rest upon return. Some develop particular dietary patterns that they find helpful, such as eating small meals oftener and drinking lots of water.

See also CIRCADIAN RHYTHMS; JET LAG; MENSTRUATION; SHIFT WORK.

birth control   The term "birth control" refers to controlling the number of children born by preventing or reducing the chance of conception by natural or artificial means. The issue is stressful for many people, including those making a choice of birth control methods or those whose religious convictions are counter to using birth control as a practical and economic plan for their families.

Methods of birth control

Each method of birth control has advantages, disadvantages, and sources of stress. They should be discussed by couples before they engage in sexual intercourse. Women and men must weigh the factors in a birth control method, including effectiveness in preventing unwanted PREGNANCY, protection from a sexually transmitted disease, freedom from side effects, costs, and spontaneity of use.

According to the 1995 National Survey of Family Growth by the National Center for Health Statistics, the most popular method of birth control is female sterilization (29.5%), followed by the birth control pill (28.5%), male prophylactics (17.7%), vasectomy (12.5%), the diaphragm (2.8%), the IUD (1.4%) and all other methods (4.9%). The numbers total more than 100% because some women use more than one method.

See also SEXUALLY TRANSMITTED DISEASES; UNWED MOTHERS.

FOR FURTHER INFORMATION:
American College of Obstetricians and
   Gynecologists
409 12th Street SW
Washington, DC 20024-2188
Phone: (202) 638-5577

METHODS OF BIRTH CONTROL

- The "pill" contains hormones that prevent conception.
- Norplant involves matchstick-size synthetic rods, which are inserted in the skin of a woman's upper arm. For five years at a slow, nearly steady rate, the rods release the hormone levonorgesterol, a form of progestin, which inhibits ovulation and thickens cervical mucus.
- Depo-Provera, an injectable form of progestin administered every three months, has been used by 15 million women worldwide.
- A diaphragm is a rubber disk with a flexible metal rim that is inserted to fit around the cervix. Spermicide placed inside the diaphragm kills most of the sperm in the area. The cervical cap is smaller and more rigid than the diaphragm but works the same.
- Placed inside the uterus, intrauterine devices (IUD) are 97% to 98% effective and are believed to set up a mild, harmless inflammation that impedes sperm and keeps any fertilized egg from implanting.
- The CONDOM, one of the oldest forms of birth control, is a simple sheath that covers the penis, blocking sperm from the uterus.
- Available since 1993 in the United States, the female condom is a long polyurethane sheath that is anchored between the cervix and the vagina.
- Medications known as the "morning after" pill can be used by women who engage in unprotected sex or who fear pregnancy. These medications are oral contraceptives taken in prescribed dosage no longer than 72 hours after intercourse, followed by another dose 12 hours later.
- Sterilization involves clamping or severing a woman's two Fallopian tubes, which otherwise carry eggs from her ovaries to the uterus.
- For men, a vasectomy involves clamping, severing, or plugging each of the two tubes in the scrotum that convey sperm from his testicles to his penis.
- *(No one method of birth control has proven to be 100% effective.)*

SOURCES:
Franklin, Deborah. "The Birth Control Bind." *Health,* July/August 1992.
Kahn, Ada P., and Linda Hughey Holt. *The A-Z of Women's Sexuality.* New York: Facts On File, 1990.

birth order   Studies of birth order have led to some generalizations about how a child's position in relation to his parents and siblings may affect his stress level, personality, and view of the world.

The first child born to a FAMILY has the advantage of undivided attention and resources. Whether that child becomes the only child of the family or the oldest child with a sibling(s) to follow, he or she may tend to be more adult in behavior and more interested in goals and personal achievement. As a group, first children are strongly represented in the ranks of the successful and powerful. They also tend to score highest on intelligence tests.

Only children often have characteristics and resulting stresses of their own. Having been the center of their parents' attention, they are in danger of becoming selfish and spoiled. Likewise, their parents' expectations for them to succeed at anything they do may be unreasonably high. With more exposure to adults, they may not relate well to other children and may have problems with sharing.

For older children, the arrival of a sibling, even though happily anticipated, has the ultimate effect of making them feel dethroned. They often assume a certain amount of responsibility for younger children in the family and may be responsible for setting a good example, showing younger children how to do things and baby-sitting. Older children are frequently more aware of family difficulties and problems and their own parents' insecurities. As a result, they tend to be more anxious, conservative, and responsible than younger brothers and sisters.

The middle child position in the family has more variables since the age and sex of siblings may have a profound effect on him or her. Middle children usually become good at sharing, but also guard their privacy. They may perceive that they are too young for the privileges of the oldest and too old for the coddling of the youngest. As a result, middle children may show off to get attention and may also seek rewarding relationships outside the family. The need to belong to a peer group is strong in middle children and they are team players, frequently quite popular. To compete with an older sibling, a middle child will develop his abilities in an area quite different from the talents of his older brother or sister.

The youngest child of a family never has the experience of having his position usurped. Younger children tend to preserve and use childish characteristics such as crying, acting cute, or emphasizing their dependence and inadequacy to get what they want. Younger children frequently have very positive feelings about themselves because of their position in the family and tend to be charming and popular. They have the best sense of humor in the family. Their disadvantage is that they often obtain information and opinions from other children rather than from adults and therefore lack the wisdom and realism they might gain from adult contact.

A very specific type of younger child is the "change of life" baby who arrives several years after the other siblings. This younger child is really more in the position of being the only child, but with several parents, since usually one or more of his or her siblings acts as a parent. These children grow up with a great deal of attention and support, but may also have the additional stress of a confused sense of themselves, from a variety of images and ideas from siblings they perceive as adult but who are, in fact, children.

Other positions in the family that can have long-lasting effects on personality are the "only daughter" or "only son" syndromes.

Only daughters have traditionally had the "feminine" chores of the family and, in many cultures, are expected to take care of the parents as they grow old, even if it means a personal sacrifice. "Only sons" were expected to enter the family business or succeed at some profession.

See also COMMUNICATION; SIBLING RELATIONSHIPS.

SOURCES:
Brownstone, David, and Irene Franck. *The Parent's Desk Reference.* New York: Prentice-Hall, 1991.
Franklin, Deborah. "Why Are Siblings So Different?" *In Health,* March/April 1991.
Richardson, Ron, and Lois A. Richardson. *Birth Order and You: How Your Sex and Your Position in the Family Affects Your Personality and Your Relationships.* Bellingham, Wash.: Self-Counsel, 1990.

bisexuality   See SEXUAL PREFERENCES.

bladder difficulties   See BEDWETTING; URINARY INCONTINENCE.

bloating   See INDIGESTION.

blood pressure   See HIGH BLOOD PRESSURE.

body image   The mental picture an individual has of his or her body at any moment. Many people are stressed by their own body image, thinking that one or more parts are too big, too small, or misshapen. Perception of their own body often determines their level of SELF-ESTEEM and self-confidence. Misperception of their body image can lead to avoidance of social or sexual activities and EATING DISORDERS, such as anorexia nervosa or bulimia.

When a normal-appearing individual becomes preoccupied with some imagined defect in appearance, the individual is said to have dysmorphic disorder. Any slight anomaly evokes a grossly excessive concern. This is often associated with anorexia nervosa and other eating disorders in which the person perceives herself or himself as obese.

See also ACNE.

SOURCE:
Hillman, Carolynn. *Love Your Looks: How to Stop Criticizing and Start Appreciating Your Appearance.* New York: Simon & Schuster, 1995.
Kahn, Ada P. and Sheila Kimmel. *Empower Yourself: Every Woman's Guide to Self-Esteem.* New York: Avon Books, 1997.

body language   A form of COMMUNICATION through facial expression, posture, gestures or movements, accompanied with or without words. Both the communicator and the listener may employ body language. It can be a device used to express emotion or a reaction to the meaning of communication.

Body language may be an indicator of the stress that the communicator and the listener are experiencing. According to Gay Turback in *The Rotarian* (April 1995), "Without uttering a syllable, it's possible to communicate love, hate, fear, rage, deceit, and virtually every other emotion in the human repertoire." The article goes on to describe how body signals have been around for more than a million years, with some researchers having catalogued 5,000 hand gestures and 1,000 postures, each with its own message. Says

---

EXAMPLES OF BODY LANGUAGE THAT ARE INDICATORS OF STRESS

Action	Meaning
Toes pointed outward	Confidence
Toes pointed inward	Submission
A jutting chin	Belligerence
Lip and nail biting	Disappointment
Lip licking	Nervousness
Foot tapping	Impatience
Leaning backward	A relaxed attitude
Leaning forward	Interest
Open palms	Honesty
Rubbing hands together	Excitement

Turback, "Although some body language is nearly universal, much of it is an accoutrement of one culture or another. Certain actions may have one meaning in Mexico, a different meaning in the United States, and no relevance in Canada. Other examples given in the article that are especially common among North Americans are shown in the table.

body therapies   Body therapies encompass ancient Eastern traditions of spirituality and cosmology along with contemporary Western neuromuscular and myofascial systems of skeletostructural and neuroskeletal reorganization. They postulate that the traumas absorbed by the psyche from "false understanding" are simultaneously absorbed as traumas in specific areas of the body. The body remembers after the mind forgets. Thus body therapies facilitate clarification of these traumas through the use of physical manipulations, movement awareness training, energy-flow balancing, and emotional release techniques. Body therapies are used by many people to prevent effects of stress as well as relieve them.

Ancient disciplines in the category of body therapies include YOGA, T'AI CHI, Zen, Taoism Tantra and Samurai. In the 20th century, Wilhelm Reich observed that clinical patients with emotional disturbances all demonstrated severe postural distortions. This observation helped to uncover more connections between the body-psyche and led to the development of the Reichian school of body therapy.

Another modern pioneer in the field was Moshe Feldenkrais, who postulated that the human organism began its process of growth and learning with one built-in response, the "fear of falling." All other physical and emotional responses were learned as the human organism grew and explored. To attain the full potential of the body-mind-emotions-spirit, there must be, according to Feldenkrais, "reeducation of the kinesthetic sense and resetting of it to the normal course of self-adjusting improvement of all muscular activity." This would "directly improve breathing, digestion, and the sympathetic and parasympathetic balance, as well as the sexual function, all linked together with the emotional experience." Feldenkrais believed that reeducation of the body and its functions was the essence of creating unity of the being. His method has helped many people with problems of BACK PAIN, whiplash, and lack of coordination. The method is also used to help people who have TEMPOROMANDIBULAR JOINT SYNDROME (TMJ), which is a collection of symptoms including pain, that affect the jaw, face, and head, often brought about by stress and tension.

Four systems of body therapies

Although many systems overlap and encompass aspects of the others, body therapies can be divided into four general categories, based on their methods.

Physical manipulation systems include the connective tissue work of the Ida Rolf school (*Rolfing*) and the deep tissue release systems such as myofascial release used by John Barnes, an American physical therapist.

Energy balancing systems include Chinese ACUPUNCTURE and ACUPRESSURE, polarity, and Jin Shin Jystu.

Emotional release systems include bioenergetics, primal therapy, and rebirthing.

Movement awareness systems include those of Aston, Feldenkrais, Trager, and Aguado.

See also ALTERNATIVE THERAPIES; AYURVEDA; MASSAGE THERAPY; MIND-BODY CONNECTIONS.

FOR FURTHER INFORMATION:
The Feldenkrais Foundation
P.O. Box 70157
Washington, D.C. 20088
Phone: (301) 656-1548

North American Society of Teachers of the
  Alexander Technique
P.O. Box 517
Urbana, IL 61801
Phone: (217) 367-6956

Rolf Institute
P.O. Box 1868
Boulder, CO 80306
Phone: (303) 449-5903

SOURCES:
Feldenkrais, Moshe. *Awareness Through Movement.* San Francisco: Harper & Row, 1972.
———. *Explorers of Humankind.* San Francisco: Harper & Row, 1979.
Feltman, John, ed. *Hands-On Healing.* Emmaus, Pa.: Rodale Press, 1989.

boredom According to Hans SELYE (1907–82), Austrian-born Canadian endocrinologist and psychologist, as well as pioneer researcher in the field of stress, boredom is not a defense against stress. Instead, as he reported in a research project, "bored subjects experienced an intense desire for extrinsic sensory stimuli and bodily motion, increased suggestibility, impairment of organized thinking, DEPRESSION, and in extreme cases, HALLUCINATIONS, delusions and confusion."

Normal function of the brain, Selye said, depends on constant arousal generated by continuous sensory input. Hallucinations, which may cause accidents, have been noted in pilots and long-distance truck drivers, presumably because the monotony of their work acts as a form of sensory deprivation.

What is boredom?
Boredom can be a self-imposed prison that keeps people from trying new things or having new, life-enriching experiences. An essential characteristic of boredom is that it is almost always the creation of the person who is bored. As a result, there are those who are bored by everything while many others are never bored.

Some people view things as boring because they really are afraid of failure. In his book, *A New Guide to Rational Living,* Dr. Albert Ellis said: "Viewing failure with fear and horror, some people avoid activities that they would really like to engage in." The rationale of such people is: If life is boring, nothing is worth doing. Thus, if nothing is worth doing, a person can hardly fail.

Overcoming boredom

Overcoming boredom depends on whether people are bored because they cannot live without excitement or because they have chosen to remain in a shell of inaction. Life is not supposed to be thrilling all the time. If people crave continuous thrills, they should reduce their expectations for excitement. If people are experiencing stress because of boredom, they should try to face reality. They should get out and do one new thing each day, such as talking to unfamiliar people, volunteering in a non-profit organization, learning a new skill, or writing letters. Boredom carried to the extreme can be a threat to health and lead to depression.

See also GENERAL ADAPTATION SYNDROME; HOBBIES; VOLUNTEERISM.

FOR FURTHER INFORMATION:
The Boring Institute
P.O. Box 40
Maplewood, NJ 07040
Phone: (201) 763-6392

bowel movements   See CONSTIPATION; DIARRHEA; INDIGESTION; IRRITABLE BOWEL SYNDROME.

brainstorming   A specialized approach to problem-solving, by group or team effort. It is based on the concept that a person alone may not be able to arrive at a solution to a problem because of a block in the thinking process or external distraction, but several people working together will be more likely to reach a solution.

When properly conducted, brainstorming sessions can be an important management tool. Employees who take part in a brainstorming session feel a part of the company. Furthermore, by giving employees entree to problems and solutions, they develop a feeling of CONTROL and ownership in what they do. As such, employee participation in brain-storming sessions may help to alleviate stress in the WORKPLACE.

In a typical brainstorming session, the coordinator who is in charge of collecting the ideas indicates that there should be a free flow of ideas, with no right or wrong answers or suggestions. All participants are encouraged to be a part of the process. However, if this brainstorming rule is not established, participants can be made to feel self-conscious and may experience a great deal of stress and anxiety .

The basic proposition of brainstorming is that one idea can lead to another and thus increase the creative output. When successful, this approach generates enthusiasm and a large number of suggestions, as one person expands upon ideas of others. Often, brainstorming sessions backfire. Participants never see the results of a brainstorming session carried out. This leads to an increase of employee stress and the lowering of morale.

See also CREATIVITY.

brainwashing   Form of mind control related to propaganda or political indoctrination. It is an extremely stress-provoking situation in which all of a person's COPING skills are called into use. Although situations and techniques of brainwashing vary, there are common elements that are used to change thought patterns and deeply held values.

For example, subjects of brainwashing can be made to feel totally out of CONTROL and to know that their needs and actions are subject to an authority before which they are powerless.

They may be subjected to mental or physical harassment and experience ridicule of deeply held beliefs. As much as possible, their persecutors make them feel that their future is uncertain. If they feel that one of the group who is controlling them is somewhat kinder than the others, they may begin to feel somewhat dependent on that person. Since subjects of brainwashing are usually kept in isolation, kept as inactive as possible and deprived of food and sleep, their bodies weaken, their thought processes become disorganized, and they will agree to almost anything. As their suggestibility increases, their SELF-ESTEEM decreases. They begin to feel guilty about past behavior that is at odds with their captors' standards.

An example of brainwashing is the treatment given American prisoners held captive by the Vietnamese during the Vietnam War. Another example is the religious CULTS that flourished in the years following the 1960s. Members of religious cults showed evidence of brainwashing techniques, such as changed speech and behavior patterns, obedience to an authoritarian leader, and rejection of friends and family outside of the cult.

See also ADVERTISING; AUTONOMY.

SOURCES:

Johnson, Joan. *The Cult Movement.* New York: Franklin Watts, 1984.

Kahn, Ada P., and Jan Fawcett. *The Encyclopedia of Mental Health.* New York: Facts On File, 1993.

Somit, Alters. "Brainwashing" in Sills, David, ed., *International Encyclopedia of the Social Sciences,* vol 1. New York: Macmillan, 1968.

breast cancer The anxiety, fear, and apprehension each woman faces when she discovers a lump in her breast is the beginning of a long, stressful period in her life, and one that deeply affects her family as well. According to an article in *National Women's Health Report,* "It (finding a lump) may well be the reason that women resist establishing a routine for examining their breasts each month."

Once a lump has been discovered either through self-examination or mammography, the woman enters a world of baffling terminology in which she must depend on others for understanding. Next, she must deal with the stress of tests and procedures used to identify a breast symptom and the time lapse before a final diagnosis is made. If a malignancy is found, she must select from a variety of treatment options and find the right resources to assure that the best decision is made. The more information she has, the easier it may be to determine the advantages and disadvantages of various therapies. Inherent at this point is the tremendous physical and emotional adjustments a woman must make regarding removal of a breast(s). Finally, when treatment is completed, she is faced with the fear that the CANCER is out of control and she must deal with the continuing anxiety over recurrence of the disease.

More aggressive therapy wanted

According to a report in *Y-ME Hotline* (November-December 1995) final results of a survey of women with advanced breast cancer reveal that 77% are willing to do whatever it takes to get more aggressive drug therapy, despite the financial, emotional, and physical side effects of the treatment. In addition, 93% of the women surveyed believed that the Food and Drug Administration is too slow in approving treatment options. The findings were announced in 1995 by three national information and advocacy organizations participating in the Roper Search mail survey: the National Alliance of Breast Cancer Organizations (NABCO), the Susan G. Komen Foundation, and the Y-ME National Breast Cancer Organization. The survey was conducted by sending questionnaires to women with advanced breast cancer; results were tabulated from 256 responses.

The majority of women (53%) in the Roper survey stated that they themselves are the most influential party in selecting their medical treatments. Seventy-seven percent felt that the chance for a favorable response (shrinking of the tumor) is the most important consideration in their treatment decision, 11 times the number for whom side effects are most important. The most encouraging aspect of chemotherapy, according to 41% of respondents, is feeling hope for their future.

According to another survey conducted by the Gallup Poll, 80% of 1,500 women receiving chemotherapy want their chemotherapy treatment to be as aggressive as they can tolerate. Sixty-one percent said that chemotherapy is worth the discomfort and inconvenience.

Role of psychoneuroimmunology

In the early 1980s, researchers in the Behavioral Medicine Branch of the National Cancer Institute tested an observation on breast cancer patients. They believed that women with better survival rates were also those who were fighters, or those who had an aggressive attitude toward conquering the disease and were active in choosing their physicians and their treatments.

Even before that, in the 1970s, British researchers followed the health of breast cancer patients. They found that breast cancer patients often seemed to hold their emotions, especially ANGER, in check. Those women who survived longest with no recurrence of disease were also those who initially reacted to the news that they had cancer in one of two ways: denying there was anything seriously wrong with them or showing "fighting spirit," a determination to do everything possible to conquer cancer. In contrast, women who succumbed had reacted to the news of their cancer either by demonstrating a stoic attitude and living their lives as though nothing had changed or having a helpless, hopeless response.

Studies conducted at Stanford University during the 1980s demonstrated that breast cancer patients who were in SUPPORT GROUPS while undergoing therapy lived longer than those who received medical treatment alone. Although there are no hard scientific data that other complementary treatments, such as RELAXATION, BIOFEEDBACK, massage, herbal remedies and many others similarly extend survival, there is little evidence that they are harmful. They can be helpful supplements to, but not substitutes for, conventional therapy.

Choosing to use an "alternative" therapy in addition to the prescribed medical therapy also gives a woman more of a sense of control over her situation.

See also ALTERNATIVE THERAPIES; CHRONIC ILLNESS; PSYCHONEUROIMMUNOLOGY.

FOR FURTHER INFORMATION:
Susan G. Komen Breast Cancer Foundation
5005 LBJ (Suite 370)
Dallas, TX 75244
Phone: (214) 450-1777

Y-Me National Breast Cancer Organization
212 W. Van Buren St.
Chicago, IL 60607
Phone: (312) 986-8338

SOURCES:
Love, Susan M. *Dr. Susan Love's Breast Book,* 2nd ed. Reading, Mass.: Addison-Wesley, 1995.
Merz, Beverly, ed. "Breast Cancer." *Harvard Women's Health Watch,* October 1995.
———. "The Mammography Muddle." *Harvard Women's Health Watch* 4, no. 7 (March 1997).
"Patients Want Aggressive Therapy," *Y-ME Hotline,* 534 (November/December 1995).

breast reconstruction Depending on their prognosis after removal of a breast (or breasts), women can choose an additional procedure during which the breast is reconstructed with artificial substances or with tissue from another body part, such as the abdomen. For those who are candidates for reconstruction, making the choice of methods can be a very stressful situation.

"Preserving the breast after CANCER can reduce stress and increase the quality of life," said plastic surgeon John Bostwick, M.D., in a clinical study released by the American Society of Plastic and Reconstructive Surgeons (ASPRS) in October 1995. The study explored immediate partial breast reconstruction using endoscopic surgery. It recommended such construction after lumpectomy and radiation treatments for women with smaller breasts when primary tumors are 2.5 cm., as well as for women who had large portions of their breasts removed leading to considerable deformity and asymmetry of the breast. "The ability to examine the breast with a mammogram is extremely important," said Dr. Bostwick. "Since women have elected to keep as much of the breast as possible, they need to know that reoccurrence of the cancer can be detected." However, just as in women who have very dense breasts, detecting early cancerous changes behind an implant with mammography may, in some cases, be difficult. There is some controversy regarding the effectiveness of mammography following reconstruction with an implant.

Because women do not always choose or have a choice of reconstruction after surgery, they return to a society that places a high value on the breast as a sex symbol and fashion statement. Marriages or relationships can be put under a terrific strain and often do not last. For these women, the stress of maintaining a sense of BODY IMAGE and self-worth follows them throughout their lives.

On the other hand, many women who are able to make a choice of breast reconstruction find that their sense of SELF-ESTEEM is enhanced. They have fewer concerns about looking attractive in clothing, entering relationships, or preserving their marriages.

See also BREAST CANCER; CHRONIC ILLNESS; SUPPORT GROUPS.

breathholding spells Childhood breathholding spells, a common and frightening phenomenon that occurs in healthy, otherwise normal children, are a source of stress for parents and child alike. Treatment of children with breathholding spells has largely focused on providing reassurance to families after a diagnosis has been made.

Some children use breathholding as an act of rebellion or a demonstration of AUTONOMY. When children know that they can terrify their parents with this behavior, the behavior becomes somewhat reinforced. According to Francis DiMario, Jr., M.D., Department of Pediatrics, University of Connecticut Health Center, Farmington, "It is neither feasible nor helpful for parents to attempt to avoid circumstances that may provide emotional upset in their child. Even though pain and fear may serve as provocatives, simple frustration and the expression of autonomy are both normal and expected in young children."

If parental stress leads to continuous attempts at appeasement, the child may soon learn to manipulate the parent with the threat of crying. This does not imply a willful attempt at breathholding, since in some cases these spells are reflexive and unpredictable. There is, nonetheless, the potential for parents to reinforce behavioral outbursts if appropriate, calm firmness is not displayed at times of customary disciplining.

Breathholding spells pose no physical danger to the child. If spells are causing anxiety to the parents, a physician should be consulted.

See also BREATHING; PARENTING.

SOURCES:
Brownstone, David, and Irene Franck. *The Parent's Desk Reference.* New York: Prentice-Hall, 1991.
Kahn, Ada P., and Jan Fawcett. *The Encyclopedia of Mental Health.* New York: Facts On File, 1993.

breathing The major features of breathing are respiration and ventilation. Respiration puts oxygen into body cells and ventilation removes the excess carbon dioxide. Poor breathing habits diminish the flow of gases to and from the body, making it harder for individuals to cope with stressful situations. With increased awareness of how people breathe and by incorporating certain controlled breathing techniques into relaxation practice, they will be able to quiet thoughts, calm emotions, deepen relaxation, and control blood pressure and other physical functions. Although breathing seems very easy and very normal, relearning breathing techniques can help many individuals who suffer from STRESS, PHOBIAS, anxieties, and panic attacks. Some performers and athletes learn this technique in order to combat STAGE FRIGHT or PER-FORMANCE ANXIETY.

Breathing is controlled by the autonomic or involuntary nervous system. Breathing patterns change during different psychological states. For example, in a state of calm and relaxation, breathing becomes deeper and more rhythmic. Under stress, breathing is shallow and irregular. When frightened, an individual may even hold the breath. However, breathing patterns can be consciously controlled in order to influence the autonomic system toward relaxation, thereby interrupting the physiological arousal that can lead to stress-related disorders and high blood pressure.

Breathing styles

Most people breathe in one of two patterns: One is chest or thoracic breathing; the other is abdominal or diaphragmatic breathing. Chest breathing, which is usually shallow and often rapid and irregular, is associated with anxiety or other emotional distress. When air is inhaled, the chest expands and the shoulders rise to take in air. Anxious people breathing in this manner may experience breath holding, HYPERVENTILATION or constricted breathing, shortness of breath, or fear of passing out. When an insufficient amount of air reaches the lungs, the blood is not properly oxygenated, the heart rate and muscle tension increases, and the stress response is triggered.

Abdominal or diaphragmatic breathing is the natural breathing of sleeping adults. The diaphragm contracts and expands as inhaled air is drawn deep into the lungs and exhaled. When breathing is even and unconstricted, the respiratory system performs efficiently in producing energy from oxygen and removing waste products.

Symptoms of inefficient breathing

Many people who feel stressed also have breathing-related complaints. Some can't seem to catch their breath or get enough air. Others may frequently sigh, yawn, or swal-low. Some breathe too deeply and hyperventilate. Symptoms associated with hyperventilation resemble those of PANIC DISORDER. Researchers have noted the overlap between hyperventilation, anxiety, and stress symptoms. It has been found that patients will hyperventilate just by asking them to think back on unpleasant or stressful events.

Physical conditions associated with breathing difficulties, particularly hyperventilation, include hypertension, ALLERGIES, anemia, angina, ARTHRITIS, ARRHYTHMIAS, ASTHMA, colitis, diabetes, gastritis, HEADACHES, heart disease and IRRITABLE BOWEL SYNDROME.

Deep, diaphragmatic breathing is a cornerstone for many relaxation therapies. Many therapeutic techniques (many known as ALTERNATIVE THERAPIES) and BEHAVIOR THERAPIES incorporate control of breathing as a basis because the cycle of stress can be altered with

---

TIPS FOR DIAPHRAGMATIC OR ABDOMINAL BREATHING FOR STRESS REDUCTION

- Lie down comfortably on your back on a padded floor or on a firm bed, with eyes closed, arms at your sides and not touching your body, palms up, legs straight out and slightly apart, and toes pointed comfortably outward.
- Focus attention on your breathing. Breathe through your nose. Place your hand on the part of your chest that seems to rise and fall the most as you inhale and exhale.
- Place both of your hands lightly on your abdomen and slow your breathing. Become aware of how your abdomen rises with each inhalation and falls with each exhalation.
- If you have difficulty breathing into your abdomen, press your hand down on your abdomen as you exhale and let your abdomen push your hand back up as you inhale.
- Observe how your chest moves; it should be moving in synchronization with your abdomen.

breath control. Individuals who have mastered these techniques find that as soon as they are aware of a stressor, they become aware of their breathing, and try to control their stress by deep, slow breaths. By contrast, holding the breath, as well as shallow, irregular breathing, can initiate as well as augment many stressful feelings and physiological responses. Posture can also affect breathing. Keeping the body in alignment allows greater lung capacity.

Breathing, yoga and language

YOGA is a more than 2,000-year-old method for developing and unifying mind, body and spirit. Yoga practitioners have long recognized the relationship between breathing and health and maintain that the life force is carried in the breath. Exercises to control breathing are incorporated into yoga postures (asanas) and practices. Yoga practitioners believe that extending and deepening the breathing process draws breath all the way down to one's heels and that deep and slow breathing can increase longevity.

See also BIOFEEDBACK; GUIDED IMAGERY; MEDITATION; PANIC ATTACKS AND PANIC DISORDER.

FOR FURTHER INFORMATION:
American Lung Association
1740 Broadway
New York, NY 10019
Phone: (212) 315-8700

SOURCES:
Kerman, D. Ariel. *The H.A.R.T. Program: Lower Your Blood Pressure Without Drugs.* New York: HarperCollins, 1993.
"RX: Breathing for Health and Relaxation." *Mental Medicine Update* 4, no. 2 (1995): 3–6.

bronchial asthma See ASTHMA.

bruxism See TEETH GRINDING.

bulimarexia See EATING DISORDERS.

bulimia See EATING DISORDERS.

bureaucracy Bureaucracy involves organizations that are made up of tightly structured hierarchies bound up in structured procedures marked by delay or inaction. Examples of bureaucracies are government agencies, insurance companies, academia and higher education, banks, health care providers and hospitals, pharmaceutical and chemical companies, utilities, and most heavily regulated industries. They have been criticized by modern management theorists as rigid and easily co-opted by power structures to serve ends other than economic efficiency. In a bureaucracy, management's expectations for employees can be stressful.

Employees valued in bureaucracies play by the rules and are punctual and detail-oriented. They do not question authority. They follow orders and procedures regardless of the consequences, and they spend long hours in meetings in which the most trivial as well as the most important decisions are made. They do not know if they are doing a good job until someone blames them for something. As a result, employees often suffer from the stress of covering for themselves regarding how the job was done rather than what the final outcomes were.

Doing business with a bureaucracy as a citizen, client or customer can be equally frustrating and stressful. Finding the right person who knows the answer to questions or can give information and getting through to him/her, particularly when "voice mail" is giving directions, has become a major feat.

See also AUTONOMY; BOREDOM; CONTROL; WORKPLACE.

burnout Contemporary term for a progressive loss of energy, purpose, and idealism resulting from overexposure to a job or other stimulus that leads to STRESS, stagnation, FRUSTRATION, and BOREDOM. It may result from ongoing, chronic stress, and it is also a cause of stress for the sufferer as well as his or her family and coworkers. It can strike anyone,

TIPS FOR COPING WITH THE STRESS OF BURNOUT

• Recognize that no one job (or personal relationship) is a total solution for life. Strive for variety in work, avoid routine.
• Put priorities into perspective; stop trying to be "all things to all people."
• Take responsibility for change.
• Set personal goals by answering these vital questions, "Where am I going?" "What do I want to achieve?" and "How am I going to do it?"
• Learn a new skill to enhance your optimism.
• Create an "outside life," interest and activities unrelated to your work.
• Develop a support system, people you can turn to for help in problem solving.
• Consider switching careers.
• Learn how to manage your personal time.
• Take breaks during the workday; go out for lunch, take walks, etc.
• Establish an exercise program at least three times a week.
• Look into alternative therapies such as relaxation techniques.
• Take mini-vacations.

from top executives, surgeons, defense attorneys, and airline pilots, to occupiers of such monotonous positions as assembly-line worker and postal employee. Burnout has no relationship to intelligence, money, or social position.

Burnout victims are often high achievers, workaholics, and idealists and are competent, self-sufficient, and overly conscientious individuals. Their common denominator is the assumption that the real world will be in harmony with their ideals. They often hold unrealistic expectations of themselves, their employers, and society, and often have a vague definition of personal accomplishment.

Burnout begins slowly and progresses gradually over weeks, months, and years to become cumulative and pervasive. Physical symptoms of burnout include excessive sleeping, eating, or drinking, physical exhaustion, loss of libido, frequent colds, headaches, backaches, neck aches, and bowel disorders. The burnout victim desires to be alone, is irritable, impatient, and withdrawn, and complains of boredom, difficulty concentrating, and burdensome work. Fellow workers may notice indecisiveness, indifference, impaired performance, and high ABSENTEEISM. Intellectual curiosity declines and interpersonal relationships deteriorate. "Overloaded," "tired of thinking," and "I don't know what I'm doing anymore" are some phrases that express the inner agony and stress of burnout sufferers.

See also AUTONOMY; CHRONIC FATIGUE SYNDROME; CONTROL; DEPRESSION; HOBBIES; RELAXATION; WORKPLACE.

SOURCES:
Kahn, Ada P., and Jan Fawcett. *The Encyclopedia of Mental Health.* New York: Facts On File, 1993.
Riess, Dorothy Young. *Better Health Newsletter* 3, no. 1 (February 1987).

butterflies in the stomach   The uneasy sensation people refer to as "butterflies in the stomach" is caused by a contraction of the abdominal blood vessels and is a response to STRESS. It is a common sensation experienced by people who must perform in front of an audience, go for a job interview, or participate in any type of activity that causes ANXIETY.

The feeling can be overcome, at least in part, by appropriate and adequate preparation for the performance, speech, or interview. Paying attention to BREATHING by taking regular and deep breaths before the event can also provide relief.

See also ALTERNATIVE THERAPIES; RELAXATION; YOGA.

caffeine One of several stimulants that affect the central nervous system by causing a rise in heart rate, blood pressure, and muscular tension. Drinking caffeine-containing drinks—such as coffee, tea, cola, and cocoa—or taking over-the-counter medications such as Nodoz or Vivarin and certain headache and diet pills may actually increase the individual's stress level because of caffeine's stimulating effect on all organs and tissues. Peak blood levels are reached in about 30 minutes after consumption. Caffeine directly affects individual cells by causing chemical reactions within them. It acts indirectly on the adrenal glands by increasing the release of epinephrine (adrenaline) and norepinephrine (noradrenaline), hormones that stimulate cell activity into the circulation system.

When taken in small amounts, caffeine can stimulate brain cells, helping reduce drowsiness and fatigue. Concentration may be improved and reactions speeded up. However, taken in large amounts, caffeine is known to cause overstimulation, ANXIETY, irritability, and restlessness. Many people who consume caffeine before going to bed complain of having INSOMNIA, which is a delay in the onset of SLEEP, a shortened sleep time, or a reduction of the average "depth of sleep." Caffeine also may increase the amount of dream sleep (REM) early in the night, while reducing it overall. People who feel stressed by insomnia should consider the amount of caffeine that they consume in the course of a day.

Additional effects of caffeine
While caffeine, in moderate doses, may increase alertness and decrease fatigue for some individuals, regular use of 350 mg or more a day may result in a form of physical dependence. Coffee contains 100 to 150 milligrams of caffeine per cup; tea contains about half, and cola about one-third that amount. Interruption of this physical dependence on caffeine can result in withdrawal symptoms such as severe HEADACHES. Many people who drink large amounts of coffee on weekdays have headaches on weekends because they may be consuming less caffeine.

Caffeine has been known to produce panic attacks in susceptible individuals. About half of the people who suffer from panic disorder have attacks after consuming the caffeine equivalent of four to five cups of coffee. Research has yet to determine whether caffeine has a direct or causative effect on panic or whether it simply alters the body to a state that triggers a panic cycle. It may be that caffeine produces its effects by blocking the action of a brain chemical known an adenosine, a naturally occurring sedative.

Caffeinism is a disorder caused by an individual's recent consumption of over 250 milligrams of caffeine. Symptoms of caffeinism may include restlessness, increased anxiety, increased phobic reactions in people with that diagnosis, nervousness, excitement, insomnia, frequent and increased urination, gastrointestinal complaints. rambling thoughts and speech, and cardiac arrhythmia.

See also PANIC ATTACKS AND PANIC DISORDER.

SOURCE:
Kahn, Ada P., and Jan Fawcett. *The Encyclopedia of Mental Health.* New York: Facts On File, 1993.

cancer It is not easy today to live without the fear of cancer. Changing reports of things in our diet, lifestyle, or environment that do or do not cause or cure cancer have placed a great deal of stress on many people. Yet in the last few decades, the outlook for those with cancer has improved considerably.

Cancer is a condition in which abnormal body cells reproduce uncontrollably. The defective cells grow slowly and are open to attack by macrophages, large cells in the IMMUNE SYSTEM that characteristically consume foreign debris and foreign bodies. When they are successful in taking over the invading cells, cancer is averted. When they fail, a tumor grows.

The defensive cells are inhibited by corticosteroids, biochemicals released under stress. Research on stress and coping shows that generally people who do not cope well in stressful situations have a decline in the activity of their natural killer cells. Many individuals with TYPE C PERSONALITY also may fall into this category.

According to an article in *World Health* (March–April 1994), physicians have recognized significant associations between stress and development of malignancies for as long as 2,000 years. In the 19th century, British physicians believed that emotional distress was the most powerful cause of cancer, and increased rates of the disease were subsequently correlated with the psychosocial stresses that have progressively developed along with lifestyle changes.

As reported in *Stress,* the newsletter of the American Institute of Stress, studies since 1950 have demonstrated that stress accelerates development and growth of different malignancies without actually causing them. Similarly, stress reduction strategies have been shown to retard tumors in laboratory animals and to prolong life in cancer patients.

In the summer edition of *Awareness,* a publication of the EHS Hospital and Medical Center, Oak Lawn, Illinois, strategies were listed that can "make a difference." An adaptation follows:

STRESS AND CANCER: HOW TO MAKE A DIFFERENCE

- Change or modify your lifestyle. Since 75% of all cancers can be rooted in individual behavior, *prevention* is key. It is important to eat a healthy diet, not smoke, and use sun screens when outdoors.
- See your doctor for regular checkups and when symptoms arise. Cancers caught early generally require less treatment and have better odds for survival. That's why *early detection* can be crucial. Screening for colon, prostate, ovarian, breast, and lung cancer is particularly important for those over 40.
- Be sure you are receiving the most up-to-date care. The best way to do that is through *intervention,* learning about how diagnoses are made, what the latest treatments and follow-ups are, and where the best research is being done. Information on cancer is readily available for computer on-line users.

There is increasing focus on another important strategy, *affirmation.* Research reports that state of mind may be more important than the seriousness of the disease in predicting longevity. Keeping a positive attitude through strong faith, participation in SUPPORT GROUPS, and using mind/body treatments such as HYPNOSIS, GUIDED IMAGERY, visualization, and other adjunctive treatments, may improve the quality and extend the length of a cancer patient's life. Positive emotions elicited by these positive approaches seem, in some cases, to retard or even reverse malignant growths.

Stress on families of cancer patients
Family members of cancer patients are open to considerable stress as they watch their loved ones undergo uncomfortable procedures and wonder about possible outcomes. At times, family members may wonder whether or not the procedures are worth the suffering they inflict on the patient. While it

may be difficult to keep up a cheerful, optimistic outlook, doing so is usually helpful to all concerned.

Family members and friends who observe the progression of the disease in a cancer patient may have feelings of confronting their own mortality. There may be subconscious (or even conscious) fears of contagion. Support groups for family members as well as the patient can be helpful.

See also ALTERNATIVE THERAPIES; BREAST CANCER; CHRONIC ILLNESS; MIND-BODY CONNECTION; PROSTATE CANCER; PSYCHONEUROIMMUNOLOGY; SIEGEL, BERNIE.

FOR FURTHER INFORMATION:
American Cancer Society
1599 Clifton Rd., NE
Atlanta, GA 30329
Phone: (404) 320-3333; (800) 227-2345

Cancer Information Clearinghouse (NCI/OCC)
Bldg. 31, Rm. 10A18
9000 Rockville Pike
Bethesda, MD 21205
(301) 496-5583

National Cancer Institute
9000 Rockville Pike
Bethesda, MD 20982
Phone: (800) 4CANCER; (800) 422-6237

Sloan Kettering Institute for Cancer Research
1275 York Avenue
New York, NY 10021
Phone: (212) 639-2000

SOURCES:
Locke, Steven, and Douglas Colligan. *The Healer Within: The New Medicine of Mind and Body.* New York: New American Library, 1986.
McAllister, Robert M., Sylvia Teich Horowitz, and Raymond U. Gilden. *Cancer.* New York: Basic Books, 1993.
Terkel, Susan Neiburg, and Marlene Lupiloff-Brass. *Understanding Cancer.* New York: F. Watts, 1993.

cardiac arrest   See HEART ATTACK.

caregivers   In contemporary society, caregivers include family members or friends of a child, elderly adults or an ill or disabled person who cannot completely care for himself. The term also applies to individuals who are health care professionals or social workers.

Stresses of caregiving
The caregiver role can be extremely stressful because of its physical and emotional demands. For example, family members who are caregivers may feel powerless and depressed in the face of the suffering of a loved one. Professional caregivers may build a wall around themselves or go to the other extreme and allow the pain and suffering they see to overwhelm them.

Caregivers have a considerable amount of power and work in a close, personal relationship with their charges, frequently with little or no supervision. Unfortunately, some situations of abuse have occurred with elderly adults as well as with children. Children are frequently victims of sexual abuse by their caregivers, while the elderly are often subjected to neglect or emotional and financial abuse. When an elderly person, disabled person, or child is entrusted to the care of another, credentials and references should be carefully checked and verified.

Caregiving to the elderly
Even though institutional options are available, 75% of care for the elderly is still provided by a family member. Increased longevity means many spouses will be caring for each another. Social mobility and shrinking family size put some women in the sole caregiver role for both their own and their husbands' aging parents. The Older Women's League in Washington, D.C., reported that at least a third of all women over age 18 can expect to be continuously in the caregiver role from the birth of their first child to the death of their parents. At the same time, women are moving into highly responsible professional positions at the time in life that their parents need care. According to the American

Association of Retired Persons, some women turn down promotions, avoid traveling, and even take early retirement to care for aging parents, adding stress to all concerned.

Individuals who have ELDERLY PARENTS or are over the age of 65 may be able to relieve some stress by planning ahead. Planning and preparation can deter the emotional and financial stress that often accompanies caring for an elderly loved one.

Identify needs: disabled children, adults or elderly persons

When an individual realizes that she or he will be in the caregiver role, stress can be relieved by identifying the kinds of assistance the disabled or elderly person wants and needs. Some needs that can be met by a family member or by outside sources include meals, shopping, cleaning, yard work, household repairs, finances, living arrangements, personal care, and home health care.

An elderly person or disabled child or adult may need services to help him or her maintain social interaction or participation in the community. These services may include transportation to the doctor, shopping, or church; psychological support such as cutting through the red tape of health insurance carriers and Medicare, Medicaid, Social Security, and other governmental bureaucracies; and protective services such as safety devices. A disabled child may also need home tutoring or special education.

If possible, the caregiver and disabled elderly person or child can explore how needs, once identified, may best be met. They can consider the resources of other family members, and their willingness and/or ability to help. Together they may look at possibilities for blending resources within the family with those from outside the family. When caregiving is a shared responsibility among family and/or friends, it leads to greater understanding of the difficulties, sharing of stress, development of positive relationships,

and enhancement of communication. Community and social services, such as Meals on Wheels, respite programs, support groups, and elderly day care, can also supplement caregivers' efforts.

FOR FURTHER INFORMATION:
Care Options (Elder Care Management)
2012 Business Center Dr. (Suite 130)
Irvine, CA 92715
Phone: (714) 254-4140

SOURCES:
"Caregiving Solutions." *Care Options* 2, no. 3 (summer 1993).
Kahn, Ada P., and Jan Fawcett. *The Encyclopedia of Mental Health.* New York: Facts On File, 1993.

carpal tunnel syndrome   A chronic condition characterized by numbness, tingling, and pain in the thumb, index, and middle fingers, and sometimes by weakness in the thumb. It may affect one or both hands. This syndrome results from pressure on the median nerve where it passes into the hand via a gap (the "carpal tunnel" under a ligament at the front of the wrist. The median nerve carries sensory messages from the thumb and some fingers and also motor stimuli to the muscles in the hand. Damage to the nerve results in sensory disturbances, particularly the numbness and tingling sensations.

Carpal tunnel syndrome is one of several possible repetitive stress injuries (RSIs) common to certain occupations in which the wrist is subjected to repetitive stresses and strains, particularly those involving gripping or pinching with the wrist held flexed. For example, computer operators, typists, carpenters, factory workers, meat cutters (meat cleaver's elbow), violinists, and even hobbyists such as golfers or canoers may develop carpal tunnel syndrome. This injury is stressful for some sufferers because they may experience confusion over whether to continue or quit a job or activity that contributes to their discomfort. The number of workers with disorders caused by repeated trauma on the job is increasing.

Some severely injured carpal tunnel victims qualify for help under the Americans for Disabilities Act. However, proof of the source of injury may be difficult, as two people may perform the identical job with only one of them developing carpal tunnel syndrome.

Carpal tunnel syndrome is especially common among middle-aged women and in women who are pregnant or have just started using birth-control pills, as well as among people who suffer from rheumatoid arthritis, myxedema, or acromegaly.

Treatment

With appropriate treatment, the pain can be relieved and there may be no permanent damage to the wrist or hand. Resting the affected hand at night in a splint may alleviate symptoms. Some health professionals may recommend ACUPUNCTURE. If symptoms persist, a physician may inject a small quantity of a corticosteroid drug under the ligament in the wrist. If this does not help, surgical cutting of the ligament may be performed to relieve pressure on the nerve.

See also WORKPLACE.

FOR FURTHER INFORMATION:
American Physical Therapy Association/PR-IH
1111 North Fairfax Street
Alexandria, VA 22314
Phone: (703) 684-2782

Association for Repetitive Motion Syndromes
P.O. 514
Santa Rosa, CA 95402
Phone: (707) 571-0397

SOURCE:
Spooner, G. Richard, et al. "Using Pyridoxine to Treat Carpal Tunnel Syndrome." *Canadian Family Physician* 39 (October 1993).

catastrophize The habit of imagining that the worst case scenario will happen. People who frequently catastrophize have little self-confidence, low SELF-ESTEEM, and have difficulties making positive and desirable life changes. An example of catastrophizing is saying to oneself, "If I go to the party no one will know me and I won't have a good time," or "If I take this new job I'll fail because I don't have the right computer skills."

Catastrophizing causes stress because it keeps people in situations they might really prefer to change, such as improving their social life, changings job, or moving to a new city. With positive SELF-TALK and learned techniques to improve self-esteem, the habit of catastrophizing can be overcome. In severe cases, various PSYCHOTHERAPIES may be helpful.

SOURCE:
Kahn, Ada P., and Sheila Kimmel. *Empower Yourself: Every Woman's Guide to Self-Esteem.* New York: Avon Books, 1997.

chemical dependencies See ADDICTION.

childbirth The birth of a child, usually by passage through the birth canal. Individuals about to participate in the childbirth experience may find it stressful. Many women experience stress in handling some of the most practical details surrounding the birthing experience, such as recognizing the start of labor and getting to the hospital on time. Some women approach childbirth with anxieties exacerbated by reports of difficulties from friends and relatives. First-time mothers, in particular, feel stressed by the unknown aspects of childbirth. Some first-time fathers, planning to attend the birth, may be stressed by a fear of blood, as well as the uncertainties of parenthood.

Women whose babies are delivered by Cesarean section experience special stresses because they believe that the procedure denies them a natural experience for a woman. They wonder if they will be able to have subsequent children by vaginal delivery. This will depend on whether or not the reason for the Cesarean section was a one-time occurrence, such as a breech presentation; whether the Cesarean scar is strong; and whether the physician is agreeable to a subsequent normal labor, assuming that the woman's pelvis is wide enough for a baby's head.

Possible relief for some stressors: natural and prepared childbirth

The term "natural childbirth" specifically refers to a movement toward unmedicated deliveries started by Fernand LaMaze (1891–1957), a French obstetrician. Interest in "natural childbirth" began developing during the 1940s and 1950s when use of drugs for pain relief and medical procedures such as routine episiotomies and enemas required removing women from their families, who had no sense of participation in the childbirth process. While the specific methods for childbirth outlined by Lamaze and Grantly Dick-Reed (1900–59), a British obstetrician and advocate of natural childbirth, vary, they both incorporate non-medical relaxation techniques as a "natural" method of pain control during labor. In addition, they questioned the need for routine medical procedures and advocated a more active participation in labor by the woman and her lay labor coach, often meaning the father of the baby or a nurse-midwife.

The natural childbirth movement has expanded to include the use of birthing rooms (in which labor and delivery take place in a home-like setting) and the presence of extended family and friends at the delivery. Some women choose to have their babies delivered at home to assure being surrounded by family members. Some opt for delivery by specially trained nurse-midwives rather than physicians. Nurse-midwives, however, require the back-up of physicians in case of medical emergencies.

The term "prepared childbirth" became popular in the early 1990s, and includes prenatal exercise classes and a wide variety of breathing and relaxation techniques.

See also PARENTING; POSTPARTUM DEPRESSION; PREGNANCY.

FOR FURTHER INFORMATION:
Informed Homebirth/Informed Birth and
  Parenting
P.O. Box 3675
Ann Arbor, MI 48106
Phone: (313) 662-6857

American College of Obstetricians and
  Gynecologists
409 12th Street SW
Washington, DC 20024-2188
Phone: (202) 638-5577

SOURCES:
Eisenberg, Arlene, and Heidi Murkoff *What to Expect When You're Expecting.* New York: Workman Publishing, 1984.
Kahn, Ada P., and Linda Hughey Holt. *The A–Z of Women's Sexuality.* Alameda, Calif. Hunter House, 1992.

child care   See DAY CARE.

chiropractic medicine   Chiropractic medicine deals with the relationship between the skeleton and the nervous system and the role of this relationship in restoring and maintaining health. Many people visit chiropractors to relieve stress as well as physical discomforts.

According to chiropractic philosophy, the body is a self-healing organism and all bodily function is controlled by the nervous system. Abnormal bodily function may be caused by interference with nerve transmission and expression. This interference can be caused by pressure, strain or tension on the spinal cord, spinal nerves or peripheral nerves as a result of a displacement of the spinal segments or other skeletal structures.

The art of the chiropractic practitioner involves detecting and correcting problems of the vertebral subluxation complex. Subluxation refers to a slight dislocation or biomechanical malfunctioning of the vertebrae (bones of the spine). According to the International Chiropractors Association, subluxation can irritate nerve roots and blood vessels, which branch off from the spinal cord between each vertebrae. The irritation causes pain and dysfunction in muscle, lymphatic and organ tissue as well as imbalance in normal body processes.

Causes of subluxation include stress, falls, injuries, trauma, inherited spinal weaknesses, improper sleeping habits, poor posture, poor lifting habits, OBESITY, lack of rest, and exercise.

Chiropractors restore misaligned vertebrae to their proper position in the spinal cord through procedures known as "spinal adjustments" or manipulation. The adjustment itself does not directly heal the body. Rather, it is the resulting alignment of misaligned spinal vertebrae that restores balance so that the body can function more optimally.

Although chiropractic is often chosen as therapy for headache, TEMPOROMANDIBULAR JOINT SYNDROME (TMJ), whiplash, and bursitis, it may not be the treatment of choice for all medical problems or conditions.

Choosing a chiropractor

Before choosing a chiropractor, ask him to fully explain the benefits, risks, and costs of all diagnostic and treatment options. Interview more than one doctor of chiropractic medicine before making a decision on the practitioner. Chiropractors are licensed by each state's Board of Chiropractic Examiners. The American Chiropractic Association has a membership directory listing ACA members.

See also ALTERNATIVE THERAPIES.

FOR FURTHER INFORMATION:
American Chiropractic Association
1701 Clarendon Blvd.
Arlington, VA 22209
Phone: (703) 276-8800

SOURCES:
McGill, Leonard. *The Chiropractor's Health Book: Simple, Natural Exercises for Relieving Headaches, Tension and Back Pain.* New York: Crown, 1997.
Rondberg, Terry A. *Chiropractic First: The Fastest Growing Healthcare First . . . Before Drugs or Surgery.* Chandler, Ariz.: Chiropractic Journal, 1996.

chlamydia See SEXUALLY TRANSMITTED DISEASES.

choices See DECISION-MAKING.

cholesterol A complex, fat-like substance in the body, most of which is produced naturally in the liver. Cholesterol is needed to survive, but too much of the wrong kind, LDL (low-density lipoprotein) cholesterol, can be a risk to health and a source of personal stress. When LDL cholesterol builds up in the walls of the arteries, it forms plaque. The technical name for this is atherosclerosis or "hardening of the arteries." If plaque builds up, causing arteries to become thicker, harder, less flexible and less efficient at transporting blood, it can lead to a HEART ATTACK or STROKE. There are no obvious symptoms of high LDL cholesterol. The only way to find out if a person has a problem is to have cholesterol checked by a blood test and evaluated by a doctor or health care professional.

The stress of learning that a person's cholesterol level is too high can be relieved by understanding what contributes to the level and how it can be controlled. Many factors raise cholesterol, including certain inherited tendencies as well as lack of exercise. One of the most common and controllable factors is diet. Eating saturated fats can raise the LDL cholesterol. Saturated fats come from animal

---

HIGH CHOLESTEROL: ONE OF SEVERAL RISK FACTORS FOR HEART DISEASE

- High LDL cholesterol
- Smoking
- Age (a man 45 or older; a woman 55 or older)
- High blood pressure (treated or untreated)
- Hereditary (father, brother or son had heart disease before 55; mother, sister, or daughter before 65)
- Low HDL cholesterol

sources, such as meat, butter, milk, and cheese, as well as the oils in tropical plants, such as coconuts and palms.

What should your cholesterol level be?

The National Cholesterol Education Program (NCEP) recommends that those who already have heart disease should have a total cholesterol level of 160 mg/dl or less, with the LDL level at 100 mg/dl or less. For those who don't have heart disease but have two or more risk factors, in addition to high cholesterol, the level should be under 200 mg/dl, with the LDL level under 130 mg/dl. For those who don't have heart disease but have fewer than two risk factors in addition to high LDL cholesterol, the overall level should be under 240 mg/dl with the LDL under 160 mg/dl.

Reducing cholesterol level

The first step in reducing cholesterol is to follow a low-fat, low-cholesterol diet. A low-fat diet generally requires that a person eat less high-saturated fat and high-cholesterol foods, such as meats, eggs, and dairy products, and more fruits, grains, and vegetables. This diet can contain small portions of turkey and chicken without the skin, and well-trimmed lean beef. Fish, broiled or baked without butter, is another low-fat source. The American Heart Association recommends limiting the total fat in your diet to less than 30% of your calories each day.

Some people worry needlessly that they may be eating too much cholesterol. These individuals may be interested to know two important facts: (1) On average, one's body absorbs only half the cholesterol in the food eaten; and (2) when the amount of cholesterol from food increases, the body produces less of its own cholesterol and will increase the amount of cholesterol it excretes.

Regular exercise raises the level of "good" cholesterol, HDL. HDL helps remove LDL, the "bad" cholesterol from the blood. Exercise also helps keep the heart muscle active and healthy. The most commonly stated goal for a heart-healthy exercise is 20 minutes of moderate exercise three times a week.

Several types of cholesterol-lowering medications are available. Medications should always be used along with a low-fat, low-cholesterol diet. A physician will decide whether medication is necessary and which medication is best for each individual.

See also ATHEROSCLEROSIS; CORONARY ARTERY DISEASE.

SOURCES:

Giles, Wayne H., et al. "Cholesterol." *The Journal of the American Medical Association* 9 (March 3, 1993): 1133–38.

Grover, Steven A., et al. "HDL Cholesterol Level Is Important Indicator of Potential Heart Disease." *The Journal of the American Medical Association,* September 12, 1995.

Chopra, Deepak (1947–) Indian-born physician whose philosophy of healing, disseminated through books, tapes, lectures, and clinics, is based on the Indian holistic system called AYURVEDA. He was once a disciple of Maharishi Mahesh Yogi, but formed his own organization in 1993. Among his books are the best-selling *Ageless Body, Timeless Mind: The Quantum Alternative to Growing Old* (1993) and a work of fiction, *The Return of Merlin* (1995).

Since 1993 Chopra has been executive director of the Sharp Institute for Human Potential and Mind/Body Medicine in southern California. He graduated from the All-India Institute of Medical Sciences in New Delhi and moved to the United States in 1970. He completed an internship at Huhlenbert Hospital, Plainfield, New Jersey, moved to Boston in 1971 and taught at several medical schools affiliated with Tufts University, Harvard University, and Boston University. He worked for 14 years as an endocrinologist in a Boston-area hospital.

Chopra claims the MIND-BODY CONNECTION can reduce stress, facilitate healing, lead to inner peace and even reverse the aging process. His mind/body programs incorporate massage, YOGA, MEDITATION, herbal supplements, nutritional guidelines, and exercise regimens. He recommends doing something that brings joy, concentrating fully on that activity, reducing distractions at work and finding inner satisfaction in daily tasks.

In one chapter on longevity in *Ageless Body*, Chopra outlines some suggestions that may be useful for those wishing to reduce stress in their lives. Techniques include listening to your body's wisdom, living in the present, taking time to be silent, and meditating to quiet the internal dialogue.

See also ALTERNATIVE THERAPIES; IMMUNE SYSTEM; RELAXATION.

FOR FURTHER INFORMATION:
Chopra Center for Well Being
7590 Fay Avenue (#403)
La Jolla, CA 92037
Phone: (619) 551-7788

Sharp Institute for Mind/Body
3131 Berger Avenue
San Diego, CA 92123
Phone: (619) 541-6737

SOURCES:
Chopra, Deepak. *Ageless Body, Timeless Mind: The Quantum Alternative to Growing Old.* New York: Crown, 1993.
———. *Creating Health.* Boston: Houghton Mifflin, 1991.
———. *Quantum Healing.* New York: Bantam, 1989.
———. *Unconditional Life.* New York: Bantam, 1992.

chronic fatigue syndrome (CFS)   Illness characterized by fatigue that occurs suddenly, improves and relapses, bringing on debilitating tiredness or easy fatigability in an individual who has no apparent reason for feeling this way. It is stressful to the sufferer because the profound weakness caused by CFS does not go away with a few good nights of sleep, but instead steals a person's vigor over months and years. Because many individuals who have CFS experience frustration both before being diagnosed and on learning that

there is no cure, DEPRESSION often accompanies the disease.

While the illness strikes children, teenagers, and people in their fifties, sixties, and seventies, it is most likely to strike adults from their mid-twenties to their late forties. Women are afflicted about twice to three times as often as men; the vast majority of those who suffer this illness are white. Because young urban professionals were most afflicted during the 1980s, the name "yuppie flu" was attached to CFS. However, individuals regarded this name as trivializing their illness.

CFS symptoms
CFS can affect virtually all of the body's major systems: neurological, immunological, hormonal, gastrointestinal, and musculoskeletal. According to the National Institutes of Health, CFS leaves many people bedridden, or with headaches, muscular and joint pain, sore throat, balance disorders, sensitivity to light, an inability to concentrate, and inexplicable body aches. Secondary depression, which follows from the disease rather than causing it, is just as disabling. However, knowing that there is a chemical basis for mood swings and that they are directly related to illness, can be reassuring.

Symptoms wax and wane in severity and linger for months and sometimes years. Some individuals respond to treatment, while others must function at a reduced level for a long time. However, for all sufferers, the cumulative effect is the same—transforming ordinary activities into tremendously stressful challenges. They cannot tolerate the least bit of exercise, their cognitive functions become impaired, and their memory, verbal fluency, response time, and ability to perform calculations and to reason show a marked decrease.

Disruption of sleep patterns causes the CFS sufferer additional stress. Despite constant exhaustion and desire for sleep, they rarely sleep uninterruptedly and awake feeling refreshed. Some have severe INSOMNIA, while others have difficulty maintaining sleep. There is often not enough rapid-eye movement sleep (REM), which is considered necessary for a good night's rest.

Many CFS sufferers experience stressful disorders of balance, or of the vestibular system, which is modulated by the inner ear. They sometimes feel dizziness, light-headedness, or nausea. Even walking can be difficult, with sufferers tilting off balance or stumbling for no apparent reason. Some individuals who have balance disorders develop PHOBIAS, such as a fear of falling. Some who have this fear even become housebound.

CFS causes stresses on sufferers, family, and friends. Those in a sufferer's support circles can reduce their stress by being helpful, understanding, and available to listen. Sufferers are likely to feel estranged from some of their friends because they believe that no one really understands their feelings of emotional and physical exhaustion. This belief is exacerbated because many sufferers think that others do not take their illness seriously. In addition, some friends and family members may fear that CFS is contagious and try to maintain a distance from the sufferer. (Medical opinion seems to indicate that CFS is not contagious.) Spouses face the issue of reduced sexual activity, although both partners can satisfy their needs by engaging in sexual activity during peak periods of energy.

Diagnosing CFS

Diagnosing CFS is stressful for physicians as well as patients because many of the symptoms are like those of other disorders. Until the mid-1980s, many CFS patients were misdiagnosed as suffering from depression, accused of malingering, encouraged to undergo stressful, costly, and inappropriate laboratory tests, or simply pushed aside by the medical community because of lack of understanding of the disease. In recent years, however, studies on the immune system,

viruses, and the physiological effects of stress have contributed to better understanding of CFS. Individuals with CFS no longer have to feel abandoned by their physicians or fear that they are "going crazy" because no one takes their illness seriously.

Treatment for CFS

Many therapies have been tried on CFS sufferers. Usually a plan is devised for each patient, depending on symptoms. Pharmacological therapies include use of antidepressant drugs, pain relieving drugs, and muscle relaxing drugs.

Other therapies that have been tried include deep relaxation, YOGA, BIOFEEDBACK, and visualization therapy to relieve stress and chronic pain. Nutritional therapies have included emphasizing certain vitamins, such as Vitamins A, B6, B12, C and E, as well as zinc, folic acid, and selenium, all of which are said to have immune-boosting potential.

Oil extract from the seeds of the evening primrose plant is another medicine that some CFS patients have found helpful. The theoretical basis for its use (although not yet scientifically proven) is that evening primrose oil contains gamma-linolenic acid (GLA), which converts in the body to prostaglandin, a vital substance in the regulation of cellular function.

Role of support groups and self-help

Several nationwide organization encourage research and political advocacy and also provide lists of local SUPPORT GROUPS. CFS sufferers may find relief from some stressors and help with practical and emotional needs through these organizations.

See also CHRONIC ILLNESS.

FOR FURTHER INFORMATION:
Chronic Fatigue Immune Dysfunction Syndrome
    Society
P.O. Box 230108
Portland, Oregon 97223
Phone: (503) 684-5261

Chronic Fatigue and Immune Dysfunction
   Syndrome Association
P.O. Box 220398
Charlotte, North Caroline 28222
Phone: (704) 362-CFID

National Chronic Fatigue Syndrome Association
919 Scott Avenue
Kansas City, Kansas 66105
Phone: (913) 321-2278

SOURCES:
Feiden, Karyn. *Hope and Help for Chronic Fatigue Syndrome.* New York: Prentice-Hall, 1990.
McSherry, James. "Chronic Fatigue Syndrome: A Fresh Look at an Old Problem." *Canadian Family Physician* 39 (February 1993).

chronic illness   Disorder or set of symptoms that has persisted for a long time with progressive deterioration. In addition to the stresses of physical pain, chronic illness often brings with it emotional consequences that can be more far reaching than the illness itself. These affect not only the patient but also cause stress for the immediate CAREGIVERS. Some, particularly close family members, let illness-related anxieties take over their lives, and their DEPRESSION arises from COPING with illness and the threat of possible long-term disability or death of a loved one.

Reactions to illness are similar to the stages of GRIEF after the death of a loved one. First there is the patient's shock and a feeling of loss of CONTROL and of AUTONOMY and of the way things used to be. In addition, they experience physical losses ranging from having to give up their job or favorite sport to impaired speech or vision. Stress and symptoms of depression may follow, including hopelessness, self-blame, shattered self-esteem, or withdrawal. Some ill persons may develop many fears. They may fear exercise and being active again, while others may deny the realities of their condition and overdo activities too soon.

The stresses of PAIN and fears about disability and death lead some ill people to substance abuse as a form of escape. Anger, denial, or perceived helplessness lead others to abandon medical treatment or assume a "why me" attitude that gives them a pessimistic view of their world.

The crucial issue is "whether you can get past the stage of rage, sadness, and overwhelming anxiety," says Lloyd D. Rudley, M.D., an attending psychiatrist at the Institute of Pennsylvania Hospital, Philadelphia. "Will you resume the initiative for living or become psychologically paralyzed?" Many people become trapped by emotions that do not serve them well, according to Dr. Rudley.

Unfortunately, there are chronically ill people who do not comply with instructions from their physicians. This may take the form of not showing up for physical therapy, refusing medication, or driving a car against the physician's advise. Individuals with emphysema may continue to smoke. According to Dr. Rudley, "People want to think everything will be normal again if they follow the doctor's orders. When things don't work this way and there is no magic formula, a patient may give up on treatment."

Some individuals neglect medical advice as a means of getting more attention. Others who harbor shame or guilt about their condition may punish themselves, in effect, by not complying with prescribed treatment. Forces of denial may be at work, too, in those who try to "bargain with illness" by following some recommendations, but not others.

How individuals coped with life stress before the illness will determine how well they respond when illness occurs. However, even when symptoms of illness go into remission or people have adjusted to their illness, a whole new set of external stressors may arise or family dynamics can change dramatically.

"Patients need to accept that chronic illness changes them permanently, that a change in lifestyle is necessary," advises Dr. Rudley. Healthy acceptance is achieved when people come to terms with the stresses of their illness as a part of who they are, "forming a sort of coexistence with it," he says.

Some individuals feel certain "benefits" from being chronically ill. Such motivations are referred to as "secondary gains" and increase the likelihood of their continuing to be ill or to have symptoms. Common "benefits" of illness include receiving permission to get out of dealing with a troublesome problem, situation, or responsibility of life; getting attention, care, or nurturing; and not having to meet their own or others' expectations.

Every area of a person's life is affected by ill health, including marriage, family, work, financial affairs, and future plans. Professional counseling can help individuals and their families adapt to stresses brought on by chronic illness. Counseling may also help individuals who feel a need to hide their illness, to increase their use of drugs or alcohol, or who fail to follow treatment recommendations or exhibit a fear of resuming their activities. It can help those who have insomnia and disrupted sleep, who experience prolonged depression, show negative personality changes, and have obsessive anxiety or preoccupation with death.

See also ELDERLY PARENTS; GENERAL ADAPTATION SYNDROME.

SOURCE:
Rudley, Lloyd D. "Conquering the Psychological Hurdles of Chronic Illness." *The Quill,* Fall 1991.

chronic pain   See CHRONIC ILLNESS; PAIN.

circadian rhythms   Cycles of sleep and wakefulness coordinated by an inherent timing mechanism known as the body's BIOLOGICAL CLOCK. The circadian rhythm of a person's body temperature is a marker for those clocks. Body temperature rises and falls in cycles parallel to alertness and performance efficiency. When body temperature is high, which it usually is during the day, alertness and performance peak—and sleep is difficult. A lower temperature (generally during the night) promotes sleep, but hinders alertness and performance. Stress may result when tasks are attempted that are not in synchronization with circadian rhythms.

Alertness and mental capability seem to be best when people follow their internal clocks, which are synchronized to the sun's 24-hour cycle. For example, sunrise means waking and working, while sundown means dinner and sleep. However, individuals who work night shifts find that their "day" is reversed. Many shift workers go home to sleep during the day when their bodies want to be awake and they have to work at night when their bodies want to sleep, according to Charmaine I. Eastman, Ph.D., in her report, *Insights into Clinical and Scientific Progress in Medicine.*

Timothy Monk, director of the Human Chronobiology Program at the University of Pittsburgh School of Medicine, says that circadian rhythms affect many performances of mental feats. For example, different skills follow different cycles, so that at any time a person's mind is naturally sharp for certain tasks and dull for others. Memory varies though the day, and short-term memory is at its peak at nine in the morning while memorizing for the long term works best around three in the afternoon. Problem-solving peaks in the morning and falls during the afternoon and evening. However, reaction time improves throughout the day and finally peaks in the evening.

Readjusting to jet lag
Jet lag—the discrepancy between an individual's "internal clock" and the exaggerated passage of time brought on by air travel across time zones—is a well-known disruption of circadian rhythms. Physical as well as mental stress may result. Symptoms of jet lag may include insomnia, headache, loss of appetite, or nausea. A conventional rule says that each time zone passed takes one day of recovery. Generally, recovering from jet lag is

easier when one flies west, rather than east. That is because it seems easier to delay the body's schedule than force it to advance. Exposure to daylight can help the body resynchronize more quickly.

For similar reasons, most people have an easier time changing from daylight savings time back to standard time in the fall than the reverse in the spring. Setting clocks back in the fall allows an hour more of sleep. However, in the spring, when clocks are set ahead and people have to get up an hour earlier than is customary, sleep deprivation may make them tired.

Adjusting to night work
People who work at night can adjust more easily and reduce stressful effects if they have darkness during the day and bright light at night. Night workers can also adjust more quickly if they can maintain a schedule of work-sleep-leisure, rather than the work-leisure-sleep pattern of day workers.

See also AIRPLANES; SHIFT WORK.

SOURCES:
"Circadian rhythms." *Mayo Clinic Health Letter,* March 1995.
Dolnick, Edward. "Snap out of It." *Health,* February/March 1992.
Eastman, Charmaine I. "Bright Light, Dark Goggles and Circadian Rhythms." *Insights into Clinical and Scientific Progress in Medicine* 14, no. 3 (1991).

claustrophobia From the Latin word *claustrum,* meaning "lock" or "bolt"; an intense fear of being confined in spaces such as elevators, phone booths, airplane, small rooms, and very crowded areas with no perceived possibility of escaping to a safe place. Most people feel mildly stressed in closed-in spaces. However, claustrophobics experience extreme stress, fearing that they will suffocate in an elevator or that an airplane carrying them may suddenly fall.

These extremely high levels of stress may lead to PANIC ATTACKS AND PANIC DISORDER for some claustrophobics. Such individuals may experience palpitations and fear that they are having a HEART ATTACK. True phobics may tend to avoid places in which panic attacks might occur.

The origins of claustrophobia vary. For some sufferers, it begins after a bad experience involving an enclosed space, such as being locked in a closet or room, while for others, the fear develops for no known reason. Using BEHAVIOR THERAPY techniques, many people overcome claustrophobia.

See also AGORAPHOBIA; ALTERNATIVE THERAPIES; ANXIETY DISORDERS; BREATHING; PHOBIAS.

FOR FURTHER INFORMATION:
Anxiety Disorders Association of America
11900 Parklawn Drive (Suite 100)
Rockville, MD 20852
Phone: (301) 231-9350

climacteric   See MENOPAUSE.

climate   Climate influences health, work, housing, transportation, dress, sports, and leisure activities and the types of products and businesses that are necessary to satisfy basic human needs. Some people prefer to live in a warm climate; others thrive on seasonal changes. Unless there are physical reasons that make it necessary to live in a warm climate, people generally live where they can find work and where they have family and friends.

Factors of climate and changes in climate induce stress for many people. Cooler climates require the body to burn and produce energy more quickly. On the other hand, cold weather raises blood pressure, is generally hard on the circulatory system, and tends to make people crave foods high in fat and starch. Warmer climates slow the body's metabolism and, if humidity is added to the heat, produce a more languid lifestyle.

It has only been in the last quarter of the 20th century that air conditioning has been perfected and become widespread in most industrialized countries. Being able to control the environment through the use of air conditioning or heating has reduced the stress level for many individuals and given greater impetus to industriousness and change. Inhabitants of cool climates have generally been thought to be more goal oriented than those who live and try to work in very warm climates.

Stormy and changeable weather, which is usually accompanied by sudden barometric changes, may produce in individuals the stresses of irritability and mood changes because the rising and falling pressure affects body fluids. A disturbing correlation between climate and human activity that is supported by statistics is the relationship between hot weather and violence. Figures show that crimes and riots are far more likely to occur in hot weather than in cool or rainy weather.

Climate affects the elderly and those who have weakened immune systems more than other individuals. The near-record-breaking heat wave in the summer of 1995 in Chicago, during which more than 500 inner-city residents died in their homes, is a testimonial to the possibly dramatic effects of climate stress.

See also RANDOM NUISANCES; SEASONAL AFFECTIVE DISORDER.

SOURCE:
Sherrets, S.D. "Climate and Personality," in Corsini, Raymond, ed., *Encyclopedia of Psychology,* vol. 1. New York: Wiley, 1984.

clinical depression   See DEPRESSION.

clinical psychology   See PSYCHOLOGY; PSYCHOTHERAPIES.

cluster headaches   See HEADACHES.

cocaine   An addictive drug that stimulates the central nervous system and induces feelings of euphoria. Some people erroneously try to combat the stresses in their lives with this and other addictive drugs, and become further stressed if they cannot find the money for supplies of cocaine. Some, recognizing their ADDICTION, become stressed when trying to give up the drug.

Cocaine is most often used in the form of white powder and is typically ingested by inhaling, or "snorting," usually through a straw or other tube in the nose. It can also be injected into the veins. After conversion to its base form, cocaine can be smoked, which is known as "freebasing."

Different users react to the drug in different ways. However, many experience an instant feeling of enormous pleasure known as a "rush." Some users also may initially feel energetic and self-confident. However, the pleasurable feelings produced by cocaine are followed by depression and fatigue, known as a "crash." To avoid a "crash," users take more cocaine, establishing a stressful and expensive cycle of use and dependency, which is extremely difficult to end and often requires lengthy treatment.

Use of cocaine can lead to severe psychological and physical dependence. It can increases the pulse, blood pressure, body temperature, and respiratory rate. Paranoid psychosis, hallucinations, and other stressful problems can result from cocaine use, which also causes bleeding and other damage to nasal passages. Cocaine is sometimes used with other drugs. The cocaine/heroin combination is called a "speedball," and the cocaine/PCP mixture is known as "space base." Cocaine-related heart and respiratory failure can lead to death.

Crack is the street name given to tiny chunks or "rocks" of freebase cocaine in smokable form. Crack is even more rapidly addicting than powdered cocaine. Extremely high blood levels of cocaine delivered to the brain by smoking crack increase the likelihood of serious toxic reactions, including potentially fatal brain seizures, irregular heartbeat, and HIGH BLOOD PRESSURE. Congestion in the chest, wheezing, black phlegm, and hoarseness may also result from smoking crack.

Use of crack by pregnant women can cause fetal loss or damage, and lead to babies with low birth weights who are extremely sensitive to noise, touch, and other stimuli, and cry frequently. The stresses involved in parenting such babies can be eliminated by avoiding use of addictive substances.

FOR FURTHER INFORMATION:
Cocaine Anonymous
3740 Overland Avenue (Suite H)
Los Angeles, CA 90034-6337
Phone: (310) 559-5833

SOURCES:
Carroll, Marilyn. *Crack and Cocaine.* Hillside, N.J.: Enslow Publishers, 1994.
Nuckols, Cardwell C. *Cocaine: From Dependency to Recovery.* Blue Ridge Summit, Pa.: Tab Books, 1989.

codependency A RELATIONSHIP in which the participants have a strong need to be needed, as well as to create mutual needs in a detrimental, weakening manner. Such an interplay of needs is required to preserve the dependent relationship. Codependent relationships are extremely stressful on at least one or both of the partners. In many cases, an individual would like to eliminate the stressors caused by the codependent relationship but is too addicted to the situation to change.

An example of a codependent relationship is one in which the husband covers up for his wife's ALCOHOLISM. He does the household chores, drives the children to their activities, and explains her problem as an "illness." He is an "enabler," because he makes it possible for her to continue with her ADDICTION. The enabler promotes the codependent relationship by compensating for or covering up difficulties or flaws in the behavior of the other out of an addictive need to be needed and to keep the relationship going.

There are many kinds codependent relationships: a parent who continues to support an adult child who should be responsible for himself because the parent wants the child to feel dependent on him or her; a husband who does all the household chores, shopping, and driving children to activities, while explaining that his agoraphobic wife is "not feeling well." Such a husband is an enabler to his wife. It is difficult for an individual to live with AGORAPHOBIA without an enabler. Many alcoholics and drug addicts also have enablers.

When a parent continues to compensate for or cover up a child's difficulties in school or with the law, thinking that they are protecting the child, that is also a co-dependent relationship. It is often interpreted that this behavior persists because preserving the child's flaws and immature behavior will keep him or her forever dependent on the parent. Since codependency is viewed as a type of addiction, advocates of the codependent theory feel that these tendencies can be overcome with a process similar to the recovery process used by Alcoholics Anonymous.

FOR FURTHER INFORMATION:
Co-Dependents Anonymous
P.O. Box 33577
Phoenix, AZ 85067-3577
Phone: (602) 277-7991

SOURCES:
Becnel, Barbara. *The Co-Dependent Parent.* San Francisco: Harper 1991.
Rieff, David. "Victims All?" *Harper's* (October 1991), pp. 49–56.

coffee See ANXIETY; CAFFEINE; GUIDED IMAGERY; HEADACHES; INSOMNIA; MEDITATION.

cognitive therapy Centers on the concept that in some people, unwanted behaviors or moods can result from distorted patterns of thinking and that these behaviors or moods can be altered by changing thinking patterns. It is an approach sometimes used to treat individuals who experience the stresses of ANXIETY DISORDERS or DEPRESSION.

The therapy focuses on the individual's own cognitive appraisals. Stressful ideas, thoughts and perceptions are directly examined and tested to determine their validity. The therapeutic benefit is that the individual's thinking may be restructured, so that situations or circumstances that were once perceived as extremely stressful are viewed in a less stressful and more realistic light.

The cognitive therapy approach was introduced in the 1970s by Aaron Beck (1921–   ), an American psychiatrist.

See also BEHAVIOR THERAPY; PSYCHOTHERAPIES.

cohabitation   Situation of unmarried individuals living together. This arrangement can lead to stress when one of the partners desires MARRIAGE and the other does not, or when, after living together for a number of years, the couple decides to separate. As in a DIVORCE, there may be additional stress when division of property, including real estate, and consequent legal arrangements occur.

There have been dramatic increases in cohabitation during the last decades of the 20th century. Greater approval and societal acceptance of living together without benefit of marriage has resulted from general attitudinal changes, including fears of permanent commitment, effectiveness of contraception during a long-term sexual relationship, and the havoc raised by divorce.

Many couples sign a cohabitation contract that is intended to remove some of the stresses in the practicalities of the living together arrangement. The cohabitation contract is a legal document in which unmarried partners agree to specified arrangements, such as how much each partner pays toward specified expenses. It may also specify division of belongings, should the couple split up.

See also LIVE-IN.

colic   The causes for colic are unknown, although there are reasons to believe that it is due to a spasm in the newborn baby's intestines. It appears around the third or fourth week of life and usually goes away on its own by the age of 12 weeks. Signs that the baby is experiencing colic are irritability, excessive screaming, and tightening of the body.

There are few solutions to the problem, and parents are placed under the stress of trying to make the baby comfortable. Feeding, cuddling, or changing diapers doesn't seem to help. Because episodes of colic seem to be worse in the evening, both parents and baby suffer from deprivation of sleep.

Handling the colicky baby
Parental anxiety may make the infant even more irritable. Feeding the baby when he or she cries could worsen the situation by causing the stomach to bloat. Rhythmic, soothing activities, such as rocking the baby, carrying the baby in a front sling or pouch, or taking the baby for a ride in the car, usually work best.

To avoid compounding the stress caused by the situation, new parents should try to avoid fatigue and exhaustion. They may find that sleeping in shifts, where one parent deals with the baby and the other gets rest, will be helpful.

See also PARENTING.

color   Studies have determined that colors have certain psychological and physical effects on the human body. Under certain circumstances, color can produce stress or induce relaxation. For example, red is the strongest and most stimulating of colors. It has been shown to increase hormonal activity and to raise blood pressure. Red stimulates creative thought and is a good mood elevator, but is not conducive to work. Orange shares many of the qualities of red, but it is considered more mellow and easy to live with.

Blue has the opposite effect of red. It lowers bodily functions and creates a restful atmosphere, although, if used too extensively, may have a depressing effect. Participants in psychological tests, when surrounded by blue, tend to underestimate time periods and the weight of objects. Purple, a combination of red and blue, has a neutral effect. When used in large amounts, for instance as a typeface, the eye does not focus on purple easily.

Having the characteristic of visibility, yellow is useful for road safety signs. Green and blue-green promote an atmosphere of relaxation, concentration, and MEDITATION. Monotonous use of the same color has been found to be more disturbing than a variety of colors.

With age, attraction to colors and their stressful and soothing effects seems to change somewhat. Babies tend to be attracted to yellow, white, pink, and red. Older children are less attracted to yellow and tend to like colors in the order of red, blue, green, violet, orange, and yellow. As adults mature, blue tends to become a favorite color, possibly because of changes in the eye itself and the way it sees color.

Colors carry with them stressful, psychological associations, which are expressed in language. For example, we are "green with envy," "see red" and "have the blues." Certain clear shades of red, orange, and yellow are associated with food and are very appetizing, while tinting foods with blue, violet, or a mixtures of colors, has the adverse effect, making the foods unappetizing.

Throughout history, mystical and healing properties have been ascribed to color. For example, the ancients associated colors with the houses of the zodiac and with the elements. They were highly important in the practice of magic. Some superstitious people believe that blue and green divert the power of the evil eye. Part of a religious symbolism and ritual, red, blue, purple, and white have been considered divine colors in Judaism, while green, the color of life and rebirth, is important in Christianity. In many cultures,

surrounding a patient with red clothing, red furniture and coverings and giving him red food and red medicine was thought to aid the healing process.

See also COLOR BLINDNESS.

color blindness Inability to recognize any colors or certain colors; usually a genetic defect located in the cones, small color-sensitive cells in the retina of the eye. Some individuals who are color blind may not be aware of their condition and experience stress when mistaking signs and symbols. They confuse color changes with dark and light shades, not understanding the nature of colors they have never seen. People who are color blind reduce the stress of the disability by training themselves to use other visual clues. For example, they learn shapes and sizes of safety signs and memorize vital information such as that the red light is usually above the green.

Other disorders of the eye may result in temporary or permanent color blindness, including degeneration of the optic nerve due to neuritis or anemia, and also infectious diseases such as syphilis or malaria. Malnutrition and ingestion of poisonous chemicals or drugs can also cause color blindness or a limited perception of colors. While cataracts and other eye diseases that result in opacities (nontransparent areas) of the lens and cornea will reduce color vision, when underlying diseases are relieved, color vision may improve.

SOURCE:
Birren, Faber. *Color Psychology and Color Therapy.* Secaucus, N.J.: Citadel Press, 1961.

combat fatigue (battle fatigue, combat neurosis) Anxieties occurring after the extreme stresses of war or battles. The term has been replaced in contemporary usage with POST-TRAUMATIC STRESS DISORDER (PTSD). Veterans of World War I were said to have "Combat fatigue," or "shell-shock," while Vietnam veterans with the same symptoms have PTSD.

See also ANXIETY DISORDERS.

commitment   See COHABITATION; DATING; INTI-
MACY; MARRIAGE; RELATIONSHIPS; SELF-ESTEEM.

communication   Process   through   which
meanings are exchanged between individuals.
When individuals feel understood, they are
communicating effectively. They are in control
of events; other people trust and respect them;
in work settings, they feel valued. Communicating effectively enhances health and
SELF-ESTEEM, nurtures relationships and helps
people cope with stress.

Failure to communicate
When individuals do not communicate well,
they feel misunderstood, frustrated, dis-
tressed, defensive, and often hostile, which
increases their stress level. Faults and flaws in
communication habits, or communication
gaps, cause stress to many people, to those
they love and those with whom they interact
on all levels, from the most intimate to the
most distant of acquaintances. People who
don't communicate effectively are more vulnerable to disease; they can be hostile and
confrontational and are at increased risk for
heart disease. People who feel misunderstood
report more DEPRESSION and more mood disorders of the kind shown to weaken their
immune function. When communication
breaks down, heart rate speeds up, cholesterol
and blood sugar levels rise, and they become
more susceptible to HEADACHES and digestive
problems and are more sensitive to pain. In
work settings, communication gaps can
reduce productivity, make workers irritable
and even increase the risk of accidents.

**Differences in male-female
communication styles**
According to Bee Reinthaler, a personnel communications specialist, in business, differences between the communications styles of
male and female managers can cause problems in efficiency and in accomplishing goals.
Males in the corporate world often use a complex combination of business, sports, and mil-

itary jargon. Their behavior is action-oriented
and competitive. On the other hand, women
generally are more demonstrative and express
their feelings. Many women frame their
speech with qualifiers, questions, and questioning intonations. They express doubts and
uncertainties more frequently than men.

According to Reinthaler, when women
wait for men to speak first, they create an
image of incompetence. "Men may then fall
into the stereotypical role of treating women
as incompetent and the stereotypical interaction continues in a destructive way. It would
be more effective if both genders of managers
would 'speak the same' language."

"Many women attempt to crack the male
communication code in the workplace until
something happens that shows they have
underestimated its complexities," says Can-
diss Rinker, an expert in the science and practice of change management. She explains that
women have been socialized from childhood
to avoid direct communication about difficult
issues, so they often use a sugar-coated
approach that other women understand, but
men do not.

Deborah Tannen, linguistics professor, says
gender differences put women in a double
bind at work that is not as evident in personal
RELATIONSHIPS. "Workplace communication
norms were developed by men, for men, at a
time when there were very few women present. The situation is aggravated when
women hold positions of authority. If they
talk in ways expected of women, they may
not be respected; if they talk in ways expected
of men, they may not be liked," says Tannen,
author of *Talking From 9 to 5: How Women's and
Men's Conversational Styles Affect Who Gets
Heard, Who Gets Credit and What Gets Done
at Work.*

**Removing the stress from your
communication style**
Individuals should apply the old "golden rule"
in communicating with others. They should

OVERCOMING STRESS BY AVOIDING COMMUNICATION GAPS

- *Learn to cope with criticism.* Receiving criticism causes stress. The impact on our mood and body depends more on how we describe the negative feedback to ourselves. Ask yourself: Does this seem reasonable? Is it fact or opinion? Are there others who might confirm or dispute this view? How would others have behaved?
- *Learn to listen.* Listening is an active process requiring openness and receptivity. Keep your mind free of distracting reactions, responses, judgments, and questions and answers.
- *Observe your own body language.* Research shows that more than half of what we communicate is conveyed by BODY LANGUAGE. Smiling, frowning, sighing, touching, or drumming fingers give out strong messages. Women tend to smile more than men, nod their heads, and maintain more continuous eye contact while listening and speaking than men. Under stress or in new situations, this tendency becomes even more pronounced.
- *Recognize and respect differences in conversational styles.* Styles of conversing play a major role in triggering misunderstandings. For example, women tend to ask more personal questions than men. Men more often give opinions and make declarations of fact.
- *Become more assertive.* Speak and act from choice and stand up for your rights without being aggressive.
- *Learn to say no when you want to.* Avoid feeling resentful, frustrated, or guilty. Take time before you respond to a request. You need not give lengthy explanations for saying no.
- *Try to resolve conflicts when you recognize them.* Use "I" statements whenever possible, rather than attacking the other person with a "you" statement. Make sure you understand each other's concerns, positions, or feelings by summarizing what you heard.

speak in the way in which they would like to be spoken to and listen to others the way they hope others will listen to them. It is important that they learn to express their likes and dislikes in a tactful and diplomatic way. They will find that when they are more direct, other people will be more responsive. With slight adaptations, these suggestions may be useful in communicating with children, siblings, parents, coworkers, bosses, or acquaintances and should be helpful in most situations.

See also ASSERTIVENESS TRAINING; IMMUNE SYSTEM.

SOURCES:

Reardon, Kathleen Kelley. *They Don't Get It, Do They?: Communication in the Workplace—Closing the Gap Between Women and Men.* Boston: Little, Brown, 1995.

Reinthaler, Bee. "Verbal Communications." *The Professional Communicator,* Fall 1991.

Sobel, David S. "Rx: Prescriptions for Improving Communication." *Mental Medicine Update* 3, no. 2 (1994).

Tannen, Deborah. *Talking From 9 to 5: How Women's and Men's Conversational Styles Affect Who Gets Heard, Who Gets Credit and What Gets Done at Work.* New York: William Morrow, 1994.

Tingley, Judith C. *Genderflex, Men and Women Speaking Each Other's Language at Work.* New York: Amacom, 1995.

commuter marriage   See MARRIAGE.

competition   One of the many dichotomies present in American life today that induces stress. It encourages individual achievement and the need to win. As such, it is the extreme opposite of another American concept—teamwork—which teaches us to respect others, appreciate their strengths and weaknesses, share our skills and knowledge, and help others meet their goals.

Early in life, children on the playing field experience the contradiction of competition and teamwork. Thus begins a source of stress we carry through much of our adulthood. Competition encourages comparisons between ourselves and others, both on a social and economic level; this in turn affects our feelings of SELF-ESTEEM.

See also AUTONOMY; CONTROL; TYPE A PERSONALITY.

compulsions   See GAMBLING; OBSESSIVE-COM-PULSIVE DISORDER; SHOPAHOLISM.

computers   When introduced into the work-place, computers were promoted as tools to simplify tasks and thus save time and effort and the stress related to getting jobs done the "old way."

Nominally, the computer is designed to serve as an extension of employees' skills and capabilities. Implied is that the user is in control and the computer maintains the burden of adaptation. In fact, in many cases, the opposite has occurred.

For lower-level employees, use of computers may diminish skill levels and autonomy and increase morale and health problems. While these workers report that the computer makes their work more enjoyable, they also report job changes associated with computers that involve stressors, including increased time pressures and reduced possibilities for control of the task. Added to that is the stress of having their work on the computer monitored by the computer itself, which collects all aspects of employees' activities and centralizes the information for management review.

For higher-level employees, computers seem to have increased the work done and set new standards of higher quality for doing it. With the advent of desktop and laptop computers, professionals in all fields are expected to do their own word processing, spread sheets, electronic mail, and presentation preparation. This has allowed management to cut back on staff. Although computers are a powerful technology, they are continuously changing the way we do business and, thus, have become a major stressor for employees at all levels.

See also AUTOMATION; INFORMATION EXPLOSION; REPETITIVE STRESS INJURY.

conditioning   Frequently used in BEHAVIOR THERAPY as a technique to reduce stress in unwanted conditions, such as phobias and anxieties.

Conditioning occurs in two major ways: classic and operant. In classic or Pavlovian conditioning, two stimuli are combined: one adequate, such as offering food to a dog to produce salivation (an unconditioned response), and the other inadequate, such as ringing a bell, which by itself does not have an effect on salivation. After the two stimuli have been paired several times, the inadequate or conditioned stimulus comes to elicit salivation (now a conditioned response) by itself.

In operant conditioning, consequences are introduced that strengthen or increase the rate or intensity of the desired activity (reinforcement) or weaken or decrease the rate or intensity of the undesired activity (punishment). Partially reinforcing or punishing the activity will increase its resistance to extinction.

condom   A cylindrical sheath of rubber, placed on the penis prior to sexual intercourse, which catches seminal fluid and prevents sperm from entering a woman's vagina and impregnating her. For some individuals, the use of a condom becomes a stressful issue. Some couples say a condom interferes with their enjoyment of sexual intercourse; in some cases, the man refuses to wear one.

In the 1980s and throughout the 1990s, during the escalation of the AIDS (ACQUIRED IMMUNODEFICIENCY SYNDROME) epidemic, condoms were promoted as a SAFE SEX measure and means of reducing the risk of the spread of AIDS and SEXUALLY TRANSMITTED DISEASES (STDs) between partners.

So that no sperm enter the vagina, the condom should be put on the penis before any contact and should be properly removed after ejaculation. If correctly used, condoms are more effective than other forms of BIRTH CONTROL. However, if the male scrotum is infected, condoms are not always effective in preventing the spread of certain sexually transmitted diseases.

Advantages of use of a condom as a contraceptive include relatively low cost, availability without a physical examination or prescription, and some protection against STDs. Disadvantages may be the possibility of a dulling sensation in the penis and the care in which condoms must be used.

Invention of the condom is often attributed to Dr. Condom (1650–85), a physician in the court of Charles II. However, the first published report of use of a condom to prevent venereal disease was in the work of the Italian anatomist Fallopius in 1564.

SOURCE:
DiClemente, Ralph J., and Gina M. Wingood. "Sexual Assertiveness Training Produces More Consistent Condom Use." *Journal of the American Medical Association,* October 25, 1995.

conflict resolution Deals with the ability of people to come out of an encounter respecting and liking each other. This a win-win situation in which the stress of anger and confrontation is minimized and those involved are able be heard, to express their position and their needs.

See also COMMUNICATION.

congestive heart failure The end result of many different types of heart disease where the heart cannot pump blood out normally. This results in congestion (water and salt retention) in the lungs, swelling in the extremities, and reduced blood flow to body tissues. Living with congestive heart failure is a very stressful situation for the sufferer as well as those around him or her. Medical treatment can improve the quality of life for many of these patients.

See also CHOLESTEROL; CHRONIC ILLNESS; CORONARY ARTERY DISEASE; HEART ATTACK; HIGH BLOOD PRESSURE.

FOR FURTHER INFORMATION:
American Heart Association
7320 Greenville Avenue
Dallas, TX 75231
Phone: (214) 373-6300

constipation Abnormally delayed or infrequent passage of hard, dry feces. Many people feel very stressed because they do not have a bowel movement every day. Parents become anxious and cause their children to be stressed. Yet, many healthy people may not have a bowel movement for several days and suffer no ill effects.

Today, advertising seems to have created an "illness" called "irregularity" for which laxatives are the cure. A better approach to solving the constipation problem is through diet and regular exercise. At any age, a persistent change in the pattern of bowel movements should be investigated by a physician to rule out a serious disorder.

Causes of constipation
Emotional factors, such as frustration and resentment may result in constipation. Tension may cause the muscles of the intestine to tighten, or contract, in what is called spastic constipation. This is often part of the syndrome known as IRRITABLE BOWEL SYNDROME. Constipation is also caused by lack of fiber in the diet. Fiber is found in foods such as whole-grain breads, fresh fruit, and vegetables. It provides the bulk that the muscles of the large intestine needs to stimulate propulsion of the fecal matter along its way.

TECHNIQUES TO AVOID STRESS IN CONFLICT RESOLUTION

- Think before speaking.
- Say what you mean and mean what you say.
- Listen carefully to the other person.
- Do not put words in the other person's mouth.
- Stick to the problem at hand.
- Refrain from faultfinding.
- Apply the same rules to handling personal and business conflicts.

Some individuals who have continuously ignored the urge, have trouble with bowel movements. Disabled and elderly people often suffer from constipation, in some cases because of the diminishing tone of intestinal and other muscles, slowing down of body signals from reduced efficiency of the nervous system, and immobility. Hemorrhoids or an anal fissure result in pain and may inhibit an individual's efforts to begin a bowel movement. Atonic constipation may be the result of constant use of laxatives and enemas. These lead to weakening of the intestinal wall, making the individual even more dependent on laxatives or enemas than ever before.

Many medications have a side effect that leads to constipation. These include medications containing morphine and codeine, verapamil (a calcium channel-blocker used in the treatment of high blood pressure, angina and cardiac rhythm disorders); any of the beta blockers (used for the same reason, but they can also cause DIARRHEA); various sedatives and tranquilizers; calcium supplements (especially the carbonate variety); and several antacid products. Being aware of the side effect may help reduce the stress of constipation.

Coping with constipation

If constipation is accompanied by alternating attacks of diarrhea, a physician should be consulted. This sometimes occurs in people who have diabetes. An examination will reveal if there is an obstruction, such as a polyp or a tumor in the colon, or the constipation may be a symptom of irritable bowel syndrome. In hypothyroidism, chronic constipation may result. Avoid a change in diet, such as omitting grainy products at breakfast, or eat them later in the day.

For many people, being aware of their own stress levels helps. Try to reduce stress by techniques such as MEDITATION and BIOFEEDBACK. Learn RELAXATION training techniques. With these techniques, in conjunction with diet and regular exercise, constipation should improve.

contraception   See BIRTH CONTROL.

control   A feeling of control over people's lives means that they are directing the outcomes of everyday events. While life is going well, most people do not consciously think about their level of control. However, when that sense of control is threatened, they become aware and this loss of control leads to stress, ANGER and FRUSTRATION.

Issues of loss of control involve situations in which people who could help themselves, do not do so. They may lose motivation because of previous failures or may be experiencing what sociologists call "learned helplessness." They feel that whatever they do will not make any difference. Their learned response is to not try to gain control over their lives. But they continue to feel the stress of the anger, frustration, and hostility, which may lead to physical problems.

The stress in some people's jobs is caused by no control over the pace of work, or the work environment or DECISION-MAKING. People living in institutions or other such situations are frustrated because they can't change their environments and feel that things are being done to them or for them. An example is patients in hospitals who feel that their sense of control and AUTONOMY has been taken away from them because of the hospital routine. Other people do not recognize their own options for making decisions and feel trapped by invisible forces. People who always try to please others in an effort to gain validation and self-esteem are an example of this. Those who fear flying do so because, when they put themselves in the hands of the pilot, they feel totally out of control.

Although individuals cannot always control all events happening around them, they can learn healthier responses to these stressful situations. RELAXATION, BREATHING, or BIOFEED-

BACK techniques can help a person gain a feeling of control.

See also HARDINESS.

coping The psychological as well as practical solutions that people must find for extremely distressing as well as everyday situations. Examples of these situations are dealing with cancer, caring for an aging relative, readjusting after the death of a loved one, facing unemployment, and dealing with RANDOM NUISANCES. Different individuals develop different ways of coping and learn to adapt their responses and reduce their stress and anxieties.

Stone and Porter, writing in *Mind/Body Medicine* (March 1995), defined coping as "constantly changing cognitive and behavioral efforts to manage specific external and/or internal demands that are appraised as taxing or exceeding the resources of the person."

To some, "coping" means getting on with life and letting things happen as they may. To others, it is consciously using the skills they have learned in the past when facing problem situations. Coping can mean anticipating situations, or it can mean meeting problem situations head-on. For example, managers who are able to handle employees in everyday situations become nervous and jittery just anticipating giving a public speech. In a serious medical crisis, some people cannot cope with their own illness but manage to muster strength when they need to care for a loved one.

Individuals can learn new coping skills from psychotherapists as well as those who practice alternative or complementary therapies such as MEDITATION and RELAXATION training. Relaxation and deep BREATHING techniques can help overcome the stress involved in a difficult situation.

Better coping for better health

When Hans Selye (1907–82), an Austrian-born Canadian endocrinologist and psychologist, wrote his landmark book *The Stress of Life*, he described the GENERAL ADAPTATION SYNDROME. The secret of health, he said, was in successful adjustment to ever-changing conditions.

Research studies have shown that people who cope well with life's stresses are healthier than those who have maladaptive coping mechanisms. In his book, *Adaptation to Life,* George Valliant, a Harvard psychologist, summarized some insights about relationships between good coping skills and health. He found that individuals who typically handle the trials and pressures of life in an immature way also tend to become ill four times as often as those who cope well.

Stone and Porter reported that coping efforts may have direct effects upon symptom perception and may have indirect effects on physiological changes and disease processes, as well as on mood changes, compliance with physician's instructions, and physician-patient communication.

See also ALTERNATIVE THERAPIES; BEHAVIOR THERAPY; COMMUNICATION; EXERCISE; HARDINESS.

SOURCES:
Locke, Steven, and Douglas Colligan. *The Healer Within.* New York: Mentor, 1986.
Selye, Hans. *The Stress of Life.* New York: McGraw Hill, 1956.
———. *Stress Without Distress.* Philadelphia: Lippincott, 1974.
Stone, Arthur A., and Laura S. Porter. "Psychological Coping: Its Importance for Treating Medical Problem." *Mind/Body Medicine* 1, no. 1 (March 1995).

coronary artery disease Caused by ATHEROSCLEROSIS (hardening) of the arteries that supply blood and oxygen to the heart. The disease is a source of stress to the sufferer as well as those who are caregivers. It is preventable to a great extent by lifestyle modifications and dietary changes.

See also CHOLESTEROL; CONGESTIVE HEART FAILURE; HEART ATTACK; HIGH BLOOD PRESSURE; TYPE A PERSONALITY.

corporate buyout The purchase of a controlling interest in a company by either the employees or another company. The word originated in the mid-seventies when there was a marked increase in company takeovers and tender offers. When corporate buyouts occur, employees are under stress due to the possibility of downgrading of their jobs, duplication of their job functions, and loss of jobs that may come during and following reorganization.

See also DOWNSIZING; LAYOFFS; WORKPLACE.

cortisol See DEPRESSION.

cosmetic surgery Procedures performed by plastic and reconstructive surgeons to improve appearance in a healthy person. Many people undergo cosmetic surgery to overcome negative and stressful feelings about parts of their face or bodies.

In a society that worships beauty, being beautiful has long been a goal of women of all ages and, in the 1990s, men as well. At the same time, older adults are waging their battles against wrinkles and other signs of aging. Nearly 400,000 cosmetic procedures were performed in 1994. The stress of maintaining looks and appearing younger has created a multibillion-dollar market for cosmetic, clothing, food, and health care products.

For plastic and reconstructive surgeons, the increase in patient demand for cosmetic surgery has been both a blessing and a curse. According to the American Society for Plastic and Reconstructive Surgery, "The 1990s have changed the way the media—and the public—view PLASTIC SURGERY and its practitioners. From the breast implant coverage to health care reform to chemical face peels, the profession has moved farther into the public eye, with all the opportunities—and drawbacks—that entail."

Choosing a cosmetic surgeon
The consumer considering cosmetic surgery can remove some of the stress from the situation by following a few guidelines. First, find a physician who has a great deal of experience in performing the procedures; be sure the surgeon is certified by the American Board of Plastic Surgery. This certification means that the surgeon has had at least five years of surgical training after medical school, including a minimum two-year plastic surgery residency. To determine the doctor's experience, talk with the doctor and with other patients and look at the diplomas. A reputable doctor will not only allow prospective patients to interview him/her, but will question them as well as to what their motives are and, if appropriate, offer alternative non-surgical procedures.

New techniques and surgical tools such as lasers now being used for facelifts, liposuction, breast reduction and augmentation, and "nose jobs" alleviate much of the stress connected to aesthetic surgery and herald a new century in which such procedures will become even more commonplace.

See also BODY IMAGE; SELF-ESTEEM.

FOR FURTHER INFORMATION:
American Academy of Facial Plastic & Reconstructive Surgery
1101 Vermont Avenue NW (Suite 404)
Washington, DC 20005
Phone: (202) 842-4500; (800) 332-FACE; (800) 332-3223
American Society of Plastic and Reconstructive Surgeons
444 E. Algonquin
Arlington Heights, IL 60005
Phone: (708) 228-9900
Referral Service: (800) 635-0635

SOURCES:
Elson, Melvin L., and John H. Harley. *The Good Look Book: Today's Options for Prolonging the Prime of Life.* Atlanta: Longstreet Press 1992.
Willis, Jan. *Beautiful Again: Restoring Your Image and Enhancing Body Changes.* Santa Fe: Health Press, 1994.

cost-cutting A goal in many organizations; means reducing employee head count and getting rid of superfluous job functions. It may be relatively easy for top management but extremely stressful for employees. Cost-cutting particularly occurs when the economy is poor and consumers are not buying products. It also occurs when management believes that stockholders want a better return on their investment dollars.

See also DOWNSIZING; LAYOFFS; WORKPLACE.

co-therapy   See PSYCHOTHERAPIES.

counseling   Many varied professional services available to individuals seeking help in some area of their life, including stress. These services may range from those of a trained social worker to a psychiatrist. Individuals, couples and families can find appropriate counseling services. They may be provided in situations such as a school, the workplace, a hospital, clinic, or a community center.

To seek counseling assistance, call a local hospital or look in the yellow pages of the telephone directory under psychologists or psychiatrists. Some listings have the heading "counselors." There are also many community self-help and SUPPORT GROUPS in which members share their experiences. For participants in these groups, sharing means they are not alone with their problems, and they learn from one another to problem-solve.

Before beginning therapy with any counselor, ask what his or her credentials are and whether they are certified by any state agency or professional board. As with any other professional, some may meet an individual's needs better than others. Individuals should not be afraid to change counselors if they are not meeting their needs.

See also BEHAVIOR THERAPY; MARITAL THERAPY; PSYCHOTHERAPIES.

Cousins, Norman (1915–90)   American author, professor of medical humanities, and leader in biobehavioral healing. Cousins managed to heal himself of a life-threatening disease and a

massive coronary attack. Both of these times, he used his own regimen of nutritional and emotional support systems as opposed to traditional methods of treatment. The experiences are detailed in his books, including *Anatomy of an Illness as Perceived by the Patient,* a worldwide best-seller, and *The Healing Heart: Antidotes to Panic and Helplessness.*

Cousins is sometimes described as the man who laughed his way to health, a simplified description of the controversial healing method he employed when he was diagnosed in the mid-1960s as having ankylosing spondylitis. This degenerative disease causes the breakdown of collagen, the fibrous tissue that binds together the cells of the body. Almost completely paralyzed and given only a few months to live, Cousins checked himself out of the hospital and moved into a hotel room. While maintaining a positive mental outlook, he took massive doses of Vitamin C and exposed himself to high doses of HUMOR, including old movies and books by James Thurber, P.G. Wodehouse, and Robert Benchley. In *Anatomy of an Illness,* Cousins wrote: "I made the joyous discovery that ten minutes of genuine belly LAUGHTER had an anesthetic effect and would give me at least two hours of pain-free sleep."

In 1980, about 15 years after his major illness, Cousins suffered a near-fatal heart attack in California. According to an article in the *Saturday Review,* Cousins told his physicians at the UCLA Intensive Care Unit that they were "looking at what is probably the darndest healing machine that has even been wheeled into the hospital." The article said that "Cousins makes his body a personal laboratory and befriends the society within his skin. He refused morphine; he asked for a change in the visiting routine to ensure rest. Gradually he improved."

When facing the treadmill stress test with fear, Cousins realized that his fear was a factor in slowing his progress, so he adopted a more relaxed lifestyle, changed his diet, and specifically avoided stress-producing situations. When he did the treadmill test again, he approached it in a relaxed manner, listened to classical music and comedy tapes, and had a better result.

A *Saturday Review* article commenting on *The Healing Heart* said that "It was not a medical textbook, but a study of awareness, listening, trust, choice, and intention about the intelligent use of a benevolent, centering will. It is about communication and partnership between the healer and the healed. It addresses as complementary the art of medicine and the science of medicine, the person and the institution, and freedom of choice and professional responsibility. The book affirms hope and belief as biologically constructive forces, with belief guided by knowledge and tempered by reason."

At one point, Cousins interviewed 600 people with malignancies and found that in many cases their disease took a sharp turn for the worse when they received their diagnoses. He determined that a physician can activate the healing process by building up both his or her and the patient's confidence and creating a partnership for healing.

See also ALTERNATIVE THERAPIES; IMMUNE SYSTEM; RELAXATION.

SOURCES:
Cousins, Norman. *Anatomy of an Illness as Perceived by the Patient.* New York, Bantam, 1981.
———. *The Healing Heart: Antidotes to Panic and Helplessness.* New York: Norton, 1983.

covert modeling   Imagining or observing another person performing a behavior or action and then imagining the particular consequences. For example, a person who feels extremely stressed about speaking in public can imagine another person getting up on the stage, delivering a talk, answering questions, and feeling successful about the situation. The next step in the concept is when the individual imagines himself or herself doing the same thing at a reduced stress level.

See also BEHAVIOR THERAPY; COVERT REHEARSAL; PSYCHOTHERAPIES.

covert rehearsal   An imagery technique in which an individual in therapy is asked to imagine himself or herself effectively doing a stressful task. The individual may repeat the visualization many times, and consider different alternatives. This procedure often follows COVERT MODELING. The goal of the technique is to motivate the individual to believe that he or she can face the situation or do the task at a reduced level of stress.

See also BEHAVIOR THERAPY; COVERT REINFORCEMENT; PSYCHOTHERAPIES.

covert reinforcement   A technique used in psychotherapy in which the individual imagines two responses to an action or situation, one stressful and another less stressful. For example, the person who first imagines seeing another give a public speech (COVERT MODELING) and then practices COVERT REHEARSAL (imagining giving the speech), now imagines that the speech has been given and that there was a favorable audience response without an undue level of stress.

See also BEHAVIOR THERAPY, PSYCHOTHERAPIES.

coworkers   The quality of a person's work relationships, particularly with colleagues, relates to his/her level of job stress. Colleagues who don't pull their weight and complain constantly can make work life miserable. Backstabbers, gossips and tattletalers damage reputations and can bring innocent people's careers to a halt.

One of the stresses relating to the unemployed worker today is lack of companionship. The day-to-day interactions with coworkers are gone, and the unemployed worker often becomes withdrawn, spending less and less time with peers. On the other side of the coin are the coworkers who are left

TIPS FOR AVOIDING STRESS WHEN WORKING WITH TROUBLESOME COWORKERS

- Tell them, in a non-confrontational manner, how their actions affect your work.
- Avoid providing the complainer with an audience and the bully with a target.
- Consider talking to your supervisor about the problem, but be prepared for possible negative results.
- Remember that you can't change someone else's behavior, but you can change how you react to that behavior.

in the corporation after DOWNSIZING or LAY-OFFS have occurred. Research has shown that their productivity is reduced, they develop poor work attitudes and they often seek new positions. Factors influencing these reactions include: when the layoff is seen as unnecessary, when workers receive information about termination in a degrading or unfair way, when criteria used to select workers in a layoff is perceived as politically motivated or biased in any way, and when termination benefits and compensation are not considered adequate.

See also CORPORATE BUYOUT.

crack   See COCAINE.

creativity   Creativity involves unusual association of ideas or words and ingenious methods of problem solving. It may involve using everyday objects or processes in original ways or may involve using an imaginative skill to bring about new thoughts and ideas. Some creative ideas are ahead of their times and may never be appreciated or are not appreciated until after their creator's death. These creative people may be stressed by feelings of inadequacy and lack of self-esteem. On the other hand, there are those who overestimate their creativity and feel stress from thinking they are undervalued and under-appreciated.

Creativity and work
While creativity is strongly associated with the arts, it is equally important in fields such as science, business, or manufacturing. People who try to be creative and cannot, feel stressed. This is particularly true of people who were hired because of their creativity. Fortunately, in corporations today, a free and voluminous flow of ideas is thought to be an important part of the creative process, even though many of the ideas may not be truly creative. Techniques such as brainstorming and other group approaches encourage the flow of ideas. These techniques bring in new people who have never been a part of the creative process and encourage a fresh viewpoint.

The creative process
Biographers and researchers of creative individuals have identified certain stages in the creative process. Often the scientist or artist identifies an area of work or a project but, after approaching it, feels dissatisfied and returns to less creative endeavors. Suddenly during this incubation period, a solution or artistic concept emerges. It then must be fleshed out, elaborated or tested.

Creativity has been found to correlate with certain personality and intellectual characteristics. Although intelligence and creativity are thought to be separate mental gifts (and not all intelligent people are creative), intelligence does seem to be necessary for creativity. Creative people have been found to be leaders and independent thinkers. They are self-assured, unconventional and have a wide range of interests. Since they are frequently involved in their own thoughts and inner life, they tend to be introverted and uninterested in social life or group activities. Passion for their field of work and a sense that what they do will eventually be recognized and make a difference are also qualities that support creativity.

The creativity theory

Many behaviorists have adopted the position that there is no such thing as a creative act, that what appears to be new is, in fact, "old wine in new bottles" or arrived at by luck and random experimentation. For example, Shakespeare created dramatic masterpieces without using original plots. Others have come up with the theory that a necessary element of creativity is a relationship with reality. A work of art may be original, but not truly creative unless it relates somehow to experiences, feelings, or thoughts, even though previously undefined, of the observer.

Mental health professionals have been interested in creativity for years. For example, J.P. Guilford (1897–1987), who explored this area in the 1960s, described two areas of thinking: convergent, or narrow, focused thinking, and divergent thinking, which allows the individual to let his or her mind roam and explore a broad spectrum of ideas. Guilford felt that the latter type of thinking was most creatively productive. Under his direction, the Torrance Tests of Creative Thinking were developed at the University of Southern California.

Stimulation to increase creativity also is of interest to researchers. It has been found that people's creativity may increase or decrease according to their environment and work habits. For example, certain people can be more or less productive at work depending on the atmosphere, the time of day and even the clothing they wear.

See also BRAINSTORMING.

SOURCES:
Benson, P.G. "Creativity Measures," in Corsini, Raymond J., ed., *Encyclopedia of Psychology*, vol. 1. New York: Wiley, 1984.
Weisberg, Robert. *Creativity, Genius and Other Myths.* New York: W.H. Freeman, 1986.
Wilmer, Harry A. *Creativity: Paradoxes and Reflections.* Wilmette, Ill.: Chiron Publications, 1991.

crime, witnessing   People witnessing a crime can be subjected to stress on many levels. First, they may be faced with a decision to come to the aid of the victim. Once the decision for involvement has been made, they may face the stress of being questioned by the police, exposed to threats or harassment from the associates or family of the criminal, and harried by postponement and rescheduling of the trial with no regard for their work schedule and other personal responsibilities.

A decision not to become involved is often made. These people may feel that there are other witnesses to the crime, and they want to avoid a difficult and personally dangerous situation. Some of them may later feel the guilt of doing nothing and they will experience extreme stress.

Watching a violent crime may also result in POST-TRAUMATIC STRESS DISORDER, with symptoms of anxiety, nightmares, insomnia, and other fears. Recovery can be aided with a variety of PSYCHOTHERAPIES administered by professionals. Victim/witness assistance programs, whose services include psychological counseling, have been initiated in some areas of the United States. During a trial, program administrators may make arrangements for witnesses to get in and out of court buildings with minimum public and media exposure and intervene with the court on behalf of the witness when he or she is a victim of stressful threats or intimidation.

See also ANXIETY DISORDERS.

crisis   A turning point for better or worse in an acute disease, or an emotionally significant event or radical change in status in a person's life. The stress involved in a crisis situation may result from a combination of the individual's perception of an event as well as his or her ability or inability to cope with it. Some people will cope with a crisis situation better than others.

Crisis intervention is often necessary to provide immediate help, advice, or therapy to individuals with acute stress or psychological or medical problems. Many crisis intervention centers utilize telephone counseling. For example, in cities throughout the United States, there is a SUICIDE hotline for those contemplating ending their lives. In some cases, a RAPE victim's first step toward seeking professional assistance is to call a rape crisis hotline. When a bombing or shooting occurs in a public place, crisis intervention services are provided for survivors who witnessed the event in an effort to prevent the onset of, or ameliorate, POST-TRAUMATIC STRESS DISORDER (PTSD).

The goal of crisis intervention is to restore the individual's equilibrium to the same level of functioning as before the crisis, or to improve it. Many different types of therapists and SELF-HELP GROUPS provide crisis intervention. Therapy may include talking to the stressed individual and appropriate family members or short-term use of appropriate prescription medications. However, crisis intervention is not a substitute for longer-term therapy. The individual may learn to immediately modify certain environmental factors as well as interpersonal aspects of the situation causing the crisis. Emphasis should be on reducing stress and anxiety, promoting self-reliance and learning to focus on the present. Longer-term therapy is helpful after the individual has regained some degree of composure and COPING skills.

See also CRIME, WITNESSING; GENERAL ADAPTATION SYNDROME; SUPPORT GROUPS.

criticism   Comments directed to individuals regarding behavior, appearance, performance, quality of work, or other characteristics that reflect on their SELF-ESTEEM. Criticism may be favorable, but usually is regarded as the opposite of praise and, as such, can be very stressful.

Fear of being criticized makes many individuals reluctant to do or try certain activities. For example, when children receive negative criticism regarding singing ability from a teacher, they may carry this message for the rest of their lives. Self-criticism can be just as harsh. After judging themselves a failure at public speaking, some adults will not try it again. Often, criticism can be stressful for the critic as well. In employment settings, for example, there are supervisors who find it difficult and very stressful to criticize employees.

An ability to accept criticism that is appropriate, and then alter behavior associated with that criticism, is considered self-improvement. Children thrive on encouragement, even when it is tinged with criticism, particularly when they receive it from a parent or teacher. On the other hand, some people take criticism very badly, and the stress of the experience results in defensiveness or feelings of helplessness and low self-worth. Constant criticism can lead to an INFERIORITY COMPLEX, which are feelings of inadequacy in most social situations.

Constructive criticism should genuinely explain and define what is desirable as well as what is not. Focusing criticism on the task or skill rather than on the person is useful. Comparing children with their siblings should be avoided to prevent further stressful situations.

See also ANXIETY DISORDERS; PHOBIAS; SOCIAL PHOBIA.

SOURCE:

Kahn, Ada P., and Jan Fawcett. *The Encyclopedia of Mental Health.* New York: Facts On File, 1993.

crowding   The gathering of large numbers of people or animals in a mass. In Hans SELYE's landmark book, *The Stress of Life* (1976), he suggested that in humans, crowding may make men more competitive, somewhat more severe and to like each other less, whereas women tend to be more cooperative and lenient and like each other more.

Selye speculated that residential crowding in itself does not produce psychological or physical symptoms of STRESS. In fact, under certain conditions, interpersonal contact is supportive, as long as the people know they have the space to get away from each other when they want to. His studies, however, did not reflect such later 20th-century stresses as heavy traffic, high-rise living, air pollution, and noise, associated with contemporary Western society urban life.

See also AUTONOMY; CONTROL; GENERAL ADAPTATION SYNDROME; PERSONAL SPACE.

crying   Vocal expression of emotion, accompanied by tears. It is both a cause of stress and a stress reliever, depending on the situation. For example, at funerals, it is a normal response to express GRIEF; at weddings, it is a response to happiness. As a natural reaction based in social custom and personal experience, people cry when they are very sad or very glad. Some movies are known as "tear-jerkers," and no sight rouses more tears than soldiers returning home. Sometimes, people cry because they cannot cope any longer with stressful situations. There may be stress from pain or from real or anticipated loss of status, security, or friendship.

According to William Frey, a biochemist, giving in to a good cry is cathartic. "Emotional tears contain a higher protein concentration than tears that are shed when the eye is irritated by onion vapor. We are quite literally crying it out, removing chemicals that have built up in the body due to stress."

Certain emotional disorders include crying as a symptom. In a depressive state, an individual may cry easily and without cause. In severe DEPRESSION, an individual may lose the capacity to cry or weep, despite a feeling of profound sadness. In a newborn baby, crying serves to inflate the lungs and clear secretions from both the eyes and the lungs. For them, hunger and pain stimulate crying.

See also COLIC.

cults   Groups of people who frequently have a religious philosophy and are often started by religious leaders or self-appointed, pseudoreligious individuals. Cults also may have social and political reform or terrorism as their goals. Family and friends of cult recruits are usually very stressed by their affiliations. Some new cult members sever all close ties and disappear without warning.

Cults share certain similarities. They seem to have arisen from a time period in the 1960s when social values were questioned and considered inadequate. Depending on the cult, new recruits are people who may not be emotionally stable, may lack family and close friends, and are searching for relief from the confusion and emotional stress of modern life. Cult leaders welcome new members with an attitude of caring and acceptance, creating a strong emotional experience for them. The moral behavior and attitudes of the cult are dictated by strong peer pressure. Members are made to feel that there are continually higher levels of commitment or sanctity that they can attain. Leaving or questioning the values of the group are looked upon as evil or sinful. Members are reminded that to return to the outside would be to return to the confusion and stress they had formerly faced.

Deprogrammers who specialize in trying to extricate cults members are often hired by their families. These deprogrammers may use force or coercion to remove members from the cult environment, and then implement BRAINWASHING techniques similar to those used by the cults in their training.

FOR FURTHER INFORMATION:
Cult Hotline and Clinic

1651 Third Avenue
New York, NY 10028
Phone: (212) 860-8533

Task Force on Cults
711 Third Avenue (12th Floor) New York, NY 10017
Phone: (212) 983-4977

SOURCES:

Johnson, Joan. *The Cult Movement.* New York: Franklin Watts, 1984.

Kahn, Ada P., and Jan Fawcett. *The Encyclopedia of Mental Health.* New York: Facts On File, 1993.

culture shock   See ACCULTURATION; MIGRATION.

D

dance therapy Dance therapy permits release of stress and expression of emotion through body movement. It can be used effectively with a wide variety of individuals, from those who have mild stress symptoms to those who have severe mental health disorders. Many individuals who will not speak about their stressful concerns will indicate something about them with movement.

Therapists who use this technique are usually trained in dance and body movement as well as psychology. Dance therapy alone does not relieve symptoms of extreme stress, but may be used in conjunction with other therapies or medication.

See also ALTERNATIVE THERAPIES; CREATIVITY.

FOR FURTHER INFORMATION:
National Dance Association
1900 Association Drive
Reston, VA 22091
Phone: (703) 476-3436

Center For Dance Medicine
41 East 42nd Street (Room 200)
New York, NY 10017
Phone: (212) 661-8401

dating A social process by which individuals become acquainted with each other and develop a RELATIONSHIP that may lead to friendship, romance, a sexual relationship, and/or marriage, is stressful for participants of all ages.

For young people, dating is a rite of passage from childhood to adulthood. Some young people begin dating during their teen years while others wait until their college years. There are often issues of SELF-ESTEEM, and many are often held back from dating because of negative feelings about themselves. Others may have the additional stres-

---

> ### TIPS TO REDUCE STRESS IN DATING
>
> - Know something about the person's background before the date.
> - Accept "blind" dates arranged only by people you know and trust.
> - Seek out people who treat others with respect.
> - Date people who agree with your values.
> - Avoid people who are overly critical or abusive.

---

sors of CRITICISM of their dates by their parents. Additionally, peer pressure can make young people drink, smoke, or enter sexual relationships before they are ready and they may suffer the stresses of pain and guilt because of their actions.

Individuals who are divorced or widowed find themselves back in the dating scene. Many of the young people's issues also hold true for older people, such as concern about self-esteem and appearance. For single parents, dating presents particular stresses as young children often "screen" their parents' dates. Some children ask embarrassing questions, such as "are you going to marry my Daddy?"

Despite the stresses inherent in dating, the process allows people a socially acceptable way of getting acquainted with others.

See also DIVORCE; INTIMACY; PUBERTY; REMARRIAGE.

SOURCE:
Vedral, Joyce L. *Boyfriends; Getting Them, Keeping Them, Living without Them.* New York: Ballantine, 1990.

day care System of caring for children or other dependents in other people's homes, in churches, and in other community centers while parents work. Changes in the economy, employment and family patterns during the last years of the 20th century have made day care an important yet stress-filled issue for many people.

Today, when both parents need or want to work, they are faced with the dilemma of seeking day care. Some parents, traditionally the mother, feel some degree of guilt about seeking day care for their children. However, as a practical matter, it has become more difficult to support a family on one income. Additionally, wives and mothers who are not forced to work for financial reasons have been encouraged by contemporary media and the Women's Movement to believe the position of housewife and mother is not rewarding. Still others, faced with the specter of a high divorce rate, may want to keep up their skills and have their own employment benefits "just in case." For the single working parent with small children, some type of child care is a necessity.

Many children whose parents work are still cared for by a relative or sitter in their own home; however, the day-care alternative does offer certain benefits. Children learn to socialize with their peers before entering school. Day care may offer educational programs, toys, and equipment. Day-care centers are licensed and run by professionals.

However, there have been some cases of abuse and negligence in day-care centers. Parents should take extreme care in choosing a day-care facility by checking it out with local authorities, interviewing families that have children at the facility, and closely monitoring the facility when their children are enrolled.

Social mobility has also increased the need for some type of daytime child care. At one time, stay-at-home mothers depended on grandmothers when they needed child care. Now, grandmothers may be hundreds of miles away and may be working themselves.

To meet the needs of sick children, some day-care centers have separate areas. Also, some day-care centers specifically for sick children have been set up either independently or in pediatric wards of hospitals.

Among some employers, day care has become a corporate responsibility. A day-care center in the mother or father's place of employment solves transportation problems and allows the parent to visit with the child during the day. The Stride Rite Corporation in Cambridge, Massachusetts, is an example of a company that started a program that combines for care small children and elderly dependents of employees in the same facility.

Studies of the effect of day care on children have not shown that children suffer any real difficulties from participation in day care and that, in some cases, children from deprived backgrounds benefit from day care; however, putting children in the hands of CAREGIVERS may lessen the extent to which mothers can influence their child with their own values and standards.

day care for the elderly
At the end of the 20th century, a trend in day care has been the establishment of facilities for care of elderly persons, whose condition does not necessitate institutional care, but who need assistance that their family cannot provide during the day. Although many midlife children experience the stress of guilt about placing an elderly parent in day care, they understand that there are benefits. For example, senior day care offers socialization, learning opportunities, and encouragement of better nutritional patterns for the midday meal.

See also AGING; DIVORCE; ELDERLY PARENTS; WORKING MOTHERS.

SOURCES:
Deutsch, F. "Day Care Centers," in Corsini, Raymond, ed., *Encyclopedia of Psychology*, vol. 1. New York: Wiley, 1984.
Edmundson, Brad. "Where's the Day Care?" *American Demographics* 12 (July 1990) 17–19.

Gallo, Nick. "Too Sick for School?" *Better Homes and Gardens,* September 1990, 62–65.

Kantrowitz, Barbara. "Day Care Bridging the Generation Gap." *Newsweek,* July 16, 1990, 52.

daydreaming   When people daydream, they are awake and experiencing a pleasant reverie, usually of wish fulfillment. Daydreaming occurs during idle moments or when people are unconcerned about the activity around them. In these ways, daydreaming, which may be a form of stress relief, differs from serious, logical, and controlled thinking which is done in a more deliberate manner.

Some people may daydream about developing great ideas or inventions, or taking new directions in life; in daydreaming, their mind is free to roam without inhibition and self-censorship. Different views of work and family situations are often developed during moments of daydreaming, because daydreams are usually concerned with ends, not means.

People of all ages daydream. Young and old may be caught staring out the window, putting down a book and gazing at nothing in a trance-like state. Unless they share their dream, it is difficult to tell if they are lost in their reveries or just bored.

See also BOREDOM; CREATIVITY.

deadlines   Most people have experienced stress in meeting or failing to meet a date or time at which something must be done. Once they have fallen behind, it is difficult to catch up. They find that rushing tends to add to the stress and decrease effectiveness. Ineffectiveness leads to frustration. Some people become moody and emotional and blame themselves or others for the deadline failure.

The key to avoiding the stress produced by deadlines is setting realistic time schedules, enlisting the help needed when deadlines go awry, and negotiating new deadlines when it appears that, for one reason or another, deadlines are going to be missed. For individuals to keep a positive outlook, they should break deadlines down to a series of small steps. As each step is completed, they will feel some success, and that success, in turn, will keep them motivated toward their final goal.

See also AUTONOMY; CONTROL; WORKPLACE.

deafness   Loss of hearing, either complete or partial. Hearing loss becomes a stressor for many individuals who begin to lose their hearing and try to draw attention away from their loss or cover it up. While hearing aids help many individuals, some are embarrassed to wear them or find them uncomfortable. Some people associate loss of hearing with AGING, and hence postpone getting a hearing aid to preserve their image of youthfulness.

Deafness and hearing loss is a major societal problem. Estimates are that about a quarter of a million persons in the United States are completely deaf, and about three million have major hearing problems.

Causes of hearing difficulties

Hearing difficulties are related to many things, including problems within the ears themselves, overall body health, emotions and external environment. People tend to shut off certain sounds at certain times and will hear only what is interesting or significant. For example, a man may hear all of a sports newscast but not hear a request to fix something around the house. In some nursing homes, it has been observed that individuals say they cannot hear, but when asked whether they want ice cream they are able to answer. The term "psychogenic deafness" pertains to such mental "shutting off" of hearing carried to an extreme. Some patients may have such a strong subconscious desire not to hear that they become completely deaf, yet have physically normal ears.

The term "psychosomatic deafness" relates to situations in which actual physical deterioration occurs in the ear as a reaction to a mental or emotional problem. There also may be combinations of both physical and psychologically induced hearing difficulties.

See also DISABILITIES.

FOR FURTHER INFORMATION:
American Speech-Language-Hearing Association
10801 Rockville Pike
Rockville, MD 20852
Phone: (800) 638-8255; (800) 638-TALK

SHHH (Self-Help for Hard of Hearing People, Inc.)
7800 Wisconsin Avenue
Bethesda, MD 20814
Phone: (301) 657-2248

death   One of the most stressful life experiences an individual faces is the death of a spouse, parent, child, close relative, or beloved friend. Another serious source of stress is when we are told that our own death is imminent. On a scale of life-stressing events, death rates a top position. People of all ages fear death as well as the process of dying.

Included in the specific sources of stress related to death are shock, GRIEF, necessity for making funeral arrangements, and perhaps the practicalities of handling the deceased person's personal affairs. How people deal with the stressors brought on by another's death vary. Many factors influence individual responses. For example, when a series of losses have occurred or if the death is sudden and unexpected, the reaction may be more extreme. If the deceased had been ill and the survivor regards the death as the loved one's liberation from pain and suffering, the grief may be somewhat tempered with those thoughts, although the loss nevertheless creates an irreplaceable void in the survivor's life.

Making funeral arrangements is extremely stressful. In the midst of extreme emotional upheaval, the survivor is faced with choosing funeral arrangements, selection of a casket, heavy expenses, and contacting friends and relatives. Calling upon relatives or friends to assist in these tasks can lighten the burden.

The stress of making funeral arrangements can be alleviated somewhat by developing a pre-need plan, which may include selection of type of funeral and burial, selection of casket, and written wishes for a service. In some cases, the individual herself/himself makes these arrangements, while these arrangements can also be made by another when a death seems imminent. Making these arrangements ahead of time relieves some of the stress during a heavily emotion-laden time.

Mourning, the period of grief that follows the loss of a loved person, is a stressful period. The mourner may have a period of feeling numb. Gradually, one's personality reestablishes itself, but during mourning the intensity of grief may lead to psychological disturbances, such as depression, and physiological disturbances, such as headaches or digestive disturbances. The mourner may withdraw from others and be almost completely preoccupied with thoughts of the loss, spending a great deal of time recalling experiences, meanings, and the emotional significance of the lost relationship.

To help a grieving person, friends should encourage the survivor to express emotions and talk about the deceased. It is important for the survivor to maintain adequate nutrition and do some physical exercise during the grief process. A strong body contributes to clearer thinking and an improved emotional state. Encourage the person to stay involved with family and friends and to reconnect with familiar routines and interests.

Those who have lost a spouse need to begin to learn to do the things for themselves that their spouse may have done before. This may mean learning new skills, such as cooking, maintaining the car, balancing the checkbook, and paying the bills. As one does these things, a new and healthy sense of mastery over life can be gained.

When facing the stressors brought on by the death of a loved one, many people find relief in their personal faith, PRAYER, or SUPPORT GROUPS.

Facing one's own death

When one is faced with the fact of his own approaching death, reactions, and sometimes those of family member, may follow a pattern. Many people go through a serious of emotional stages at such times. The initial reaction is denial, which usually lasts a short time in a mentally healthy person. After the initial shock, the patient becomes angry and asks, "Why me?" If these feelings cannot be expressed, the anger may turn inward and the patient may become extremely depressed. The next stage is negotiation, and one may try to make a deal with the doctors, or with his God, hoping that if he cooperates or devotes himself to noble causes, he will survive. As he becomes aware that his demise is inevitable, the patient will admit what is happening and either give up to hopelessness or try to discover some sense of meaning and purpose. Next comes a stage of commitment, characterized by acceptance; at this point, many patients find new courage. As death nears, one has either a sense or fulfillment or a feeling of forlorness and depression. If one has adequately worked though the first stages and reacts with fulfillment, one's last moments can be peaceful and tranquil.

Ethical, moral, and legal aspects

Death as an ethical and legal issue and how people die can be stressful for health care professionals as well as the individuals concerned and their families. Some patients who are near death may ask for a death-inducing potion or instrument. Physicians are stressed by the dilemma of providing assistance in such cases. There have been instances in which family become involved in a loved one's death, sometimes incriminating themselves in subsequent unpleasant legal situations. The question of assisted suicide is both a moral and legal issue.

Legal definitions of death vary, causing stress for family members, physicians, lawyers, and courts. At one time death was simply when the heartbeat and breathing stopped. Now it is recognized that the brain is the basis for life. People whose hearts and lungs have stopped working can be maintained for years on machines, but no one is really "alive" when they are brain dead. Brain death means an unconscious state, in which the person has no reflexes and cannot breathe or maintain a heartbeat. The electroencephalogram (EEG) of the person would be flat, without any regular oscillations indicating function of the brain. Brain death occurs naturally within a few minutes after the heart stops, because oxygen necessary for life is not carried through the blood to the brain.

In most states a physician must certify death, and indicate the time, place, and cause. In some cases, circumstances of death play a major role in insurance payments; when there are suppositions of homicide or SUICIDE, the death takes on additional stressful dimensions for the family.

In the latter part of the 20th century, many individuals choose the place for their death. Some who have terminal illnesses opt to go home, rather than stay in the hospital with its impersonal surroundings.

"Advance directives" and dying with dignity

While medical science has created ways to prolong life even in terminal cases, an increasing number of people are beginning to "take charge" of their own deaths by advance directives so that they will not be kept alive on respirators or by other artificial means. On these legal documents, they can specify the types of life support systems they do and do not want. For example, one man may say he will not tolerate being tube-fed when he can no longer keep food down in the normal way, while another will want nutrition provided but not assistance in breathing. This permits a physician to omit heroic treatment efforts without civil or criminal liability.

Dying with dignity is a term that gained popularity during the 1980s and 1990s when high technology enabled health care practitioners to maintain terminally ill people on life support systems. Wanting to "die with dignity," individuals can plan ahead by executing a document known as an advance directive, in which they make treatment wishes known while still healthy. In 1991, the federal Patient Self-Determination Act was enacted, under which health care providers must give patients information about advance directives, including living wills and durable power of attorney for health care.

Living will. A living will allows people to specify when and under what conditions they want treatment to be withheld, should a terminal illness be suffered. They can spell out, for example, that if an irreversible coma occurs, they do not want heroic lifesaving measures to be taken. In some states, the living will must be signed by the person executing it, as well as two witnesses who are at least 18 years old.

When the physician determines and notes in the medical record that the patient has met four specific conditions, a living will goes into effect. The four criteria are that the patient has a condition that is terminal, incurable, and irreversible, and death is imminent. Additionally, some state laws regarding living wills do not recognize the withdrawal of hydration and nutrition. Individuals who do not wish fluids and nutrition to be administered when they meet the four conditions required for a living will, either cross those items off from the living will document or execute a durable power of attorney for health care, spelling out this wish.

Durable power of attorney for health care. This document allows people, as principals, to appoint another person, known as the agent, to make medical care decisions in case they become mentally or physically incompetent. The document permits one to determine at what point the power of attorney becomes

effective and the scope of the agent's decision-making powers. Durable powers of attorney enable people to give very specific directions about what treatment they want and do not want.

Advance directives may be revoked at any time while one is still competent. If it is necessary to revoke a durable power of attorney after individuals become incapacitated, legal action may be necessary. Advance directives become part of the permanent medical record. However, health care providers are not bound to carry out an advance directive that conflicts with state legislation, and it is important for concerned individuals to check the laws of each state involved for optimal peace of mind.

See also END OF LIFE CARE.

SOURCES:
Kübler-Ross, Elisabeth. *On Death and Dying.* New York: Macmillan Company, 1996.
Logue, Barbara. *Last Right: Death Control and the Elderly in America.* New York: Lexington Books, 1993.

decision making   Some decisions are made easily, while others are arrived at after considerable struggle. Decision making is stressful because it involves addressing alternatives, options, and possibilities for reassessment at a later time.

The most important decisions people can make usually focus on their health and well-being, affect other people, involve large amounts of money, and require risk taking. Because many people are uncomfortable taking risks, doing so may generate stress and, in turn, that stress can interfere with making the best decisions.

Information used in making decisions is extremely important. How people perceive a situation, past experiences with like situations, as well as their own background and culture, play a large part in the decision-making process. Problems may occur when complete information is not gathered or not carefully analyzed in terms of where it is has come from.

See also COPING; GENERAL ADAPTATION SYNDROME.

defense mechanisms   Part of an unconscious mental process that individuals use to reach compromise solutions with stressful problems. Individuals have a wide variety of defense mechanisms, ranging from projection, which is blaming someone else for one's situation, and rationalization, which is justifying questionable behavior by defending its propriety, to sublimation, which is rechanneling energy into creative projects. DENIAL is another defense mechanism. The presence of pathological denial (for example, of a drinking problem) is often seen in people with alcoholism or substance abuse problems.

In cases of extreme child abuse, dissociation (splitting of one's mind from the physical circumstance) becomes a defense mechanism. While defense mechanisms can be helpful in coping with daily life, excessive use of such devices and dependence on them can lead to higher levels of STRESS for the individual.

In follow-up studies of the Harvard University class of 1934, Dr. George Vaillant found that, though virtually all of his subjects had significant life crises, those who overcame them tended to have "mature" defenses such as suppression (the capacity to focus on only the most important issue at the time, suppressing thought or worry about other problems until the one of high priority is solved) and a good sense of HUMOR. Those who were overwhelmed by the stresses of life crises tended to employ "less mature—more primitive" (blaming others) and denial (not admitting the presence of a problem to oneself).

See also COPING; GENERAL ADAPTATION SYNDROME.

denial   A DEFENSE MECHANISM in which individuals do not admit to themselves that a problem or event produces STRESS and ANXIETY. Additionally, a denial of a situation by some people can be a source of stress to others.

See also CHRONIC ILLNESS; COPING; ELDERLY PARENTS; GENERAL ADAPTATION SYNDROME.

dentists   Many people experience stress when going to a dentist or even thinking about it. In fact, many people are so fearful of dentists and dentistry that they wait until they have a severe toothache or other dental problem before seeking help.

Stress relating to dentistry is fairly common. According to the American Dental Association, 35,000,000 Americans experience moderate to high anxiety about dentistry. Estimates are that possibly 12,000,000 people experience such severe anxiety that they avoid going to the dentist, some for many years.

Some people may have had bad experiences in a dental chair as a child and developed a fear of dentistry. Others are afraid of pain and blood, of having a shot, or of the sound of the dentist's drill. Others fear being out of CONTROL while seated in the dental chair. Some are truly dental phobics and experience queasy feelings in their stomach, trembling hands, sweaty palms and increased pulse rate; others may fear having a panic attack while in the chair.

Fears surrounding dentistry that are most frequently expressed by individuals include (in descending order) the injection needle, seeing the local anesthetic syringe, feeling vibrations from the drill in their mouths, the dentist using a probe to examine their teeth, seeing the dentist walk in, being taken into the dental chair, hearing the drill sounds while in the waiting room, entering the waiting room, driving to the dentist's office, seeing the calendar showing one day left before an appointment, calling for an appointment, and being reminded that a dental appointment is needed.

Managing dental stress

Many people overcome their stressful feelings with complete explanations of procedures that will be done, how anesthetics will be administered, and of how long the procedure will take. Knowing that they can ask the dentist to stop a procedure for a moment helps many people feel more CONTROL about their situation. Some individuals choose to use deep BREATHING and RELAXATION techniques, including their own audio tapes, BIOFEEDBACK devices or HYPNOSIS. BEHAVIOR THERAPY helps many who are phobic about dentistry.

See also ANXIETY DISORDERS; PANIC ATTACKS AND PANIC DISORDER; PHOBIAS.

FOR FURTHER INFORMATION:
American Dental Association
211 East Chicago Avenue
Chicago, IL 60611
Phone: (312) 440-2500

depression   A mood or AFFECTIVE DISORDER characterized by a wide range of symptoms, including hopelessness, helplessness, personal devaluation, and extreme sadness. Some depressions are marked by extreme stress, anxiety, withdrawal from others and changes in sleep patterns. The person suffering from depression may exhibit lethargy or agitation, loss of appetite or compulsive eating, loss of sexual desire, an inability to concentrate and make decisions, exaggerated guilt feelings, and thoughts about SUICIDE.

Depression causes stress for family members as well as the sufferer. Symptoms may change or increase over days or weeks. Depressed persons may withdraw from human contact but not admit to symptoms. Others are so disabled by their condition that they cannot call a friend, relative, or medical help. If another person calls a doctor for them, they may refuse to go because they do not believe that they can be helped. Many depressed persons will not follow a doctor's advice, and may refuse help and comfort. Persistence on the part of family and friends is essential, although stressful, because in many cases depression is the illness that underlies suicide.

Defining depression

The term depression applies to a condition on a continuum of severity; it can be a temporary mood fluctuation, a symptom associated with a number of mental and physical disorders, or a clinical syndrome encompassing many symptoms, such as major depression or dysthymic disorder.

Clinical depression refers to a depression that lasts for more than a few weeks or includes symptoms that interfere with job performance and the ability to handle everyday decisions and routinely stressful situations. Clinical depression is a term that overlaps with the terms *major depression, dysthymia, unipolar depression,* and *exogenous depression.*

Seasonal moods disorder (SEASONAL AFFECTIVE DISORDER). Some individuals have mood symptoms related to changes of season, with depression occurring most frequently during winter months and an improvement in the spring. Many of these individuals experience periods of increased energy, productivity, and even euphoria in the spring and summer months. This type of depression often responds well to light therapy.

Melancholia. Melancholia is a severe form of depression that may originate without any precipitating factors, such as stress. This is in contrast to a reactive depression, which occurs after some stressful life event such as loss of a job or divorce.

Age of onset and incidence

People of all ages can become depressed, although major depressive episodes peak at age 55 to 70 in men and at age 20 to 45 in women. About 20% of major depressions last two or more years, with an average of eight months. About half of those experiencing a major depression will have a recurrence within two years.

Estimates are that 2% to 3% of men and from 4% to 9% of women in the United States suffer a major depression. The lifetime risk may be as high as 10% for men and 25% for women. Unfortunately, about 66% of those who suffer from depression fail to recognize the illness and do not seek treatment.

Some individuals may have only one episode of clinical depression during their lifetimes. Others have episodes that are separated by several years or suffer clusters of episodes over a short time span. Between episodes, such individuals function normally. However, 20% to 35% of sufferers have chronic depression that prevents them from functioning totally efficiently. For these people, it is a recurrent disorder that may require maintenance on medication to prevent additional episodes.

Depression is the most common mental health disorder among the elderly. According to the National Institute of Mental Health (NIMH), estimates of depression among elderly people ranges from 10% to 65%. Other estimates indicate that 20% of geriatric outpatients are depressed.

Causes of depression
Many factors can lead to depression, including a family history of depression, psychosocial stressors, diseases, alcohol, drugs, and anxiety disorders. Individuals who have personality disorders, especially obsessive-compulsive, dependent, avoidant, and borderline personality disorders, may tend to be more susceptible to depression than other individuals.

Psychosocial factors. Depression can come from an individual's lack of confidence in his or her interpersonal skills, overdependency on others, perfectionism, unrealistic expectations, and psychosocial events, such as the death of a spouse, loss of a job, or, for some, the stresses of urban living.

Environmental influences. Researchers view depression as the result of an interaction of environmental and biological factors. Historically, depression has been viewed as either internally caused (endogenous depression) or externally related to environmental events (exogenous or reactional influences). Major changes in the individual's environment, such as a move or job change, or any major loss, such as a divorce or death of a loved one, can bring on depression. Feeling depressed in response to these changes is normal, but when depression lasts over one month and interferes with effective functioning, treatment can be helpful.

Some environmental factors relating to depression include being unemployed, elderly, alone, poor, and having financial problems.

Illness. Psychological stressors caused by chronic illness can lead to depression. For example, a debilitating disease that severely restricts usual lifestyle or any illness that impinges on cerebral functioning and

---

SIGNS AND SYMPTOMS OF DEPRESSION

Psychological
- Loss of interest
- Unexplained anxiety
- Inappropriate feelings of guilt
- Loss of SELF-ESTEEM
- Worthlessness
- Hopelessness
- Thoughts of death and suicide
- Tearfulness, irritability, brooding

Physical
- Headache, vague aches and pains
- Changes in appetite and changes in weight
- Sleep disturbances
- Loss of energy
- Psychomotor agitation or retardation
- Loss of libido
- Gastrointestinal disturbances

Intellectual
- Slowed thinking
- Indecisiveness
- Poor concentration
- Impaired memory

impairs blood flow to the brain can produce depression. Such illnesses may include adrenal cortex, thyroid, and parathyroid dysfunctions, and many neurologic, metabolic, and nutritional disorders, as well as infectious diseases.

Medications. Some medications can cause depression. For example, during the 1950s, doctors learned that some people taking reserpine, a medication for high blood pressure, suffered from depression. Since then, depression has been noted as a side effect of some tranquilizers and hormones and, of a number of medications. However, alcohol is more likely to cause depression than any medication.

Social learning theory. Stress can disrupt involvement with others, resulting in less positive reinforcement, which in turn leads to more negative self-evaluation and a poor outlook for the future. Depressed people view themselves and their world negatively; this leads to a further sense of low self-worth, feelings of rejection, alienation, dependency, helplessness, and hopelessness.

Cognitive theory. Unrecognized negative attitudes toward oneself, the future and the world can result in feelings of failure, helplessness, and depression. Especially under stress, such attitudes may activate a prolonged and deepening depressive state. Negative attitudes are usually distorted; learning what they are can help reverse both depression and a tendency for future depression.

Interpersonal theory. This theory emphasizes the importance of social connections for effective functioning. An individual develops adaptive responses to the psychosocial environment at an early age. When early attachment bonds are disrupted or impaired, the individual may be vulnerable later on to depression. An example is a young child who loses a parent to death or through divorce.

Psychoanalytic theory. A psychoanalytical position regarding depression is that a loss, or a real or perceived withdrawal of affection in childhood, may be a predeterminant for depression in later life.

Other theories suggest that unrealistic expectations of self and others and loss of self-esteem are essential components leading to depression. Depression that arises following a loss may result from failure to fully come to terms with the reality of the loss.

Genetic factors. Some individuals may be biologically predisposed to develop depression, based on genetic factors that researchers do not yet fully understand. There are genetic markers that indicate susceptibility to manic-depressive illness, and there has been considerable research in the last decades of the 20th century focused on understanding the biochemical reactions influenced by these genes.

Evidence indicates that depression runs in families; among more severe depressives, family is a more significant factor. For example, if one identical twin suffers from depression or manic-depression, the other twin has a 70% chance of also having the illness. Research studies looking at the rate of depression among adopted children support this finding. Depressive illnesses among children's adoptive family have little effect on their risk for the disorder; however, among adopted children whose biological relatives suffered depression, the disorder is three times more common than the norm.

Neurotransmitter theory. Recent research indicates that people who have depression have imbalances of NEUROTRANSMITTERS, natural biochemicals that enable brain cells to communicate with each another. Biochemicals that often are out of balance in depressed people include SEROTONIN, NOREPINEPHRINE, and dopamine. An imbalance of serotonin may cause anxiety, sleep problems, and irritability. An inadequate supply of norepinephrine, which regulates alertness and arousal, may contribute to fatigue and lack of motivation. Dopamine imbalances may relate to a loss of sexual interest and inability to experience pleasure. Researchers continue to find other neurotransmitters that may be important in clinical depression.

Cortisol. Another body chemical that may be out of balance is cortisol, a hormone produced by the body in response to extreme cold, fear, or anger. In most people, cortisol levels in the blood peak in the morning, then decrease later in the day. In people who have depression, however, cortisol peaks early in the morning and does not level off or decrease in the afternoon or evening.

Psychotherapies for depression

Estimates are that between 80% and 90% of all depressed people can be effectively treated for depression by a variety of types of therapist. In general, therapists use "talk" treatment to try to understand the individual's personal and social relationships that may have caused or contributed to the depression. Depression, in turn, may make these relationships more stressful.

Psychoanalysis. Treatment of depression with psychoanalysis is based on the theory that depression results from past conflicts pushed into the unconscious. Psychoanalysts work to help the patient identify and resolve past conflicts that led to depression.

Short-term Psychotherapy. In the mid-1980s, researchers reported effective results of short-term psychotherapy in treating depression. They noted that cognitive/behavior therapy and interpersonal therapy were as effective as medications for some depressed patients. Medications relieved patients' symptoms more quickly, but patients who received psychotherapy instead of medication had as much relief from symptoms after 16 weeks, and their gains may last longer. Data from this and other studies may help researchers better identify which depressed patients will do best with psychotherapy alone and which may require medications.

Behavior and cognitive therapy. These therapies are based on the understanding that people's emotions are controlled by their views and opinions of themselves and their world. Depression results when individuals constantly berate themselves, expect to fail, make inaccurate assessments of what others think of them, CATASTROPHIZE, and have negative attitudes toward the world and their future. Therapists use techniques of talk therapy to help the individual replace negative beliefs and thought patterns with positive ones.

Electroconvulsive therapy (ECT). Use of ECT to treat depression declined in the last two decades of the 20th century as more effective medications were developed. However, ECT is still used for some individuals who cannot take medications due to their physical condition, or who do not respond to antidepressant medication. ECT is considered as a treatment when all other therapies have failed or when a person is suicidal.

If psychotherapy is not helpful or the depression is at such a severe level that there is a loss of work or of function, or persistent and increasing suicidal ideation over one to three months, medications may be needed to lift the depression in conjunction with therapy.

Pharmaceutical approach to treating depression

Effectiveness of medication depends on overall health, metabolism and other unique characteristics. Results are usually not evident right away; antidepressant medications usually become fully effective in about 10 to 20 days after an individual begins taking them. Approximately 70% of patients will improve or recover while taking antidepressant medications, but some may need to continue medication over a six-month or year-long period to prevent relapse or recurrence.

The major types of medications used to treat depression are tricyclic antidepressants, MAO inhibitors (MAOIs), lithium, and "novel antidepressants."

Tricyclic antidepressants are often prescribed for individuals whose depressions are marked by feelings of hopelessness, helplessness, fatigue, inability to experience pleasure, and loss of appetite and resulting weight loss.

Monoamine oxidase inhibitors (MAOIs) are often prescribed for individuals whose depressions are characterized by anxiety, phobic and obsessive-compulsive symptoms, increased appetite and excessive sleepiness, or those who fail to improve on other antidepressant medications.

Lithium is sometimes prescribed for people who have manic-depressive illness (a severe affective disorder characterized by a predominant mood of elation or depression, and in some cases an alternation between the two states). Sometimes it is prescribed for people who suffer from depression without mania. Those most likely to respond to treatment with lithium are depressed individuals whose family members have manic-depression or whose depression is recurrent rather than constant.

"Novel antidepressants." During the 1990s, more specifically active antidepressant drugs with less propensity for side effects were developed. Serotonin reuptake inhibitors (SRIs), for example, fluoxetine (Prozac) and sertraline (Zoloft), are one class; buproprion (Wellbutrin) is another class. Many other new medications are under development to treat depression.

Anticonvulsants as antidepressants. For patients with manic-depressive illness (bipolar disorder) where lithium is not effective, drugs used to prevent temporal lobe seizures are sometimes used.

Side effects of antidepressant medications. Some people experience side effects from antidepressant medications, which in themselves may be stressful. Common side effects include dry mouth, constipation, drowsiness, and weight gain; these effects usually diminish somewhat or disappear as the body makes adjustments. The more recently developed "novel antidepressants" have a lower incidence of these side effects.

RECOGNIZING ADOLESCENT DEPRESSION

- Sadness; feelings of helplessness or hopelessness
- Poor SELF-ESTEEM and loss of confidence
- Overreaction to criticism
- Extreme fluctuations between boredom and talkativeness
- Sleep disturbances
- Anger, rage, and verbal sarcasm; guilt
- Intense ambivalence between dependence and independence
- Feelings of emptiness in life
- Restlessness and agitation
- Pessimism about the future
- Refusal to work in school or cooperate in general
- Increased or decreased appetite; severe weight gain or loss
- Death wishes, suicidal thoughts, suicide attempts

Depression in adolescents

Depression in teenagers may be somewhat different from that in adults. Some adolescent symptoms may be overlooked as part of growing up. Teenagers may be depressed because of being in trouble, or in trouble because of being depressed. Their depression is sometimes linked to poor school performance, truancy, delinquency, alcohol and drug abuse, disobedience, self-destructive behavior, sexual promiscuity, rebelliousness, GRIEF, and running away. They may feel a lack of support from family and other significant people, and a decrease in their ability to cope effectively.

Adolescence is a period of demanding and complicated conflicts that lead many young people to develop anxieties, negative self-esteem, and fears about their future. Some develop depression when overwhelmed by the stresses of peer pressure, feelings of loneliness, powerlessness, and isolation. Low performance in school can lead to a feeling of rejection, social expectations may be unrealistic, and conflicting messages from family may magnify struggles for independence and assertiveness.

Contributing factors to adolescent depression may include exaggerated concerns, misperceptions and continual self-criticism. The lack of ability to embrace what life has to offer results in boredom, which may be an indicator of vulnerability to depression.

Self-help for individuals and their families

Self-help and support groups allow individuals of all ages to share ideas for effective COPING and self-care. Benefits of these groups include increasing contacts with other people, for example, by participation in special interest groups; learning to cope with exaggerated thoughts; and following regular exercise programs.

The National Depressive and Manic-Depressive Association is a national self-help organization, with chapters throughout the country that meet locally to help members cope effectively with depression.

The Depression and Related Affective Disorders Association (DRADA) is a nonprofit organization focusing on manic depressive illness and depression. DRADA distributes information, conducts educational meetings, and runs an outreach program for high school counselors and nurses. DRADA helps organize support groups and provides leadership training programs and consultation for those groups (see below).

See also AGORAPHOBIA; DEFENSE MECHANISMS; PHARMACOLOGICAL APPROACH: PSYCHOTHERAPIES; PUBERTY.

FOR FURTHER INFORMATION:
Depression and Related Affective Disorders Association (DRADA)
Johns Hopkins Hospital (Meyer 3–181)
600 N. Wolfe Street
Baltimore, MD 21287
Phone: (410) 955-4647

National Alliance for the Mentally Ill
2101 Wilson Blvd. (Suite 302)
Arlington, VA 22201
Phone: (703) 524-7600

National Depressive and Manic Depressive Association
222 South Riverside Plaza (Suite 2812)
Chicago, IL 60606
Phone: (312) 993-0066

National Institute of Mental Health
Office of Scientific Information
Public Inquiries Section
5600 Fishers Lane (Room 15C-17)
Rockville, MD 20857
Phone: (301) 443-4513

National Mental Health Association
1020 Prince Street
Alexandria, VA 22314
Phone: (703) 684-7722

SOURCES:
Garland, E. Jane. "Adolescent Depression." *Canadian Family Physician* 40, (September, 1994).
Greist, John H., and James W. Jefferson. *Depression and Its Treatment: Help for the Nation's #1 Mental Problem.* Washington, D.C.: American Psychiatric Press, 1984.
———. *Depression and Its Treatment.* New York: Warner Books, 1994.
Kahn, Ada P., and Jan Fawcett. *The Encyclopedia of Mental Health.* New York: Facts On File, 1993.
Karp, David Allen. *Speaking of Sadness: Depression, Disconnection, and the Meanings of Illness.* New York: Oxford University Press, 1996.
Klerman, Gerald. *Suicide and Depression Among Adolescents and Young Adults.* Washington, D.C.: American Psychiatric Press, 1986.
Robb-Nicholson, Celeste. "Depression." *Harvard Women's Health Watch,* March 1995, 2–3.
Warneke, Lorne. "Management of Resistant Depression." *Canadian Family Physician,* (October 1996): 1973.

dermatitis Inflammation of the skin, sometimes due to allergy, but sometimes occurring without any known reason. It can result in painful itching and the distress of extreme discomfort. For some individuals, if the itching persists without relief, dermatitis leads to a feeling of helplessness and DEPRESSION.

Many types of dermatitis are better known as eczemas, such as atopic, common in babies; nummular, which occurs in adults, cause unknown; and dermatitis of the hand, the result of household detergents and cleansers.

Other types of dermatitis include seborrheic, which appears on the face, scalp, and back, develops during stress, and is a reaction to something that comes in contact with the skin.

See also ALLERGIES; CHRONIC ILLNESS; HIVES; POISON IVY.

FOR FURTHER INFORMATION:
American Academy of Dermatology
930 N. Meacham Road
Schaumburg, IL 60168
Phone: (708) 330-0230

desensitization, systematic See BEHAVIOR THERAPY; PHOBIAS.

diabetes (diabetes mellitus) Disorder in which the pancreas produces too little or no insulin for the body's needs. Insufficient insulin results in an abnormally high glucose level in the blood, leading to excessive urination, constant thirst, and hunger. When the body cannot store or use glucose, there is weight loss and fatigue, and accelerated degeneration of small blood vessels.

Diabetes is not contagious, although it tends to run in families. While there is no cure for it, with appropriate medical care and patient compliance, the disease can be kept under control.

Coping with the stresses and treatment of diabetes

Diabetes brings with it the stresses and consequences of a CHRONIC ILLNESS for the individual as well as the family. When diabetes is diagnosed, many highly charged feelings enter into its acceptance. There may be ANGER,

GUILT, or anxieties, both expressed and unexpressed, and these feelings should be discussed with family members. If it is a child who is diabetic, encourage discussion so that the child understands that having such feelings is part of the COPING process. Stable mental health is important for proper control of diabetes because emotional stresses affect secretions of hormones that may counteract or interfere with the helpful effects of insulin.

Diabetic health care teams will have suggestions to help individuals reduce their stress levels. They may suggest ALTERNATIVE THERAPIES, such as RELAXATION exercises and BIOFEEDBACK. They may encourage participation in group therapy sessions with other families to learn how others cope with diabetes. Such groups foster exchanges of helpful ideas concerning the practical aspects of diabetes. They may suggest use of the "buddy system," working with another diabetic to reinforce support and provide a model for adjustment to life with diabetes. There are groups run by local affiliates of the American Diabetes Association, hospitals, and community health departments. Awareness of existing services is the first step toward obtaining assistance and maintaining a good mental attitude about the disease.

The health care team of the diabetic will consider individual emotional needs along with menu and exercise plans, and therapy with insulin and other medications. Problems such as mishandling the food plan, refusing to take insulin injections, consciously overeating, and DEPRESSION occur in some diabetics, and compound their stress levels. These situations can be successfully handled with the support of health care professionals, parents, spouses or significant others.

The personal role in the treatment of diabetes is important. For example, diabetic individuals need to devote more time to personal care than may have been done before, particularly giving specific attention to skin, feet, and teeth, and promptly treating minor injuries such as burns, cuts, and bruises. Keeping diabetes under control can help diabetics avoid later stresses such as difficulties in the vascular system and eye and kidney disease.

Individuals afflicted with diabetes face not only a shortened life span but also the probability of incurring acute and chronic complications. People who have diabetes are two and a half times more likely to suffer from strokes than those without diabetes; people with diabetes are two to four times more likely to develop cardiovascular disease. Diabetes is the leading cause of new cases of blindness in adults from 20 to 74 years of age and is the leading cause of end-stage kidney disease.

Prevalence, causes, and types of diabetes

In the United States, about two persons per 1,000 have insulin-dependent diabetes by the age of 20; the insulin-dependent form (Type I) affects about 150 to 200 persons per 100,000. Non-insulin-dependent (Type II) diabetes is more common; approximately 2,000 persons per 100,000 are affected. With age, the risk for developing diabetes increases. People of middle or older age are more likely to develop diabetes than younger people, and women are more likely to have diabetes than men.

Heredity, obesity, and stresses such as emotional shocks, family disturbances, or surgery can lead to diabetes. Researchers have emphasized the power of disruptive and stressful life events as influencing the course of the disease. Pregnancy also places extra stresses on the body, and diabetes is often diagnosed in pregnant women or women who have repeated miscarriages. People who have diabetes, especially Type II, often have high blood pressure too.

Type I, insulin-dependent diabetes, can occur at any age, though it most commonly occurs during youth. Type I diabetes used to be called juvenile-onset diabetes and is still called that by some health care professionals. About one of every 2,500 children has this dis-ease. Because the pancreas produces little or no insulin, such patients become dependent on outside sources of insulin. The disease can be controlled with insulin, proper diet, exercise, and careful monitoring.

Type II is non-insulin-dependent diabetes. Estimates are that between 60% and 90% of those with non-insulin-dependent diabetes in Western societies are obese. Thus it is important for obese individuals to lose weight. This type of diabetes used to be called maturity-onset diabetes and may still be called that by some health care professionals. Type II is much more common than Type I; more than five million Americans have the disease. This type is less severe than insulin-dependent diabetes and starts more slowly. Often it can be controlled by diet alone or by a combination of diet, exercise and oral medication.

See also IMMUNE SYSTEM; SUPPORT GROUPS.

FOR FURTHER INFORMATION:
American Diabetes Association
National Service Center
1660 Duke Street
Alexandria, VA 22314
Phone: (703) 549-1500; (800) 232-3472

National Diabetes Information Clearinghouse
Box NDIC
Bethesda, MD 20892
Phone: (301) 468-2162

SOURCES:
Eastman, Richard. "Prevalence of Diabetes Increasing in U.S." *Journal of the American Medical Association,* November 2, 1995.
Kahn, Ada P. *Diabetes.* Chicago: Contemporary Books, 1983.
Schade, David S. "The Stress Factor." *Diabetes Forecast,* March-April 1982.

diaphragmatic breathing   See BREATHING.

diarrhea   Refers to fluidity, frequency, or volume of bowel movements when compared with the usual pattern for a particular person. It is not a disorder, but a symptom of a problem. In some individuals, stress and ANXIETY bring on diarrhea. Individuals who have IRRI-TABLE BOWEL SYNDROME may suffer bouts of diarrhea.

While diarrhea may be the result of anxiety, it also causes stress and anxious moments. The traveler who has a sudden attack must quickly find a public restroom. The speaker or performer about to go onstage must take time to deal with the personal emergency.

Acute diarrhea affects almost everyone at some time, often as a result of eating contaminated food or drinking contaminated water. Usually attacks clear up within a day or two with or without treatment; many effective treatments are available as over-the-counter medications. Chronic diarrhea may be symptomatic of more serious conditions requiring medical attention.

FOR FURTHER INFORMATION:
American Gastroenterological Association
6900 Grove Road
Thorofare, NJ 08086
Phone: (609) 848-9218

dieting Generally refers to following a special or modified diet for the purpose of losing weight. Motivation to be as thin as models unrealistically motivates many people, particularly women, to begin dieting. Dieting is stressful because losing weight is not easy; it means setting realistic goals. It requires time—often a year for positive results—for some people; it means hard work, both losing the weight and keeping it off. It is also stressful because many people perceive themselves as overweight, whether this is the case or not.

Some dieting approaches involve extensive behavior modification. These programs offer SUPPORT GROUPS and education about good NUTRITION and exercise. Most important, they offer help in altering the individual's behavior in order to limit food intake, increase physical activity, and reduce the stress of the current social pressures to be thin.

There are dangers involved in dieting. Donna Ciliska, in *Canadian Family Physician* (January 1993), said: "The drive for thinness in women as they strive to be what our culture demands has contributed to poor nutrition, an increase in EATING DISORDERS, a decrease in SELF-ESTEEM, discrimination against overweight people, and a diminished bank account. Paradoxically, overweight is more common in men and poses more of a health risk; the social pressure for them to be thin is less severe than for women. Fewer men seek weight loss programs."

Individuals who believe they are overweight should have a physical examination from their family physician to determine whether they are actually overweight or are weight-, shape- or food-obsessed. If overweight, further assessment is necessary; if not overweight, they need supportive strategies to help them feel better about themselves and referral to community resources to help them with their concern.

See also BODY IMAGE; OBESITY.

FOR FURTHER INFORMATION:
American Dietetic Association
216 W. Jackson Blvd. (Suite 800)
Chicago, IL 60606
Phone: (312) 899-0040

Food and Nutrition Information Center
National Agricultural Library Bldg. (Room 304)
Beltsville, MD 20705
Phone: (301) 504-5414

SOURCES:
Ciliska, Donna. "Women and Obesity." *Canadian Family Physician,* January 1993.
Hamilton, Michael, et al. *The Duke University Medical Center Book of Diet and Fitness.* New York: Fawcett Columbine, 1991.
Thomas, Patricia, ed. "Dieting May Be a Losing Proposition." *Harvard Health Letter* 19, no. 10 (August 1994).

disabilities A disability refers to a temporary or permanent loss of faculty. It may refer to physical disabilities, such as loss of a leg or of hearing, or mental capabilities, such as retardation or autism. COPING with a disability causes stress for the one who has the disability and also for parents, siblings, and children who face caring for the disabled person.

Persons who become disabled often struggle with the anxiety of trying to be like everyone else. Because of their disability they may feel a loss of SELF-ESTEEM compounded, in many cases, by the limitations of the living situations they encounter. According to Reverend John A. Carr of the Yale-New Haven Medical Center, who was born with the congenital absence of both hands and one foot, "Coping with a handicap will depend on how human interactions occur, to allow more or less progress toward meaningful life." In the book, *Coping with Crisis and Handicap,* Reverend Carr recommends that open dialogue between those who are disabled and those who are not is essential because, "In denying our efforts to fight for a world more open to the handicapped, whether we refer to architectural or attitudinal barriers, we may be denying ourselves accessible avenues we will need later."

Coping with a disability in the family

Mary S. Challela, director of nursing and training at the Eunice Kennedy Shriver Center for the Mentally Retarded, defines *parental coping* as "managing the day-to-day activities of meeting the disabled child's needs, the parents' needs, and those of other children in the family, in a realistic manner. Before parents can be expected to assume any of these tasks effectively, they must be allowed and encouraged to respond emotionally to the crisis of disability." How parents react, she explains, is influenced by how and when they are told of the abnormality, their degree of social isolation, the type and severity of the disability, social class and education, attitudes of families and friends, and information received from and attitudes of professionals. Parents need emotional support and counseling in dealing with the initial and subsequent crises, education in learning how to care for the

child's special needs, guidance in dealing with other family members, and continued interest and encouragement.

According to Allen C. Crocker, Children's Hospital Medical Center, Boston, there are many emotions generated in the sister or brother of a disabled child, including "concern, curiosity, protectiveness, frustration, sorrow, grief, anxiety, longing, unhappiness, jealousy, and resentment. The elements of stress assuredly exist and are troubling to consider."

Many professionals urge special support for siblings, and value the role of self-help groups for parents, siblings, and other family members. Such groups can help resolve problems and feelings, serve as a socializing agency for all concerned, and provide a way to reach out to others in similar situations. Also, these SUPPORT GROUPS provide an important exchange of resources and often become an important force for obtaining services through legislation and social pressure.

In some cases, it may be an ELDERLY PARENT who becomes disabled. Coping mechanisms for relieving the stresses of the situation include obtaining professional guidance and social support.

See also GENERAL ADAPTATION SYNDROME; PARENTING.

FOR FURTHER INFORMATION:
Architectural and Transportation Barriers Compliance Board
1331 F Street, NW (Suite 1000)
Washington, DC 20004-1111
Phone: (202) 272-5434; (800) 872-2253;
　(800) USA-ABLE

Mobility International, U.S.A.
P.O. Box 3551
Eugene, OR 97403
Phone: (503) 343-1284

National Information Center for Children and
　Youth with Disabilities
P.O. Box 1492
Washington, DC 20013
Phone: (202) 884-8200

SOURCE:
Milunsky, Aubrey, ed. *Coping with Crisis and Handicap.* New York: Plenum Press, 1981.

dis-stress Hans SELYE (1907–82), an Austrian-born Canadian endocrinologist, differentiated between the unpleasant or harmful variety of STRESS called *dis-stress* (from the Latin *dis* = bad, as in dissonance, disagreement) and *eustress* (from the Greek *eu* = good, as in euphonia, euphoria). During both distress and EUSTRESS the body undergoes virtually the same nonspecific responses to various stimuli acting upon it. However, certain emotional factors, such as frustration and hostility are particularly likely to turn stress into dis-stress.

See also COPING; GENERAL ADAPTATION SYNDROME.

SOURCES:
Selye, Hans. *The Stress of Life,* rev. ed. New York: McGraw Hill, 1978.
———. *Stress Without Distress.* Philadelphia: Lippincott, 1974.

diversity Relates to any group of people that is mixed in terms of race, religion, ethnicity, or gender. Because diversity may be perceived as an approach to quotas in schools or in the WORKPLACE, the concept can be a source of stress for those involved. Stress can also arise between individuals from diverse backgrounds because of cultural differences. Respect for, and understanding of, these differences can make diversity a successful concept in business, religious, or community activities.

Conducting diversity awareness workshops is one way in which companies have introduced the idea of valuing personal differences. However, these workshops are only a first step in creating an environment in which previous prejudices, a major source of stress, will be erased and a true sensitivity to diverse employee needs will prevail.

See also ACCULTURATION; COMMUNICATION.

divorce The legal ending of a MARRIAGE and a situation in which all involved experience stressful times. Husband, wife, children, and even grandparents are affected by the dissolution of a marriage in the family. Divorce is a serious social problem in the United States—during the 1990s, about half of all marriages ended in divorce.

Women and men who seek divorce do so because they have any one or more of many stressors in their marriage, such as a poor sexual relationship, difficulties in communicating with each other, differences in goals, or financial problems. Feelings of failure are common when a marriage breaks up; lack of success in a marriage should not reflect on a sense of SELF-ESTEEM, but it does. While many divorced individuals learn from their experiences and bring new insights to new relationships, some of these will end in second or third divorces.

Divorced people are commonly angry with each other, feel that perhaps they have been exploited or treated badly, and suspect infidelities. Depending on what triggered the anger, it may not be easy to forget. However, if appropriately contained, one's anger will not interfere with adjusting to a new life.

According to Ada P. Kahn, in "Divorce: For Better Not For Worse," published by the Mental Health Association of Greater Chicago, studies show that when parents are unhappy, children do not feel that keeping the marriage together on their behalf is a gift. There is no advantage for children when parents stay in a marriage in which they are constantly stressed and cannot resolve basic issues.

Kahn advises telling children why you are getting a divorce, that it was a rational decision by both parties, deliberately and carefully undertaken with reluctance and with full recognition of how stressful it would be. Children have the right to know why, with an explanation suited to their age and level of understanding. Parents should try to communicate what divorce will mean for the children, specifically, how it will affect their visiting and living arrangements. They should be assured that they have parental support, permission to love both parents, and that both parents will continue to love them. Assurance that the children are not responsible for the rupture and that they are not responsible to heal the rupture should come from both parents. More complex explanations are in order in case of desertion or abuse.

As a consequence of divorce, many children feel a diminished sense of being parented, because their parents are less available, emotionally, physically, or both. Children may feel that they are losing both parents. This is an expected part of the divorce experience. In most instances, it is temporary, but in a significant number of families, unfortunately, it is a feeling that lasts a long time.

The most serious long-range effect is that children feel less protected in their growing-up years and become concerned that they will repeat their parents' mistakes of a failed man-woman relationship. To address this issue, parents should talk about it or be ready to talk when children ask questions. They should not continue to fight the battles after their divorce, and should never criticize former mates in front of the children. Parents should realize that they are role models after the divorce just as they were in the marriage.

Divorced individuals do marry again. However, according to the Center for the Family, Corte Madera, California, 60% of second marriages fail, particularly if one or more of the mates bring children into the marriage.

DATING and meeting new people after divorce brings stress and anxieties about acquiring a sexually transmitted disease, because of the prevalence of AIDS (ACQUIRED IMMUNE DEFICIENCY SYNDROME) and STDs (SEXUALLY TRANSMITTED DISEASES).

Rebuilding life after divorce may be stressful, complicated, and difficult. The best advice is to take one step at a time and start by choosing one step you really need or would like to take. Newly divorced people can seek out resources for their particular needs in their community where there are churches, synagogues, and community mental health agencies that may be able to help.

Divorce differs from annulment, in which a court declares that a marriage has been invalid from its beginning; reasons for annulment vary among states and countries.

See also COMMUNICATION; COPING; SEXUALLY TRANSMITTED DISEASES.

FOR FURTHER INFORMATION:
Center for the Family
5725 Paradise Drive (#300B)
Corte Madera, CA
Phone: (415) 924-5750

SOURCES:
Kahn, Ada P., and Linda Hughey Holt. *The A–Z of Women's Sexuality*. Alameda, Calif.: Hunter House Publications, 1992.
Wallerstein, Judith S. *Second Chances: Men, Women, and Children a Decade After Divorce*. New York: Ticknor & Fields, 1989.

dizziness A feeling of being unsteady, lightheaded, or faint and a sensation of spinning, turning, falling in space, or of standing still while objects around are moving. Some individuals experience dizziness in extremely stressful situations or as a phobic reaction. People who come into contact with an object that they fear may react with dizziness, weak knees, and sweaty palms; they also may fear fainting, falling, having a HEART ATTACK, or otherwise embarrassing themselves. Dizziness, as a result of a PHOBIA, usually disappears when the phobic object is removed or when the person gets to a place of safety.

During a phobic reaction or a panic attack, an individual may hyperventilate (breathe more than they need to). This results in a drop in the carbon dioxide in the blood, causing constriction of blood vessels in the brain, leading to dizziness or fainting. HYPERVENTILATION is sometimes caused by a physical condition, but is often the result of stress, anxiety, worry, or panic attacks.

Dizziness also may accompany seasickness. Some sailors advise keeping one's eyes on the horizon to give one a steady spot to watch. In most cases, dizziness disappears when the individual sets foot on land. Dizziness as a result of intoxication with alcohol usually subsides after a period of sleep.

There are prescription drugs as well as some over-the-counter remedies available to help control dizziness. When dizziness occurs often, a physician should be consulted, as it may be a symptom of a condition in need of medical treatment.

See also AGORAPHOBIA; PANIC ATTACKS AND PANIC DISORDER.

doctors   See PHYSICIANS.

domestic violence   Abuse of spouses, children, or parents in the home. This may take the form of wife-battering, child abuse, INCEST, or abusing elders. All of these situations are extremely stressful to the victims as well as others in the family. The abuser may behave violently as a response to particular stressors in his or her life.

Domestic violence happens in all strata of society, and there are many more cases than official records indicate because it is a subject often covered up out of fear and shame. Characteristics of persons who are victims of family violence include ANXIETY, powerlessness, GUILT, and lack of SELF-ESTEEM.

Professionals who treat victims of family violence are concerned with getting the victims, usually women or children, away from the abuser and into therapy before the abuse becomes too severe and additional stressors arise. Some perpetrators as well as victims of family violence compound their difficulties with use of alcohol or drugs.

Battered women

Battered women are victims of physical assault by husbands, boyfriends, or lovers. Battering may include physical abuse, some-times for purposes of sexual gratification, such as breaking bones, burning, whipping, mutilation, and other sadistic acts. Generally, however, battering is considered part of a syndrome of abusive behavior that has very little to do with sexual issues. Drug and alcohol-related problems are more common among families with battering behaviors. Women who select and choose to remain in abusive relationships were also often abused as children. Many women stay in such relationships without reporting the abuse and without seeking counseling. Batterers often were abused themselves as children.

Women who are abused by their husbands or boyfriends not only sustain injuries from physical beatings but also suffer from many mental and emotional scars, including POST-TRAUMATIC STRESS DISORDER (PTSD), DEPRESSION and anxiety.

Help for battered wives is available. First, physical protection, often provided by women's shelters within the community, must be assured for the woman and her children. Second, social support services must provide economic protection, since women often stay in abusive relationships due to lack of practical economic alternatives. Finally, psychotherapeutic intervention should be aimed at both batterer and victim to trace antecedents of the violent behavior, correct substance abuse problems, and substitute positive COPING mechanisms for violent behavior patterns.

Most abused women do not seek help until beatings become severe and have occurred over a period of time, often two to three years. Some women are too embarrassed or believe that if they report the beating to police they will not be taken seriously. The majority of women who seek help because of family violence are between ages 20 and 60. In 75% of households in which abuse takes place, the husband or boyfriend is an alcoholic or on drugs.

A study at the University of California-San Francisco during 1992 indicated many details about living conditions and circumstances surrounding battered women. According to the study, the battered women who were interviewed did not depend on their violent partner for most of their financial support; almost 30% had jobs and many had income from families, welfare, social security, and other sources.

Among other findings, 40% of the women had to be hospitalized for injuries. One in three of the women had been attacked with a weapon, most often a knife or a club; four had been shot. One in 10 was pregnant when beaten; 30% of the group said they had been abused before they were pregnant. In about half the cases, the husbands or boyfriends drank heavily or abused drugs; 86% of the women had been beaten at least once before.

According to Kevin J. Fullin, M.D., St. Catherine's Hospital, Kenosha, Wisconsin, as many as one in two women has suffered from an episode of domestic violence sometime in her life. Due to such a high rate, physicians and healthcare workers are developing new approaches to domestic violence in order to increase its detection. The goal is to properly identify anyone who comes to a hospital with a domestic abuse situation. The woman, child, or adult who is suspected of being abused is questioned in a non-threatening, non-judgmental manner without any other family members present. The goal of this confidential questioning is to find the real cause of the problem and do something to stop the abuse.

Battered child syndrome
Battered child syndrome includes rough physical handling by caregivers resulting in injuries to the baby or child. This can result in failure to grow, a disability, and sometimes death of the baby or child. Studies have shown that parents who repeatedly injure or beat their babies and children have poor CONTROL of their own feelings of AGGRESSION, or may have been abused or psychologically rejected as children.

WHAT BATTERED WOMEN CAN DO

- Leave the scene of the abuse; stay with a friend or family member who will be supportive emotionally and provide a safe haven.
- To eliminate confrontation, leave the home when the abuser is absent.
- Take bank records, children's birth certificates, cash, and other important documents along with clothing and personal items.
- If possible, photograph or videotape any consequences of abuse, such as injuries to yourself or damage to the home. These could be important for possible later court proceedings.
- Call the police and file a police report. Obtain an order of protection as soon as possible.
- Seek counseling for yourself and your children; join a SUPPORT GROUP along with others who have been victims of family violence.

The syndrome is found among people with stable social and financial backgrounds as well as in parents who are mentally unstable, alcoholic, or drug-dependent. In most states, laws require physicians to report instances of suspected, willfully inflicted injury among young patients. When it appears that the child will continue to be battered, steps are taken to remove the child from the home.

Legal rights of domestic violence victims
Until the latter years of the 20th century, police and the legal system often viewed domestic violence as a private matter and not a crime. Now, in many states, the police may arrest a batterer if there is evidence of abuse. Civil actions might include legal separation, child custody, child support, and divorce. One common civil action in cases of domestic violence is the temporary restraining order, which involves making a complaint and going to a hearing to obtain a legal document that limits how close a person may come to a woman and her children.

A criminal complaint can be filed in addition to or instead of civil actions. A criminal complaint involves a police investigation, and if enough evidence is found, may lead to an arrest and involvement of the judicial system.

See also ADDICTION; ALCOHOLISM; CODEPENDENCY.

FOR FURTHER INFORMATION:
Batterers Anonymous
1269 N.E. St.
San Bernardino, CA 92405
Phone: (714) 355-1100

National Coalition Against Domestic Violence
P.O. Box 34103
Washington, DC 20043-4103
Phone: (212) 638-6388

National Council on Child Abuse and Family
  Violence
1155 Connecticut Avenue NW
Washington, DC 20036
Phone: (202) 429-6695

SOURCES:
Kahn, Ada P., and Jan Fawcett. *The Encyclopedia of Mental Health.* New York: Facts On File, 1993.
Shannon, Kari. "Domestic Violence Detection at St. Catherine's." *Chicago HealthCare,* December 1991.

Dossey, Larry (1940–) Dallas, Texas, physician, lecturer, and author of *Healing Words (The Power of Prayer and the Practice of Medicine), Meaning and Medicine (Lessons from a Doctor's Tales of Breakthrough and Healing),* and other books. Much of his writing is directed toward helping readers relieve stress in their lives.

He believes that American society is in the grip of a "time sickness" epidemic. He defines this as a disorder in which we feel so overloaded and stressed by schedules that our bodies rebel and we respond to all ringing bells—alarm clocks, telephones—as signals to get ready for action. Our bodies pump stress hormones, which in turn suppress immune response. Cholesterol and stomach acidity is increased. "The end result," he says, "is frequently some form of 'hurry' sickness, expressed as heart disease, high blood pressure, insomnia, irritable bowel syndrome."

About Dossey's best selling books, a reviewer in *Whole Earth Review* (Fall 1993) said: "Modern medicine is based on standardization, the assumption that the criteria for symptoms, prognoses and curative practices can be measured and objectified. Individuals with a set of symptoms are expected to be helped by the same course of treatment, and the percentage who will recover can be predicted. Dossey brings us quite a different perspective, one which taken to its extreme would create a totally different and ultimately individualized medicine."

Dossey emphasizes that meaning, or the significance that one attaches to an interpretation of an event, has been overlooked in modern medical practice. Significant life events that are highly stressful and are known to contribute to susceptibility to disease, such as death of a spouse or loss of a job, can have a very different subjective meaning. Each interpretation of a similar event will bring about stress in different ways.

In his writings, Dossey suggests many possible avenues toward stress reduction and relief, including PRAYER and MEDITATION. He believes that therapies should be judged according to their effects and under conditions in which they work. For example, experiments with people have shown that prayer and meditation positively affected HIGH BLOOD PRESSURE, wounds, heart attacks, HEADACHES and anxiety. He believes in utilizing our powers of intuition and telepathy as well as meditation to deepen RELAXATION. Also, he encourages becoming aware of the unconscious part of ourselves in order to summon all the healing powers within ourselves and others, when we need them to overcome stressful situations.

Dossey suggests that prayer and standard medical approaches can be used together; he does not suggest that prayer be relied on instead of other therapies. He insists that science and religion stand side by side, respecting the domain of each other and preserving the highest aims of each.

His view of the mind is that it is not localized or confined to the body, but extends outside it. This suggests that mind is capable of affecting not only one's own body but also other bodies that may be far away; this lends an explanation to Dossey's concept of the effectiveness of distant prayer.

He has co-chaired a panel on MIND-BODY CONNECTIONS at the National Institutes of Health's OFFICE OF ALTERNATIVE MEDICINE. When referring to several eras of medical practice, he says Era I was and remains based on the materialist theory of disease and its treatment. Era II discovered the mind/body link; it conceives mind as implicated in healing, though it understands mind as local, existing within the body and limited by the body's position in time and space. Era III medicine, he continues, expands this understanding by focusing on how the powers of the mind work between people.

See also ALTERNATIVE THERAPIES; FAITH; PLACEBO EFFECT.

SOURCES:

Dossey, Larry. *Healing Words: The Power of Prayer and the Practice of Medicine.* San Francisco: Harper, 1993.

———. *Meaning and Medicine: Lessons from a Doctor's Tales of Breakthrough and Healing.* New York: Bantam/Doubleday, 1991.

———. *Prayer Is Good Medicine.* San Francisco: Harper, 1996.

downsizing Refers to employee cutbacks (LAYOFFS) and not rehiring for jobs that employees have vacated. Downsizing is stressful for the managers who make the decision as to who will go and who will stay and for the employees who are asked to leave.

In many cases, the stress involved in downsizing leaves workers with ANGER and is a possible trigger for DEPRESSION. To help workers avoid and/or handle anger, such issues as job category, seniority, and performance must be addressed. Equally important issues include treatment of dismissed employees, positive employee recommendations, and dealing with surviving employees.

Most companies now consider downsizing or employee cutbacks as a routine part of business. As they become more and more an everyday occurrence, the very idea of downsizing brings stress to many workers. In 1994, an American Management Association (AMA) survey of 713 companies showed that 30% of companies reporting a downsizing planned to repeat the exercise. Respondees gave business downturn, improved staff utilization, transfer of production or work, automation or other new technology, merger or acquisition, and plant or office obsolescence as reasons for downsizing.

With downsizing, workers at all levels are affected, no matter how long they may have worked for the organization, no matter how well they perform their jobs or how effectively they have managed their budgets and staffs. Of the 430,000 identified jobs eliminated by AMA respondents since July 1988, half belonged to hourly workers and half belonged to salaried workers.

Signs of impending downsizing include a hiring freeze, pessimistic budget projections, closed-door meetings, decreasing sales, and consolidation of operations. Middle managers should be particularly alert to requests for department justification and work plans based on budget reductions.

See also JOB CHANGE; WORKPLACE.

SOURCE:

Meyer, G.J. *Executive Blues: Down and Out in Corporate America.* New York: Franklin Square Press, 1995.

dreams Mental activity that occurs when one is asleep. Some people enjoy their dreams while others find them stressful, particularly if they are scary or otherwise unpleasant.

Dreaming usually involves many vivid sensory images, such as sight, sound, motion, touch, and even smell or taste. For many people, dreaming at night is a continuation of mental impressions, ideas, and thoughts from that day, and there are no deeply hidden meanings. They may be sorting out events from the day in a distorted way because the mind is not conscious and awake. For others, images in dreams may be symbols of unconscious thoughts that may mean nothing, or may refer to many things. For example, for some people, water may symbolize birth. There are individuals who believe that through interpretations of symbols in a dream, people can have a better understanding of how best to cope with life's stresses. However, symbols are highly individual matters.

Dreaming occurs during periods of rapid eye movement (REM) sleep, which last for about 20 minutes and occur four or five times a night. SLEEP deprivation, stress, DEPRESSION, and drug abuse often interfere with REM time. Necessary biochemical changes occur at REM and non-REM times that are essential for normal daytime functioning. People who are awakened during periods of REM sleep usually can report their dreams clearly. Those who awaken normally may not remember dreams at all, or only in a fragmentary way.

People have tried to give meanings to dreams for thousands of years. Many interpretations of dreams have come forth, from Joseph in Egypt to Sigmund Freud in Vienna. Much folklore has developed around the subject of dreams, some of which may add to or relieve the dreamer's stress.

See also JOURNALING.

FOR FURTHER INFORMATION:
Association for the Study of Dreams
P.O. Box 1600
Vienna, VA 22183
Phone: (703) 242-8888

Community Dream Sharing Network
P.O. Box 8032
Hicksville, NY 11802
Phone: (516) 735-1969; (516) 796-9455

SOURCES:
Delaney, Gayle. *Living Your Dreams.* San Francisco: Harper & Row, 1988.
Faraday, Ann. *The Dream Game.* New York: HarperCollins, 1990.

driving   See AUTOMOBILES; RANDOM NUISANCES.

drug therapy   See DEPRESSION; PHARMACOLOGICAL APPROACH.

durable power of attorney   See DEATH.

dysfunctional family   This term indicates that the developmental and emotional needs of one or more members of a FAMILY are not being met, leading to STRESS for all concerned.

Research has shown that people raised in dysfunctional families—where alcohol or drug abuse, emotional or physical abuse, neglect, incest, marital conflict, or severe workaholism were present—carry varying vestiges of these problems well into adulthood. These issues generally surface in intimate RELATIONSHIPS and on the job. Since these are places where other kinds of stress can be found, unresolved family issues can compound the stressors.

People from dysfunctional families usually are excellent employees. They are hard workers, dependable, resourceful, loyal, kind—attributes that have helped them survive their earlier experiences. However, because people from dysfunctional families have often not learned to feel good about themselves, they may have poor SELF-ESTEEM, compensate by working longer hours than others, try for PERFECTION, and take on more than they can handle. This leads to even more stress, which impacts their job performance and physical health.

Causes of dysfunctional relationships
Often, the basic problem is lack of COMMUNI-CATION or poor communications between family members, even though they live in the same household. An example of a dysfunctional family is one in which there is marital conflict between the parents that results in their young son showing signs of aggressive behavior in school. The family may come to the attention of a school nurse because of the behavior problems of the child, which may be a symptom of the dysfunction of the family at home. The parents may be unaware that their behavior is causing a great deal of stress for the child.

In a dysfunctional family, there is little emphasis on encouraging each child to develop AUTONOMY. An example is a family that expects its adolescent child to obey curfew rules appropriate for a younger child.

Dysfunctional families usually do not communicate constructively when they are having difficult times. For example, when a child becomes seriously ill, there may be little communication about the illness between family members, and this leads to unexpressed feelings of guilt. ALCOHOLISM and substance abuse tends to be a characteristic of dysfunctional families, as the substance abuser cannot be depended on to fulfill expectations.

Family therapy is helpful in improving life situations for members of dysfunctional families. In therapy, family members learn to improve their communication skills and learn new coping skills to deal with everyday problems as well as major life events.

See also AGGRESSION; COPING; INTIMACY; PSY-CHOTHERAPIES.

dysmenorrhea   See MENSTRUATION.

dyspareunia   Sexual intercourse that is painful for the woman. It causes extreme stress for both partners and may lead to avoidance of sexual intercourse and ultimately to the breakup of a relationship.

The first step in reducing the stress of pain during sexual intercourse for a woman is to discuss it with her partner. For some women, psychological factors play a part; once the pain has been experienced, the woman may fear recurrence of the pain. This happens to some women who have been abused as children or raped. Some of these women may fear pregnancy or acquiring a SEXUALLY TRANSMITTED DISEASE (STD) and are not able to relax during intercourse. Tension and anxiety, or a lack of adequate stimulation before actual penetration, may also contribute to pain during intercourse.

Psychological counseling or SEX THERAPY may be helpful. Medical diagnosis may reveal that the pain occurs for any of several reasons, including dryness of the vagina, tightness of the vaginal muscles, a vaginal infection, an infection of the urethra or urinary tract, or from a local irritation, such as from a spermicide or the material of a condom or diaphragm.

During foreplay (stimulation) before intercourse, the vaginal walls secrete a lubricating fluid that makes intercourse more comfortable. However, during breast feeding and after MENOPAUSE, many women find that secretions are not sufficient and a water-soluble jelly may be helpful as a lubricant. Hormone replacement therapy postmenopausally also helps to increase lubrication and thicken the skin of the vaginal wall.

A change in position during intercourse can help relieve pain for some women. They may feel discomfort when the penis contacts the cervix (the neck of the uterus) and can avoid discomfort by less deep penetration. A pain felt deep in the pelvis may be caused by endometriosis, ovarian tumors or cysts, or by some other condition that should be investigated and treated by a physician.

See also SEXUAL DIFFICULTIES; SEXUALITY; SEX-UAL RESPONSE CYCLE.

SOURCE:
Kahn, Ada P., and Linda Hughey Holt. *The A-Z of Women's Sexuality.* Alameda, Calif., Hunter House, 1992.

dysthymia A chronic and persistent mood disturbance that has been present for at least two years and is characterized by relatively mild symptoms of DEPRESSION, such as low SELF-ESTEEM, difficulty in concentrating, feelings of hopelessness, loss of appetite, and difficulty in sleeping. This disturbance is a source of stress for the individuals and their families, employers, and coworkers because it limits participation and productivity.

Individuals who have dysthymia are usually chronically unhappy. Some develop major depression, improve, and then return to the milder state of dysthymia. The coexistence of these mild and severe forms of depression is referred to as double depression. This condition is treatable; help is available from trained social workers, psychologists, and psychiatrists. In some cases, medications may be prescribed.

See also AFFECTIVE DISORDERS; PHARMACOLOGICAL APPROACH.

E

eating disorders Eating disorders involve compulsive misuse of food to achieve some desired physical and/or mental state. They are characterized by an intense fear of being fat and severe weight loss and may result in ill health and psychological impairments.

People with eating disorders may be experiencing stress in some aspect of their lives, which they think will be improved by dieting in excess. They have low SELF-ESTEEM and a fear of fatness. When sufferers acknowledge their compulsive behavior, their stress is often expressed in feelings of DEPRESSION and a wish to commit SUICIDE. Sufferers typically hide their illness; when family, friends, or coworkers discover their illness, they try to help. Typically, people with eating disorders feel they don't deserve to be helped, and this creates a great deal of stress for all concerned.

Eating disorders share common addictive features with alcohol and drug abuse, but unlike alcohol and drugs, food is essential to human life and proper use of food is a central element of recovery.

Estimates indicate that there are eight million reported victims of eating disorders in the United States—seven million of them women (although the number of males is increasing) between the ages of 15 and 30. Eating disorders can be cured when the sufferer accepts treatment; an estimated 6% of all reported cases die.

Anorexia nervosa

Anorexia nervosa is a syndrome of self-starvation in which people willfully restrict intake of food out of fear of becoming fat, resulting in life-threatening weight loss. Anorexics (people who suffer from anorexia nervosa) "feel fat" even when they are at normal weight or when emaciated, deny their illness, and develop an active disgust for food. Deaths from anorexia nervosa are higher than from any other psychiatric illness.

Causes of anorexia vary widely. Many anorexics are part of a close family and have special relationships with their parents. They are highly conforming, anxious to please, and may be obsessional in their habits. There is speculation that girls who refrain from eating wish to remain "thin as a boy" in an effort to escape the burdens of growing up and assuming a female sexual and marital role. Another contribution to the increase in anorexia is contemporary society's emphasis on slimness as it relates to beauty. This is particularly prevalent in the fashion industry with its overly thin models. Most women diet at some time, particularly athletes and dancers, who seem more prone to the disorder than other women. In some cases, anorexia nervosa is a symptom of depression, personality disorder or even schizophrenia.

Symptoms include severe weight loss, wasting (cachexia), food preoccupation and rituals, amenorrhea (cessation of the menstrual period), and hyperactivity (constant exercising to lose weight). The anorexic may suffer from tiredness and fatigue, sensitivity to cold, and complain of hair loss.

Eating disorders sometimes result in other mental health disorders as well as depression. Individuals may suffer from withdrawal, mood swings, and feelings of shame and guilt. Both anorexics and bulimics develop rituals regarding eating and exercise. They often are perfectionists in habits, such as clothes and personal appearance, and have an "all or nothing" attitude about life.

Bulimia

Bulimia is characterized by recurrent episodes of binge eating followed by self-induced vomiting, vigorous exercise and/or laxative, and diuretic abuse to prevent weight gain. Most people view vomiting as a disagreeable experience, but to a bulimic, it is a means toward a desired goal.

Another eating disorder is bulimarexia, which is characterized by features of both anorexia nervosa and bulimia. Some individuals vacillate between anorexic and bulimic behaviors. After months and perhaps years of eating sparsely, the anorexic may crave food and begin to binge, but the fear of becoming overly fat leads her/him to vomit.

Bulimics may be of normal weight, slightly underweight, or extremely thin. Binging and vomiting may occur as much as several times a day. In severe cases, it may lead to dehydration and potassium loss, causing weakness and cramps.

A cycle of addiction

Behaviors of anorexics and bulimics are driven by the cycle of addiction. There is an emotional emptiness that in turn leads to the psychological pain of low self-esteem. The individual looks for a way to dull the pain by using addictive agents (starvation or bingeing), which usually results in the need to purge or medical problems. Finally, suffering from guilt, shame and self-hate, the individual goes back to a routine of starvation and/or bingeing and purging.

Treatment

Medical problems caused by the disorder should be diagnosed and managed first. When the medical complications are severe, an individual may be hospitalized to stabilize physical functions and monitor nutritional intake. Often, small feedings are carefully spaced because the patient cannot handle very much food at one time. In some cases, antidepressant medications are begun during the hospital stay.

In the late 1990s, treatment of eating disorders can cost an excess of $30,000 a month. Many patients need repeated hospitalizations and can require treatment extending two years or more. Some therapists believe that anorexia/bulimia is never cured but merely arrested. However, some behaviorists believe that weight gain indicates a cure. There are several therapies used in treating the eating disorders; these should be discussed with the individual's therapist. A major part of therapy for eating disorders involves helping the individual rethink her/his perception of BODY IMAGE, because often it is perceived flaws that led to the eating disorder in the first place.

Many people with eating disorders are treated on an outpatient basis. There may be weekly counseling that includes individual and group sessions for outpatients and family, marital therapy, and specialized support for eating disorders.

FOR FURTHER INFORMATION:
National Association of Anorexia Nervosa and
    Associated Disorders (ANAD)
Box 7
Highland Park, IL 60035
Phone: (847) 831-3438

Anorexia Nervosa and Related Eating Disorders
P.O. Box 5102
Eugene, OR 97405
Phone: (503) 344-1144

BASH (Bulimia Anorexia Self Help)
c/o Deaconess Hospital
6150 Oakland Avenue
St. Louis, MO 63139
Phone: (800) 762-3334

SOURCE:
Kasvikis, Y.G., et al. "Past History of Anorexia Nervosa in Women with Obsessive-Compulsive Disorder." *International Journal of Eating Disorders* 5, no. 6 (1985).

ejaculation   The emission of semen from the penis at orgasm, usually during intercourse or masturbation. Ejaculation disorders are conditions in which ejaculation occurs before or very soon after penetration, does not occur at all, or in which the ejaculate is forced back into the bladder. Because ejaculation disorders interfere with the completion and enjoyment of sexual intercourse, they are very stressful for men as well as for their partners, who do not always know how to help and may feel some blame.

Early ejaculation is ejaculation occurring within 10 to 60 seconds after penile penetration of the vagina and is also known as premature ejaculation. It is the most common sexual problem in men, often because of overstimulation or anxiety and stress about sexual performance.

Inhibited ejaculation is a rare condition in which erection is normal but ejaculation does not occur. It may be psychological or it may be a result of a complication of other disorders or drug use.

Retrograde ejaculation occurs when the valve at the base of the bladder fails to close during an ejaculation. This forces the ejaculate backward into the bladder. Retrograde ejaculation may be the result of a neurological disease or can occur from pelvic surgery, surgery on the neck of the bladder, or after a prostatectomy.

Treatment for ejaculation difficulties may begin with a visit to a physician, a urologist, or a sex therapist.

See also SEX THERAPY; SEXUAL DIFFICULTIES; SEXUAL RESPONSE CYCLE.

elderly parents   By the year 2050, estimates indicate that the elderly population age 85 and over will be 18.9 million, equaling those at present age 65 to 69. While people are living longer, healthier lives, care for the very elderly has become a common and stressful issue for society at large and for families. The decision to take a more active role in their par-

ents' lives is one of stress for many middle-aged children.

Role reversal
Adult children should be attentive to changes in their parents' judgment and ability to take care of themselves and their affairs. To overcome the awkwardness of the role reversal, children should talk to their parents, find out how they perceive their circumstances, and discuss mutual concerns. They can agree to explore the situation further and work together toward a mutually agreeable approach. If the parents do not acknowledge problems, the adult children can keep the dialogue going by asking how they would advise a friend in similar circumstances. This technique may help everyone focus more clearly on immediate needs and solutions as well as longer-range solutions.

The more elderly the parent becomes, the more dependent he or she becomes. Adult children may face a range of other more stressful emotions, and possibly the reappearance of long-forgotten feelings. In some families, they may have always felt grateful to their parents and welcome the opportunity to repay them. In other families, they may find their parents' dependency too stressful to accept and feel overburdened, resentful, or guilty about their inability or unwillingness to help.

Taking on more responsibility for one's parents is an evolving process. Sometimes it may be one or another sibling who does not want to accept the fact that the parent is becoming dependent or differs with the way problems are approached. In time, children and parents will become more comfortable with the role reversal and move toward new patterns of meeting everyday situations.

Physical care
As people age, they are more susceptible to a variety of physical disorders. Some conditions such as anemia often result from a poor diet or an underactive thyroid gland; both conditions can be diagnosed and treated. Failing

vision and hearing, also thought to be attributable to old age, may be rectified by removing a cataract or using a hearing aid. It is necessary, but stressful, that CAREGIVERS remain alert to signs of illness and find the time to take their elderly parent in for regular checkups and visits to the doctor when symptoms appear.

Emotional care

In general, the elderly as a group are as mentally healthy as the general population. Still, there are some illnesses specific to this age group that can affect their behavior, judgment, and memory. For example, elderly parents may be overly fearful of losing CONTROL of what is going on around them. Symptoms may be mild, such as sadness, loneliness, irritability, or confusion, or they may be severe, such as DEPRESSION, agitation, or delusions. Common causes of depression in the elderly are isolation and feelings of not being wanted or needed. They are afraid of being a nuisance and at the same time fear being put away in a nursing home even more.

Elderly parents, feeling the stress of losing their independence, may direct their HOSTILITY toward the adult child. Making them a part of family plans and activities, and encouraging them to attend a senior citizen or day-care centers, can provide the socialization they need and, at the same time, make them feel like useful members of society.

Adult children should watch for mental health symptoms such as forgetfulness and paranoia in their elderly parent and get appropriate help. There are specialists in geriatric mental health who can be consulted.

Living arrangements

As parents age, they may decide that it is in their own best interest to discuss and review their living options. Most older people, despite increased physical or mental frailty, want to live independently as long as possible. They may want to live near family members so that help with daily activities and personal care is at hand. While this type of arrangement may be ideal for the elderly person, it places a great deal of stress and strain on the family. Others may want to live with their families, ideally in a separate part of the house where they can maintain their independence. Two or three (maybe four) generations living under one roof can prove to be very stressful for most families.

Today, there are many other living arrangements for the elderly, ranging from independent residential living in adult communities, assisted living in apartments where some meals and health and social programs are provided, shared housing in the elderly person's own home or in a communal living arrangement, plus skilled nursing and rehabilitation centers. Social workers usually advise not rushing changes in living, unless needs are immediate and obvious.

When difficult questions such as choosing living arrangements arise, all people, the elderly included, may not be ready to make decisions. They may want more time before talking about the problem again. Adult children should consider involving others, such as grandchildren, trusted friends, or their doctor in discussions.

Advance directives

As parents age, they may begin to think about DEATH and whether doctors should use life-prolonging interventions when they are ill. Advance directives are arrangements that can help ease the ethical dilemma of decision making when facing a parent's major illness or prolonged disability. Advance directives are legal documents signed by the parent that direct adult children to do what the parents desire in the matter of using life-prolonging medical technology.

Reducing stress as a caregiver

Many adult children find that they cannot cope with their elderly parents alone. They may have few or no other family members with whom to share the caregiving responsi-

---

PREVENT FUTURE STRESS: TIPS FOR TALKING WITH AN ELDERLY PARENT

- Be patient in starting your discussion.
- Set goals for each discussion. Be realistic.
- Discuss his/her wishes; permit parents to maintain their dignity and keep a sense of control.
- Use specific examples: "I've been concerned about your safety at home since your neighbor, Maggie, broke her hip."
- Suggest some options; explain advantages and disadvantages.
- Make some specific short-term as well as long-term plans to give both of you peace of mind.

---

bilities. If there are siblings, they may live too far away or have heavy demands on their time.

The idea of sharing responsibilities can be important for the major caregiver. It also increases the number of people to whom parents continue to relate. To get some ideas about available services in the community, such as day care, meals, recreation, living arrangements, and respite help, consult the local Office on Aging. Many such programs feature sliding-scale fees. Additionally, community mental health programs have specialists in the care of older adults who can provide counsel and references to SUPPORT GROUPS to help share concerns and practical approaches.

For adult children whose parents live away from them, local social workers are affiliated with networks that can help them arrange for long-distance care.

See also AGING.

SOURCE:
Kahn, Ada P. "Becoming a Parent to Your Parents." Chicago: Mental Health Association of Greater Chicago, 1988.

electroconvulsive therapy (ECT)   See DEPRESSION.

ELISA test (enzyme-linked immunosorbent assay)   Laboratory test commonly used in the diagnosis of infectious diseases; a highly sensitive screening test for evidence of the presence of HIV antibodies, considered a causative agent of AIDS (ACQUIRED IMMUNODEFICIENCY SYNDROME). Tests found positive by this procedure are usually subsequently tested with another confirmatory assay (after the late 1980s, the Western blot confirmatory assay). Waiting for test results is a stressful time. Learning about a positive test result causes considerable stress and increasing dilemmas for many individuals. Therefore, appropriate counseling and expert interpretation should be done before and after test results are known.

See also CHRONIC ILLNESS; HUMAN IMMUNODEFICIENCY VIRUS.

FOR FURTHER INFORMATION:
CAIN (Computerized AIDS Information Network)
San Francisco AIDS Foundation
54 Tenth St.
San Francisco, CA 94103
Phone: (415) 864-4376

SIECUS (Sex Information and Education Council of the U.S.)
130 W. 42nd St. (Suite 2500)
New York, NY 10036
Phone: (212) 819-9770

National AIDS Information Clearinghouse
Centers for Disease Control
Box 6003
Rockville, MD 20850
Phone: (800) 458–5231

emotions   A range of feelings that humans experience. These may include joy, happiness, sadness, gladness, despair, loving, disgust, fear, surprise, or many others. These feelings are unique to each individual, and in periods of stress, many emotions may become evident.

Researchers say that emotional feelings begin before the age of two months (when the baby first smiles) and continue to develop as the infant advances into childhood. Developing emotional feelings is an important factor in having good mental health in later life. Researchers have found that lack of loving attention and a trusting relationship during infancy may result in emotional deprivation. Children who are emotionally deprived often crave attention and experience a great deal of stress in COPING with their frustration.

As individuals grow older, their emotional reactions are influenced by past experiences. For example, before a job interview, there may be feelings of stress and nervousness; before a happy occasion there may be feelings of joy or gladness mixed with the stress of not knowing what lies ahead. Sweaty palms, red face, nervous tic, weak knees, or rapid heartbeat are some of the indications that individuals are under stress from their emotions.

The term "emotional problem" or "emotional disorder" is applied to many mental health concerns; how people express their emotions is an important aspect of mental health. For example, many emotional responses such as nervousness, LAUGHTER, CRYING, and elation are considered within the range of normal. However, when responses are out of the range of normal, such as pervasive sadness in DEPRESSION, mental health is threatened.

The term "emotional charge" refers to a stressful build-up of feelings stored in the body and mind. An emotionally charged discussion is one in which one or more of the participants have a built-up store of emotions and "let loose" those feelings; often the feelings have nothing to do with the discussion at hand.

Self-help for emotional problems

Emotional Health Anonymous is a national self-help program that provides support to men and women who experience emotional problems and illnesses. The self-help groups of EHA use a modified version of the 12 steps to recovery of Alcoholics Anonymous to help participants during and after their crisis periods. Founded in 1970, there are SUPPORT GROUPS throughout the United States as well as in other countries.

FOR FURTHER INFORMATION:
Emotional Health Anonymous
General Service Office
2430 San Gabriel Blvd.
San Gabriel, CA 91779
Phone: (818) 573-5482

SOURCE:
Padus, Emrika, ed. *The Complete Guide to Your Emotions and Your Health.* Emmaus, Pa.: Rodale Press, 1992.

emphysema   A chronic, obstructive lung disease that causes its victims to struggle for every breath they take. Because their lungs have lost much of their natural elasticity, people suffering from this disease cannot completely exhale the carbon dioxide that is trapped in their lungs. They experience extreme stress as they fight to replace the stale air with fresh oxygen. Family members who wish to be helpful feel useless and frustrated.

Emphysema develops over time. A chronic cough, often called a "smoker's cough," and a general shortness of breath are warning signs of emphysema. Sufferers do not realize they have it until the first signs of breathlessness appear, and by then delicate lung tissue may have been damaged excessively. Emphysema is a CHRONIC ILLNESS; there is no cure.

Some people who have emphysema require use of a portable oxygen tank, making traveling complicated and stressful because of the need to make arrangements to replenish their supplies periodically. For these individuals, because of the constant use of oxygen, eating out in restaurants or going to movies or concerts is also a stressful experience for them as well as their companions.

There is no known cause for emphysema, but most cases are related to cigarette SMOKING. Other contributing factors are air pollution and certain dusts and fumes. The disease is not caused by a germ or a virus and it is not an infectious or contagious disease.

Easing the stress of emphysema

Physicians can prescribe medications to relieve the feeling of breathlessness that accompanies this disease. There are also medicines that help clear mucus from the lungs and that can ward off chest infections. Also, emphysema patients can be taught by physical therapists to use their abdominal, chest, and diaphragmatic muscles to help them breathe more easily.

See also BREATHING.

FOR FURTHER INFORMATION:
Chicago Lung Association
1440 West Washington Blvd.
Chicago, IL 60607
Phone: (312) 243-2000

Employee Assistance Programs (EAPs) EAPs are designed to provide employees with help for stressful problems they face on or off the job; having an EAP in one's company is an important employee benefit. From the employer's point of view, whatever EAPs can do to help reduce stress for the employee, helps with the stress of running a business.

Employee Assistance Programs (EAPs) have been in existence for the past 50 years. Most authors trace their origin to the founding of Alcoholics Anonymous in 1935. In the 1960s and 1970s the scope of EAPs began to include help for employee problems such as DEPRESSION and other mental health concerns, drug abuse, DIVORCE, and other family difficulties. In the 1980s and 1990s, these programs have been expanded to include issues such as environmental stress, corporate culture, managing rapid technological change, and retraining.

According to the Employee Assistance Professional Association (Arlington, Virginia), in the early 1990s, about one-third of the nation's workers were covered by some form of an EAP and about 75% of the "Fortune 500" companies have EAPs.

How EAPs work

There are two types of EAP: internal and external. The majority of EAPs use indepen-dent companies that provide EAP services under a contract with the employer.

While the programs are geared to identifying employees whose personal problems may adversely affect their job performance, they also take a proactive stance in helping employees avoid problems before they occur. For example, companies are offering their employees seminars on stress reduction, PARENTING, adolescents and drugs, exercise, health, and diet.

EAPs provide referrals to appropriate professional services for employees and their immediate families. Confidentiality is assured; most employees would not use an EAP if they thought their problems would be revealed.

Employers implement EAPs for a variety of reasons. One is the skyrocketing costs related to providing a medical benefits program; another is the huge cost attributed to downtime due to employee alcohol addiction and mental illness. A four-year study of mental health care received by employees of the McDonnell Douglas Corporation estimated that the company could have saved $5.1 million over three years if those employees who did not seek treatment had done so. Employees who used the EAP for chemical dependency also lost 44% fewer workdays and filed fewer medical claims than those who did not.

Through its EAPs, Hewlett-Packard offers stress management courses to its 56,000 U.S. employees. Programs range from learning coping skills to dealing with teenage drug abuse. Additionally, Hewlett-Packard offers its employees physical activities—membership in health clubs and on-site weight rooms, basketball courts, jogging tracks, and Nautilus equipment—as a means of stress reduction and an avenue toward healthier lives. Saturn Corporation, an automobile manufacturer headquartered in Tennessee, provides one-on-one counseling by specially trained health care specialists, much of which is stress-related. E.I. Dupont, the Delaware chemical manufacturer, takes an individualized approach to helping its employees deal with stress.

See also JOB CHANGE; JOB SECURITY; WORKPLACE.

empty nest syndrome Situation in which children have grown up and left home; a source of stress experienced by many middle-aged parents. Typically, the syndrome seems to affect women more than men, and particularly women whose lives have focused on their children at the expense of engaging in activities for themselves. For these women, the empty nest syndrome can be a mild form of DEPRESSION that occurs after the children have left. Such women (and men, too, to some extent) no longer feel needed and feel a void in their life.

On the other hand, there are many middle-aged couples who view their children leaving home with a sense of relief and fulfillment at having accomplished a major life task. Many empty nesters, particularly women, return to work, take on volunteer activities in their community, enroll in classes, or engage in new HOBBIES for which they previously had no time.

See also MENOPAUSE.

enabler See CODEPENDENCY.

end-of-life care There is need for discussion and physician education in the area of health care at the end of life, according to a report of a study by the Robert Wood Johnson Foundation released in 1995. Persons near DEATH and their family members often experience extreme stress because of use or nonuse of medical procedures and lack of communication with their health care practitioners.

Also in 1995, the American Medical Association established the Task Force on Quality of Care at the End of Life, "To aid physicians in identifying when in the care-giving process, a transition in care needs may occur, and to identify actions that can be taken to improve the quality of life for those facing the end of life."

Ethical considerations
In a background paper, the American Medical Association's Task Force reported that end-of-life issues have always been fraught with problems that society as a whole has not yet addressed. Through their close relationships with their patients, physicians continue to hold a significant role in how people address these issues. Assuming patients do not misunderstand the prognosis and treatment options and they are not suffering from a treatable form of DEPRESSION, physicians in virtually all cases are morally obligated to abide by the competent patient's directions in the provision or stoppage of life-sustaining treatment. Physicians have an obligation to relieve pain and suffering and to promote dignity and AUTONOMY of dying patients in their care. This includes providing effective palliative treatment, even though it may foreseeably hasten death.

The AMA also is developing a working definition of "futile treatment" that physicians will be able to use in consultation with patients and their families when intensive care is requested and the physician does not believe such treatment has a reasonable chance of benefiting the patient.

Euthanasia and physician-assisted suicide
While competent patients generally retain autonomy in end of life decisions, this does not extend to requests for euthanasia or physician-assisted SUICIDE. Dire social implications are inherent in these issues, and they pose a serious risk of abuse that is virtually uncontrollable, according to the AMA background paper. Such practices are ethically prohibited. They are fundamentally inconsistent with the physician's role as healer, and they could contribute to erosion of the patient/physician relationship.

Importance of end-of-life issues
Patients deserve full information about their clinical status, honest assessment of prognosis, and education about potential treatment options, including palliative and hospice care. Physicians should encourage patients to consider their attitudes and beliefs about health care and quality of life prior to a crisis. They should advocate completion of advance directives, a signed paper that states the patient's wishes as to prolonging life. At the same time, medicine recognizes its responsibility to take actions to enhance the decision-making ability of the medical/health care team that is ethically, morally, and professionally trained and can be entrusted to provide care for patients at the end of life.

To increase understanding and use of advance directives, in late 1995 the AMA took action to familiarize physicians with the patient guide jointly released in October 1995 by the AMA, the American Association of Retired Persons (AARP) and the American Bar Association (ABA): *Shape Your Health Care Future and Health Care Advance Directives.*

See also ELDERLY PARENTS.

SOURCE:
Background paper, American Medical Association, November 21, 1995.

endogenous depression See EXOGENOUS DEPRESSION.

endorphins Group of substances formed within the body that relieve PAIN and STRESS. Endorphins have a chemical structure similar to morphine. Since the early 1970s, researchers have understood that morphine acts at specific sites called opiate receptors in the brain, spinal cord, and at other nerve endings. From this knowledge, they identified small peptide molecules produced by cells in the body that also act at opiate receptors. These morphine-like substances were named endorphins, short for endogenous morphines.

Effects of endorphins are noted, for example, in accident victims, who feel no initial pain after a traumatic injury, or in marathon runners, who do not feel muscle soreness until they complete their race. In addition to their effect on pain, endorphins are considered involved in controlling the body's response to stress, regulating contractions of the intestinal wall, and in determining mood.

Addiction and tolerance to narcotic analgesics, such as morphine, are thought to be due to or to cause suppression of the body's production of endorphins. Withdrawal symptoms that occur when effects of morphine wear off may be caused by a lack of these natural analgesics. Conversely, ACUPUNCTURE is thought to produce pain relief partly by stimulating release of endorphins. LAUGHTER and EXERCISE are also said to promote endorphins.

See also MEDITATION; RUNNER'S HIGH.

enuresis See BEDWETTING.

environment The stresses caused by the environment are a reality of life today. In cities throughout the United States, there is a rising number of days when the Pollution Standard Index (PSI), which is a combined reading of five major pollutants—particulate matter, sulfur dioxide, carbon monoxide, ozone, and nitrogen dioxide—goes beyond acceptable standards. In fact, PSI can fluctuate from as few as three to a high well over 200 in any given year. Difficulties in breathing, runny eyes, and light-headedness, all sources of STRESS for the sufferer, are just some of the symptoms caused by bad air.

Inside the home or WORKPLACE, environmental hazards continue to prevail. It is estimated that up to 15% of the population is sensitive to indoor pollutants, which may be 10 times more concentrated than in nearby outdoor air. Some chemicals found in and around the household and workplace are pesticides, permanent press fabrics, gas stove fumes, car exhaust, and particle board. Even water causes environmental illnesses; symptoms range from mild to disabling and are often nonspecific. Every part of the body can be affected by flu-like headaches, muscle aches, and fatigue, or more debilitating food intolerance and central nervous system problems such as memory loss, confusion, and DEPRESSION.

See also CLIMATE: RANDOM NUISANCES; SICK BUILDING SYNDROME.

FOR FURTHER INFORMATION:
National Coalition Against the Misuse of
  Pesticides
530 Seventh Street SE
Washington, DC 20003
Phone: (202) 543-5450

National Pesticide Telecommunication Network
Texas Tech University Health Sciences Center
School of Medicine (Room S-129), Thompson Hall
Texas Tech University
Lubbock, TX 79409
Phone: (800) 858-7378

National Safety Council
1121 Spring Lake Drive
Itasca, IL 60143-3201
Phone: (708) 285–1121

National Safe Workplace Institute
1121 Spring Lake Drive
Itasca, IL 60143–3201
Phone: (708) 285-1121

SOURCE:
Altman, Roberta. *The Complete Book of Home Environmental Hazards.* New York: Facts On File, 1990.

envy At one time or another, most people experience envy, a sense that something that others have is lacking in their lives. It is a stressful emotion and people usually are unwilling to admit to this feeling.

Envy can spring from many types of RELATIONSHIPS. However, it is the situations close at hand, involving FRIENDS, relatives, neighbors, or colleagues, that are generally more intense and generate envy. An ability to imagine or identify with an admired person's strengths is an intellectual asset, which may enable individuals to progress and better themselves. However, it becomes negative when the envious person remains fixated on another person's life and does not try to better his own life in a constructive way. Low SELF-ESTEEM produces envy, which often does not improve by the attainment of material things, status symbols, or fame. Healthy self-esteem makes envy unlikely and allows for creative identification with admired traits in others.

Modern American life is full of elements that create envy. For example, the mobile quality of society deemphasizes social class and creates the feeling that all things are possible for all people. This can create stressful feelings of FRUSTRATION, failure, and envy when expectations are thwarted. Mass media, especially TELEVISION, allows Americans to view "lifestyles of the rich and famous." ADVERTISING plays on feelings of envy with situations of "keeping up with the Joneses." The "Me Decade" of the 1980s, with its narcissism and "yuppie" lifestyle, created a climate in which envy flourished. Faced with a wide array of consumer products made available by high technology, it is always possible for individuals to feel that someone else has more than they do.

Because feelings of envy imply that someone is in a superior position and because most religions regard envy as sinful, people develop various ways of masking or suppressing it. To avoid expressing envy, some people develop superior and snobbish attitudes and gossip, criticize, or imply that the person to be envied is really the envious one.

See also HOSTILITY; JEALOUSY.

epinephrine Hormone secreted by the adrenal gland; also called ADRENALINE. It is a powerful stimulant and is sometimes referred to as the "emergency" hormone, as it effects the entire body. Epinephrine is responsible for reactions to FEAR and ANGER during stressful times, such as rapid heartbeat and the feeling of nervousness and agitation. Release of epinephrine throughout the body is part of the human body's FIGHT OR FLIGHT readiness response to danger or threat of danger.

As a last resort in cases of cardiac arrest, epinephrine is injected into the heart to start it beating again.

See also NEUROTRANMITTERS; STRESS.

ergonomics Ergonomics issues arise from particular jobs and include the repetitiveness of chores and the use of body force or posture to perform tasks, plus the environment in which the job is being done, such as poor lighting and ventilation, chair and desk heights, and level of noise. These issues can be viewed as stress carriers in the WORKPLACE and may be a cause of illness and injury resulting from job tasks.

See also CARPAL TUNNEL SYNDROME; REPETITIVE STRESS INJURY.

SOURCES:
Brown, Stephanie. *The HandBook: Preventing Computer Injury.* New York: Ergonomne, 1993.
Donkin, Scott W. *Sitting on the Job: How to Survive the Stresses of Sitting Down to Work—A Practical Handbook.* Boston: Houghton Mifflin, 1986.

estrogen replacement therapy See MENOPAUSE.

eustress Hans SELYE (1907–82), pioneer researcher in the field of STRESS, coined the term *eustress* to refer to "good stress." During eustress and DIS-STRESS (bad stress), the body undergoes virtually the same nonspecific responses to the various positive or negative stimuli acting upon it. However, he explained, the fact that eustress causes much less damage than dis-stress demonstrates that "how you take it" determines whether one can adapt successfully to change.

Examples of "good stress" include starting a new romance, getting married, having a baby, buying a house, getting a new job, or getting a raise at work. All these situations, as well as others, demand adaptations on the

part of the individual. Both *eustress* and *dis-stress* are part of the GENERAL ADAPTATION SYNDROME (G.A.S.), which Selye described as being the controlling factor in how people cope with stresses in their lives.

Later researchers (Holmes and Rahe) included several "good stress" situations in their Social Readjustment Rating Scale, which was designed to be a predictor of ill health. Sources of good stress included marriage, marital reconciliation, retirement, pregnancy, buying a house, and outstanding personal achievement.

See also COPING; HOMEOSTASIS; LIFE CHANGE SELF-RATING SCALE.

SOURCES:
Selye Hans. *The Stress of Life,* rev. ed. New York: McGraw Hill, 1978.
———. *Stress Without Distress.* Philadelphia: Lippincott, 1974.

euthanasia See END OF LIFE CARE.

exercise When individuals exercise to reduce their STRESS, they are usually participating in such cardiovascular activities as walking, jogging, weight lifting, using aerobic machines, and engaging in aerobic programs or sports such as skiing, swimming, cycling, or rowing. They participate in daily workouts and in weekends devoted to sports to combat the stress-related, physical tension in their lives at work or at home.

In addition to relieving stress and muscle tension, exercise helps boost energy levels, improves posture, lowers blood pressure, and helps control BREATHING. All of these things have a calming effect on individuals because they raise their pulse rate, increase the supply of blood and oxygen to muscles and vital organs, raise ENDORPHIN and metabolism levels, and rev up the immune system.

Exercise can have positive benefits that serve as a way to raise SELF-ESTEEM and increase CREATIVITY. According to Jeff Zwiefel, M.S., director of the National Exercise for Life

Institute, physical strength and stamina and a confident attitude are the main by-products of exercise. A study at Baruch College, New York, found that people who are stronger and more muscularly fit have a significantly better self-image than their peers. Psychological tests have indicated that those who exercise are more confident and emotionally stable, and outlive those who are sedentary.

The same positive effects of exercise on creativity were found by Joan C. Gondola at Baruch College, when she administered a test on female college students. One group had exercised 20 minutes before the test and the other group had not; the exercise group had more imaginative responses than those who had not. The boost in creativity may be attributed to the release of ADRENALINE and ENDORPHINS during exercise. The right side of the brain is stimulated by these chemicals, which control creative and intuitive processes.

See also BODY IMAGE.

FOR FURTHER INFORMATION:
Aerobics and Fitness Association of America
15250 Ventura Blvd. (Suite 310)
Sherman Oaks, CA 91403
Phone: (800) 445-5950

National Fitness Foundation
2250 E. Imperial Hwy. (Suite 412)
El Segundo, CA 90245
Phone: (213) 640-0145

exogenous depression Exogenous (reactive) DEPRESSION is a type of depression that originates outside the body. It is often caused by emotional factors, such as BURNOUT, GRIEF, or STRESS. Exogenous depression is contrasted with endogenous depression, which researchers believe may be caused by a chemical imbalance in the body.

exposure therapy   See BEHAVIOR THERAPY.

extramarital affairs   See ADULTERY.

extroversion   See INTROVERSION.

F

faith   See PRAYER; RELIGION.

faith healing   The essence of faith healing, for those who believe in it, is the strong conviction of "mind over matter." For some people, belief in faith healing contributes to relief of stress.

Historically, some faith healing takes place with the assistance of a "healer" who places hands on the individual who is then healed. For example, faith healing was and still is an accepted phenomenon of Roman Catholicism, where certain saints have been thought to have healing powers. The Catholic shrine at Lourdes has gained the reputation for causing miraculous recoveries. Native American religious practice includes rituals intended to promote healing of mental and physical ills. Faith healing is a central doctrine of Christian Scientists, who actively discourage reliance on doctors and conventional medicine. Today, there is a renewed interest in faith healing brought about by the resurgence of the fundamental and Pentecostal religious movements. Some of the movements' ministers seem able to cure their congregants' afflictions by arousing in them a religious fervor or hysterical response.

Psychosomatic illnesses are thought to lend themselves best to the faith healing process. To counter the claim that faith healing has succeeded where conventional medical treatments have failed, some skeptics take the position that patients resort to faith healing only when desperate. Feeling that something must work, a person gets into a state of mind in which psychosomatic symptoms disappear, or if the problem is genuinely physical, patients at least feel better.

Research methods are difficult to apply to faith healing, in part because of the question-

able psychosomatic aspects of many diseases. Also, many spontaneous remissions or recoveries from serious or hopeless conditions without benefit of the faith healing process have been recorded. A psychological study of individuals who had a physical stress condition relieved by faith healing showed that, while there was little indication of mental illness, they had strong DENIAL mechanisms. These denial mechanisms could have kept them from recognizing continuing symptoms of their stress.

See also ALTERNATIVE THERAPIES; IMMUNE SYSTEM; MIND-BODY CONNECTIONS; PLACEBO EFFECT; PRAYER; RELIGION.

SOURCES:
Galanter, Marc. *Cults, Faith, Healing and Coercion.* New York: Oxford University Press, 1989.
Oxman, T.E., et al. "Lack of Social Participation or Religious Strength and Comfort as Risk Factors for Death after Cardiac Surgery in the Elderly." *Psychosomatic Medicine* 57(1995): 681–89.
Rose, Louis. "Faith Health," in Cavendish, Richard, ed., *Man, Myth and Magic*, Vol. 4 New York: Marshall Cavendish, 1983.
Sobel, David, and Robert Ornstein, eds. "Faith Heals." *Mental Medicine Update* 4, No. 2 (1995).

family   Family and other RELATIONSHIPS sometimes buffer the stresses faced by individuals during their lifetime. However, for many people, families can also be a source of stress. As an example, men and women going through marital problems are especially vulnerable to the effects of relationship conflict. They may suffer from emotional consequences such as DEPRESSION and can have a compromised immune function leading to an increased rate of physical illness. CAREGIVERS who provide support for family members who are ill are another example of a highly stressed group. A decreased immune function has been observed in spouses caring for mates with ALZHEIMER'S DISEASE.

George R. Parkerson, M.D., and colleagues at Duke University Medical Center reported in the *Archives of Family Medicine* (March 1995) that individuals who see themselves as enduring high family stress are likely to have greater health problems than those reporting low family stress. Patients completed several different surveys that looked at SELF-ESTEEM, life events and changes, DEPRESSION, and family-induced stress. In addition, information on the number of physician visits, referrals to other physicians, hospitalizations, severity of illness, and cost of treatment incurred by these patients was tabulated. Results showed that family stress often had a stronger impact on health outcomes than other types of stress such as social or financial stress. Those with high family stress scores had more frequent follow-up visits to the clinic, more referrals to specialists, more hospitalizations, a higher severity of illness, and incurred higher charges for clinical health care than did those with low family stress. They also had fewer social support systems.

In evaluating family stress, researchers used the Duke Social Support and Stress Scale (DUSOCS), a 24-item questionnaire; patients indicated personal stress and/or support from each of six different types of family member and four different types of non-family member. In their report, researchers note: "It is important to remember that the study examines only the effect of family stress as perceived by the patient and does not measure family stress in terms of the family as a total system, nor does it measure perceptions of other members of the patient's family."

The Duke University researchers recommended that family physicians identify patients with high family stress and give them the special care they may require to prevent unfavorable outcomes. They suggested that questionnaires such as those used in the study can help identify patients who are at high risk of adverse health-related outcomes and who may not be recognized as such through standard medical history reports, physical exams, and medical tests.

Having patients bring family stress issues out in the open with their physicians can be useful. The researchers said that one randomized, controlled trial showed that when family physicians discussed details about stressful and supportive family members with their patients after reviewing questionnaire results, patients said they felt generally better and the process helped them to improve relationships with their families.

See also COMMUNICATION; DYSFUNCTIONAL FAMILY; INTIMACY.

SOURCES:
Burg, M.M., and T.E. Seeman. "Families and Health: the Negative Side of Social Ties." *Annals of Behavioral Medicine* 16 (1994): 109–15.
Parkerson, George R., et al. "Perceived Family Stress as a Predictor of Health-Related Outcomes." *Archives of Family Medicine* 4 (March 1995).

family therapy   See PSYCHOTHERAPIES.

family violence   See DOMESTIC VIOLENCE.

farming   Stressful occupation because farmers have little CONTROL over their lives; weather affects their yield, international trade dictates their prices, and government subsidies affect their income. For many families, farming is a way of life and comes with a whole set of values, standards, mores, and characteristics.

Currently, farming as a vocation is also threatened by a lack of respect from the public because many farmers have to rely on government subsidies to make their livelihood. This lack of respect, added to the farmer's stress, pressure, and frustration, can result in physical violence, first focused on the spouse and then on the children. This is a major social problem, but one that cannot be really addressed because of the private, independent nature of farmers, who live in relative isolation and have few options on how to change their lot.

According to an article in *Canadian Family Physician* (February 1992), farmers are disadvantaged by rural society traits, such as pride and inability to express EMOTIONS, that are barriers to seeking help for their stress.

See also DOMESTIC VIOLENCE.

SOURCE:
Haverstock, Linda. "Stress in Farming." *Canadian Family Physician* 38 (1992): 405–06.

fathering, older   Fathering later in life is less stressful than fathering at an earlier age, according to economist Martin Carnoy, a Stanford University professor of education. In his book, *Fathers of a Certain Age,* Carnoy and his co-author son David argue that men in their late 40s, 50s and even 60s, secure in their careers and ready to make time for families, are more nurturing and willing to share in child-care responsibilities than their younger counterparts. As a result, they find fatherhood less stressful at their age.

The Carnoys reviewed literature comparing fathering experiences at different ages and interviewed many older fathers, exploring how they feel about PARENTING small children late in middle age. "These older fathers are more stable financially and better able to provide for a child," the elder Carnoy said. "But more important, they are usually willing to spend a great deal of time on the FAMILY. They have fought the workplace wars and are much less sanguine about the rewards of long work days. Almost everyone we interviewed who was raising second families was spending more time with their children than they did as 30-year-old fathers trying to climb career ladders. Family plays a much more important everyday role in older fathers' lives."

Fathers of a Certain Age suggests that middle-age fathering is on the increase after many years of decline, and that this is no accident. As college-educated women seek to build their professional careers and postpone childbearing to their early 30s and beyond, they are much more likely to end up marrying a man who is in his mid-40s or older. This has resulted in "fathers at a certain age," and census data indicate that more than 350,000 men in the United States over age 45 fall into this category.

Although the Carnoys found that older fathers are intensively involved with their children, the book discusses some of the major pitfalls of later fatherhood. Not only do many middle-aged fathers have to deal with their disapproving older children from a previous marriage, they also face the sheer energy requirements of raising a young child, the possibility of paternal death early in a child's life, and the financial difficulties of facing RETIREMENT and paying for a college education.

SOURCE:
Carnoy, Martin, and David Carnoy. *Fathers of a Certain Age.* Boston: Faber and Faber, 1995.

fatigue   See CHRONIC FATIGUE SYNDROME.

fear   An emotion that results in an intense and unpleasant stress that comes about because of a real threat. In fear, there may be intense feelings of wanting to escape, together with physiological reactions including weakness, DIZZINESS, rapid breathing, rapid heartbeat, nausea, muscle tension, and weakness in the knees. Different individuals have different physiological responses to fear.

The terms "fear" and "phobia" are often misused and are improperly interchanged. Fear is a real and knowable danger, and usually can be recognized by others. Phobia on the other hand, is an inappropriately fearful response to a situation and is out of proportion to the real danger, if there is danger at all. Real fear is normal. Chronic PHOBIAS that cause avoidance behavior are considered ANXIETY DISORDERS.

At times, fear can be a helpful emotion. For example, the fear reaction enables people to get out of the way when they hear the whistle of a train. It signals the hypothalamus, which triggers a release of ADRENALINE into the body. Adrenaline acts immediately to prepare the body for FIGHT OR FLIGHT. Breathing deepens, perspiration increases to cool the body, pupils dilate to sharpen vision, the face may turn pale, and the heart beats noticeably faster.

See also AGORAPHOBIA; ANXIETY; SOCIAL PHOBIA.

feedback Involves objective information given by a therapist, teacher, or parent, or by others in a SUPPORT GROUP, to an individual who is seeking comments about his feelings or actions. It is a sharing of feelings or thoughts and ideally should be given without evaluating consequences to the individual or demanding that he make a change. Negative feedback, even when given with complete objectivity, can be stressful and generally arouses defensiveness in the individual. Positive feedback, on the other hand, enhances SELF-ESTEEM and makes the individual feel good.

See also COMMUNICATION; LISTENING.

feldenkrais method   See BODY THERAPIES.

feng shui One way to reduce chances for stress is to practice a philosophy that ensures harmony and good fortune. Such is the Chinese art of geomancy, or feng shui, which involves the proper alignment of objects with geographical features. In *Hemispheres* magazine (November 1993), John Goff translates feng shui as "wind and water" and defines it as "a product of a culture that honors the spirits of mountains and rivers and views the landscape as a living thing with cosmic currents."

Practiced first in Hong Kong, where it influenced the design of many corporate

---

USE FENG SHUI TO REMOVE STRESS WHEN BUILDING OR FURNISHING A HOUSE

- Entryways and windows should be wide enough to allow light, which symbolizes the sun and allows good energy to come in.
- Mirrors are particularly useful in cramped spaces and over furniture that does not face windows or doors because they reflect positive energy and deflect negative forces.
- Buildings near water are good because water is an element of wealth, insight, and motivation. Avoid building near tall buildings because they block positive energy and on cul de sacs because negative energy has no place to escape.

---

buildings, including Citicorp International and Motorola Semiconductors Hong Kong, Ltd., feng shui has spread to other parts of the world as well. In addition to corporate offices, there are factors that can remove stress from a household (see above).

fertility   See INFERTILITY.

fibromyalgia Form of "soft-tissue" or muscular rheumatism that causes PAIN in the muscles and fibrous connective tissues (ligaments and tendons). It is an accepted clinical syndrome that causes stress for the sufferer, not only because of the pain and discomfort, but also because of the difficulty in having it diagnosed properly.

According to Barry M. Schimmer, M.D., chief of the section on rheumatology at Pennsylvania Hospital, "For a long time we thought that their problems were psychosomatic and these patients were referred for psychiatric help. Today we know that this condition is very real and needs to be dealt with and treated like any other chronic illness."

The exact cause of fibromyalgia is unknown and there is no known cure. Many different factors trigger the pain, including an illness, such as the flu, hormonal changes, or physical or emotional trauma.

Symptoms

The ailment, which affects three to six million Americans, primarily Caucasian, middle-class women between the ages of 45 and 55, results in muscles becoming tight and tense, and the person feeling emotionally drained. Other symptoms of the disease in addition to pain and constant fatigue are feeling "down" and anxious; numbness and tingling in the hands, feet, and legs; sleep disturbance, tension headaches, subjective swelling, bladder spasms, and irritable bowel. Cold weather, extremes of activity, fluctuation of barometric pressure, and stress often aggravate the symptoms of fibromyalgia.

Diagnosis and treatment

Since diagnosis of fibromyalgia is so difficult, a rheumatologist does extensive detective work in sorting out the patient's medical history and performing a thorough examination. Said Dr. Schimmer, "When we examine the patient we will find tender 'trigger points' in certain patterns over the neck, shoulders, chest, lower back, and hips and this helps to separate fibromyalgia from other conditions."

Nonsteroidal anti-inflammatory agents are used, as are coricosteroids, but they often do not help. Efforts are made to improve sleep. Non-pharmacologic treatment emphasizes aerobic exercise, particularly water aerobics. Light sports, such as swimming, bicycling, and walking, are encouraged. Some people find BIOFEEDBACK, hypnotherapy, massage, and SUPPORT GROUPS helpful. Many patients, in an acute stage of their disease, worry about having bone cancer or other ominous disorders; some become very anxious. Psychotherapy can help certain individuals overcome the attendant stresses of this disorder.

See also MASSAGE THERAPY; PSYCHOTHERAPIES.

SOURCES:

McIlwain, Harris H., and Debra Fulghum. *The Fibromyalgia Handbook.* New York: Henry Holt, 1996.

Starlanyl, Devin. *Fibromyalgia and Chronic Myofascial Pain Syndrome: A Survival Manual.* Oakland: New Harbinger Publications, 1996.

Williamson, Miryam Ehrlich. *Fibromyalgia: A Comprehensive Approach: What You Can Do About Chronic Pain and Fatigue.* New York: Walker and Company, 1996.

fight or flight response   This is an innate reaction present in humans as well as animals to a stressful or threatening situation in which the SYMPATHETIC NERVOUS SYSTEM (SNS) mobilizes the body for maximum output and use of energy. When facing a stressful situation, the SNS causes many physiological reactions, including a rapid heartbeat, deep breathing, slowing down of digestion, and an increase in blood pressure. These physical functions enable the person (or animal) to quickly flee the dangerous situation or fight back against an aggressor.

An example of the fight or flight response is when an individual realizes that he is on a railroad crossing and the train is coming closer than he thought. Fast flight ensues. Also, when a mother animal's cubs are threatened by a predator animal, her instincts take over and the fight or flight response follows.

See also ANXIETY DISORDERS; FEAR; PANIC ATTACKS AND PANIC DISORDER; STRESS.

financial stressors   See MONEY.

fitness   See EXERCISE.

flashbacks   See POST-TRAUMATIC STRESS DISORDER.

flatulence   The expulsion of air, usually swallowed when eating, from the stomach or intestine but can also be induced by ANXIETY in times of stress. Fear of passing wind or gas is a common SOCIAL PHOBIA and can cause stress or embarrassment.

Certain foods are well known as tending to cause flatulence; the list includes beans, cabbage, onions, peppers, cucumbers, celery, and dairy products.

See also INDIGESTION; IRRITABLE BOWEL SYNDROME.

flooding   See BEHAVIOR THERAPY.

flying   See AIRPLANES.

folk medicine   See ALTERNATIVE THERAPIES; FAITH HEALING; PRAYER.

forgetting   An inability to retrieve stored long- or short-term memories. It is a common occurrence and a source of stress to many people. Most people forget short-term as well as long-term memories, particularly the elderly who experience MEMORY loss as they grow older. But forgetting is a sign not just of old age. Many people consciously block out stressful memories and many are simply forgetful. They may forget recently made appointments, forget what their boss told them earlier in the day, or forget occurrences that happened in childhood.

Scientific studies have concentrated primarily on two factors, inhibition and loss of retrieval clues. Inhibition is the theory that similar kinds of learning, either before or after the event to be remembered, interfere with later recall of that event. Loss of retrieval clues is based on the theory that recall is easier when the individual is dealing with familiar people, things, and situations. Other theories hold that individuals have "selective" memories, and may forget events or situations previously encountered that were unpleasant, stressful, or even traumatic. This concept is related to repression, which suggests that forgetting is a COPING mechanism.

See also ALZHEIMER'S DISEASE; POST-TRAUMATIC STRESS DISORDER.

Framingham Type A   See TYPE A PERSONALITY.

friends   Friends are unique among human RELATIONSHIPS. While individuals have little or no choice in family or neighbors, they can choose their friends. Some friendships evolve from shared interests or values, some simply from a shared history, and some from compatible personalities. Qualities most appreciated in friends include loyalty, trust, and an ability to keep a confidence. People want to feel that they can rely on their friends and can have an open and honest friendship during good as well as stressful times.

When friends are supportive, they help relieve the stress during periods of turmoil or crisis. Individuals who experience DEPRESSION often report a lack of friends, although having a wide circle of friends is not a preventive factor for depression. Some reports have indicated that individuals who have many friends may be healthier and actually live longer than those who do not.

Friends can also be a source of stress because they may challenge or be challenged by other relationships in the individual's life. For example, a friendship may be broken or changed when one friend marries. A friend of the opposite sex frequently is unsettling to a spouse or lover. Friends who do not meet with parents' approval can be a source of family conflict. Friends who decide to share housing or enter into a business partnership sometimes discover undesirable facets of the other person's personality that could be ignored when the relationship was less formal. In the WORKPLACE, a friendship may dissolve when two people are vying for the same promotion.

A 1990 Gallup poll reported that the typical American places much importance on friendship. It also indicated some frustrations about the time and flexibility needed to form friendships. The survey showed that women and men approach friendship quite differently. Women tended to form more intimate relationships with other women than men with men. One-on-one activities that promote conversation are more popular with women, whereas men are more likely to get together in groups for sports, cards, or other such activities. Men rely on their wives for emotional support, but many women, even those who are married, often rely on women friends. Women are more likely than men to have a best friend of the same sex, but a third of the men surveyed said a woman was their best friend.

People make friends in many ways. In the Gallup report, 51% of the 18- to 29-year-olds made most of their friends at school. Of the 30- to 49-year-olds, 51% said they made most of their friends through work. From the age of 50 up, friends came from a greater variety of sources, including church, work, clubs, or other organizations.

When participants were asked about arguments with friends, those under age 30 reported more disagreements. Friendship evidently becomes more tranquil with age, possibly because friends settle their differences and learn to recognize sore spots, or possibly because age enables people to recognize and discard difficult and stressful relationships.

See also INTIMACY.

SOURCE:
Kahn, Ada P., and Jan Fawcett. *The Encyclopedia of Mental Health.* New York: Facts On File, 1993.

frigidity An old term that refers to the inability of a woman to obtain satisfaction (usually orgasm) during sexual intercourse. Sex researchers Masters and Johnson coined the term "female orgasmic dysfunction" to replace this term. Regardless of the label, the situation may be a cause of stress for the woman as well as her partner.

Lack of satisfaction during sexual intercourse may result from a combination of many factors, including the desirability of one's partner, poor COMMUNICATION between the partners concerning sexual behaviors

and desires, and cultural rejection of certain sexual practices. Other factors necessary to the woman's arousal—stimulation and satisfaction—vary widely between individuals. Also, the fear of desertion, acquiring a SEXUALLY TRANSMITTED DISEASE (STD) or pregnancy may interfere with satisfaction for some women.

In some cases, interest in sexual activity and sexual satisfaction depends on the woman's physical and mental health. DEPRESSION, STRESS, fatigue, or alcohol may reduce sexual satisfaction. Narcotics and some tranquilizers may also reduce interest in sexual activity. Counseling, therapy, and special exercises outlined by a sex therapist may help many women who have orgasmic dysfunction to become more physically responsive and emotionally free to enjoy sexual pleasures.

See also ANORGASMIA; DYSPAREUNIA; SEX THERAPY; SEXUAL DIFFICULTIES; SEXUAL RESPONSE CYCLE.

frustration Interference with an individual's impulses or desired actions of internal or external forces. Internal forces are inhibitions and mental conflict, and external forces can come from a parent, teachers, and friends, as well as the rules of the society. There are deep feelings of discontent and tension because of unresolved problems, unfulfilled needs, or roadblocks to personal goals. Regardless of the cause, frustration causes stress for most people.

Modern life is filled with frustrations from birth to old age. Crying babies may be frustrated because of hunger, school-age children may be frustrated by high expectations of their parents, parents may be frustrated by their jobs, and the elderly may be frustrated by their increasing lack of independence.

People who are repeatedly and constantly stressed by frustrations respond in many ways. A person who is mentally healthy usually deals with frustration in an acceptable way, sometimes with HUMOR. Others react with ANGER, HOSTILITY, AGGRESSION, or DEPRESSION, while still others become withdrawn and passive. Many children and adults who are constantly frustrated show regressive behavior—going back to childlike behavior, particularly aggression or depression—and

may become unable to cope with problems on their own.

See also CONTROL; COPING; GENERAL ADAPTATION SYNDROME; STRESS MANAGEMENT.

funeral arrangements   See DEATH.

G

galvanic skin response (GSR) Use of an electronic device attached to an individual's fingertips that measures minute amounts of perspiration in the skin in response to emotional or psychological stressors. The more tense the individual is, the more perspiration is on his skin; as the individual becomes calmer, there is less perspiration.

The device converts its electrical information to an easily observable form, such as light or a buzzing sound, and can be used in conjunction with BIOFEEDBACK or as a test after an individual has learned the biofeedback technique to reduce effects of stress.

See also RELAXATION.

gambling Playing a game (such as cards or slot machines and roulette) for money or other stakes or betting on an uncertain outcome (such as a horse race or football game). The fascination with gambling and the prospect of winning can reduce stress for certain individuals by helping them forget their problems. This is particularly true when they are able to control their gambling by setting a dollar limit on their losses and stopping their gambling at that point. However, for many people, gambling becomes an ADDICTION and a compulsion, and they play on and on.

People gamble for many reasons. Some simply enjoy the sociability of the event while others find the risk and unpredictability of the game exciting and stimulating. Some derive a sense of power and importance from winning; others may gamble out of rebellion. To gamble is still illegal in some situations or considered sinful or immoral by some religious groups.

A compulsion or an addiction
Gambling may be considered a compulsion or addiction when the gambling activity becomes the most important aspect of people's lives. Such individuals will direct all of their efforts toward obtaining money to gamble. Seeking funds to enable gambling can become a stressor. For family and friends of the addicted gamblers who may not be able to pay household bills and provide a living, it becomes a source of stress as well.

Although gambling does not involve ingesting substances, compulsive gambling has many characteristics in common with alcoholism. Both the National Council on Compulsive Gambling and Gamblers Anonymous have estimated that there are six million compulsive gamblers in the United States. Typically, the compulsive gambler is a married man in his early to mid-thirties, employed in a field involving money and high risks, such as investment, business, or the law. Usually, compulsive gamblers are outgoing, generous, and gregarious, but are prone to sudden negative mood swings. Even in serious stages of compulsive gambling, gamblers will express concern about their health, but not about their addiction to gambling and the stress caused by it.

National attention was focused on the problem of compulsive gambling in the late 1980s with the well-publicized problems of baseball star Pete Rose. Shortly afterward, a Gallup Poll showed a somewhat ambivalent public attitude toward gambling. Survey results indicated that gambling as an activity, both legal and illegal, is on the upsurge and extremely popular. Public sentiment ran toward increasing legalized gambling, although 61% of those surveyed said they thought legal gambling encouraged excessive gambling.

Historically, there have been underworld aspects surrounding gambling. Films frequently depict expensively dressed, glamorous men and women gambling in casinos in exotic locations all over the world, or seedy, down-on-their-luck characters playing cards or shooting craps and about to get raided by the police. Today, when more and more states are passing laws that allow gambling and lotteries have become an American way of life, gambling has become completely accessible to people in all walks of life.

Gamblers Anonymous offers a recovery program similar to Alcoholics Anonymous. The Council on Compulsive Gambling offers a crisis intervention hotline for compulsive gamblers and their families.

See also SELF-HELP GROUPS.

FOR FURTHER INFORMATION:
Gamblers Anonymous
3255 Wilshire Blvd. (Suite 610)
Los Angeles, CA 90010
Phone: (211) 386-8789

National Council on Compulsive Gambling
John Jay College of Criminal Justice
445 W. 59th St.
New York, NY 10019
Phone: (212) 765-3833

SOURCES:
Hugick, Larry. "Gambling on the Rise; Lotteries Lead the Way." *The Gallup Poll,* June 1989.
Kahn, Ada P., and Jan Fawcett. *The Encyclopedia of Mental Health.* New York: Facts On File, 1993.

gender role A collection of attitudes and behaviors that are culturally and socially associated with maleness or femaleness. Along with many societal changes, gender roles have also changed significantly, particularly during the last half of the 20th century. The gender role for many women in Western cultures was historically passive and submissive, until the "women's liberation" movement and "sexual revolution." Child care is no longer exclusively the woman's role; and earning the larger part of the family income is no longer exclusively the man's role. These changes have not occurred without stress. Women try to handle motherhood and a

career at the same time or sacrifice one for the other, while some men fear that wives will advance more rapidly in their career than they will, and others have mixed emotions about their role as fathers.

Stressors from gender roles also occur when individuals have persistent feelings of discomfort about their sexual identity. Transsexualism is the most common example of this situation. When people have internal conflicts regarding gender identity, and do not accept their biological designation, stressful anxieties may develop, leading them into practices such as "cross dressing" and adopting the role of the other sex. Many individuals who believe that they are men or women in the body of the other sex experience stressful anxieties to the extent that some of them seek surgical sex change operations.

See also HAVING IT ALL; SEXUAL DIFFICULTIES.

general   adaptation   syndrome   (G.A.S.)
Refers to a term we now know as STRESS; it was coined by Hans SELYE (1907–82), an Austrian-born Canadian endocrinologist and psychologist, in his landmark book, *The Stress of Life* (1956). The G.A.S. is the manifestation of stress in the whole body as it develops over time. It is through the G.A.S. that various internal organs, especially the endocrine glands and the nervous system, help individuals adjust to constant changes occurring in and around them and to "navigate a steady course toward whatever they consider a worthwhile goal."

Dr. Selye was a pioneer in an area that has continued to look at stress as a threat to wellness. The secret of health, he contended, was in successful adjustment to ever-changing conditions. Life, he said, is largely a process of adaptation to the circumstances in which we exist. He viewed many nervous and emotional disturbances, such as high blood pressure and some cardiovascular problems, gastric and duodenal ulcers, and certain types of allergic problems, as essentially diseases of adaptation.

Selye called his concept the general adaptation syndrome because it is produced only by agents that have a *general* effect on large portions of the body. He called it *adaptive* because it stimulates DEFENSE MECHANISMS. He used the term *syndrome* because individual manifestations are coordinated and interdependent on each other.

There are three stages in the G.A.S., Selye said. Individuals go through the stages many times each day as well as throughout life. Whatever demands are made on us, we progress through the sequence. The first is an alarm reaction, or the bodily expression of a generalized call for our defensive forces. We experience surprise and anxiety because of our inexperience in dealing with a new situation. The second stage is resistance, when we have learned to cope with the new situation efficiently. The third stage is exhaustion, or a depletion of our energy reserves, which leads to fatigue. Adaptability, Selye continued, was a finite amount of vitality (thought of as capital) with which we are born. We can withdraw from it throughout life, but cannot add to it.

See also COPING; DIS-STRESS; EUSTRESS; HARDINESS; HOMEOSTASIS; PSYCHONEUROIMMUNOLOGY.

SOURCES:
Selye, Hans. *The Stress of Life.* New York: McGraw Hill, 1956.
———. *Stress without Distress.* Philadelphia: J.B. Lippincott, 1974.

generalized anxiety disorders (GADs) See ANXIETY.

generation gap See BABY BOOMERS; COMMUNICATION; INTERGENERATIONAL CONFLICTS; LISTENING.

generation X At the end of the 20th century, many young people under the age of 30 who had no definite career plans or jobs were referred to as members of Generation X. These young people experience stress because of a lack of jobs and the necessity of moving back to their parents' homes. Parents who had thought they were going to be empty nesters also find the situation stressful.

About two-thirds of the returnees are college educated. Their length of stay at home is 2.5 years, according to a 1995 study at Brown University. Because of a tight job market and low pay raises, the adult children have had to postpone marriage. They are not able to afford independent housing or a car.

Parents may have to put their own plans on hold until their children can be financially independent. They want to help their children out but in many cases cannot afford to totally subsidize them. Parents and returning children may find it useful to sit down with an independent third party to iron out details of their new living arrangements. The young people may also benefit from psychological career counseling.

See also COMMUNICATION; INTERGENERATIONAL CONFLICTS; LISTENING.

SOURCE:
Hornblower, Margot. "Great Expectations." *Time,* June 9, 1997.

geriatric depression See DEPRESSION.

geropsychiatry See PSYCHOTHERAPIES.

glass ceiling An invisible barrier that keeps many working women from rising to the top of their field despite good qualifications, experience, and hard work. This frustration leads to stress and anxiety and, for many individuals, DEPRESSION.

There are many variations of the effects of the glass ceiling. For example, men in high-level posts may be brought from outside the organization to provide a fresh outlook while qualified women already in the organization are passed over. Also, in discussions involving teamwork and negotiations, women are often kept on the periphery of the decision-making process.

Teasing and harassment of women may discourage them from seeking a promotion. Women in lower-level positions are sometimes given responsible, demanding work, which is not reflected in title or salary. As women attempt to progress in an organization, they may find that performance standards are higher for them than for men. Women may also be inhibited by assumptions that a feminine management style is more passive and nurturing toward fellow workers and less goal oriented and driven than the masculine management style.

Women who do make it past the glass ceiling frequently credit the influence of a mentor, spouse, or parent. Some women avoid the glass ceiling by striking out on their own. In the late 1980s, the number of self-employed women was growing faster than the number of men.

See also SEXUAL HARASSMENT; WOMEN'S MOVEMENT.

global warming   The idea that human activities can rapidly change Earth's climate is a cause for concern and stress for people all over the world.

Global warming is not a new concept. Jean Fourier, a French physicist, was the first to understand the "greenhouse" effect. In 1824 he suggested that Earth stays warm at night because its atmosphere traps sun-warmed gases in the same way a greenhouse holds heated air. In 1892, Svante Arrhenius, a Swedish physical chemist, predicted that, if levels of carbon dioxide in the atmosphere doubled, the average temperature of Earth would rise between 1.5 and 4 degrees Celsius, close to the prediction most climatologists share today.

Stresses arise for many people who become overly concerned about the increased incidence of more intense cold during winter and more intense heat during summer, as well as flooding, landslides, tornadoes, and hurricanes. Additionally, some people are concerned about the use of products such as aerosol sprays and chemical pollutants, which may contribute to global warming. Many environmental activists take on global warming as a personal crusade.

globus hystericus   See LUMP IN THE THROAT.

goals   See HARDINESS.

gonorrhea   See SEXUALLY TRANSMITTED DISEASES.

grief   An intensely powerful, painful, and stressful emotional reaction caused by the loss of a loved one or of something with very important personal significance in an individual's life. While the expression of grief is unique to each individual, there are recognized stages of grief (bereavement), which include some common characteristics as well as sources of STRESS for most people.

Many individuals call into play their own DEFENSE MECHANISMS. These mechanisms may help an individual cope with the pain of the loss.

Numbness is a pervasive feeling that enables the mourner to get through the first few days following the DEATH of the loved one; it may last from a few days to a few months. HALLUCINATIONS are also common among the recently bereaved; in some cases, they believe that the dead person walks into the room or they see him/her in a crowd. In the case of a deceased infant or child, a parent may hear his/her cry or voice.

As the initial feeling of numbness begins to wear off, the individual may feel anger and despair and feel overwhelmed by the circumstances; these feelings can lead to DEPRESSION. In some cases, such as death or divorce, people may feel angry that the person deserted them.

Physical symptoms are fairly common, including HEADACHES, INSOMNIA or gastrointestinal complaints. Attempted SUICIDE is an abnormal expression of grief, but is not uncommon. There may be an increase in use of tranquilizer drugs and alcohol at this time.

The individual may experience intense feelings of helplessness. Questions arise: "Could I have prevented this from happening? Why wasn't I powerful enough to do something more?" Such thoughts are part of the human condition. People like to feel that they are in CONTROL at all times, and with grief they feel the loss of that control.

Many people who have experienced loss say that it can take up to two years to adjust and get on with life. However, overwhelming feelings of loss do recur. In the long run, a positive attitude can help overcome depressed feelings and the stresses of adjustment.

A support system often influences how well an individual adjusts after a period of grief. The recovery process may be accelerated with friends and family nearby. Widowed persons with no relatives and few friends seem to have the most stressors and the most difficult time adjusting to the death of a loved one. Some parents who have lost an infant try to have another baby within a few years; however, the feeling of loss of the first one never really goes away. Many divorced people remarry but others do not.

Overcoming the stresses of grief

Individuals who continue to suffer from the stresses of grief for a long period of time may find mental health counseling helpful. Getting help when it is needed is a sign of strength and wisdom; appropriate referrals for mental health help can be obtained from a social worker or a physician. SUPPORT GROUPS for widows and widowers, parents and divorcees are effective for many people. Knowing that others had the same emotional reactions can help participants cope better with their grief stressors. Those grieving for the loss of a child may also find help in appropriate support groups.

The Bereavement and Loss Center in New York is an organization that provides professional counseling services for individuals who have suffered loss or who anticipate a loss, such as loss of a spouse, child, relative, or friend. The center is nonsectarian and provides psychiatric social workers and psychiatrists with an advisory staff, including other medical specialists, financial advisers, and attorneys. Other sources of help can be found through many organizations that offer telephone information and referral services. Crisis telephone lines and centers and hospital social service departments are sometimes a fast way of getting help; these numbers should be listed in a special section of local telephone books.

Another's grief as a stressor

One person's grief is often a source of stress for another. Some individuals are at a loss for what to say or what to do. Despite these feelings, there are some supportive activities that might be helpful. For example, offering a quiet supportive presence; encouraging the bereaved person to talk and share happy as well as sad memories; avoiding being judgmental of any comments the bereaved person might make; encouraging him or her to remain connected to former support systems, such as social or church groups; and being available in a proactive way to get the person back into the cycle of a mentally healthy lifestyle.

See also PREGNANCY; SUDDEN INFANT DEATH SYNDROME.

FOR FURTHER INFORMATION:
Bereavement and Loss Center of New York
170 East 83rd Street
New York, 10028
Phone: (212) 879-5655

Elisabeth Kübler-Ross Center (workshops, regional groups)
So. Rte. 616
Head Waters, VA 24442
Phone: (703) 396-3441

Mental Health Association of Greater Chicago
104 South Michigan Avenue
Chicago, IL 60603-5901
Phone: (312) 781-7780

Parents of Murdered Children
100 E. Eighth St. (Suite B41)
Cincinnati, OH 45202
Phone: (513) 721-LOVE

Pregnancy and Infant Loss Center
1415 Wayzata Blvd. (Suite 105)
Wayzata, MN 55391
Phone: (612) 473-9372

Theos (groups in the U.S. and Canada for
   widowed people)
1301 Clark Building
717 Liberty Ave.
Pittsburgh, PA 15222
Phone: (412) 471-7779

SOURCES:
Kahn, Ada P. "Living With the Death of a Loved
   One," (brochure). Chicago: Mental Health
   Association of Greater Chicago, 1989.
Kahn, Ada P., and Jan Fawcett. *The Encyclopedia of
   Mental Health.* New York: Facts On File, 1993.
Kübler-Ross, E. *On Death and Dying.* New York:
   Macmillan, 1971.
Ramsay, R.W., and R. Noorbergen. *Living With Loss.*
   New York: William Morrow, 1981.

group therapy   See PSYCHOTHERAPIES.

grudges   See HOSTILITY.

GSR   See GALVANIC SKIN RESPONSE.

guided imagery   A technique to help the
individual generate vivid mental images that
help reduce STRESS. It creates positive mental
pictures and promotes the relaxation necessary for a healing process. The individual pictures an image, such as a calm, serene lake
with sailboats slowly moving along, breathes
in a relaxed manner, and becomes more
relaxed. The individual gradually learns to
notice every detail of the imagined scene and
how the sense of RELAXATION deepens with
this self-talk. He learns, too, that this sense of
calm can be created at any time by BREATHING
and imagining the positive vision.

Some case studies and clinical reports suggest that the guided imagery technique may be
helpful in the treatment of chronic PAIN, ALLER-
GIES, hypertension, autoimmune diseases, and
stress-related gastrointestinal, reproductive,
and urinary symptoms. In addition to direct
effects, imagery may augment the effectiveness of medical treatments and help people
tolerate discomforts and side effects of some
medications or invasive procedures.

Imagery has qualities that make it valuable
in mind/body medicine and healing; it can
bring about physiological changes, provide
psychological insights and enhance emotional
awareness. Use of imagery, in some cases,
changes the need for medication. Depending
on an individual's medical condition, imagery
is best used under the supervision of a physician in conjunction with holistic medicine.

Guided imagery can be used alone or
together with other relaxation techniques. It is
often used in conjunction with HYPNOSIS,
although the two techniques are distinct.
While hypnosis serves to induce a special
state of mind, imagery consists of a focused,
intentional mental activity.

See also ALTERNATIVE THERAPIES; IMMUNE
SYSTEM; IRRITABLE BOWEL SYNDROME.

FOR FURTHER INFORMATION:
The Academy for Guided Imagery
P.O. Box 2070
Mill Valley, CA 94942
Phone: (800) 726-2070

SOURCES:
Goleman, Daniel, and Joel Gurin, eds. *Mind Body
   Medicine: How to Use Your Mind For Better Health.*
   Yonkers, N.Y.: Consumer Report Books, 1993.
Kerns, Lawrence. *Chicago Medicine* 97, no. 22
   (November 21, 1994).

guilt   Emotional response to a perceived or
actual failure to meet expectations of the self
or others. Guilt is a stressor for many people
because guilt feelings can be destructive if
carried to an extreme. It can destroy people's
sense of SELF-ESTEEM and feeling of capability.
However, these feelings can also be construc-

tive when people begin to understand their sources of guilt and learn to cope with this very common aspect of the human condition.

Some individuals, depending on differences in conscience, can steal or commit crimes against others and not feel any guilt, while others will suffer from stressful guilt feelings over incidents that occur all their lives. Many individuals may experience guilt feelings for not remembering the birthday of a parent or spouse. Middle-aged adults may experience guilt feelings when dealing with their aging parents. Some individuals who are bereaved over a death of a loved one may feel some guilt about not having done enough for the person when they were alive. Parents of infants who die of SUDDEN INFANT DEATH SYNDROME (SIDS) suffer stress because of feelings of guilt over not preventing the death of their child. Spouses and relatives of people who commit SUICIDE may have guilt feelings for years, wondering if they could have prevented the death.

For some individuals, mental health counseling or participation in an appropriate support group can help relieve some of these uncomfortable feelings of guilt.

See also COPING; DEPRESSION.

SOURCE:

Kahn, Ada P., and Jan Fawcett. *Encyclopedia of Mental Health.* New York: Facts On File, 1993.

habits Learned responses that one performs automatically and frequently. They may include useful procedures, such as knowing how to use a computer keyboard, taking a shower in the morning, or always leaving a key in a certain place. Habits can also be responses to stressful situations, such as scratching the head, NAIL BITING, HAIRPULLING, or reaching for a cigarette. These unwanted or undesirable habits, if continued, can contribute to people's stress levels.

Habits can include certain repetitive and ritual behaviors such as those practiced by sufferers of OBSESSIVE-COMPULSIVE DISORDER. These habits that usually cause the individual stress can be changed by BEHAVIOR THERAPY, psychotherapy, and the substitution of more constructive habits. RELAXATION therapy, GUIDED IMAGERY, HYPNOSIS, and BIOFEEDBACK may also be helpful techniques in overcoming these habits.

See also ANXIETY DISORDERS.

hair loss Hair falling out, extremely thinning hair, and baldness. Hair loss is stressful for people because they associate their "crowning glory" with SELF-ESTEEM and BODY IMAGE. For many, hair loss is also symbolic of aging. Sufferers of hair loss may resort to so called magic potions, which are megavitamins, and scalp massage and treatments to encourage new hair to grow.

More recently, several hair loss products have been developed and are selling as over-the-counter products. They have proved successful for some people but must be used on a continuous basis to be effective.

Hair loss is common; nearly two out of three men develop some form of balding. An even higher percentage of men and women combined have some form of hair loss during their lives.

With appropriate diagnosis, many people suffering from hair loss can be helped. Diagnosis is the first step. Hair loss can be due to many different causes, such as pregnancy, high fever, severe infection, or severe flu. It may also be due to thyroid disease, inadequate protein in the diet, certain prescription drugs and cancer treatment drugs, birth control pills, low serum iron, major surgery, chronic illness, or ringworm of the scalp. After some forms of hair loss, hair will regrow. Individuals undergoing chemotherapy experience hair loss; expectations are that hair will grow back some time after completion of chemotherapy. Other forms can be treated successfully by dermatologists.

About 90% of a person's scalp hair is continually growing. Shedding 50 to 100 hairs a day is considered normal. When a hair is shed, it is replaced by a new hair from the same follicle located just below the skin surface. Scalp hair grows about a half-inch a month. As people age, their rate of hair growth slows down, and thinning hair may be noticeable.

See also AGING.

FOR FURTHER INFORMATION:
American Academy of Dermatology
930 North Meacham Road
P.O. Box 4014
Schaumburg, IL 60168-4014
Phone: (708) 330-0230

American Hair Loss Council
4500 South Broadway
Tyler, TX 75703
Phone: (214) 581-8717

National Alopecia Areata Foundation
714 C Street (Suite 216)

San Rafael, CA 94901
Phone: (415) 456-4644

hair pulling   A habit that involves pulling out scalp hair and sometimes hair on eyebrows, eyelashes, and body; men may pull out beard and mustache hairs. For many people, hair pulling is a mechanism for COPING with STRESS. They do it when they are feeling nervous or tense; or it is a compulsion, known as trichotillomania.

Some individuals pull hair in front of others, but most often the activity is pursued in secret. The hairs are carefully hidden or disposed of. The hairless areas have distinctive features and help distinguish trichotillomania from other forms of hair loss and disease. The patches are irregular in outline, not sharply defined, and the hair loss is never complete. Many of the hairs will break off rather than be completely pulled out, so that variable amounts of stubble remain. There are usually no signs of inflammation, and the scalp elsewhere is normal.

The habit can be treated with BEHAVIOR THERAPY or other forms of PSYCHOTHERAPIES.

See also ANXIETY DISORDERS; HAIR LOSS; HYPNOSIS; OBSESSIVE-COMPULSIVE DISORDER.

FOR FURTHER INFORMATION:
The Obsessive Compulsive Disorder (OCD)
   Foundation
P.O. Box 9573
New Haven, CT 06535
Phone: (203) 772-0565

Hakomi   Form of body-centered psychotherapy based on principles that show individuals ways to live in harmony with themselves and others. It teaches individuals to enter a state of awareness in which spontaneous and often nonverbal information becomes available and from which basic and unconscious beliefs stem and direct their lives. Many people use Hakomi as a way of preventing the harmful effects of stress.

The body stores and expresses what the mind and heart believe. Trained to look at nuances of voice and body language, posture and gesture, Hakomi therapists help individuals study these avenues to unexpressed feelings and past trauma, and gain release from the past. Hakomi teaches how to observe oneself from a step away (witnessing) as well as from inside one's present experience. Individuals learn to have a choice of responses. Through the use of witnessing, unwanted defenses can be studied and willingly yielded.

Hakomi is a blend of many philosophies and ideologies, including Eastern philosophy, Western psychology, Taoism, Feldenkrais, Reichian, Rolfing, and other structural bodywork therapies, Ericksonian hypnosis, focusing, and neurolinguistic programming.

See also ALTERNATIVE THERAPIES; BODY THERAPIES.

hallucinations   Feelings that a person is seeing, hearing, smelling, tasting, or feeling something that is really not there. They are sources of stress because these perceptions cannot be reinforced by anyone else. Hallucinations may be disturbing to sufferers as well as those who are trying to understand what they are feeling.

Hallucinations sometimes occur as a reaction to certain medications, to high fevers and serious illnesses. They also occur in some severe mental disorders, such as schizophrenia.

Reactions to hallucinogens
Hallucinogens are drugs and agents that produce profound distortions to one's senses of sight, sound, smell, and touch, as well as the senses of direction, time, and distance. Although some individuals may resort to hallucinogens for relief from stress, there are no acceptable medical uses for hallucinogens.

People may experience a "high" associated with use of hallucinogens, which may last as long as eight hours. However, there are aftereffects, including acute ANXIETY, restlessness, and sleeplessness. Long after the hallucinogen is eliminated from the body, the user may experience "flashbacks," which are fragmentary recurrences of hallucinogenic effects.

Hallucinogens occur naturally but are primarily created synthetically. The most common hallucinogens are LSD (lysergic acid diethylamide), mescaline, peyote, psilocybin mushrooms, MDMA 3,4-methylenedioxymethamphetamine, and phencyclidine PCP.

See also ADDICTION.

FOR FURTHER INFORMATION:
American Society on Addiction Medicine
5225 Wisconsin Avenue NW (Suite 409)
Washington, DC 20015
Phone: (212) 244-8948

handedness   See LEFT-HANDEDNESS.

handicap   See DISABILITIES.

hangover   A disagreeable physical effect that occurs after consuming too much alcohol, or disagreeable aftereffects from the use of drugs. Sometimes sleeping medications cause hangover-like symptoms. A hangover is a source of stress as it produces physical as well as emotional symptoms that differ between individuals. Some may experience nausea, vomiting, or DIZZINESS, while others may have HEADACHES, sleepiness, unsteadiness, blurred vision, depression, or self-pity. For many individuals, symptoms do not occur until several hours after drinking the alcohol, when they awaken from sleep. They may blame the mixing of drinks, but drinking any one alcoholic beverage alone can cause a hangover.

The distinctive headache experienced as part of a hangover may be due to toxic substances that are released into the bloodstream and cause irritation of the brain membranes. Headaches may also come from the pressure of swollen blood vessels, which is an effect of alcohol. When alcohol promotes excessive urination, the resulting loss of fluid may reduce spinal fluid pressure, which has been known to bring on a headache.

Usually individuals recover from hangovers without medical assistance. Recommendations from physicians generally include aspirin (unless one is aspirin intolerant), bed rest, and solid food as soon as possible. A cup of coffee and a meal helps most people feel better.

See also ALCOHOLISM AND ALCOHOL DEPENDENCE.

harassment   See SEXUAL HARASSMENT.

hardiness   Term coined by Salvatore Maddi, Ph.D. (a University of Chicago psychologist), and relating to stress-buffering characteristics of people who stay healthy. People with hardiness are able to withstand significant levels of STRESS without becoming ill; those who are more helpless than hardy develop more illnesses, both mental and physical.

In working with executives at a major American employer, Dr. Maddi and colleagues determined three techniques that can augment hardiness as well as happiness and health.

Focusing is a technique developed by Eugene Gendlin, an American psychologist. It is a way of recognizing signals from one's body that something is wrong, such as tension in the neck or a mild headache. With stress, these conditions worsen. Maddi suggests mentally reviewing where things are not feeling just right and reviewing situations that might be stressful. Focusing increases one's sense of CONTROL over stress and enables one to make changes.

Reconstructing stressful situations. This is a technique in which you think about a recent stressful episode and write down three ways in which it might have gone better and three ways in which it might have gone worse. If you can't think of what you could have done differently, focus on a person you know who deals with stress well and what he or she would have done. Realize that things did not go as badly as they could have. Also, realize that you can think of ways to cope better with the same situation.

Self-improvement. In this technique, you know there are some situations you cannot control; you cannot avoid some situations, such as a serious illness or illness of a member of your family. To regain your sense of control and achieve more effective COPING, choose a new task to master, such as learning how to swim, dance, or develop a new hobby.

Suzanne Kobasa, a City University of New York psychologist, also used the term hardiness to identify and measure a style of psychological coping. Some of the characteristics people with hardiness exhibited included viewing life's demands as challenges rather than threats, responding with excitement and energy to change, and having a commitment to something they felt was meaningful, such as their work, community, and family. A third trait was a sense of being in control. Having the right information and being able to make decisions can make an important difference in coping with stress.

Issue of control in hardiness

A study reported in the *Journal of Personal and Social Psychology* (April 1995) detailed how 276 Israeli recruits completed questionnaires on hardiness, mental health, and ways of coping at the beginning and end of a demanding, four-month combat training period. Two components of hardiness, commitment and control, measured at the beginning of the training, predicted mental health at the end of the training. Commitment improved mental health by reducing the appraisal of threat. Control improved mental health by reducing appraisal of threat and by increasing the use of problem-solving and support-seeking strategies.

See also GENERAL ADAPTATION SYNDROME; LEARNED HELPLESSNESS.

Sources:

Floria, V., et al. "Does Hardiness Contribute to Mental Health during a Stressful Real-life Situation? The Roles of Appraisal and Coping." *Journal of Personal and Social Psychology* 68 (April 1995): 687–95.

Goleman, Daniel and Joel Gurin, eds. *Mind Body Medicine. How to Use Your Mind for Better Health.* Yonkers, N.Y.: Consumer Reports Books, 1993.

Padus, Emrika, ed. *The Complete Guide to your Emotions and your Health* Emmaus, Pa.: Rodale Press, 1992.

"having it all"   Expression that became popular during the 1980s; refers to career WOMEN who follow their chosen business or profession, get married, and raise a family. For many, this has become a satisfying way of life, but others have experienced many stressors, such as frustrations and anxieties. Some women feel that they are not giving adequate attention to their MARRIAGE and children, are constantly tired, and feel some guilt over having their children in DAY CARE centers.

Nevertheless, an increasing number of women do opt to enter business and professions. Those who are most successful say it is due to the helpfulness and understanding of their spouses as well as an adequate day-care situation.

See also WOMEN'S MOVEMENT; WORKING MOTHERS.

headaches   Headaches include pains in the head, from the outer linings of the brain and from the scalp and its blood vessels and muscles; headaches occur due to tension in or stretching of these structures. They are a source of stress because of their discomfort and unpredictability. They may be caused by a reaction to stressful situations as well as to overindulgence in alcohol, extreme fatigue, and certain infections. Headaches are fairly common in DEPRESSION, sleep disorders, and in individuals who have many anxieties, as well as those suffering from BOREDOM. The National Headache Foundation estimates that more than 80 million Americans develop headaches each year that are serious enough to warrant treatment by a physician. They are the most frequent complaint that physicians treat and may indicate a more serious condition.

Types of headaches
Tension or muscle contraction headaches, caused by tightening in the muscles of the face, neck, and scalp, may result from stress or poor posture; they may last for days or weeks and can cause variable degrees of discomfort. About 90% of all headaches are classified as tension headaches.

Cluster headaches. The term refers to a characteristic grouping in a series of attacks. The pain is generally very intense and severe and is almost always one-sided; during a series, the pain remains on the same side. In a new series, it can occur on the opposite side. Cluster headaches are not associated with the gastrointestinal disturbances or sensitivity to light that typically accompany other vascular headaches, such as migraine.

Temporomandibular joint (TMJ) headaches cause a dull ache in and around the ear that gets worse when one chews, talks, or yawns. Sufferers may hear a clicking sound on opening the mouth and feel soreness in the jaw muscles. Stress, a poor bite, or grinding of the teeth may bring on the headache.

Caffeine headaches occur in some individuals who drink too much CAFFEINE in coffee, tea, and soft drinks. Some people can relieve their symptoms by eliminating drinks containing caffeine from their diet. Others, however, who drink large quantities of such liquids and stop abruptly, may suffer caffeine withdrawal symptoms, including headaches, irritability,

depression, and sometimes nausea; relief may occur with ingestion of a caffeinated beverage.

Migraine headaches
Migraine or vascular headaches are characterized by the throbbing sensation that occurs when blood vessels in the head dilate or swell. Migraine is an often debilitating disease that occurs in periodic attacks, with each attack lasting from four to 72 hours. Symptoms may include intense pain, often associated with nausea, vomiting, appetite loss, and an unusual sensitivity to light and/or sound. Migraines generally start on either side of the head and usually remain one-sided. Of the 23 million American migraine sufferers, 60% are women. Men and women between the ages of 35 and 45 years suffer most from migraine headaches, according to a study reported in the *Journal of the American Medical Association* (December 31, 1991). More than three-fourths of migraine sufferers come from families in which other members have the same disorder. The *JAMA* researchers reported that 8.7 million females and 2.6 million males suffer from migraine headache with moderate to severe disability. Of these, 3.4 million females and 1.1 million males experience one or more attacks per month.

Common migraine headaches start unexpectedly, while *classic* migraine is usually preceded by a warning symptom known as an aura, which occurs five to 30 minutes prior to the headache. Typically, the aura includes HALLUCINATIONS of jagged light or color, speech impairment, perception of strange odors, confusion, and tingling or numbness in the face or limbs.

Why migraine headaches are so stressful
Because migraine headaches usually recur, sufferers become concerned that an attack will happen at an unfortuitous time, such as on the day of a graduation, a wedding, or important appointment. Migraine headaches often begin during a period of time filled with anxi-

eties, such as during adolescence or MENO-PAUSE, or around the time of a DIVORCE or death of a mate. When a physician diagnoses headaches, the individual's anxieties and COPING styles will be considered.

Migraine headaches, which often occur in members of the same family, may result from a predisposing genetic biochemical abnormality. Also, personality traits may play a role in determining who gets migraines. Although there is no typical personality associated with these headaches, some migraine sufferers have characteristics of compulsivity and PERFECTION.

Emotional tension and stress may lead to migraine attacks, because under extreme stress, the arteries of the head and those reaching the brain draw tightly together and restrict the flow of blood. This in turn may result in a shortage of oxygen to the brain. When blood vessels dilate or stretch, a greater amount of blood passes through, putting more pressure on the pain-sensitive nerves in and close to the walls of the arteries.

Common migraine triggers
In a susceptible person, the migraine trigger might be something seen, smelled, heard, eaten, or experienced; it may be one particular trigger or a combination of factors.

Approximately 20% of all migraine sufferers have a sensitivity to a specific food or

---

DIETARY FACTORS: POSSIBLE MIGRAINE ATTACK TRIGGERS

- Caffeinated foods and drinks: coffee, tea, chocolate, cocoa, colas/soft drinks
- Alcohol: especially red wine, vermouth, champagne, beer
- Dairy products: aged cheeses, sour cream, whole milk, buttermilk, yogurt, ice cream
- Breads: sourdough, fresh yeast, and some types of cereals
- Vegetables: some types of beans (broad, Italian, lima, lentil, fava, soy), sauerkraut, onions, peas
- Snacks: nuts, peanuts, peanut butter, pickles, seeds, sesame
- Meats: organ meats, salted meats, dried meats, cured meats, smoked fish, meats with nitrites (such as hot dogs, sausages, lunch meat)
- Fruits: most citrus fruits, bananas, avocados, figs, raisins, papaya, passion fruit, red plums, raspberries, plantains, pineapples
- Monosodium glutamate (MSG): a flavor enhancer often used in restaurants and also in seasoned salt, instant foods, canned soup, frozen dinners, pizza, potato chips
- Soups: particularly those containing MSG; soups made from bouillon cubes
- Desserts: chocolate, licorice, molasses, cakes/cookies made with yeast
- Seasonings and flavorings such as soy sauce, some spices, garlic powder, onion powder, salt, meat tenderizers, marinades
- Hunger; missing meals, fasting, dieting

COMMON MIGRAINE TRIGGERS

- Dietary habits (see detailed listing following)
- Environmental factors, such as weather, bright lights, glare or noise
- Emotional factors, such as depression, anxiety, resentment, or fatigue
- Activity, such as motion from riding in a car or airplane, lack of sleep, too much sleep, eyestrain, and a fall or head injury
- Hormonal, such as menstrual cycle or use of oral contraceptives or estrogen supplements
- Medications, such as overuse of over-the-counter pain relievers and some prescription medications

---

foods. Knowing that certain foods may trigger migraines is an additional source of stress. Many individuals find that certain foods (such as cheese, chocolate, and red wine) containing a substance known as tyramine trigger migraine attacks. Sodium nitrite, a preservative used in ham, hot dogs, and many other sausages, is a trigger for some people. Although some migraine researchers have recommended that all migraine sufferers avoid these foods, only about 30% of people who have migraine headaches experience this reaction to some foods. Not eating or missing meals can cause low blood sugar levels, which are also a migraine trigger.

Identifying and avoiding the triggers that cause headaches is one of the most significant management techniques for controlling headache frequency and stress.

**Migraine headaches, hormones
and pregnancy**

Although migraine headaches are more common in young boys than in young girls, the number of girls affected increases sharply after the onset of MENSTRUATION. Certain hormonal changes that occur during PUBERTY in girls and remain throughout adulthood may be implicated in the triggering and frequency of migraine attacks in women.

The link between female endocrine changes and migraine headaches is reinforced by the finding that 60% of women sufferers involved in a clinical study related attacks to their menstrual cycle. Individual differences exist: attacks may occur several days before, during, or immediately after the woman's menses.

In females with migraine, about 77% find that their attacks disappear completely, occur less often, or are milder during pregnancy. In others, attacks either worsened or remained unchanged.

Oral contraceptives also affect the incidence of migraine attacks. Some migraine sufferers find their attacks are worsened while they are on the Pill. Others find that they are not affected, and a small percent report improvement. Yet some women, even without any predisposition to migraine, develop it while on the Pill, and nearly three-quarters find their headaches disappearing after they stop taking the Pill.

Diagnosis

When a headache does not respond to RELAXATION, rest, sleeping, simple self-medication such as aspirin or non-steroidal anti-inflammatory drugs available over-the-counter, cold compresses on the head, or relaxation in a dark room, medical assistance should be sought. During a complete physical and neurological examination, the physician will ask about the history of the headaches, the period of time in which they have been occurring, when they occur, the circumstances at the time, and how long they last.

Diagnostic techniques may include use of computerized tomography scanning (CT scanning) or magnetic resonance imaging (MRI).

Diagnosis is necessary before an individual takes any medication for headaches. Medications that help tension headaches will not help severe migraine headaches, and drugs targeted to relieve migraine headaches may not help any other type. Also, it is important that one does not overmedicate for headaches and bring on other side effects from medications.

Therapies for headaches

Treatments for headaches include non-pharmacological treatments, such as BIOFEEDBACK, MEDITATION, and relaxation techniques, as well as prescription medications. In the mid-1990s, a medication became available in tablet form (sumatriptan succinate) that is a highly selective serotonin receptor-agonist for the treatment of migraine with or without aura. It is not indicated for cluster headache.

For migraine or vascular headaches, medication is targeted toward altering responses of the vascular system to stress, hormonal changes, noise, and other stimuli. Such medications affect the dilation reaction of the blood vessels. Ergot, a naturally occurring substance that constricts blood vessels and reduces the dilation of arteries, has historically been a popular medication. Ergot may be given by inhalation, injection, orally, or rectally. Some people find that if they take the ergot medication early enough in prepain stages of an attack they can abort their headaches or at least reduce their intensity.

Some vascular headaches are helped with prophylactic (preventive) measures. The drug of choice for prevention of migraine in carefully selected patients is propranolol. Propranolol is a vasoconstrictor that can be taken daily for as long as six months. This drug may slow down the vascular changes that occur during the migraine attack; it is frequently prescribed for some individuals who have headaches more than once each week. Propranolol has an advantage over ergot medications in that rebound headaches are not brought on by discontinuance of propranolol.

Medications for muscle contraction headaches are directed toward relieving muscular activity and spasm. Analgesics (pain relievers) commonly used are aspirin, dextropropoxyphene, and ethoheptazine. Injection with anesthetics and corticosteroids may be helpful.

For treating cluster headaches, choice of medications depends on the frequency and severity of headaches, as well as response to previous treatments. Some drugs used include ergotamine, methysergide, cyproheptadine, lithium, and steroids, as well as oxygen inhalation and histamine desensitization. These treatments should be used only under the careful guidance of a physician who is familiar with their use.

In depressed individuals, some antidepressant drugs may provide relief from headaches including migraine; examples are the monoamine oxidase inhibitors (MAOIs) such as phenelzine sulfate.

Alternative therapies
A wide variety of ALTERNATIVE THERAPIES may be helpful for headache sufferers. Some individuals experience relief with their use and without medication while others use them in conjunction with medication. When individuals consider alternative therapies, they should be discussed with the attending physician. Although some people can relieve their headache pain with alternative therapies, for others these therapies act as an adjunct or complement to the PHARMACOLOGICAL AP-

PROACH, making the sufferer more receptive to medical treatment.

Biofeedback involves teaching a person to control certain body functions through thought and willpower, with feedback from an electronic device.

Meditation (also known as transcendental meditation) is a technique of inward contemplation that helps some people relieve anxieties and in turn relieve some headaches, by relaxation. During meditation, the mind, as well as other organs in the body, slows down; heart rate decreases, breathing becomes slower, and muscle tensions diminish.

ACUPUNCTURE has been successfully used to treat some headache sufferers. Acupuncture probably works because the needle insertions somehow stimulate the body to secrete ENDORPHINS, naturally occurring hormone-like substances that kill pain. ACUPRESSURE involves pressing acupuncture points with the hands, and can be done by a professional as well as by a trained lay person.

See also ANXIETY; GUIDED IMAGERY; HANGOVER; HYPNOSIS; TEMPOROMANDIBULAR JOINT SYNDROME.

FOR FURTHER INFORMATION:
American Association for the Study of the
    Headache
P.O. Box 5136
San Clemente, CA 92672
Phone: (714) 498-1846; (800) 255-ACHE

National Headache Foundation
5252 N. Western Avenue
Chicago, IL 60625
Phone: (773) 878-7715

SOURCES:
Diamond, Seymour. *The Hormone Headache: New Ways to Prevent, Manage, and Treat Migraines and Other Headaches.* New York: Macmillan, 1995.
Inlander, Charles B., and Porter Shimer. *Headaches: 47 Ways to Stop the Pain.* New York: Walker, 1995.
Maas, Paula, and Deborah Mitchell. *The Natural Health Guide to Headache Relief: The Definitive Handbook of Natural Remedies for Treating Every*

Kind of Headache Pain. New York: Pocket Books, 1997.

healing touch   See THERAPEUTIC TOUCH.

health communications   The public is constantly bombarded by stressful messages about health; it happens in the newspapers and magazines, on TV and, if using the Internet, while sitting at the computer. On any given day, CANCER is (or is not caused) by "blank," and you take "blank" vitamins and you will (or will not) grow old.

STRESS and ANXIETY surround almost every health communication, including the ADVERTISING of medical products. A session at the February 1995 meeting of the American Association for the Advancement of Science was devoted to "The Public, the Media, and Scientific Controversies." One perspective presented showed that "the emphasis on bad news, compounded by the media's ability to disseminate such information quickly, globally, and graphically, is a major factor in destroying trust. Good news, such as further testing that fails to show a health hazard is often fuzzy and carries little weight in forming an opinion." Thus consumers are left confused and frustrated by news about health that is intended to be useful.

See also ARTHRITIS; CHRONIC ILLNESS; HEART ATTACK.

hearing loss   See DEAFNESS.

heart attack   Known medically as myocardial infarction; the sudden death of a part of the heart muscle, characterized, in most cases, by severe, unremitting chest pain. Contributory factors to a heart attack include STRESS, HIGH BLOOD PRESSURE and TYPE A PERSONALITY.

The onset of a heart attack is extremely stressful for the sufferer as well as onlookers. The individual may be short of breath, restless, feel nauseated or vomit, or lose consciousness. *It is crucial to respond immediately to a suspected heart attack.* In mild cases, pain and other symptoms are very slight or do not develop at all, in which case the attack is known as a "silent heart attack." Such an episode may be discovered only by subsequent tests.

Fear of having a heart attack is a common sources of stress, because many symptoms of anxieties and PHOBIAS (including HYPERVENTILATION, PALPITATIONS, and faintness) mimic some of the symptoms of a heart attack. Such fears are not unfounded; heart attack is the leading cause of death for both men and women in the United States. Every year, 1.5 million Americans have a heart attack; one-third of them die as a result. However, from 1981 to 1991, death rates from heart attack decreased over 30%, due partly to better diagnosis and advancements in prevention, treatment, surgery, and medication. Treatment of heart attacks with clot-dissolving drugs, for example, has helped reduce the death rate dramatically.

Once the coronary artery gets blocked by a clot, a heart attack can occur quite suddenly. Within minutes of a heart attack, the heart muscle begins to change. Deprived of oxygen, the affected portion of the heart muscle deteriorates and dies; surrounding tissue may also be damaged. The longer the artery remains blocked, the greater the damage and possibility of death. According to the American Heart Association, about 60% of all heart attack deaths occur within the first hour. Fear, unfamiliarity with the symptoms, and DENIAL are some of the reasons why individuals and their families delay getting help. Many deaths from heart attack can be prevented with proper and prompt treatment.

Symptoms of a heart attack
If the warning signs listed in the box on page 166 occur, individuals should get help immediately.

Symptoms may be mild, or severe, or even completely absent. Often, older individuals have the fewest or mildest symptoms of heart attack. Few people have all the classic signs.

WHAT TO DO IF A HEART ATTACK IS SUSPECTED

Seventy percent of heart attacks occur in the home; family members can assist immensely if they know what to do in response to the emergency, including cardiopulmonary resuscitation (CPR) procedures. Also:

- Do not spend time trying to reach your physician. Have someone call your local emergency number (911 in many urban areas) or an ambulance service. Tell the dispatcher that heart attack is suspected.
- If getting to a hospital is faster by car, have someone drive you there instead of waiting for an ambulance.
- Ask to be taken to an area hospital equipped with 24-hour emergency cardiac care.
- Try to stay calm. Lie down, propped up with pillows. Agitation can increase the likelihood of abnormal, life-threatening heart rhythms.
- Have someone call your personal physician.

The sooner a person receives appropriate medical treatment, the greater the chances of surviving a heart attack and avoiding permanent damage to the heart. Some potent new drugs that can prevent the death of the heart muscle, for example, work only if they are given within the first few hours after the heart attack.

HEART ATTACK WARNING SYMPTOMS

- A crushing chest pressure or pain in the center of the chest that lasts more than a few minutes or goes away and comes back. The discomfort may be felt as a burning sensation that can be mistaken for severe heartburn.
- Chest pain that spreads to the shoulders and arms or the left or both sides, as well as to the neck or back
- Accompanying nausea, vomiting, sweating, cold sweats, shortness of breath, palpitations, light-headedness, or faintness
- A sensation of impending doom

Diagnosis and treatment for heart attack in an emergency room may be stressful for the sufferer. One may be fearful and anxious about the surroundings, expectations for life, and hopes for recovery.

Stresses after a heart attack
Individuals who have suffered a heart attack have an increased risk of suffering another one in the following few years. They live with the stress of ANXIETY about this probability. Many such individuals benefit from psychological counseling. The chances of surviving for many years can be improved by attention to life-style changes, including more RELAXATION, increased exercise, better diet, reduction of OBESITY, and cessation of SMOKING. An individual who has had a heart attack should have regular check-ups by a physician. Support and exercise groups can be helpful.

See also ATHEROSCLEROSIS; BIOFEEDBACK; CHOLESTEROL; HEARTBURN; MEDITATION.

FOR FURTHER INFORMATION:
American Heart Association
7320 Greenville Avenue
Dallas, TX 75231
Phone: (214) 373-6300

National Heart, Lung and Blood Institute
9000 Rockville Pike
Bethesda, MD 20892
Phone: (301) 496-4236

heartburn Burning sensation in the upper part of the abdomen or under the breast bone. It is a cause of STRESS for many people who may fear that it is related to heart disease. Heartburn is also a symptom of stress, because it can be brought on by nervousness or overeating. The burning sensation is actually associated with the esophagus, a muscular tube that connects the throat with the stomach. The tube passes behind the breastbone alongside the heart, which is why irritation or inflammation here is known as heartburn.

Heartburn and distress in the digestive tract is frequently a response to emotional stress. Tense, nervous people who worry about their jobs and family problems often complain of "acid INDIGESTION" and heartburn. The list of foods that disagree with heartburn sufferers includes just about anything a person would want to eat. When things go smoothly for these people, everything agrees with them. When they are upset or frustrated, nothing does. Heartburn usually starts slowly, about an hour or so after they have eaten a heavy or spicy meal. The pain can sometimes be quite intense and may last a few hours.

Coping with heartburn

In some cases, the pain is due to irritation (esophagitis) from hydrochloric acid in the stomach juice that has backed up into the esophagus; relaxation of the valve between the stomach and the esophagus is one cause of esophagitis. Hiatus hernia, in which part of the stomach slips up into the chest, is another. This type of heartburn is often brought on by lying down, especially after overeating. It may be helped by raising the head of the bed, by avoiding certain foods, especially sweets, and by a low-fat, low-calorie diet.

TIPS FOR RELIEVING THE STRESS OF HEARTBURN

- Avoid certain foods that are spicy, acidic, tomato-based or fatty, such as sausages, chocolate, tomatoes, and citrus fruits.
- Avoid alcohol, tea, colas, and coffee, even decaffeinated.
- Eat moderate amounts of food to avoid overfilling your stomach.
- Stop or at least cut back on smoking.
- Don't try to exercise immediately after eating or before lying down.
- Elevate the head of your bed or use extra pillows to raise the level of your head above your feet.
- Avoid tight belts and other restrictive clothing.
- Learn relaxation techniques.
- If none of these help, see your doctor.

People whose heartburn is brought on by stress and emotional factors may not have abnormal amounts of hydrochloric acid in their stomachs. They are probably oversensitive to normal acidity, just as they may overreact to the ordinary stressors of daily life. Adequate rest and RELAXATION and occasional use of antacids may be helpful. Individuals who suffer frequent heartburn should be checked by a physician. If there are no medical problems, a change in mental attitude toward the stressors in the individual's life should be considered. Relaxation training and medication may be helpful.

See also ALTERNATIVE THERAPIES; MEDITATION; PEPTIC ULCER.

help lines See HOT LINES; SELF-HELP GROUPS; SUPPORT GROUPS.

hemorrhoids Enlarged veins at the lowest part of the intestine. Hemorrhoids may be painful or bleed, causing stress for the sufferer. The word literally means a blood (*hemo*) flow (*rhoid*), describing one of the characteristics of the disease, bleeding from the anus. "Piles" is a layman's term for hemorrhoids.

Hemorrhoids are also stressful because in many cases their cause cannot be determined. CONSTIPATION, straining while defecating, sitting for long periods, and infections can aggravate the condition once it starts. The disorder usually is mild, but if neglected, may result in annoying or painful complications such as itching, protrusion outside the anus, or fissures in the anus, and possibly secondary infection.

Treatment consists of warm sitz baths, soothing ointments, antibiotics for infection, measures such as laxatives or stool softeners to relieve constipation, and a diet of digestible foods. Any bleeding from the anus should be investigated by a physician.

See also IRRITABLE BOWEL SYNDROME.

hepatitis B See SEXUALLY TRANSMITTED DISEASES.

herbal medicine   Use of a plant or portion of a plant valued for its medicinal, savory, or aromatic qualities. Herbalism gained popularity in the United States toward the end of the 20th century. Estimates are that Americans spend over a billion dollars on herbal remedies in a year; many people seek these alternative remedies to relieve stress.

Herbal medications are deeply rooted in most folk medicine traditions and have played an important role in the evolution of modern medicine and pharmacology. For example, when the Pilgrims landed in Plymouth in 1630, they set up herb gardens that contained the medicinal varieties brought from the Old World. The settlers soon discovered that the Native Americans had their own healing plants, including cascara sagrada and goldenseal. According to the World Health Organization, 80% of Earth's population uses some form of herbal therapy.

Many contemporary medications are based on specific herbs but are manufactured from synthetic substances believed to be more effective than the natural herbs Still, herbal therapies remain a major component of Ayurvedic, homeopathic, and other alternative approaches.

Herbal products are marketed in the United States as foods, and are permitted by the Food and Drug Administration provided that the products do not make any therapeutic claims. Herbal products are sold "over-the-counter" and are not subject to the same safety and efficacy standards that apply to over-the-counter medications. Herbal packaging labels rarely contain guidelines regarding indications for proper use. As with any medication, herbal remedies are best used under the guidance of a knowledgeable individual, in this case, an herbalist.

See also ALTERNATIVE THERAPIES; AYURVEDA; HOMEOPATHY.

FOR FURTHER INFORMATION:
The Herb Research Foundation
1007 Pearl Street (Suite 200)
Boulder, CO 80302
Phone: (303) 449-2265

SOURCES:
Chevallier, Andrew. *The Encyclopedia of Medicinal Plants.* Boston: Houghton Mifflin, 1996.
National Women's Health Report. "Alternative Therapies and Women's Health," Washington, D.C.: National Women's Health Resource Center, May/June 1995.
Schar, Douglas. *The Backyard Medicine Chest: An Herbal Primer.* Washington, D.C.: Elliott & Clark, 1995.

herpes simplex virus   HSV can cause blister-like sores almost anywhere on a person's skin. It usually occurs around the mouth and nose or the buttocks and genitals. Herpes is a name used for some 50 related viruses. Herpes simplex is related to the risk for infectious mononucleosis, chicken pox, and shingles (varicella zoster virus). HSV infections can be very stressful because they can reappear without any predictability; also, the sores may be painful and embarrassing.

Two types of HSV
Type 1. Studies show that most people get Type 1, which affects the lips, mouth, nose, chin, or cheeks during infancy or childhood. It is transmitted by close contact with family members or friends who carry the virus. It can be transmitted by kissing, or by using the

---

HERBAL REMEDIES FOR STRESS RELIEF

- See a physician first for serious conditions. Do not attempt to self-medicate.
- Consider the sources of your products; select reputable brands.
- Choose reliable forms such as tinctures or freeze-dried, as powdered forms may lose potency upon exposure to air.
- Overdosing can have harmful effects. Take recommended dosages at suggested intervals.
- Watch for reactions; if unwanted reactions occur, stop the medication.

same eating utensils and towels. A rash or cold sores on the mouth and gums appear shortly after exposure. Symptoms may be barely noticeable or may need medical attention for relief of pain.

Type 2. Type 2, which includes genital herpes, one of the many diseases caused by the herpes virus, most often appears following sexual contact with an infected person. It has reached epidemic numbers, affecting anywhere between five to 20 million persons in the United States, or up to 20% of all sexually active adults. Genital herpes, although relatively uncommon in the United States until the late 1960s, may be the most common sexually transmitted disease in the late 1990s. The chronicity of the disease and the fact that no cure exists is a source of significant stress in the lives of its sufferers. Stress and anxiety associated with having this SEXUALLY TRANSMITTED DISEASE can be reduced with education, counseling, and supportive physical care.

Herpes is particularly stressful because once the virus invades the body, it remains for life, although it may be dormant most of the time. In different individuals, episodes recur with more or less frequency.

Although genital herpes is not usually a medically serious disease, it can lead to DEPRESSION and other emotional conditions. Many victims tend to resent the sex partner from whom they contracted the disease, often leading to divorce or the breaking up of a relationship. Others consider themselves damaged for life, fearing that they are unfit for marriage or a lasting relationship.

The disease is most commonly spread by direct contact, meaning that to get herpes, uninfected skin must come in contact with an active herpes sore. However, the virus may be shed without noticeable symptoms and may thus be transmitted. As herpes sores may be hidden in the internal parts of the female genitalia or may not be painful, one victim may unwittingly infect another.

Once the herpes virus has entered the skin, it multiplies rapidly. First symptoms are usually itching or a tingling sensation, followed by the eruption of unusually painful sores or blisters. Typically, in the first attack the sores appear two days to two weeks after exposure and last two to three weeks. Subsequent attacks, which may occur in a few weeks or not for years, generally last about five days. When an attack subsides, the virus lies dormant and travels along the nerve fibers until it reaches a resting place.

Complications

In rare cases, the herpes virus may travel to the brain and cause a serious, often fatal, form of encephalitis. More commonly, herpes may infect the cornea of the eye; if untreated, the infection can lead to visual damage and even blindness. None of these complications, however, is as common as periodic recurrences at the original site of infection.

A serious complication of genital herpes affects infants born to women who have active infections at the time of birth. Some infants who contract disseminated herpes infections die, and half of those who survive may suffer brain damage or blindness. Many doctors recommend that the baby be delivered by Cesarean section if the mother has an active infection near the time of delivery.

Prevention

The most effective way of preventing genital herpes is avoiding all sexual contact with an infected person. Use of a condom and spermicidal agent will reduce the risk, but this is not absolutely foolproof, particularly when the lesions are on the skin of the perineum and not on the penis or in the vagina.

Treatment and self-help

There is no way to rid the body of the herpes virus. However, antiviral agents developed during the 1990s shorten the duration of an active infection, relieve discomfort, and speed healing. By halting the virus from reproducing itself and spreading to other cells, these agent stops the formation of new herpes blisters and help existing sores heal faster.

Many herpes sufferers learn to recognize patterns of recurrence and factors that trigger subsequent episodes. RELAXATION techniques to reduce stress are indicated if stress is a factor in recurrent disease. There are a number of herpes counseling centers and groups throughout the country to lend support and help to victims of the disease. The American Social Health Association maintains a National Herpes Information Hotline number: (919) 361-8488. The toll-free number to request free literature is (800) 230-6039.

FOR FURTHER INFORMATION:
The Herpes Resource Center
260 Sheridan Avenue (Suite 307)
Palo Alto, CA 94306
Phone: (800) 227-8922; (415) 328-7710

American Academy of Dermatology
930 N. Meacham Road
P.O. Box 4014
Schaumburg, IL 60168-4014
Phone: (708) 330-0230

SOURCES:
Nourse, Alan Edward. *Herpes.* New York: Franklin Watts, 1985.
Sacks, Stephen L. *The Truth About Herpes,* 3rd ed. Seattle: G. Soules Book Publishers, 1988.

high blood pressure The term "blood pressure," as used in medicine, refers to the force of blood against the walls of one's arteries, created by the heart as it pumps blood through the body. As the heart pumps or beats, the pressure increases; as the heart relaxes between beats, the pressure decreases. High blood pressure (hypertension) is the condition in which blood pressure rises too high and stays there.

High blood pressure is an important individual as well as public health issue because it affects as much as 25% of the adult population in the United States. High blood pressure has been associated with the stresses resulting from certain negative emotions or aggressive and hostile behaviors. Although the degree of stress is difficult to assess objectively, acute and probably chronically stressful situations can result in an elevation of the blood pressure. Certain individuals are overreactive to stress and may suffer more than others when confronting certain situations. Individuals with high blood pressure have higher irritability levels, more GUILT feelings, and more psychic distress.

There are many studies of the effects of psychological factors such as stress, psychological or PERSONALITY characteristics, and life events on blood pressure. A problem with these studies has been the difficulty of assessing psychosocial factors and determining whether they are causes or consequences of high blood pressure. It is possible that the process of labeling or treating a person with blood pressure elevation can induce a stressful psychological change.

Diagnosing high blood pressure
According to the National Heart, Lung and Blood Institute, high blood pressure is more likely to develop in people with a family history of high blood pressure, those who are overweight, eat a high-salt diet, drink excessively, and/or are physically inactive.

In its early stages, high blood pressure does not usually produce any symptoms; thus it is sometimes called "the silent killer." Many people who have high blood pressure feel just fine. Regular check-ups are the only way to detect high blood pressure.

High blood pressure is usually diagnosed during an office visit to a physician. The physician uses a stethoscope and a sphygmomanometer, an inflatable cuff attached to a device that measures blood pressure. With each heartbeat, blood is pumped through the arteries and veins. The force with which blood pushes against the artery walls creates blood pressure, which is represented by two numbers. The top number, systolic pressure, indicates the maximum pressure with which blood pushes against the arteries during a heartbeat. The lower number, diastolic pressure, indicates pressure against the arteries when the heart is at rest. Normal or healthy blood pressure is in the 120–90 range. If the reading regularly hits 140–90, one is said to have high blood pressure.

High blood pressure usually starts when arteries become too narrowed or constricted, impeding the flow of blood. High pressure in these damaged arteries makes them susceptible to a buildup of fatty, cholesterol-containing deposits, a condition known as ATHEROSCLEROSIS. If blood vessels feeding the heart become blocked and/or hardened, a person may suffer chest pain (known as angina) or may have a HEART ATTACK. When the blood supply to the brain is disrupted, STROKE may occur. Other effects may be kidney failure and eye damage.

"White coat hypertension"

Some individuals actually show elevations in their blood pressure when visiting a physician's office. Their blood pressure is generally normal but increases in the presence of physicians and other health care professionals. This is because these individuals feel stressed and fearful of doctors or the surroundings, such as laboratories, where they might encounter needles or blood testing devices. They may be diagnosed with high blood pressure.

Physicians who understand this phenomenon usually take the patient's blood pressure at the end of the visit as well as the beginning, and take a careful history to determine the effects of the patient's phobias on the blood pressure.

Treating high blood pressure

Non-drug measures can help many people control their high blood pressure. In many cases, however, these measures may be recommended along with medication because they are beneficial for overall good health. Helpful techniques include BIOFEEDBACK;

SELF-HELP FOR TREATING HIGH BLOOD PRESSURE

- *Stress control.* Training in relaxation techniques and use of biofeedback help some patients handle stressful life situations in more constructive ways.
- *Weight reduction.* Some overweight people can reduce their blood pressure by losing excess weight.
- *Salt restriction.* In combination with medication, salt restriction is often helpful.
- *Restriction of dietary cholesterol.* High blood levels of cholesterol, coupled with high blood pressure, can damage arteries.
- *Restriction of alcohol consumption.* Drinking should not exceed two ounces of 100-proof, which equals eight ounces of wine or 24 ounces of beer a day.
- *No smoking.* Nicotine directly affects the heart and blood vessels producing acute increases in blood pressure. Independent of high blood pressure, smoking can damage arteries.

BREATHING; GUIDED IMAGERY; HYPNOSIS, RELAXATION; T'AI CHI.

Role of exercise in reducing high blood pressure

Many activities that reduce stress, including aerobic exercise, running, biking, walking, and swimming, also reduce both systolic and diastolic blood pressure. The American College of Sports Medicine (ACSM) recommends aerobic activities three to five days a week for 20 to 60 minutes per workout at intensities 40% to 80% of maximum effort.

However, the ACSM advises people with high blood pressure to avoid high-intensity strength training, or weight training, because it temporarily elevates blood pressure whether one has high blood pressure or not.

Role of nutrition

Maintaining a proper diet can be beneficial in treating high blood pressure, according to a review in the *Archives of Family Medicine*

(August 14, 1995). Claude K. Lardinois, M.D, University of Nevada School of Medicine, conducted a study to determine the efficacy of nutritional factors in preventing high blood pressure as well as their role in the treatment of individuals with established high blood pressure.

The researcher found that weight reduction, sodium chloride restriction, and avoidance of excessive alcohol consumption appear to be the best nutritional approaches to the treatment of high blood pressure. "The role of dietary alterations of fiber, calcium, magnesium, potassium, dietary fats, carbohydrates, and protein is less convincing. Unfortunately, much of the available data are insufficient to make a final recommendation regarding a potential role for these alterations in the prevention and treatment of high blood pressure," said the researcher.

Weight control is important because the prevalence of high blood pressure is 50% higher among overweight adults than among adults of normal weight; 33% of people who have high blood pressure are overweight. Overweight individuals have a twofold to sixfold increased risk for developing high blood pressure. Modest weight loss can favorably affect high blood pressure.

Recommendations for a prudent diet for high blood pressure prevention and treatment, based on the current review of the literature, include modest weight loss (10% of present weight), limiting sodium intake to 100 millimoles (six grams of sodium chloride) and limiting alcohol consumption to no more than two drinks per day (30 milliliters of ethanol).

Drug treatment for high blood pressure
Taking medication for high blood pressure is stressful for some individuals because many medications cause side effects or other problems that complicate treatment. These effects may include fatigue, sexual IMPOTENCE, and DIZZINESS. A study in the *Journal of the American Medical Association* (June 14, 1985) reported that, of 3,844 patients being treated for high blood pressure, 9.3% stopped their drug treatment because of "definite" or "probable" side effects, and an additional 23.4% stopped drug treatment because of "possible" side effects.

In some cases, one drug will maintain pressure control over time. More often, one drug controls it for a time; then a second or third may be needed. High blood pressure can be controlled, as long as appropriate medicines are taken:

- *Diuretics* act on the kidneys, causing them to flush out salt and water. As fluid in the blood vessels goes down, pressure goes down.
- *Beta blockers* act on the heart, reducing the rate at which it beats and the amount of blood it pumps; with less output, pressure drops.
- *Vasodilators* relax the small arteries, reducing their resistance to blood flow, causing blood pressure to go down.
- *Sympathetic inhibitors* act on the sympathetic nervous system and also relax the arteries, keeping pressure down.
- *Calcium channel blockers* lower the levels of calcium in the blood vessel muscle cells. This relaxes the vessels, and pressure drops.
- *ACE inhibitors* work in a unique way in the body, and have been shown to be effective in controlling high blood pressure, usually without causing some of the troublesome side effects caused by older drugs. ACE inhibitors interrupt a chemical chain reaction in the body that causes blood pressure to rise. The kidney triggers the process by releasing an enzyme called "renin" into the bloodstream. As part of the chain reaction, the lungs produce an enzyme called ACE (angiotensin-converting enzyme). The presence of ACE leads to production of another chemical that raises pressure. ACE inhibitors bind up ACE, interrupting the chemical chain and maintaining more normal pressure.

- *Alpha blockers and central alpha agonists* keep blood vessels open by blocking the action of certain nerves.

  See also ALTERNATIVE THERAPIES; EXERCISE; NUTRITION; PETS; TYPE A PERSONALITY.

FOR FURTHER INFORMATION:
American Heart Association
7320 Greenville Avenue
Dallas, TX 75231
Phone: (214) 373-6300

National High Blood Pressure Education Program
National Institutes of Health
Bethesda, MD 20014
Phone: (301) 496-1051

SOURCES:
Kerman, D. Ariel. *H.A.R.T. Program: Lower Your Blood Pressure Without Drugs.* New York: HarperCollins, 1992.
Lardinois, Claude K. "Role of Nutrition in Treating Hypertension." *Archives of Family Medicine,* August 14, 1995.
Pickering, Thomas G., et al. "How Common Is White Coat Hypertension?" *Journal of the American Medical Association*, January 8, 1988, 225–28.

HIV/AIDS Treatment Information Service (ATIS)   This is a free telephone reference service for health care providers as well as people living with HIV disease. Many people find relief from some of the psychological stresses of living with HIV disease when they get answers to their questions and sources for further information. During 1995, its first year, the staff responded to more than 10,000 calls.

The HIV/AIDS Treatment Information Service is sponsored by the Agency for Health Care Policy and Research, Centers for Disease Control and Prevention, Health Resources and Services Administration, National Institutes of Health, and the Substance Abuse and Mental Health Services Administration. The service is offered through the Centers for Disease Control National AIDS Clearinghouse.

Reference specialists answer questions about the latest treatment options, provide customized database searches, and link callers to other HIV/AIDS information resources. Through the service, callers can acquire copies of the latest federally approved treatment guidelines, including recommendations for HIV counseling and voluntary testing for pregnant women, guidelines for prevention of opportunistic infections in persons infected with HIV, and study results concerning anti-HIV therapy, which lowers risk of AIDS and death in patients with intermediate-stage HIV disease.

In late 1995, the treatment service developed the *Glossary of HIV/Aids-Related Terms* to help people understand the technical terms related to HIV, its associated treatments, and the medical management of related conditions. To obtain a copy of the *Glossary* or to obtain information on new treatment guidelines, phone: (800) HIV- 0440.

See also HUMAN IMMUNODEFICIENCY VIRUS.

hives   Pink swellings called "wheals" that occur in groups on any part of the skin. They are stressful to the sufferer because, as they are forming, they usually are very itchy and may also burn or sting. Until they are diagnosed, the sufferer may be bewildered about the cause and possibilities for relief. Hives usually go away within a few days to a few weeks. Occasionally, a person will continue to have hives for many years. About 10 to 20% of the population will have at least one episode in their lifetime.

When hives form around the eyes, lips, or genitals, the tissue may swell excessively. Although frightening in appearance, the swelling usually goes away in less than 24 hours. Dermatologists may use the term "angioedema" to describe this type of swelling, which is also used to describe very deep large hives on other areas of the body.

In the commonest kind of hives, each individual wheal lasts a few hours before fading away, leaving no trace. New hives may continue to develop as old areas fade. They can vary in size from as small as a pencil eraser to as large as a dinner plate and may join together to form larger swellings.

Causes of hives
Hives are produced by blood plasma leaking through tiny gaps between the cells lining small blood vessels in the skin. Histamine, a natural chemical, is released from cells called "mast cells," which lie along the blood vessels in the skin. Many different things, including allergic reactions, chemicals in food, or medications, can cause a histamine release. Sometimes it is impossible to find out why histamine is being released and hives are forming.

The most common foods that cause hives are nuts, chocolate, fish, tomatoes, eggs, fresh berries, and milk. Fresh foods cause hives more often than cooked foods; food additives and preservatives may also be responsible. Hives may appear within minutes or up to two hours after eating, depending on where the food is absorbed in the digestive tract.

Almost any prescription or over-the-counter medication can cause hives. Some of these drugs include antibiotics (especially penicillin), pain medications, sedatives, tranquilizers, and diuretics. Antacids, vitamins, eye and ear drops, laxatives, vaginal douches, or any other non-prescription item can be a potential cause of hives.

Many infections can cause hives. Viral upper respiratory tract infections are a common cause in children. Other viruses including hepatitis B may also be a cause, as well as a number of bacterial and fungal infections.

Some people develop hives from sunlight, cold, pressure, vibration, or EXERCISE. Hives due to sunlight are called "solar urticaria." This is a rare disorder in which hives come up within minutes of sun exposure on exposed areas and fade within one to two hours. Reaction to the cold is more common. Hives appear when the skin is warmed after exposure to cold. If the exposure to cold is over large areas of the body, large amounts of histamine may be released, which can produce sneezing, flushing, generalized hives, and fainting. A simple test for this type of hives can be done by applying an ice cube to the skin.

Diagnosis and treatment of hives
Diagnosis depends on each individual's medical history and a thorough examination by a dermatologist. The best treatment for hives is to find the cause and then eliminate it, which is not always an easy task. While investigating the cause of hives, or when a cause cannot be found, dermatologists often prescribe antihistamines to provide some relief to the sufferer. Antihistamines work best if taken on a regular schedule to prevent hives from forming.

In cases of severe hives, an injection of epinephrine (adrenaline) or a cortisone preparation, may bring relief.

See also ALLERGIES.

FOR FURTHER INFORMATION:
American Academy of Dermatology
930 N. Meacham Road
Schaumburg, IL 60172-4965
Phone: (708) 330-0230

HIV positive See ACQUIRED IMMUNODEFICIENCY SYNDROME; HUMAN IMMUNODEFICIENCY VIRUS.

hobbies Activities people engage in because they want to, not because they must for economic reasons. They are sources of satisfaction, RELAXATION, and relief from the stresses of everyday life for many people. People who look forward to RETIREMENT do so because they will have more time for hobbies. Choosing hobbies is up to each individual, although in many cases they bring people with common interests together. For many people, collecting antiques or other collectibles is a hobby.

According to Allen Elkin, Ph.D., director, Stress Management and Counseling Center,

New York City, "people who derive most of their identity from their profession are going to need other sources of SELF-ESTEEM when they leave that profession behind." People who have hobbies usually have a consuming interest in their chosen activity. Many former workaholics find satisfaction in a hobby that forces them to concentrate and be patient, such as building a model train, bird watching, or producing clay sculptures.

Winston Churchill is said to have commented on hobbies: "The cultivation of a hobby and new forms of interest is a policy of first importance . . . to be happy and really safe, one ought to have at least two or three hobbies." Churchill painted and also wrote a book, *Painting as a Pastime*.

See also VOLUNTEERISM.

SOURCES:
Godbey, Geoffrey, and John Robinson. *Time For Life: The Surprising Ways Americans Use Their Time.* University Park: Pennsylvania State University Press, 1997.
Kanfer, Stefan. "The Art of Having Fun." *Modern Maturity,* October 1995.

holiday depression   Many individuals experience DEPRESSION as a low mood swing during periods of the year in which holidays occur or on holidays themselves. They can be stressful times, particularly for some single and widowed individuals who may feel alone and lonely, and see the rest of their world in a celebratory mood surrounded by families. The anticipation of holidays induces some people to drink, eat, or smoke more.

The stresses of holiday depression often occur when individuals have been uprooted from their families and moved elsewhere for employment or other reasons. The stresses of moving and relocation are compounded by their being alone. Some individuals in family settings experience mood shifts out of nostalgia for lost loved ones or for circumstances that existed earlier in their lives.

COPING WITH HOLIDAY STRESS

- Have realistic expectations so that you will not place too many demands on yourself. Be assertive and learn to say no when you want to.
- Consider your support system. If you don't have one, devote some time and energy to developing a support system by reaching out to others.
- Identify your major annoyances at this time of year. Be aware of when they happen and plan to have alternative responses if you usually become depressed.

Avoiding holiday depression
People who know that they will be alone on holidays and will feel stressed should avoid their holiday depressive episodes by planning ahead. They can take a trip to an interesting place, engage in some enjoyable activity with a group, or invite other people without families to share holiday activities together. Other individuals who know they will be alone on holidays may volunteer their services to hospitals or shelters for the homeless. Feeling that they will be helpful to others is a way of combating the stressful feelings associated with these times.

Usually the depressed mood brought about by holidays under such circumstances goes away after the holiday season. However, when the depressive mood does not improve as the calendar rolls on, individuals should seek professional help.

See also AFFECTIVE DISORDERS; SEASONAL AFFECTIVE DISORDER.

holistic medicine   Holistic medicine involves a shift in belief systems from the dualistic mind/body split toward a view of mind, body, and spirit as being closely connected. It has come to mean a specific way of thinking and practicing the art and science of medicine and for dealing with illness as well as relieving stress. Practitioners of holistic medicine view the individual as a totality, rather than as a headache to be relieved or a backache to be cured.

See also ALTERNATIVE THERAPIES; AYURVEDA; HERBAL MEDICINE; HOMEOPATHY; MIND-BODY CONNECTIONS; PSYCHONEUROIMMUNOLOGY.

Holmes, Thomas H., M.D. (1918–) Neuropsychiatrist who researched effects of stressful life change events on health status. He is known for devising a social adjustment rating scale along with Richard H. Rahe, M.D., another researcher in the area of life changes, as a predictor of illness.

See also LIFE CHANGE SELF-RATING SCALE.

homelessness Stresses of homeless people range from solving everyday practical problems such as finding shelter and enough food, to serious disorders such as substance abuse, DEPRESSION and schizophrenia. The stresses of physical as well as mental health problems are intensified by homelessness and, conversely, homelessness precipitates health problems. Because of the nature of the population, it is difficult to assess the numbers of homeless people and their characteristic stressors.

The difficulties in providing medical and mental health care for the homeless are related in part to the reluctance of some of the people to present themselves for care, as well as insufficiencies of community health centers. Many of the psychiatrically impaired homeless avoid contact with the health care system. Community mobile outreach services are an important way to help these individuals obtain food, clothing, and medical and mental health care.

For many of the poor and homeless populations, emergency department physicians are their source of primary care. These physicians often provide care for families that are in dire financial shape, the elderly, victims of rape and domestic violence, and drug abusers.

A survey of homeless adults living in beach areas near Los Angeles revealed a high rate of prior psychiatric hospitalization. The survey covered 529 people who had spent the previous night outdoors, in a shelter, in a hotel, or in the home of a relative with whom they did not expect to stay very long. Sixty-four percent of the people interviewed were white; 73% were men. They had been homeless for an average of two years. Altogether, 44% had been in hospitals for psychiatric reasons, including ALCOHOLISM and drug dependence. Twenty-one percent had made an outpatient visit for a mental or emotional problem within the past year. Forty-one percent had never used mental health services.

The worst symptoms were noted in the hospitalized group. There were more SUICIDE attempts, more daily drinking and delirium tremens. Seventy-six percent of the hospitalized group and 48% of the others had been arrested. People who had been hospitalized were more likely to be living in shelters. The 41% who had never used mental health services had been homeless about half as long as the rest and were least likely to be sleeping outdoors. Surprisingly, they scored at the same level as the general population on a questionnaire estimating well-being.

According to mental health professionals, to address the complex needs of those categorized as homeless persons requires a multidisciplinary approach. Social services are needed for short-term and long-term food, housing, and entitlement services. Networks should be developed to enable access for those people to specialty medical services, emergency food pantries, transportation, overnight shelter, and respite care for children while the parent negotiates the systems. Churches often provide for emergency needs and long-term support. Legal services are needed to advocate for the rights and entitlements. Children who are homeless require interaction with school systems, health care providers, day-care centers, and, often, child protective services to promote health and prevent further illness or trauma.

SOURCES:

Kahn, Ada P., and Jan Fawcett. *Encyclopedia of Mental Health.* New York: Facts On File, 1992.

McFarland, Gertrude K., and Mary Durand Thomas. *Psychiatric Mental Health Nursing.* Philadelphia: J.B. Lippincott, 1991.

homeopathy A system to promote healing based on a philosophy of not bombarding the body with medications, but stimulating and assisting the body to heal itself, using the smallest amount of medication possible. Many people use homeopathic remedies to prevent, reduce, and alleviate stress. Homeopathy is considered an alternative therapy.

Homeopathy uses medicines made from plants, minerals, animals, animal substances, and chemicals. Whereas some conventional medications suppress symptoms and the body's immune response, and occasionally unfortunate reactions to drugs or drug interactions occur, homeopathic practitioners prescribe only one medication at a time and claim that there are rarely, if ever, unwanted side effects. Homeopathic medicines are produced in accordance with processes described in the *Homeopathic Pharmacopoeia of the United States.*

A person-oriented instead of disease-oriented system, homeopathic practitioners treat patients based on their symptoms rather than relying solely on diagnostic techniques. Homeopathic practitioners seek to find *causes* as well as treat symptoms; this is often done in a holistic way by talking extensively with the patient to obtain a complete health and psychosocial history. In this regard, homeopathy has a characteristic in common with the Chinese belief that the best doctors do not use medicine; they heal by giving guidance for healthful living.

Homeopathy is used for a wide variety of chronic and acute problems. These include (but are not limited to) anxieties, ALLERGIES, digestive problems, gynecological conditions, and skin diseases. Many homeopathic remedies can be self-prescribed and purchased over the counter. However, as with any medication, it is prudent to consult a practitioner who is knowledgeable about the subject. Such individuals can be located through reputable local homeopathic pharmacies or the National Center of Homeopathy, Alexandria, Virginia, or the International Foundation for Homeopathy, Seattle.

Historical background of homeopathy

The history of homeopathy goes back about 250 years. Samuel Hahneman, M.D., a German physician, noted that Peruvian bark cured malaria. To test his theory that the bark might *cause* as well as *cure* malaria, he ingested small amounts of the bark and developed symptoms of malaria. He termed this effect a "proving" of symptoms. Another example of a "proving" of symptoms is that poisons in large doses are fatal; moderate doses can cause symptoms, but small doses can stimulate the body toward reduction of symptoms. Homeopathy is based on the law of similars, or "let like cure like." What has the power to cause also has the power to cure.

There is a parallel in Western medicine, where vaccines and allergy shots are used that contain tiny amounts of killed virus, or allergens, to stimulate the body's immune system and prepare it for actual challenge.

The practice of homeopathy came to the United States in the early 1800s. By the mid-1800s, several medical colleges taught homeopathy. Around 1900, there were 22 homeopathic medical colleges and one out of five doctors used homeopathy. However, by 1920, only 15 colleges remained. The decline in the use of homeopathy in the United States coincided with medical science's increasing view of the body as a mechanistic device, the advent of medical specialization, development of other prescription drugs and medicinal technology, and opposition by the American Medical Association.

The American Foundation for Homeopathy began teaching homeopathy as a postgraduate course for doctors in 1922. Today, courses are offered by the National Center for Homeopathy.

In recent years, interest in homeopathy has increased along with a widening interest in HOLISTIC MEDICINE and ALTERNATIVE THERAPIES. Homeopathy may appeal to many people because only natural substances are used as medications. Remedies include substances that can be dissolved in a liquid medium; metals and salts are not dissolvable. According to Hahneman's original description, remedies are ground together 10 times for 10 minutes. Subatomic energy is released. For an inexplicable reason, once diluted beyond the 12th dilution, nothing is found under a microscope. Also, because medications are so diluted, possibilities of side effects are reduced.

Some homeopathic practitioners in the United States also use other adjunctive therapies, such as spinal manipulation and nutritional counseling.

The largest use of homeopathic medications is in India. It is also popular in France and England and becoming popular in Australia and Germany. In Switzerland and Germany, homeopathic practitioners work under direction of doctors of medicine. According to Dr. Sujatha Pillai, a practitioner at Ehrhart & Karl, Chicago, 32% of family physicians in France prescribe homeopathic medicines. A survey in the *British Medical Journal* (June 7, 1986, 1498–1500) indicated that 42% of British physicians refer patients to homeopathic physicians. According to *Everybody's Guide to Homeopathic Medicines* (1991), members of the English royal family are homeopathic medicine users and the queen of England is the patron of the Royal London Homeopathic Hospital and the British Homeopathic Association.

Researchers have reported the efficacy of homeopathic medications. For example, one study reported in *Lancet* (1986) compared hay fever patients taking homeopathic preparations with those taking a placebo. The study showed that those who received the homeopathic medicine had six times fewer symptoms than those who received the placebo. Studies have been reported using homeopathic remedies for arthritis, fibromyalgia, and influenza.

Another homeopathic technique: Bach flower remedies

Bach flower remedies are so-called after Edward Bach (1886–1936), a British bacteriologist and homeopath. Flower remedies are a branch of homeopathic medicine, and said to be useful in acute situations. He developed a system of 38 flower remedies for 38 different emotional states, based only on a person's psychological symptoms. Distinct from homeopathy, more than one Bach remedy is prescribed at a time. Homeopathic practitioners believe in their efficacy.

FOR FURTHER INFORMATION:
International Foundation for Homeopathy
2366 Eastlake Avenue E (#301)
Edmonds, WA 98020
Phone: (206) 776-4147

National Center for Homeopathy
801 North Fairfax Street (Suite 306)
Alexandria, VA 22314
Phone: (703) 548-7790

SOURCES:
Cummings, Stephen, and Dana Ullman. *Everybody's Guide to Homeopathic Medicines.* New York: Jeremy Tarcher/Perigree Books, 1991.
Merz, Beverly, ed. "Complementary Therapies: Homeopathy." *Harvard Women's Health Watch* 4, no. 5, (January 1997).
Thomas, Patricia, ed. "Homeopathy: Is Less Really more?" *Harvard Health Letter* 20, no. 7 (May 1995).

homeostasis The body's tendency to maintain a steady state, despite stressful external changes. The physical properties and chemical composition of body fluids and tissues tend to remain remarkably constant. However, when our self-regulating powers fail, often because of repeated STRESS, the individual's health is threatened.

In the late 19th century, Claude Bernard, a French physiologist at the Collège de France in Paris, taught that one of the most characteristic features of all living beings is their ability to maintain the constancy of their internal milieu, despite changes in the surroundings. Subsequently, Walter B. Cannon, a Harvard physiologist, named this power to maintain constancy *homeostasis,* which can be translated as physiological "staying power or self-preservation."

Coping with stress and disease involves a fight to maintain the homeostatic balance of our tissues, despite damage. Hans SELYE, the Austrian-born Canadian pioneer in stress research, discussed the concept of homeostasis in his landmark works, *The Stress of Life* (1956) and *Stress without Distress* (1978). He said that the nervous system and the endocrine system play particularly important parts in maintaining resistance during stress. They help to keep the structure and function of the body steady, despite exposure to stress-producing or stressor agents, such as nervous tension, wounds, infections, or poisons. He explained this steady state as homeostasis.

See also COPING; GENERAL ADAPTATION SYNDROME; MIND-BODY CONNECTIONS; STRESS MANAGEMENT.

SOURCES:
Selye, Hans. *The Stress of Life,* rev. ed. New York: McGraw Hill, 1978.
———. *Stress Without Distress.* Philadelphia: Lippincott, 1974.

homesickness   Not really a sickness; happens when people are away from familiar surroundings and family to whom they feel close. Many people have experienced the stresses of homesickness as children while away at camp or visiting friends or relatives; soldiers experience it while stationed in distant lands. Homesickness may involve feelings of loneliness and confusion with the unfamiliar. How individuals adapt to such situations depends on their personal COPING skills and ability to adapt. If homesickness persists, it may lead to symptoms of mild DEPRESSION. However, in most cases of homesickness, relief occurs when individuals return to the familiar or when they adapt to the new situation.

See also ACCULTURATION; GENERAL ADAPTATION SYNDROME; INTIMACY; MIGRATION; NOSTALGIA; RELATIONSHIPS.

homosexuality   Sexual activity between members of the same sex, ranging from sexual fantasies and feelings through kissing and mutual masturbation, to genital, oral, or anal contact. The individual who practices homosexuality, if a man, is termed a homosexual; a female homosexual is referred to as a lesbian. Both men and women homosexuals are sometimes referred to as "gay." Fear of or prejudice against homosexuals is known as homophobia and is a source of stress to many in the general community.

Historically, homosexuals in the United States have faced the stresses of social discrimination but recently attitudes about homosexuality have evolved. In 1979, the U.S. surgeon general ordered that homosexuality not be classified as a mental disease and defect. The "gay liberation" movement of the 1970s brought about open discussions of homosexuality and human rights. During the 1980s, homosexual activists increased public acceptance of homosexuality as a life-style.

The term "homosexuality" was popularized during the 1960s. During the 19th century, other terms were proposed, including "homoerotic" (aroused by the same sex) and "homophile" (lover of the same sex). Cunnilingus between two women was called sapphism after the ancient Greek poet Sappho, and lesbianism was named for the Greek island of Lesbos where she lived.

homosexual panic

Homosexual panic (Kempf's disease) is a panic attack that develops from a fear or delusion that one will be sexually assaulted by an individual of the same sex. The term, coined by Edward Kempf, an American psychiatrist (1885–1971), in 1920, also applies to the fear that one is thought to be homosexual. This feeling occurs more often in males than in females.

There may be DEPRESSION, conscious GUILT over homosexual activity, agitation, HALLUCINATIONS, and ideas of SUICIDE. This type of panic attack may develop after many varied life circumstances, such as a loss or separation from an individual of the same sex to whom one is emotionally attached, or after failures in sexual performance, illness, or extreme fatigue.

See also GENDER ROLE; LESBIANISM; PANIC ATTACKS AND PANIC DISORDER; SEXUAL DIFFICULTIES; SEXUAL PREFERENCES.

SOURCES:

Kite, Mary E., and Kay Deaux. "Gender Belief Systems: Homosexuality and the Implicit Inversion Theory." *Psychology of Women Quarterly* 11 (1987): 83–96.

Marcus, Eric. *Is There a Choice? Answers to 300 of the Most Frequently Asked Questions About Gays and Lesbians.* San Francisco: Harper, 1993.

National Museum and Archive of Lesbian and Gay History. *The Gay Almanac.* New York: Berkley Books, 1996.

hopelessness   State of mind in which individuals feel that it is impossible to deal with the stresses of life and that situations they face have no possible solutions. They may see limited or no available desirable alternatives and may experience the stresses of emptiness, pessimism, and being overwhelmed. Nothing matters, and they "give up."

Hopelessness is a characteristic of DEPRESSION. A hopeless person is passive and lacks initiative. Such an individual may not be able to reach a desired goal, accepts the futility of planning to meet goals, has negative expectations of the future, perceives a personal loss of CONTROL, and sees "no way out." Successful treatment of depression with medication and certain types of psychotherapy can reverse this profound state of hopelessness.

The stress of extreme feelings of hopelessness may lead to ADDICTION or SUICIDE. Hopelessness sometimes results from false or unrealistic expectations. For example, hopeless people may feel that they should be able to accomplish anything and everything, and then descend into despair upon failure. Some individuals with depression feel that nothing they do will work out and that they are powerless.

Some people who are stressed may tend to magnify events to the extent that everything appears as an insurmountable obstacle in relation to themselves. Still another type of magnification results in despair, when they idealize other people and events. For example, a new friend may be thought to be perfect, or an upcoming vacation is planned to run a smooth course. When the friend proves to have perceived personality flaws and bad weather spoils the vacation, the individual who is the most unrealistic and idealistic may begin to lose hope about any friends or any vacation.

The stress of hopelessness may also result from a sense of being trapped in a negative set of circumstances from which there is no escape. When presented with a task that must be performed, but seems to be impossible, a sense of FRUSTRATION and futility leads to hopelessness.

The stress of confusion also leads to a sense of hopelessness, as confusion contributes to people's feelings of loss of control. It is important to understand that hopelessness is a subjective state, related to the way in which people perceive their prospects as potentially reversible.

See also COPING; PERFECTION.

SOURCE:

Kahn, Ada P., and Jan Fawcett. *The Encyclopedia of Mental Health.* New York: Facts On File, 1993.

hormone replacement therapy See MENO-
PAUSE.

hospitalization The stress of illness is often
intensified by the threat of being in a hospital,
which most people find fraught with ANXIETY
from beginning to end.

Stress starts with the need for a second
medical opinion, which, unless there is an
emergency, is often a requirement of medical
insurers before commitment to a hospital can
be made. Stress then follows patients to the
hospital registration desk where the approach
of many admissions personnel to gathering
patient information does little to make them
feel comfortable.

Loss of privacy, another key stressor,
begins at the very moment patients exchange
their clothes for hospital gowns and settle
down in rooms shared with at least one or
more strangers who may be a great deal more
or less sick than they. It is further compounded by the number of visitors they or
their roommates may have—people who talk
loudly as they spill into all corners and all
sides of what can be a too small hospital
room. In teaching hospitals, the stress continues to prevail when doctors and interns
gather around patients' beds to discuss clinical aspects of their illnesses, sometimes as if
the patients didn't exist or at least were not
right there in the bed.

Stress escalates when loss of privacy combines with the loss of CONTROL patients experience as they are thrown into the uneven
rhythm of the hospital routine—being
aroused at early hours for medication before
a change in shifts occurs, moving on stretch-
ers or in wheelchairs from one end of the
hospital to another, waiting in drafty corri-
dors for countless tests and X rays, buzzing
for nursing assistance that never comes, having unappealing meals served at hours when
they are often least hungry, and facing constantly changing caretakers and variations in
the delivery of care. The most serious

sources of hospitalization stress are being in
PAIN and having to rely on others for help in
controlling that pain. A device that allows
patients to control the intake of pain medication when they need it has alleviated this
problem for some.

Today, patients waiting to receive various
transplants—heart, lungs, kidney, and liver—
experience an additional aspect of stress
regarding when or whether the transplant
will come. The lists of those needing transplants far exceed availability, and for some
there is little likelihood of a match. Questions
also arise concerning the criteria for the lists
and for those who are given priority. An
example of that arose in 1995, when baseball
star Mickey Mantle received a transplant a
short time after a diagnosis was made.

Stress follows all patients out of the recovery room—with regulations concerning how
long their hospital stays can be. In 1995,
length of hospital stays became a major issue
in connection with the birth of babies. It was
felt by some that first-time mothers were
being sent home too soon and were often both
mentally and physically ill-prepared to take
care of a baby. For other mothers, the added
stress of taking care of older children—along
with the responsibilities of a newborn before
they have fully recovered their strength—was
awaiting them.

The shortened hospital stays of the later
1990s have increased the anxiety of most
patients. Much of the time needed for rehabilitation and recovery now is spent outside of
the hospital, which puts a good deal of the
burden of care on patients' families. For those
without families, other means of home care
must be found and questions arise about the
costs of this care.

Lastly, there is the stress on family and
friends related to hospitalization of the
dying—ethical questions relating to withdrawal of nourishment and treatment, particularly when there are no directions from the
patient.

See also ACCESS TO CARE; AUTONOMY; DEATH; END OF LIFE CARE; PERSONAL SPACE.

hostages   Victims who are subjected to the extreme stresses of isolation, confinement, and sometimes mental and physical torture. Captors frequently keep hostages in a state of uncertainty about their fate. Hostages may be individuals in a foreign country or held locally by criminals for any one of many purposes.

Hostages may be blindfolded, kept in darkness, and have their ears covered. The sensory deprivation experience may produce HALLUCI-NATIONS. Some hostages have become paranoid, depressed, and think that their country and families have forgotten them.

Readjustment to normal life after release, though welcome, is sometimes stressful for ex-hostages. Many experience nightmares, insomnia, bouts with abnormal fears, DEPRESSION, and feelings of rage and helplessness for some time. Mental health professionals are gaining an understanding of the state of mind of former hostages through experience. Current thinking is that a regulated "decompression period" helps former hostages adjust to normal life and to being back with their families.

Following the Persian Gulf war during 1991, several hostages were released after long years of captivity. Richard Rahe, M.D., director of the Nevada Stress Center at the University of Nevada School of Medicine, and a former Navy psychiatrist with extensive experience working with hostages and disaster victims, in an interview with *Psychiatric News*, said that how the individuals behaved before, during, and after the hostage experience can aid in predicting who might have difficulties upon reentry.

"People who do well have done well in the past with stress. They have had adequate-to-good childhoods. They did well in captivity. They passed through depression, and found themselves through helping others. They turned the experience into a positive one,

by reviewing their lives, making positive changes."

Rahe also said that survivor GUILT is common, as are recriminations about the way they might have behaved in captivity, and many are angry toward their families or the government for not doing enough to help them. At greatest risk of developing full-blown POST-TRAUMATIC STRESS DISORDER (PTSD) are those people who already had symptoms before being taken hostage and those without a good support system.

Elmore Rigamer, M.D., chief psychiatrist, U.S. State Department, quoted in *Psychiatric News* (January 4, 1991) regarding the "keys to staving off deterioration" in a hostage situation, commented that "mastery" and "connectedness" are the keys to overcoming psychological hurdles associated with having been a hostage. Mastery (a sense of CONTROL) and connectedness (feeling accurately informed) are both important for hostages and their families. "The ones who were able to take control of themselves will do wonderfully. The more feeling of loss of control, the worse."

Dr. Rigamer emphasized the psychological value of relaying information to hostages and families during and after the crisis. During the crisis he spent as much time as he could on the telephone with State Department hostages in Baghdad and Kuwait and their families back home, clearing up rumors and giving out information.

In *Psychiatric News* (January 4, 1991), Thomas M. Haizlip M.D., University of North Carolina, outlined seven stages of mastery applicable to both the hostages and their families:

1. Discriminating between good and bad forces
2. Coping by knowing what to do if it ever happens again
3. Putting your life back in order
4. Dealing with survivor guilt (having left some people and worldly goods behind)

5. Realizing that healthy people are willing to take advantage of a two-to-three-week "window" after the experience, when willingness to talk is greatest
6. Hooking up any symptoms with the event, rather than further repressing them
7. Recognizing that many people do not want help because they feel they themselves are important dispensers of help

Many of these stages are also applicable after other life traumas, such as domestic violence, witnessing, or being a victim of a crime.
See also AUTONOMY; BRAINWASHING.

SOURCES:
Haizlip, Thomas M. "Hostages." *Psychiatric News,* January 4, 1991, 18.
Kahn, Ada P., and Jan Fawcett. *The Encyclopedia of Mental Health.* New York: Facts On File, 1993.

hostility   A persistent attitude of deep resentment and intense ANGER. It may be the result of stressful situations or may also cause stress for the individual. The hostile person may have an urge to retaliate against a person or situation. During some situations of intense FRUSTRATION, deprivation, or discrimination, feelings of hostility may be a normal reaction. However, hostile attitudes also may occur during ANXIETY attacks, in OBSESSIVE-COMPULSIVE DISORDER, or DEPRESSION. Some people who have anti-social personalities frequently have hostile attitudes.

At best, hostile people are simply grouchy. At worst, they are consumed by hatred. A hostile person may have a tense-looking face and body. They are easily excitable. They seem to have chips on their shoulders and a bitterness toward the world. They may be sarcastic and moody and respond aggressively when challenged.

For many individuals, the stresses of hostilities can be worked out through EXERCISE, better COMMUNICATION skills, BEHAVIOR THERAPY, use of MEDITATION and RELAXATION, and psychotherapy.

See also AGGRESSION; ALTERNATIVE THERAPIES; PERSONALITY; PSYCHOTHERAPIES; TYPE A PERSONALITY.

SOURCE:
Friedman, Howard S. *The Self-Healing Personality.* New York: Henry Holt, 1991.

hot flashes   A sudden feeling of warmth occurring on the face, chest, or entire body. They are a major symptom of MENOPAUSE experienced by many midlife WOMEN. Hot flashes are sources of stress because they come on unexpectedly, and can be embarrassing as well as uncomfortable. The woman's body may become flushed, and patches of redness may appear on her chest, back, shoulders, and upper arms. She may perspire profusely; episodes may last from seconds to minutes. As sweat evaporates, the body temperature decreases, causing chills and a cold, clammy sensation. Women experience the symptoms of hot flashes in a variety of ways. Some have only a few, others continue to have them for years; some women have hot flashes several times a day, once a week, or less frequently. For most women, however, hot flashes are self-limiting symptoms and disappear without any treatment.

Effects of hot flashes
Because hot flashes may occur during the night and disrupt sleep, women experiencing hot flashes may become irritable, tired, and depressed. In a 1986 survey (Holt and Kahn), typical complaints about hot flashes included waking up at night drenched in sweat, ruining clothes from perspiration, feeling embarrassed at flushing and shivering with no control, and being intolerant of heat or cold. Many women find their bodies unable to deal comfortably with even slight temperature variations.

Some women say that the most stressful aspect of a hot flash is that it makes them feel out of CONTROL and interferes with their sense of well-being. While hot flashes are not a threat to health, they can make a woman uncomfortable and even anxious about having one in social or professional situations.

Previous generations of women were sometimes told that hot flashes were "all in their head," and that menopause was expected to be a time filled with bizarre behavior and delusions. Such comments from medical professionals no doubt added to the stress level of those women. Fortunately, this is no longer the case as medical practitioners understand the triggers for hot flashes, and supplements and medications are available to treat them.

Why hot flashes happen

Hot flashes occur because of hormonal changes. A hormone known as luteinizing hormone (LH) rises after menopause. Before menopause, it is the substance that helps trigger ovulation. LH "surges" seem to set off hot flashes by dilating surface blood vessels. Hormonal changes associated with the hot flash may also be due to nerve activity in the hypothalamic area that controls temperature and anterior pituitary function.

Medical and self-help

When hot flashes occur so often that a woman feels stressed by them, or if she cannot get a good night's sleep, if they interfere with sexual activity or work, or if they make her chronically exhausted and depressed, medical assistance should be sought. Hot flashes are often treated with hormone replacement therapy and alternative medications including sedatives and anticholinergic agents (substances that block or interfere with transmission of certain impulses in the parasympathetic nervous system).

A woman's diet may play a role in whether she suffers from hot flashes. Refined sugars, caffeine, alcohol, and spicy foods may trigger hot flashes in some women. Recognizing the potential role of diet in reducing or eliminating hot flashes, many alternative

---

> **TIPS FOR RELIEVING THE STRESS OF HOT FLASHES**
>
> - Air stuffy rooms; keep a window open if one is too warm.
> - Layer clothing. A suit with a lightweight blouse gives the wearer more flexibility than a wool dress.
> - Wear a cotton (or other absorbent material) blouse under a sweater. Avoid wearing a sweater next to the skin.
> - For desk-workers, use a small, desk-top fan.
> - During a hot flash, do not overreact. Keep calm; others will not pay attention.
> - Learn RELAXATION techniques to feel in control of the situation.
> - Regular exercise will tone the vascular system and may help a woman feel better.
> - Keep weight down. Slender women seem to have less erratic estrogen production, and hence fewer erratic experiences with hot flashes.
> - Seek homeopathic or alternative remedies; add soy products to your diet.

---

therapists recommend that women ingest foods or herbs containing "phytoestrogens." Phytoestrogens are natural-occurring sources of estrogen. Sources of phytoestrogens include soybeans, alfalfa, and rice. In addition to certain foods, nutritional supplements are frequently recommended by alternative health providers as a means of reducing the incidence of hot flashes. Vitamin E and bioflavinoids have shown some promise in this area. Herbal remedies for hot flashes include ginseng, vitex, garden sage, sarsaparilla, and don quai.

Homeopathic remedies for hot flashes include *Cimicfuga racemosa, Lachesis, Sepia,* and *Pulsatilla.* ACUPUNCTURE is emerging as a potential treatment for hot flashes. Proponents of acupuncture emphasize that this therapy has been used for centuries in China and other countries as an effective remedy for hot flashes and other menopausal symptoms.

The stresses brought about by hot flashes can be somewhat alleviated by several self-help suggestions.

See also ALTERNATIVE THERAPIES; HERBAL MEDICINE; HOMEOPATHY.

SOURCES:
Kahn, Ada P., and Linda Hughey Holt. *The A–Z of Women's Sexuality.* Alameda, Calif.: Hunter House, 1992.
———. *50 Ways to Cope with Menopause.* Lincolnwood, Ill.: Publications International, 1994.
National Women's Health Report. "Alternative Therapies and Women's Health." Washington, D.C.: National Women's Health Resource Center, May/June 1995.

hot lines   Telephone lines maintained by trained personnel to provide crisis-intervention service or information on a given topic. Throughout the United States, hot lines cover many concerns related to stress and mental health. In many cases, the numbers for information and help are toll-free and usually operate on a 24-hour basis.

Most city telephone directories list some of the available hot lines.

See also SELF-HELP GROUPS; SUPPORT GROUPS.

housework   Today, more women (and men) than ever are trying to juggle time for families, jobs, and housework. These time pressures may cause many people to experience feelings of being overwhelmed, guilty, and stressed. In her book, *Where Did the Time Go,* author Ruth Klein offers several suggestions for stress busters: a hot bath, window shopping, and exercise. She urges working people to change their situations by learning to live with the things that cannot be changed, taking time for play, and using weekends for re-energizing.

Several studies on housework since the 1920s show that, rather than eliminating tasks, small appliances designed to save time and effort can actually create more work and often stress for the person doing housework. Small appliances—also called conveniences—raise standards, motivate a desire for PERFECTION, consume more time overall, and create new tasks. While the drudgery level may have gone down, the frustrations in assembling the appliance, reading directions for its use, having it break down, and finding time to wait for the repairperson to come, may increase the stress level.

That is why Klein recommends finding a team of household helpers, such as professional house cleaners, gardeners, and carpenters, who not only assist but also come with their own equipment.

See also RANDOM NUISANCES.

SOURCE:
Klein, Ruth. *Where Did the Time Go.* Rocklin, Calif.: Prima Publishing, 1993.

human immunodeficiency virus (HIV)   The HIV virus is considered responsible for causing the infection that leads to *Acquired Immunodeficiency Syndrome* (AIDS), which continues in epidemic proportions in the United States and elsewhere in the world in the late 1990s. Many people experience stress because of concern about this virus; those who have it are anxious about their health and those who do not have it are fearful of contracting it. Many people have a misunderstanding about how it is transmitted, which adds to their stress level.

How the virus is transmitted
The virus is usually transmitted by direct exchange of body fluids, such as blood or semen, or by using contaminated needles for illicit drug use. Many individuals experience stress about contracting the virus by eating in restaurants in which infected individuals may work or by sending their children to a school that an infected child is known to attend. In most cases, these anxieties are unfounded, as the virus does not survive outside the body, according to research reports.

Individuals who suspect their partners of high-risk sexual contacts, such as homosexual men or prostitutes, should seek medical advice about screening for and preventing transmission of the HIV virus. Use of condoms during sexual intercourse is promoted as a way to prevent the transmission.

Fewer HIV-infected babies being born

Following a surge in the number of babies born with the virus in the 1980s, the numbers peaked in 1991 and leveled off in mid-1995, according to *The Journal of the American Medical Association* (September 26, 1995).

Susan F. Davis, M.D., Centers for Disease Control and Prevention (CDC), and colleagues estimated that 14,920 HIV-infected infants were born in the United States from 1978 to 1993. In 1978, 70 babies were born with HIV. The biggest increase came between 1986 and 1987 when numbers jumped from 1,100 to 1,390; the peak was in 1991 when 1,760 babies were born with HIV. Then the numbers fell slightly to 1,750 in 1992 and 1,630 in 1993.

According to the authors, "Data suggest the incidence of transmission of the HIV infection from mother to child increased markedly during the 1980s probably as a result of the growth of the HIV epidemic among women of childbearing age. After 1989, however, the observed prevalence of HIV infection leveled among childbearing women, for unknown reasons. Possible explanations include decreased fertility among HIV-infected women, an increased number of abortions among HIV-infected women, or a stable state of HIV incidence among childbearing women, with a proportional number of HIV-infected women aging beyond childbearing years."

Concerns about getting HIV from a health care professional

Some people experience stress when having blood drawn or dental and medical procedures done because they fear contracting the HIV virus. According to an article in *Health* (September 1992) the person who draws the blood presents virtually no risk. To infect a person, a health professional who is HIV positive would have to get stuck with the needle, and in turn stick that person with the contaminated needle. There is little likelihood of this happening. In the case of dental hygienists who manipulate sharp instruments inside a person's mouth, they would have to injure themselves and bleed into exposed tissue in that person's mouth.

According to an article in *Health* (September 1992), one can reduce one's stress level about this situation by being sure that one's health care professional is taking universal precautions. Look over the doctor or dentist's office. Equipment and instruments should look clean. Personnel should wash their hands before and after procedures, and should wear gloves, masks, and eye guards (during procedures where body fluids might splatter). Protective gear should be changed or discarded between patients. Needles and other sharp objects should be disposed of in secure containers. Anything that goes in your mouth or inside your body should arrive in sterile packaging, be disinfected, or be sterilized by autoclave or dry heat.

See also HIV/AIDS TREATMENT INFORMATION SERVICE; SEXUALLY TRANSMITTED DISEASES.

FOR FURTHER INFORMATION:
CAIN (Computerized AIDS Information Network)
San Francisco AIDS Foundation
54 Tenth Street
San Francisco, CA 94103
Phone: (415) 864-4368

AIDS-Hotlines National AZT Hotline
Phone: (800) 843-9388

National AIDS Information Clearinghouse
Centers for Disease Control
Box 6003
Rockville, MD 20850
Phone: (800) 458-5231

SOURCES:
Davis, Susan F. "Fewer HIV-Infected Babies Being Born." *The Journal of the American Medical Association,* September 26, 1995.

Japenga, Ann. "The Secret." *Health,* September 1992.

Kahn, Ada P., and Linda Hughey Holt. *Midlife Health: Every Woman's Guide to Feeling Good,* New York: Avon Books, 1989.

humor   A positive emotion that usually provides a helpful release of stress and anxieties for many people. Humor may actually ease PAIN and may help the respiratory system by exercising the lungs. LAUGHTER, the expression of humor, may influence the immune system, by stimulating production of certain hormones that help to ease pain and lift one's mood.

Humor is a universal language and has universal appeal. The basis for much humor is that we are prepared for one thing and something else happens. Although we are startled, we know there is no danger, and we release our surprise in laughter. Thus a story with an unexpected ending, or a game of peek-a-boo for an infant, can seem humorous and bring about a laughter response.

Shared humor relieves anxiety in stressful group situations, such as when airplanes or trains are delayed. It also relieves stresses that result from BOREDOM. At times when it seems that nothing is left to talk about, familiar topics can be renewed by employing humor.

In work situations, a humorous approach can help one face sources of stress and daily

---

PREVENT STRESS: AVOID THESE USES OF HUMOR

- Poking fun at other people's individual shortcomings
- Reflecting anger
- Offending with inappropriate use of sexual references or profanity
- Dividing a group by put-downs
- Using a stereotype to denigrate a person or group
- Creating a cruel, abusive, and offensive atmosphere

---

disappointments. Blumenfeld and Alpern, in their book *Humor at Work,* outline some characteristics of stress-reducing humor, which can be used in the workplace as well as in other settings. However, the authors warned against using humor that can be misused and actually lead to stress.

Some therapists employ humor to momentarily relieve DEPRESSION during therapy sessions. One technique is known as paradoxical therapy, in which the therapist gives the individual new perspectives on his or her problems by exaggerating them to the point of making them seem funny. The therapist might assign the individual to be depressed or anxious at a certain time of day. Sometimes the silliness of such situations helps alleviate the individual's depressed or anxious feelings.

Historical overview of humor

Ancient scholars understood the role of humor in good health. The Book of Proverbs says: "A merry heart doeth good like a medicine." Conversely, many individuals who suffer from depression lose their sense of humor and few things make them smile or laugh. Studies in the late 20th century suggested that an ability to enjoy humor and to laugh have effects on mental as well as physical health. Norman COUSINS' book, *Anatomy of an Illness* (1977), stimulated interest in the use of humor in recovery from both mental and physical ill-

---

USE OF HUMOR TO RELIEVE STRESSFUL SITUATIONS

- Reduce tension by joking about universal human frustrations and faults.
- Encourage people to relax and laugh.
- Delight in poking fun at oneself.
- Unite people by building rapport.
- Create a supportive atmosphere of fun and caring.
- Note the positive aspects of human relationships.

ness. While fighting ankylosing spondylitis, he checked out of the hospital and spent weeks watching Marx brothers movies and other comedies. He believed that the positive feelings aroused by humor and laughter helped him recover. Increasingly, hospitals and health care practitioners are bringing humor programs into their compendia of therapies.

FOR FURTHER INFORMATION:
International Laughter Society
16000 Glen Una Drive
Los Gatos, CA 95030
Phone: (408) 354-3456

SOURCES:
Blumenfeld, Esther, and Lynne Alpern. *Humor At Work.* Atlanta: Peachtree Publishers, 1994.
Fry, William F., and Waleed A. Salameh, eds. *Handbook of Humor and Psychotherapy.* Sarasota: Professional Resources Exchange, 1987.
Morreall, John. *Taking Laughter Seriously.* Albany: State University of New York, 1983.
Ziv, Avner. *Personality and Sense of Humor.* New York: Springer Publishing Co., 1984.

hypertension   See HIGH BLOOD PRESSURE.

hyperventilation   Deep and fast BREATHING; it is sometimes referred to as overbreathing. Some individuals who feel very stressed and those who have panic attacks and PHOBIAS may react with hyperventilation, which in turn makes them fear that they are dying or having a HEART ATTACK.

Hyperventilation can result in rapid heartbeat, sweating, and numbness or tingling in the hands and feet, light-headedness, DIZZINESS, fainting. These symptoms in turn exacerbate the individual's stress and anxiety level.

Individuals who are hyperventilating typically feel short of breath, and when they breathe deeply and faster to get more air into their lungs, they are really taking in too much air. This breathing pattern makes them feel even more stressed, as it removes too much carbon dioxide from the blood, where it is needed for the body to perform efficiently.

When an individual has a dizzy spell or feels the effects of hyperventilation, breathing into a paper bag for a few minutes can help restore the balance of oxygen and carbon dioxide in the blood. When some of the exhaled carbon dioxide from the bag returns to the lungs, the individual will begin to breathe more normally again.

RELAXATION therapy, including breathing instruction, helps some individuals relieve the stressful symptoms of hyperventilation.

See also COPING; MEDITATION.

hypnosis (hypnotherapy)   A type of attentive, receptive and focused concentration accompanied by an altered state of consciousness and a diminished awareness of environmental stimuli. It is considered an alternative therapy and is sometimes used to help relieve symptoms of stress, such as ANXIETY, PHOBIAS, and PAIN, and insomnia and to control habits such as SMOKING, overeating, or NAIL BITING, often in conjunction with other therapies.

Hypnosis is sometimes used for memory enhancement. While hypnosis does not help a person remember better, it relieves some of the stress and tension that may be inhibiting memory. The greater the stress the individual feels, the less likely he is to remember clearly and accurately.

Hypnotherapy utilizes the hypnotic "trance," a state of deep RELAXATION, to produce a state of high suggestibility. While in this state, suggestions are offered either by a therapist or the individual himself; such suggestions are aimed at improving some aspect of physical or mental health, or stress reduction. Often the suggestion takes the form of imagining a desired result in detail.

In that state some people gain the ability to change their perceptions of stress, anxiety, pain, memories, and feelings. "This opens up a tremendous use of hypnosis in pain control," says Peter B. Bloom, M.D., past president, International Society for Hypnosis.

Hypnotherapy has been used as a complement to medical therapy in a number of conditions and as a primary treatment modality in others. In the management of pain, for example, hypnosis has been used not only to reduce the stress and anxiety that accompany painful medical procedures, but also to reduce the discomfort and need for analgesics associated with labor and delivery, hysterectomy, coronary bypass surgery, and abdominal surgery.

Benefits of hypnotherapy include decreased nausea and pain, shorter hospital stays, and more rapid healing. Hypnotherapy has been used to decrease bleeding in hemophiliacs, to help stabilize blood sugar in diabetics, and to reduce the severity of asthmatic attacks.

Self-hypnosis

Treatment with hypnosis involves teaching self-hypnosis techniques so participants can induce a trancelike state in themselves and use suggestions to help them restructure their thinking regarding the condition for which they are seeking help. Some individuals undergo hypnotic induction by listening to a voice giving them instructions to become increasingly relaxed and focused. Many people are then taught to enter the hypnotic state on their own and to give themselves suggestions aimed at achieving their goals. For example, in management of pain, hypnosis helps to block the perception of pain by drawing the individual's attention away from it. Self-hypnosis has been shown to be effective for the control of chronic headaches.

Self-hypnosis is sometimes used to promote relaxation on cue in stressful situations. In general, autohypnosis by itself will not significantly relieve stress responses. It can, however, be used as a supplement to BEHAVIOR THERAPY to make images more vivid and to heighten one's ability to concentrate.

Contrary to popular belief, the power of hypnosis lies within the individual and not the hypnotist. In a therapy situation utilizing hypnosis, the individual cooperates with the therapist to utilize this form of intense concentration to facilitate and accelerate reaching particular therapeutic goals. Individuals cannot be hypnotized against their will, but some individuals are more or less capable of achieving a hypnotic trance.

See also ALTERNATIVE THERAPIES; HEADACHES.

FOR FURTHER INFORMATION:
American Society of Clinical Hypnosis
2200 East Devon Avenue (Suite 291)
Des Plaines, IL 60018
Phone: (847) 297-3317

International Society for Medical and
Psychological Hypnosis
1991 Broadway (18B)
New York, NY 10023
Phone: (212) 874-5290

SOURCES:
Callahan, Jean. "Hypnosis: Trick or Treatment?" *Health,* May-June 1997.
Kerns, Lawrence L. "A Clinician's Guide to Mind-body Treatments." *Chicago Medicine,* November 21, 1994.
Lehrer, Paul M., and Robert L. Woolfolk, eds. *Principles and Practice of Stress Management,* 2nd ed. New York: Guilford Press, 1993.

hypothalamus The coordinating center of the brain; plays an important part in reacting to stressful situations. It is a small area located above the pituitary gland, with nerve connections to most other areas of the nervous system; it controls the SYMPATHETIC NERVOUS SYSTEM (controls the inner body organs). During STRESS, FEAR, or excitement, the brain sends signals to the hypothalamus, which initiates a chain of activity, including faster heartbeat, faster BREATHING rate, and increased blood flow to the muscles (the FIGHT OR FLIGHT RESPONSE).

The hypothalamus also controls reactions that cause sweating or shivering, stimulates appetite and thirst, regulates sleep, motivates sexual behavior, and determines EMOTIONS and MOODS; it indirectly controls many of the endocrine organs that secrete hormones.

I

illiteracy The inability to read or write. It is a personal stressor for many people, contributing to their poor self-image and affecting their ability to obtain employment with which to support their families. People who are unable to read or write or who do one or both poorly may develop techniques to hide or compensate for their lack. Embarrassment may keep them from seeking help. For children, the illiteracy of a parent can also be a source of embarrassment and cause them a great deal of stress.

Illiteracy is a fairly common problem in the United States estimates are that 75% of unemployed Americans are illiterate. In the early 1990s, the New York Telephone Company had to give 60,000 people an entry-level exam in order to hire 3,000 employees. Some major corporations have had to use graphics on assembly lines to compensate for workers' inability to read simple phrases. As jobs have become increasingly technical and the economy has shifted from an industrial to a service base, more jobs will require skills that include reading and writing ability.

Illiteracy is strongly related to poverty, drug use, and crime. It has been reported that about 75% of adult prison inmates are functionally illiterate. According to a survey by the National Advisory Council on Adult Education, in the late 1980s, 40% of all armed services enlistees read below a ninth grade level.

A study of emergency room and clinic patients at two public hospitals reported that a high proportion of them are unable to read and understand basic written medical instructions, according to an article in *The Journal of the American Medical Association* (December 5, 1995). The study raises the question of whether the estimated 40 to 44 million adults in the United States who are functionally illiterate and another 50 million adults who are only marginally literate are leaving doctors' offices and hospitals without understanding the next steps to take to ensure their good health.

The authors commented that patients with limited literacy skills who have difficulty reading informed consent forms present a troubling ethical issue. "The ethical obligation of physicians to explain the risks and benefits of any procedure or treatment is fundamental to the physician-patient relationship. Patients unable to understand informed consent forms cannot intelligently participate in their own care."

LEARNING DISABILITIES account for some illiteracy; however, there is not always agreement among educators as to what extent. There is a growing movement in American education to reduce illiteracy by treating reading and writing problems as learning disabilities at an early stage in schooling.

At the end of the 20th century, many community organizations have taken on illiteracy as a project. Volunteers work with people who need help reading and writing.

See also SELF-ESTEEM; VOLUNTEERISM.

imagery See GUIDED IMAGERY.

immigration See ACCULTURATION; MIGRATION.

immune system A collection of cells and proteins that protect the individual against possibly harmful microorganisms such as viruses, bacteria, and fungi. It is involved in problems of ALLERGIES and hypersensitivity, rejection of tissues after grafts and transplants, and probably CANCER. Suppression of the immune system can occur as an inherited disorder or after infection with certain viruses, including HIV (the virus that causes AIDS), resulting in lowered resistance to infections and to the development of malignancies. There is evidence that severe STRESS and DEPRESSION may inhibit normal immune function, although this has not been proven.

Relationship of stress and the immune system

There are possible physiological and behavioral explanations for changes in the immune system due to stress and negative emotional states. Stress is associated with activation of several systems, including the hypothalamic-pituitary-adrenal axis and the SYMPATHETIC NERVOUS SYSTEM.

Certain life-style factors influence the immune response. For example, lack of SLEEP or EXERCISE and use of alcohol and drugs affect the immune system in adverse ways. The best ways for a person to maintain immune system health are to have a balance of exercise, rest, RELAXATION, recreation, fun, and LAUGHTER, a nutritionally healthy diet, and positive connections with family and/or friends.

Writing in *World Health* (March-April 1994), Dr. Tracy B. Herbert, Carnegie-Mellon University, reported on studies relating stress and the immune system. Factors such as bereavement, DIVORCE, UNEMPLOYMENT, and caring for a relative with ALZHEIMER'S DISEASE were investigated. Generally, studies found that there is a large decrease in both lymphocyte proliferation and natural killer cell activities in individuals who have experienced stress.

The duration of stress also affects the amount of immune change; the longer the stress, the greater the decrease in the number of specific types of white blood cells. Dr. Herbert also reported that interpersonal stress seems to produce different immune outcomes when compared with the stress due to unemployment or exams.

Researchers have also looked at relationships between ANXIETY and depression and the immune system. Results suggest that depression and anxiety are associated with decreases in lymphocyte proliferation and natural killer cell activity, changes in the numbers of white blood cells, and the quantity of antibodies circulating in the blood. It seems that the ability of the body to produce antibodies to a specific substance is related to the level of anxiety. More anxiety results in less antibody production after exposure to a potentially harmful substance.

See also AUTOIMMUNE DISORDERS; ALTERNATIVE THERAPIES; GUIDED IMAGERY; HUMAN IMMUNODEFICIENCY VIRUS; MEDITATION; MIND-BODY CONNECTIONS; PSYCHONEUROIMMUNOLOGY.

SOURCES:
Herbert, Tracy B. "Stress and the Immune System." *World Health,* March-April 1994.
Locke, Steven, and Douglas Colligan. *The Healer Within.* New York: New American Library, 1986.
Sapolsky, Robert M. *Why Zebras Don't Get Ulcers: A Guide to Stress, Stress-Related Diseases, and Coping.* New York: W.H. Freeman, 1994.

implosive therapy   See BEHAVIOR THERAPY.

impotence   The inability of a male to complete sexual intercourse due to partial or incomplete achievement of, or maintaining, an erection. Estimates indicate that 10 million American men have erectile impotence and consequently the stress of FRUSTRATION, embarrassment, and irritability. Impotence may take the form of low interest in sexual activity, premature ejaculation, coitus without ejaculation, or erectile capacity only with prostitutes. It is a stressor for men as well as their partners.

Symptoms

Sex researchers Masters and Johnson gave the label *primary impotence* to the condition of never having had an erection, and *secondary impotence* to the condition of having had an ability to have an erection in the past but not in the present.

Scientific and medical views vary regarding the number of those afflicted with psychological and physiological impotence. Research by the Surgitek/Medical Engineering Corporation indicates that nearly 50% of impotent men suffer from physiological problems, with a large number afflicted with irreversible organic impotence.

As many as half the cases of male impotence are the result of physical disorders. Serious hormonal imbalance, nerve and muscle damage, and circulatory problems can cause impotence. Although the majority of men with physically induced impotence are in the 40- to 69-year-old age group, the condition can affect the very young and the very old. In older men, physical causes of impotence include circulatory problems, neurological disorders, hormonal abnormalities, and medications.

Psychological factors such as ANXIETY, marital discord, and chronic DEPRESSION have been found to interfere with the process. In times of extreme stress in their personal or business lives or after drinking too much alcohol, men may experience temporary erectile impotence. Short episodes of erectile impotence are common and should not be a cause for undue concern by men or their partners.

Diagnosing impotence

Diagnosing the causes of impotence involves many physical and psychological tests conducted with the impotent man, and, in some cases, his partner. The physical examination includes blood, hormone and circulation tests, neurological studies, and tests on penile blood pressure and temperature, among others.

An important test to distinguish organic from psychological impotence is the Nocturnal Penile Tumescence Test (NPT), in which erections that occur during sleep are measured. Most men have between two and five erections while asleep, each lasting from five minutes to half an hour. In the test, which can be conducted in sleep laboratories or in the home, an electronic device is used to record changes in penile size. An insufficient number of nocturnal erections may indicate a physical problem for which further medical attention is necessary.

Treatment

Emotional factors, such as marital stress or depression, also affect impotence. It was once thought that psychological factors caused most impotence, but with increasing medical knowledge, the proportion that can be explained on physiological grounds is increasing. It is important for men suffering from impotence to have a thorough check-up for physical as well as emotional causes by a knowledgeable physician and/or sex therapist. Treatment may be as simple as treating the disease or eliminating the drug causing it, or as complicated as surgical implantation of a prosthesis. SEX THERAPY is helpful to many men. In 1998 the FDA approved Viagra (sildenafil citrate), the first oral pill to treat impotence.

See also PROSTATE CANCER; SEXUAL DIFFICULTIES; SEXUAL RESPONSE CYCLE.

FOR FURTHER INFORMATION:
American Urological Association
1120 N. Charles Street
Baltimore, MD 21201
Phone: (301) 727-1100

Impotence Institute of America, Impotents
  Anonymous
10400 Little Patuxent Parkway (Suite 485)
Columbia, MD 21044-3502
Phone: (800) 669-1603

National Kidney and Urologic Diseases
Information Clearinghouse
3 Information Way
Bethesda, MD 20892-3580
Phone: (301) 654-4415

SOURCES:
Church, Paul, and Peta Gillyatt. "Impotence: No Need to Suffer in Secret." *Harvard Health Letter* May 1996, 21, no. 7 (May 1996).
Frye, Christopher C., ed. "Impotence." *Mayo Clinic Health Letter,* August 1997.

incest   Generally defined as sexual intercourse between persons so closely related that they are forbidden by law to marry. When these sexual relations occur, many family members, including the victims, do not report them out of fear of reprisal or fear of being abandoned by the perpetrator. Stress and family tensions are ongoing in such situations.

In Western society, sexual intercourse between father-daughter or mother-son, between cousins, or between uncles and nieces, aunts and nephews, is prohibited.

See also DOMESTIC VIOLENCE.

SOURCES:

Kosof, Anna. *Incest: Families in Crisis.* New York: Franklin Watts, 1985.

Spies, Karen Bornemann. *Everything You Need to Know About Incest.* New York: Rosen Publishing Group, 1992.

Tritchell, James B. *Forbidden Partners: The Incest Taboo in Modern Culture.* New York: Columbia University Press, 1987.

incontinence, urinary   See URINARY INCONTINENCE.

indecision   See DECISION-MAKING.

indigestion   Refers to a variety of symptoms brought on by eating, including FLATULENCE, HEARTBURN, abdominal pain, and NAUSEA. It causes a burning discomfort in the stomach because the individual has eaten too much, too fast, or too-rich, spicy, or fatty foods. Nervous indigestion is a common cause of stress. This stress generally results from anything that causes ANGER, ANXIETY, PAIN, and FEAR. STAGE FRIGHT, going for a job interview, or going on a first date are sometimes stressful situations that can cause indigestion.

To keep stress levels in line, eat a balanced diet; do not overdo. Allow plenty of time for eating. Limit foods that cause indigestion; eat small meals four times a day instead of three larger ones. Get adequate sleep and practice deep breathing, visualization, and other stress-reducing techniques.

Belching

Belching, or common burping, comes from the swallowing of air or from gas in the stomach caused by the chemical reactions of food and digestive juices. Many individuals feel stressed by the embarrassment that results from belching in a social situation or public place. To overcome the embarrassment, as well as the source of the problem, careful attention to diet may make a difference. Also, taking more time to select foods carefully and eat slowly may reduce the incidence of this annoying reaction.

Belching may occur more frequently when an individual feels stressed because he or she either eats too fast or selects foods that contribute to heartburn, bloating, and belching. In addition to diet, RELAXATION techniques may be useful.

Bloating

The term "bloating" applies to the full, distended feeling in the abdomen, which occurs after overeating. Many people react to stressful situations by overeating, eating too fast, or eating spicy, greasy, foods, all of which contribute to bloating. The discomfort causes further stress, as bloating leads to belching or burping, which can be socially embarrassing.

See also IRRITABLE BOWEL SYNDROME; NUTRITION.

TIPS TO RELIEVE STRESS DUE TO BLOATING

- Relax before eating; eat and drink slowly.
- Limit foods/beverages that contain air, such as carbonated drinks, baked goods, whipped cream, and souffles. Don't smoke, chew gum, suck on hard candy, or drink through straws or narrow-mouthed bottles.
- Correct loose dentures.
- Eat fewer rich foods, such as fatty meats, fried foods, cream sauces, gravies, and pastries.
- Don't lie down immediately after eating.
- Don't try to force yourself to belch.

inferiority complex An individual's feeling of very low SELF-ESTEEM. He or she feels that other people are better-looking, better achievers, or more successful. Some children develop an inferiority complex because they are the victims of bullies while they are growing up. Other children do so because their parents have not encouraged them or belittle or overly criticize all their efforts. In some families one child may be compared unfavorably with another; this can lead to an inferiority complex. Inferiority complexes can haunt individuals throughout their lives and cause them stress in business and social situations. It can lead to mental and physical disorders such as sleeplessness, DEPRESSION, loss of appetite, and HEADACHES.

Some people have inferiority complexes because of their BODY IMAGE. Contemporary advertising may contribute to the negative image many people, particularly women, have of their bodies. Female models are often anorexic and compulsive about remaining thin, some to the point of interfering with their good health. They set examples that are impossible, and unhealthy, for the average person to attain.

The term "inferiority complex" was first used by Carl Jung (1875–1961), a Swiss psychiatrist and philosopher. A complex includes ideas linked together and related to feelings that affect an individual's behavior and PERSONALITY. People with serious inferiority complexes can learn to raise their self-image during psychotherapy.

See also EATING DISORDERS; PSYCHOTHERAPIES.

SOURCE:
Kahn, Ada P., and Sheila Kimmel. *Empower Yourself: A Woman's Guide to Self-Esteem.* New York: Avon Books, 1997.

infertility An inability of a couple to conceive. Usually the diagnosis of infertility is made after at least one year of sexual intercourse without contraception. Infertility is often a cause of STRESS and ANXIETY for many couples, particularly those who have delayed marriage and childbearing until their late 30s or early 40s. This frustrating and often anguishing problem affects about 15% of all couples of childbearing age, and only about one-half the couples professionally treated for infertility achieve pregnancy.

Other stresses produced by infertility can result in sexual problems, such as low or nonexistent sexual desire. Fortunately, for most couples this is usually a situational problem, and when the infertility is resolved, the lack-of-desire problem goes away.

According to William W. Hurd, assistant professor of obstetrics and gynecology, University of Michigan Medical Center, about one in 10 couples are considered "subfertile," which means that their chances of having a baby without professional intervention are slim. The infertility rate increases dramatically with age; couples between ages 30 and 35 have a 33% chance of being subfertile, and the odds jump to 50% by the time they reach 40. The probability of becoming pregnant the "old-fashioned" way is less than 10% among couples age 40 and older.

In approximately 40% of infertility cases, the problem is solely female; in another 40% it is solely male, and in the remaining cases, it involves both partners. In about 3.5% of cases, infertility is never explained.

Female infertility
Failure to ovulate is a common cause of female infertility. It may be caused by a hormonal imbalance, stress, or a disorder of the ovary, such as a tumor or a cyst. Disorders of the uterus and blocked Fallopian tubes are other reasons for infertility. It is rarely caused by a chromosomal abnormality or allergy to her partner's sperm.

Reasons why subfertility increases with time are largely based on changes that take place in a woman's body as she ages. For example, older ovaries in middle-aged women produce less fertility-enhancing hormones. Additionally, these ova are not as receptive to sperm penetration and they tend to be spontaneously aborted once fertilized.

Male infertility
Once infertility problems were considered the woman's domain. Now, however, sperm production and motility, hormonal imbalances, anatomical factors, infections, and inflammatory diseases are known to affect a man's ability to father a child.

According to Dana Ohl, M.D., assistant professor of surgery, University of Michigan Medical Center, anabolic steroids, which can lower sperm count drastically and sometimes irreversibly, will also leave an indelible mark on infertility statistics in the years to come; young men in high school who use steroids will find difficulty in impregnating their wives five to 10 years from now.

Some men perceive their condition as a stressful threat to their masculine identity, which they may associate with their sexual prowess. One of the best ways to get men to accept infertility is to encourage them to talk about their condition, both with their partners and in support groups.

Diagnosing infertility
Infertility does not always mean that conception is impossible. Today there are advances in many areas that might affect fertility: ovulatory, cervical, uterine and endometrial, tubal, pelvic, and sperm. In diagnosing infertility, physicians look at medical factors that alone or in tandem could prevent pregnancy. They want to know, for example, if the ovaries release an egg each month, and along with it, a proper amount of hormones to allow for implantation. They also want to know if the male partner's sperm is of sufficient volume, motility, and quality to fertilize an egg.

Assisted reproduction techniques
Assisted reproduction techniques, which were developed during the 1980s and 1990s,

offer hope to conceive a child, even for couples stressed by complex forms of infertility. These techniques originated in England with the birth of the first IVF (*in vitro* fertilization) baby, Louise Brown, in 1978. Since then, assisted reproduction procedures have been successfully performed worldwide, enabling thousands of couples with otherwise untreatable infertility to produce their own healthy babies.

Couples most suited for IVF are those in which the wife has a normal uterus and ovaries, but her Fallopian tubes are damaged, blocked, or absent. Many patients in IVF programs have previously been treated for tubal disease that required surgery, which proved unsuccessful, or which required complete removal of the Fallopian tubes. Women suffering from endometriosis, or adhesions affecting reproductive organs, may be candidates for IVF or GIFT (Gamete Intra-Fallopian Transfer). Couples in whom the husband has an infertility problem may also be suitable for IVF, TET (tubal embryo transfer), or ICSI (direct sperm injection into an egg cell).

Options with technology
Understanding the options with assisted reproduction techniques helps relieve the stress of infertility for many couples. IVF is essentially a tubal bypass procedure. Mature eggs are retrieved from the ovary with ultrasound guidance. The eggs are fertilized by the husband's sperm in the laboratory. In special circumstances, IVF procedures may be performed using donated egg cells, sperm, or embryos. The resulting embryos are transferred into the woman's uterus or into her tubes via laparoscopy.

Tubal Embryo Transfer (TET) is performed through laparoscopy in an operating room. GIFT (Gamete Intra-Fallopian Transfer) is similar to IVF, but the eggs and sperm, instead of being incubated *in vitro*, are placed together in the Fallopian tubes of the wife. GIFT can be performed if at least one of the tubes is healthy but an egg is unable to reach it.

Couples interested in exploring how medical technology can help them conceive should contact local medical centers and thoroughly check the credentials of the physicians who specialize in infertility or reproductive endocrinology, as well as the laboratories and facilities they are considering. Knowing that they are in the hands of experts will help relieve some of the stresses of undergoing the assisted reproduction procedures, which may be emotionally and financially costly.

A support group started by infertile couples is RESOLVE.

See also BIOLOGICAL CLOCK; IMPOTENCE.

FOR FURTHER INFORMATION:
American Fertility Society
2140 11th Avenue South (Suite 200)
Birmingham, AL 35205-2800
Phone: (205) 933-8494

Fertility Research Foundation
1430 Second Avenue (Suite 103)
New York, NY 10021
Phone: (212) 744-5500

RESOLVE, Inc.
P.O. Box 474
Belmont, MA 02178
Phone: (617) 484-2424

SOURCES:
Berger, Gary S., Mark Goldstein, and Mark Fuerst. *The Couple's Guide to Fertility,* rev. ed. New York: Doubleday, 1994.
Corson, Stephen L. *Conquering Infertility: a Guide for Couples.* New York: Prentice-Hall 1990.
"Costly Choices, No Guarantees: The Maze of Fertility Services." *Women's Health Center Management* 5, no. 7 (July 1997).
Daya, Salim. "Investigation of the Infertile Couple." *Canadian Family Physician* 35 (June 1989).

information explosion Today, all types of professionals are caught in the volume of information they need to do their jobs. This is occurring at the same time that career and family commitments are taking up more and

---

HANDLING THE STRESS OF INFORMATION EXPLOSION

• Recognize what information is most important.
• Prioritize information files and take them to read on trains, buses, planes, and in hotel rooms.
• Learn to toss what is not important; if you can, rely on someone else to do the sorting and tossing.
• Use customized on-line data bases that target the information you need.
• Depend on audiotapes to keep you informed while you drive or jog.
• Reduce your level of stress and you will find that you will retain more of the information you need.

---

more of their time. The fact that there is more to read and less time available to read it is in itself stressful.

It is not only the growing stacks of magazines and newspapers in homes and memos and reports in offices that causes the concern described by Richard Wurman in his book, *Information Anxiety.* It is also the information forced on us through COMPUTERS with their on-line programming, fax machines, electronic mail, cellular phones, voice mail, answering machines, VCRs, audio and videotapes, and through the increasing number of regular and cable TV channels.

The problem is, Wurman says, that while print and computer information envelops us, what we really need is knowledge. However, the solution for something that sifts through and synthesizes all of the data to make it usable is still a long way off. In the meantime, it is necessary to be creative in the approach to information gathering.

See also RANDOM NUISANCES.

inhibition The inner restraints within individuals that prevent them from carrying out mental or physical activities. As a psychoanalytic term, inhibition means unconsciously restraining instinctual impulses. Inhibitions cause stress for many people because they feel blocked from doing many things they might like to do. Some people who have many inhibitions are shy and withdrawn. Some, who are extremely inhibited about certain areas of their lives and activities, may develop SOCIAL PHOBIAS. They may feel inhibitions about speaking in front of a crowd, about walking into a room filled with strangers, or calling a new acquaintance to arrange a social engagement. Others have inhibitions related to sexual activity; SEX THERAPY may be helpful with these concerns.

The stresses associated with many inhibitions can be overcome with a variety of therapies, including BEHAVIOR THERAPY.

See also PHOBIAS; PSYCHOTHERAPIES.

insomnia   The inability to SLEEP or stay asleep; often a stressful situation and may be a symptom of other disorders. Among the most prevalent causes of insomnia are a history of STRESS, recent GRIEF, ANXIETY, or DEPRESSION. According to a study reported in *Canadian Family Physician* (February 1992), insomnia occurs in up to 35% of patients who have depression, anxiety, or mania. Certain prescription drugs (antihypertensives, antiasthmatics) along with CAFFEINE, nicotine, and alcohol are believed to account for another 12% of cases of insomnia. While alcohol helps some people fall asleep more easily, they often awaken in about four hours with rebound insomnia. Other causes of insomnia include tolerance to, or withdrawal from, sedative-hypnotics, restless leg syndrome (aching, burning, pricking sensations in leg muscles during the night in bed), and sleep apnea.

See also ALCOHOLISM AND ALCOHOL DEPENDENCE.

FOR FURTHER INFORMATION:
American Sleep Disorders Association
604 Second Street SW
Rochester, MN 55902
Phone: (507) 287-6006

SOURCE:
Harrison, Pam. "Insomnia not a Diagnosis but a Complaint." *Canadian Family Physician* 38 (February 1992).

intergenerational conflicts   Intergenerational conflicts resulting in stress have particular meaning within the family. Because people live longer, it is not unusual to have family members representing as many as three or four generations. Having more than two of those generations living under one roof is less likely to occur today than in earlier times, but it is generally agreed that generational conflicts are often due to living together in one residence. However, no matter how close or far apart the generations live, as long as they continue to meet and share holiday and other family celebrations, some areas of generational conflict, often labeled as a generation gap, will persist.

"Generation gap" refers to the inability to communicate, viewing the same phenomenon with opposite conclusions, insensitivity to the feelings of others, and criticism of one's feelings and beliefs. While generation gaps have always existed, the gap, which usually extended between parents and children, has broadened to include grandparents as well. In these three-generational families, issues that most often involve all three generations in areas of disagreement include behavior.

Some young people often carry a stereotype of older adults as "living in the past," overly conservative and unable to understand the young and how much things have changed since they were young. While many young people admire and love older people, and in specific instances (parents, relatives, friends, teachers) even use them as role models, the stress-filled intergenerational conflicts persist.

A good deal of stress emanating from middle-aged and older adults toward the young is, in fact, due to the overpowering youth culture of the 1990s. In addition, older people's view of the younger generation may be colored by their own feelings of self-achievement and life satisfaction. When they feel good about themselves, they are more likely to have higher expectations of the younger generation.

See also AGE DISCRIMINATION; BABY BOOMERS; COMMUNICATION; ELDERLY PARENTS; GENERATION X; LISTENING; PARENTING; PUBERTY.

intimacy   Intimacy is marked by very close association and friendship between individuals. Emotional intimacy can exist between lovers, friends, siblings, or children and parents. There is evidence that intimacy can be linked to good health, but when a relationship turns sour, it can be a source of stress for many people.

Close relationships and good health
There is evidence that suggests that when individuals have happy relationships, the likelihood of disease and complications from disease is far less, according to Len Sperry, M.D., Duke University. A five-year study found that unmarried heart patients who did not have a confidante were three times more likely to die from cardiac disease than those who were married or had a close friend. Similar findings were presented in a Canadian study of 224 women with breast cancer. Seven years after they had been diagnosed, 76% of the women with at least one intimate relationship survived. The explanation for this, Sperry says, is that feeling cared about and important helps maintain a person's optimism in times of stress. These emotional boosts translate into a strong immunity that helps fight disease.

The stress and fear of intimacy
Author of the book, *Too Close for Comfort: Exploring the Risks of Intimacy*, Geraldine Piorkowski, Ph.D., explored the theory that the fears and stress of intimacy can be healthy when they are realistic and protective of the self. To do this, Piorkowski suggests that indi-

---

TAKING THE STRESS OUT OF INTIMATE RELATIONSHIPS

- Don't plunge in. Relationships should develop slowly.
- Autonomy is important, don't lose control of your own needs.
- Don't expect perfection in yourself or the other person.
- Set boundaries and recharge, using periods of distance to strengthen your sense of self.
- Accept criticism, rejection, and disappointment as a fact of life.
- Maintain a life away from the relationship.

---

viduals reflect and learn from past experiences, schedule enough time to develop these relationships, be willing to share feelings with others, work at relationships but allow for failures, and be on intimate terms with more than one person.

Dr. Piorkowski comments, "There is a level of imperfect intimacy that is good enough to live and grow on. In good-enough intimacy, painful encounters occasionally occur, but they are balanced by the strengths and pleasures of the relationship. There are enough positives to balance the negatives. People who do well in intimate relationships don't have the perfect relationship, but it is good enough."

Developing intimacy in cyberspace
More and more people are developing relationships on-line. They meet in chat rooms, and, for more intimacy, carry on their affair using E-mail and exchange photos via the Internet. There's also an addictive quality to conversing on-line, and some people, particularly those who have not been honest, may have been wasting the other's person's time. But the real danger is that on-line relationships are not limited to consenting adults. Sexual predators use the information highway as a route to meet children and lure them to meeting places and abuse them. In 1997, a

detective was quoted as saying, "The Internet has been a dream come true for a pedophile. It has taken the playground from the street and put it into their home where they can cultivate potential victims in secrecy and in seclusion."

In 1997, a 15-year-old New Jersey boy was sexually assaulted by a man he met in a "chat room," where people type in comments under assumed screen names. After that incident, that teenager was accused of sexually assaulting and killing an 11-year-old boy.

Because not all Internet users are benign, parents should warn their children about the dangers of on-line predators.

SOURCE:
Piorkowski, Geraldine K. *Too Close For Comfort: Exploring the Risks of Intimacy.* New York: Plenum Press, 1994.

introversion A PERSONALITY characteristic marked by self-reliance and more of an interest in working alone or doing recreational activities alone than with others. The opposite personality type is characterized by *extroversion,* which involves more outgoing tendencies. Introverts may be stressed because they are preoccupied with their own inner thoughts and feelings rather than with other people. Introverts tend to be rather contemplative and sensitive people, and may seem aloof to others.

See also PERSONALITY; SELF-ESTEEM.

irritable bowel syndrome (IBS) Applies to a pattern of symptoms in the digestive tract that affect about twice as many women as men. Only rarely does IBS begin in people over the age of 50; it is a disease of young adulthood and sometimes adolescence. For many, the attacks are brought on by certain stressful life situations.

IBS is one of the most common gastrointestinal conditions seen by physicians today. The symptoms most commonly experienced include abdominal pain, CONSTIPATION or diar-

rhea, and gaseousness. Symptoms may vary in severity and may last for a day or even months, if not treated. Irritable bowel syndrome in the past was referred to as mucous colitis, spastic colitis, nervous diarrhea, and irritable colon; these terms have generally been discarded.

IBS often has been considered to be caused by emotional conflict or STRESS because doctors have been unable to pinpoint its organic cause. However, many individuals who suffer from ANXIETY DISORDERS, panic attacks, or panic disorder also suffer from IBS. While stress is a link, there are also other contributing factors. For example, eating causes contractions of the colon. Normally, this response may cause an urge to have a bowel movement within 30 to 60 minutes after a meal. In people with IBS, the exaggerated reflex can lead to cramps. Sometimes the spasm delays the passage of stool, leading to constipation. At other times, the spasm leads to more rapid passage of feces or diarrhea. While some symptoms, such as abdominal pain, may be triggered by emotional stress, the symptoms are real and not imaginary. Symptoms occur because the intestinal tract does not function properly, although no organic disease is present.

IBS can cause a great deal of discomfort, but is not serious. However, for some people it can be a source of stress and disabling. Some people may be afraid to go to dinner parties, seek employment, or travel on public transportation. However, with attention to stress management, proper diet, and sometimes medication prescribed by a physician, most people with IBS can control their symptoms effectively.

Self-help for IBS
Individuals who have been diagnosed with IBS may be advised to engage in more tension-relieving activities, such as sports or HOBBIES, and physical EXERCISE. They may be advised to concentrate on RELAXATION techniques and possibly counseling by a psychol-

ogist who can provide guidance in relaxation techniques. Also, they may be advised to eat meals at regular times and with good eating practices, such as chewing slowly, and with measures designed to keep them from swallowing air. Large meals may also cause cramping and diarrhea in some people, so that eating smaller meals more frequently, or eating smaller portions of foods may be recommended. Foods that are low in fat and rich in carbohydrates and protein may also help alleviate symptoms. Dietary fiber, present in whole grain breads and cereals and in fruits and vegetables, has also been shown to be helpful in lessening IBS symptoms. High-fiber diets keep the colon mildly distended, which helps to prevent spasms from developing. Some forms of fiber also keep water in the stools, thereby preventing hard, difficult-to-pass stools from forming. Although high-fiber diets may cause gas and bloating, over time, these symptoms may dissipate as the digestive tract becomes used to the increased fiber intake. Chewing gum, drinking carbonated beverages, caffeine, and alcohol, and smoking should be avoided.

Getting medical help

Periodic flareups of IBS symptoms are fairly common. When IBS becomes the body's habitual way of reacting against undue stress—and since most people experience some physical symptoms of stress at least occasionally—the goal should be to control these symptoms.

Individuals who have IBS may be advised to take a combination of antispasmodic drugs and tranquilizers, which may relieve symptoms. Antispasmodic medications are sometimes called anticholinergics; as painful spasms may be the primary symptom of IBS, treatment with these medications is often useful. However, in an effort to regulate colonic activity or minimize stress, some individuals become dependent on laxatives or tranquilizers. When this occurs, the physician may try to withdraw the drugs slowly and work with the individual to control specific symptoms of stress, as well as the irritable bowel symptoms, with life-style changes.

See also ANXIETY; GUIDED IMAGERY; INDIGESTION; MEDITATION; PANIC ATTACKS AND PANIC DISORDER.

SOURCES:

Cunningham, Chet. *The Irritable Bowel Syndrome (I.B.S.) & Gastrointestinal Solutions Handbook.* Leucadia, Calif.: United Research Publishers, 1995.

Tannenhaus, Norra. *Learning to Live with Chronic IBS.* New York: Dell, 1990.

isolation   See LONELINESS.

Japan, stress in See KAROSHI.

jealousy An attitude or EMOTION that encompasses a continuum of ENVY, distrust, hostility and rivalry with another person. It sometimes leads to suspicion of unfaithfulness or apprehension of a loved one's exclusive devotion. When an individual experiences jealousy, he or she has feelings of low SELF-ESTEEM and self-imposed stress.

Examples of jealousy include the feeling that some children experience when a new sibling arrives, or when one's spouse has an intimate RELATIONSHIP with another. An individual may be jealous about another's ability to afford the luxuries of life, such as elegant housing, country club memberships, expensive clothes and fur coats. Jealousies also occur when one individual perceives another as smarter, or at work when one individual is passed over for another who gets a promotion.

Stress caused by jealousy can be relieved by a realistic look at oneself and one's capabilities, whether academic, financial, or professional. An assessment of one's own good points can override feelings of envy of others. If not dealt with, jealousy can lead to inappropriate behavior such as stalking, sexual abuse, and criminal action.

See also RELAXATION.

jet lag Term given to the disruption of one's body rhythms (CIRCADIAN RHYTHM) resulting from traveling through several time zones within a short span of time. It takes many individuals several days or longer to recover from the stress of this type of travel. The sleep schedule, appetite, and ability to concentrate well while recovering from jet lag vary from individual to individual.

See also AIRPLANES.

SOURCE:
Wingler, Sharon. *Travel Alone & Love It: A Flight Attendant's Guide to Solo Travel.* Willowbrook: Chicago Spectrum Press, 1996.

job change Making the transition into a new position, whether continuing to work for the same company or for a new one, can be stressful. Both situations have pros and cons. Coming from the outside means the individual does not have to worry about managing coworkers or friends. However, when the individual does not have a mentor or friend in a new company, he has no one to rely on, to show him the ropes and to introduce him to corporate policies and politics. Starting out fresh also means not knowing what employees are good at, who are the hard workers, and who sloughs off.

Promotion, whether from within or without, can also significantly raise stress levels because it raises fear of incompetence and fear of failure. Usually these fears and stresses will go away once the new position is mastered and evidence of SUCCESS becomes visible.

See also DOWNSIZING; JOB SECURITY; LAYOFFS; NETWORKING; WORKPLACE.

SOURCE:
Snyder, Don J. *The Cliff Walk: A Memoir of a Job Lost and a Life Found.* Boston: Little, Brown, 1997.

job security Lack of job security is a major cause of instability and stress for workers throughout the world. This was not so 30 to 40 years ago. Then, many employers had implicit or explicit long-term employment contracts with their workers, contracts that emphasized management's commitment and pledge to minimize the need for LAYOFFS. Wages and job benefits increased over the years, and it was not unusual for the company to pay the total cost of employees' health care and charge minimally for family coverage. This job security led workers to expect to remain in their jobs for many years, and it was not unusual for workers to devote their entire working lives to one company, retiring with the traditional gold watch and company pension.

During the later 1990s, DOWNSIZING, layoffs, MERGERS, and other organizational changes have greatly altered the job security picture. Employers are no longer sharing their wealth; raises and employee benefits have been scaled back. Full-time jobs are harder to find.

Suggestions for improving one's job security include learning to operate one's own business, becoming a free agent or "gun-for hire," setting new professional goals, looking for new jobs while still employed, considering new fields, building portable skills; setting up a network of trusted colleagues, clients, former bosses, and other professionals who know the worker's track record and opportunities available in his/her field; creating an escape hatch (options, lateral moves, further education); and being ready to accept change.

See also JOB CHANGE; NETWORKING; WORKPLACE.

SOURCE:
Alderman, Lesley, and Karen Cheney. "Here's the Good News about Jobs." *Money,* May 1996, 111–21.

journaling   Writing down thoughts and experiences in a daily or weekly journal is a way for the individual to relieve stress, sort out confusion, and deal with problems. Writing, and reading what has been written, sometimes exposes suppressed, subconscious feelings that can be dealt with more constructively when they are recognized. In this sense, a diarist may get closer to his/her feelings and better understand self-motivations.

The cathartic effect of writing involves a distancing from negative feelings and experiences. Once the feelings or experiences are described on paper, the writer frequently has a sense of being rid of them, of being able to go on to something else. Writing may also help to bring repressed thoughts and attitudes out into the open and eliminate some of the restrictions that sap energy and limit productivity. Simply the act of writing may grant a sense of CONTROL, a way of giving some order and manageability to problems.

Symptoms such as ANXIETY, DEPRESSION, and apathy may be masks for envy, JEALOUSY, and rage turned inward at the self. Some diarists have found it useful to write a portrait of a person whom they envy or who has angered them. The portrait sometimes reveals qualities of their own that they wish to either develop or change.

Making lists in a diary can be a good way of setting goals and giving order to what may seem to be an enormous or chaotic task. Journaling also can be useful for the person who is attempting to control addictive or obsessive behavior.

Journaling is used by many SUPPORT GROUPS for overeaters, as well as those who wish to stop SMOKING or drinking. The diary not only improves self-understanding and serves as a way to record progress, but also gives the individual something to do over which he/she has complete control when he wants a drink, cigarette, or is about to give in to a desire to overeat.

See also EATING DISORDERS; SELF-ESTEEM.

SOURCE:
Adams, Kathleen. *Journal to the Self.* New York: Warner Books, 1990.

judicial proceedings   Stresses endured by individuals serving on juries range from being away from their families in the event of a sequestered jury, to the agonizing DECISION-MAKING processes in which they will have to engage.

First there is the stress of the selection process, during which an individual faces the feeling of being out of CONTROL of his destiny for the next day or, perhaps, for weeks. Then there is the concern about being sequestered for a period of time with a group of strangers. Some stress surrounds how well the individual will get along with fellow jury members. There is also the stress of making the right decision, particularly in a life or death matter, and having one's own judgment swayed by others in making a decision.

Stresses for lawyers

LAWYERS are the first to attest to the extreme stress that arises during a jury trial. This stress often is exhibited by a loss of temper on both sides of the issue. That is why stress management is a popular topic of seminars offered to lawyers nationwide. These seminars encourage lawyers to recognize the stressors such as physical separation from their families and disruption of normal routines that may occur, particularly when a trial goes on for a long period of time, and to strategize ways to handle the stress. The seminars emphasize the need for lawyers to maintain themselves physically and emotionally and to try to talk out feelings, something that can be alien to those involved in legal work.

When asked about effective ways to handle stress, many lawyers highly rate building a wall of separation between their professional and private lives. Others value a healthy regimen that includes no SMOKING or drinking, staying in shape by exercising, and establishing healthy life-style habits.

Stresses on trial judges

A study reported in the *Bulletin of the American Academy of Psychiatry Law* (1994) examined work-related stress among American trial judges. A representative sample of 88 judges completed questionnaires addressing type and magnitude of specific work-related stressors, psychological stress symptoms, and psychosocial moderators of stress.

Types of stressors noted included cases, litigating parties, purposes and consequences of decisions, conflicts between professional and personal values, and seriousness of a criminal offense. The most stressful aspect of work related to poorly prepared or disrespectful counsel, exercising judicial management and discretion, and highly emotional cases under public scrutiny.

SOURCES:
Eells, T.D., and C.R. Showalter. "Work-related Stress in American Trial Judges." *Bulletin of the American Academy of Psychiatry and Law* 22 (1994): 71–83.
Kahn, Ada P. "Win the Case Against Stress." *Record* (Chicago Bar Association), May 1994.

K

Kabat-Zinn, Jon, Ph.D. Founder and director of the Stress Reduction Clinic, University of Massachusetts Medical Center, Worcester, where he is also an associate professor of medicine. He is the author of popular books about coping with STRESS including *Mindfulness Meditation in Everyday Life, Meditation for Daily Living,* and *Full Catastrophe Living: Using the Wisdom of Your Body and Mind to Face Stress, Pain and Illness.*

Dr. Kabat-Zinn is a proponent of mindfulness MEDITATION, a more than 2,000-year-old Buddhist method of meditation, and living fully in the present. This approach offers a unique way to cope with stress and illness. Mindfulness meditation can help induce deep states of RELAXATION and, at times, directly improve physical symptoms.

Other forms of meditation involve focusing on a sound or the sensation of breath leaving and entering the body. Anything else that interferes in the mind during these types of meditation is seen as a distraction to be disregarded. Mindfulness, on the other hand, is *insight* meditation and encourages the meditator to note any thoughts as they occur and observe them intentionally but non-judgmentally, moment by moment. This practice of observing thoughts, feelings, and sensations can help the meditator to become calmer and have a broader perspective regarding life. Kabat-Zinn teaches readers to reflect on the beauty of the present and emotional and spiritual applications of meditation.

In his writings, Kabat-Zinn shows readers meditation postures and ways to meditate, including concentrating on walking or standing, and visualizing mountains and lakes. Typically, the training program for mindfulness meditation is eight weeks long.

Like many mind-body techniques, mindfulness meditation has just begun to be explored scientifically. Controlled studies are investigating whether mindfulness meditation can influence the healing process and help in treating many diseases.

See also ALTERNATIVE THERAPIES; GUIDED IMAGERY; MIND-BODY CONNECTIONS.

FOR FURTHER INFORMATION:
Stress Reduction Clinic
University of Massachusetts Medical Center
Worcester, MA 01655
Phone: (508) 856-1616

SOURCES:
Kabat-Zinn, Jon. *Full Catastrophe Living: Using the Wisdom of Your Body and Mind to Face Stress, Pain and Illness.* New York: Delacorte, 1991.
―――. *Wherever You Go, There You Are: Mindfulness Meditation in Everyday Life.* New York: Hyperion, 1993.

karoshi "Death from overwork"—synonymous with stress in Japan. An article by C. Frank Lawlis in *Alternative Therapies* (July 1995) reports that "People (in Japan) are literally dying at their workstations. It appears that their entire physiological system collapses or shuts down."

Lawlis draws from a 1989 study by Chiyoda Fire and Marine Insurance, Ltd., one of the top insurance carriers in Japan. Chiyoda, which covers over 100,000 Japanese corporations, conducted a major study on health problems Japanese people are likely to encounter. One important conclusion of the study was that in 40% of the health problems, stress played a major role.

As a result, Chiyoda established N.C. Wellness, a company that developed programs integrating Oriental medicine into health promotion for employees. Buildings housing the programs were constructed to focus on tranquil space and function in a similar fashion to that of a "cocoon." At the same time, they were designed as places for nonordinary pleasure where "interference from everyday affairs is barred" and where the environment to practice the mind-body and awareness elements of balance is enjoyable and protective.

The first prototype center was opened in Kichjoji, Musashino-shi, Tokyo, in June 1994. The core program offered at this site incorporated six "directions": self-management, self-promotion, self-discovery/purpose of life, fun and pleasure, interpersonal skills, and community.

See also ACCULTURATION; ALTERNATIVE THERAPIES; MIND-BODY CONNECTIONS.

kinesics The study of COMMUNICATION as expressed through facial expression and other body movements. Theories and techniques of studying this type of nonverbal communication were developed by Ray L. Birdwhistell (1918–), who found that certain gestures and expressions were specifically male or female and also related to regional and national groups. BODY LANGUAGE changes with age, health, mood, and the degree of STRESS or RELAXATION experienced by the individual. Birdwhistell developed his theories with the use of photography and a notation system of symbols called kinegraphs to describe gestures and expressions.

SOURCE:
Birdwhistell, Ray L. *Kinesics and Context.* Philadelphia: University of Pennsylvania Press, 1970.

kleptomania   See SHOPAHOLISM.

Kohut, Heinz   See SELF-PSYCHOLOGY.

kundalini   See YOGA.

L

laughter   An individual's response, a smile, chuckle, or explosive sound, to something that inspires joy or scorn. The ability to laugh, and its companion, a sense of HUMOR, can provide psychological relief from stress, tension, ANXIETY, HOSTILITY, and emotional pain. Laughter helps individuals deal with stressful situations, whether at work, in social situations or in health care settings.

Laughter may be a defense against personal feelings of self-consciousness or embarrassment. An ability to laugh at oneself can be an important COPING mechanism against these stresses. However, many people find it difficult to poke fun at themselves and to acknowledge that they have made a mistake. Individuals suffering from DEPRESSION often lose their ability to laugh and see no humor in their lives or in the world around them.

The curative powers of laughter

Maintaining a sense of humor can help most people stay healthy. It causes the body to have a physiological response, and the IMMUNE SYSTEM gets the benefit. For example, when one laughs, various muscles tense, then relax, which can result in toning. BREATHING gets faster, allowing the body to take in more oxygen and to get rid of more carbon dioxide. Heart and pulse rate and blood pressure also increase to promote more vigorous circulation, and an increase in the brain's chemical transmitters aids mental alertness.

Research shows that laughter, like exercise, can stimulate the brain to produce secretions known as ENDORPHINS. Endorphins increase one's sense of physical and mental well-being and, to some extent, relieve pain.

The curative power of laughter is not a 20th-century discovery. In the Book of Proverbs, it says: "A merry heart doeth good

like a medicine." Norman Cousins (1915–90), former editor of the *Saturday Review* and later a member of the faculty of the medical school at the University of California at Los Angeles, used the curative power of laughter to help himself recover from a degenerative disease of the body's connective tissue. Following are a few excerpts from Cousins' *Anatomy of An Illness,* in which he described the benefits of laughter:

> I made the joyous discovery that ten minutes of genuine belly laughter had an anesthetic effect and would give me at least two hours of pain-free sleep . . . Exactly what happens inside the human mind and body as the result of humor is difficult to say. But the evidence that it works has stimulated the speculations not just of physicians but of philosophers and scholars over the centuries.

Cousins checked out of the hospital and spent weeks watching the Marx Brothers' movies and other comedies. He attributed his recovery to the positive feelings that laughter aroused in him.

Research in laughter

In an article titled "Laughter" in *American Scientist* (January-February 1996), University of Maryland psychologist Robert R. Provine attempted to shed some light on laughter as a stereotyped, species-specific form of COMMUNICATION. Among other things, Provine's research provides a novel approach to the mechanisms and evolution of vocal production, speech perception, and social behavior.

The laugh tracks of television situation comedies—attempts to stimulate contagious laughter in viewers—and the difficulty of extinguishing "laugh jags" or fits of nearly uncontrollable laughter are familiar phenomena. "Rather than dismissing contagious laughter as a behavioral curiosity," Provine suggests, "we should recognize it and other laugh-related phenomena as clues to broader and deeper issues. Clearly, laughter is a powerful and pervasive part of our lives."

Provine and his assistants observed human laughter in various natural habitats, such as shopping malls, classrooms, sidewalks, offices, and cocktail parties. Among other things, they found that, contrary to their expectations, most conversational laughter is not a response to structured attempts at humor, such as jokes or stories. Spontaneity, mutual playfulness, in-group feelings, positive emotional tone, and not comedy, mark the social settings of most naturally occurring laughter. They also found that the average speaker laughs about 46% more often than the audience, and that females, whether they are speakers or audiences, laugh more often than males. "In some respects laughter may be a signal of dominance/submission or acceptance/rejection," Provine concluded. "In some situations, laughter may modify the behavior of others by shaping the emotional tone of a conversation."

See also PSYCHONEUROIMMUNOLOGY.

FOR FURTHER INFORMATION:
International Laughter Society
16000 Glen Una Drive
Los Gatos, CA 95030
Phone: (408) 354–3456

SOURCES:
Peter, Laurence J. *The Laughter Prescription. The Tools of Humor and How to Use Them.* New York: Ballantine Books, 1982.
Provine, Robert R. "Laughter." *American Scientist* 84, no. 1 (January-February 1996).
Roach, Mary. "Can You Laugh Your Stress Away?" *Health,* September 1996.

lawyers Individuals whose profession is to conduct lawsuits and provide advice regarding legal obligations for clients. Under constant pressure to win, there are extremely high levels of STRESS associated with practicing law. Lawyers are frequently in adversarial situations and face deadlines and pressures from many people, including clients, partners, and opposing lawyers.

Litigators, lawyers who represent clients in JUDICIAL PROCEEDINGS, must have a tough exterior to dominate the situations that they encounter and to win. In private life, some find it difficult to switch to a more equal role with personal partners or family, resulting in still another level of stress and tension.

Lawyers as individuals tend to be high achievers. Usually they have high expectations of themselves and others; often these expectations are unreasonable, causing a disparity. "Most lawyers are by nature compulsive people," said Nancy Weisman, general counsel, Rush North Shore Medical Center, Skokie, Illinois, in an article in the Chicago Bar Association's journal, *Record* (May 1994). "Lawyers are often the bringers of news, both good and bad. We bear the burden of delivering answers from other lawyers or the courts. It's easy to explain a win. Explaining a lost motion or case is a stressor lawyers face at times," said Weisman.

Additionally, lawyers must be good listeners and watch for BODY LANGUAGE and unspoken signals to try to anticipate the opposing lawyer's responses. Body language plays an equally important role in anticipating feelings of the judge or jury. At the same time, lawyers usually make efforts to hide signs of their vulnerability, which in itself is a stressful posture to take.

Different stressors at different career stages
Lawyers face different stresses that may threaten their mental and physical health at various career stages. Just out of law school, in midcareer, and when nearing RETIREMENT they face particular tension-producing factors. Personal stressors compound the tension levels they face throughout their lives.

Most young lawyers begin careers as associates and are single. Hoping to meet a mate, they try to maintain an active social life, but find it difficult while working 80 hours a week or more. The added pressure of a new social relationship when they do enter into one, while meeting the demands of their bosses and clients, can be overwhelmingly stressful.

Married lawyers, particularly those who have children, are often torn between wanting to do their jobs well and enjoying family life. They may have experienced feelings of resentment about being absent from family events because of clients' needs. They want to have time and energy for their children's needs and for their partners. They have to factor these stressors into already stressful days.

As careers advance, there is the COMPETITION to become a partner as well as comparison with the careers of former classmates. Some law firms' new family leave policies have great appeal for young lawyers; still they worry that they will be on a slower track than their peers.

Lawyers who are solo practitioners or in very small firms face the constant challenge of bringing in enough business to stay afloat. Lawyers whose firms have reorganized or merged with another firm may find the prospect of being downsized out of the firm a serious stressor. Those who do stay find that they have a new boss to report to, a new internal structure to adjust to, and new or additional responsibilities beyond their full workload.

As they near retirement, some lawyers feel threatened by younger partners in their firms. Others may regret not reaching the top echelon of their firm. They become concerned about what they will do after they retire from their positions, which have centered on their practice and their clients. Some face the stressful situation of having had too little time to develop outside interests or HOBBIES, which are usually the key to making a smooth transition from career to retirement.

See also DOWNSIZING; JOB SECURITY; LAYOFFS; MERGERS.

SOURCE:
Kahn, Ada P. "Win the Case Against Stress." *Record* (Chicago Bar Association), May 1994.

layoffs   Layoffs or reductions in force (RIFs) have become everyday occurrences for companies. The potential for this occurrence affects everyone and is a cause for stress. Today, more than ever, there is no JOB SECURITY, and the big organization that took care of its workers is a thing of the past.

An example of a major national corporation implementing massive layoffs is AT&T. Early in January 1996, AT&T announced that it would eliminate 40,000 jobs by 1998. In November 1996, AT&T offered buyouts to more than 70,000 workers, but only 6,500 accepted. Of the 40,000 jobs to be eliminated, about 75% will have to be cut by layoffs.

The AT&T cutback was the third-largest in corporate America in three years. In 1993, IBM did away with 63,000 jobs and Sears, Roebuck and Co. announced the demise of 50,000 jobs as well as jobs connected to its catalog, known as the Big Book.

During the recession years of the 1980s, job reduction was blamed on national or international business conditions. At the end of the 20th century, more and more companies are reducing their workforces in order to save money (after merger or acquisition) or realize productivity gains.

Layoffs also are due to plant closings, work slowdowns, corporate DOWNSIZINGS or MERGERS, and acquisitions. Being laid off is different from being fired, though the individual will probably feel the same stress. When workers are fired, it is because their performance is lacking; when layoffs occur, performance is rarely cited.

Typically, there are five emotional stages that follow a termination, and they are not unlike those felt at the time of any major loss:

Stage One: Denial. *It must be some mistake, this can't be happening to me.*

Stage Two: Self-Blame. *I must have done some-thing wrong. How did I screw up?*

Stage Three: Anger. *Why did management do this to me?*

Stage Four: Depression. *It's not worth getting out of bed in the morning.*

Stage Five: Acceptance. *What happened may be all for the best.*

On virtually every indicator of mental and physical health, job loss due to layoffs has a negative impact. People who lose their jobs are often anxious, depressed, unhappy and, in general, dissatisfied with their lives. They have lowered SELF-ESTEEM, are short-tempered, and are fatalistic and pessimistic about the future. Thus, job loss is clearly hard on one's health, and it is important to get CONTROL over one's life and one's stress after a job loss.

See also WORKPLACE.

learned helplessness   According to Martin E.P. Seligman, an American psychologist (1942–   ), learned helplessness refers to a feeling of helplessness and stifling of motivation brought about by exposure to aversive events over which people have no CONTROL. Such stressful situations lead to feelings of powerlessness, BOREDOM, and DEPRESSION, and the individual becomes passive and non-assertive.

In experiments, Seligman and Steven Maier, another psychologist, exposed animals to pathologic amounts of psychological stressors. Those stressors included loss of control and predictability within certain contexts, a loss of outlets for FRUSTRATION, a loss of sources of support, and a perception of life worsening. The animals had trouble COPING with many varied tasks, such as competing with other animals for food or avoiding social AGGRESSION. Such animals have a motivational problem; they are helpless because they do not even attempt to cope with a new situation.

The condition that the animals experienced was a condition very similar to depression in

humans. Later on, Seligman coined the term LEARNED OPTIMISM to refer to the opposite behavior, in which an individual does not give up but persists toward a goal.

See GENERAL ADAPTATION SYNDROME.

SOURCE:
Seligman, Martin E.P. *Learned Optimism.* New York: Alfred A. Knopf, 1991.

learned optimism   A term coined by Martin E.P. Seligman in his book *Learned Optimism* (1991), describing attitudes and behaviors people exhibit when they face the stress of failures and disappointments that inevitably are a part of life's experience. According to Seligman, in childhood, individuals learn to explain setbacks to themselves. Some are able to say and believe: "It was just circumstances; it's going away quickly, and there is much more in life." Scientific evidence has shown that this optimism is vitally important in overcoming defeat, promoting achievement and maintaining or improving health. He documents the effects of optimism on the quality of life.

In his book, Seligman shows how to stop automatically assuming GUILT, how to get out of the habit of seeing the direst possible implications in every setback, and how to be optimistic.

The opposite is LEARNED *HELPLESSNESS*, a term he coined earlier, which relates to an attitude of hopelessness about the future and future activities.

See also COPING; GENERAL ADAPTATION SYNDROME.

SOURCE:
Seligman, Martin E.P. *Learned Optimism.* New York: Alfred A. Knopf, 1991.

learning disabilities   A group of physical and psychological disorders that interfere with learning. Because they may be taunted by their peers, young people who have such disabilities may also suffer stress from a loss of

SELF-ESTEEM and motivation. Learning disabilities are also a source of stress to parents who have high expectations for their children. Even when the disabilities are diagnosed, they may wonder why their children are not doing well in school and urge them to do better.

Learning disabilities include problems in learning caused by defects in speech, hearing, and memory; they do not include disabilities due to emotional or environmental deprivation or to poor teaching.

Children with minimal or borderline MENTAL RETARDATION generally have difficulty learning. Other children suffer from *hyperactivity,* which lowers the attention span; *dyslexia,* which is difficulty in reading; *dyscalculia,* an inability to perform mathematical problems; and *dysgraphia,* referring to writing disorders. Specific learning difficulties in children of normal intelligence may be caused by forms of *minimal brain dysfunction,* which may be inherited and untreatable.

Generally difficult to diagnose, children with learning disabilities should be observed and taught by teachers who have a degree in special education. Stresses of learning difficulties faced by children, parents, or adults can best be handled by obtaining help from social workers or psychologists specializing in learning disabilities. In addition to diagnostic testing, these professionals can provide necessary psychological support.

See also ATTENTION-DEFICIT HYPERACTIVITY DISORDER; PARENTING.

SOURCES:

Grey House Publishing. *The Complete Learning Disabilities Directory.* Lakeville, Conn.: Grey House Publishing, 1994.

Hall, David. *Living With Learning Disabilities: A Guide for Students.* Minneapolis: Lerner Publications, 1993.

left-handedness   In religious symbolism and folklore, the left side is associated with the devil, and this attitude has permeated outlooks held by many people for centuries. Left-handers often deal with subtle attitudes reflected in such phrases as a "left-handed compliment" that imply that something is wrong with being left-handed. Left-handed people are a minority in the United States, comprising about 13% of the population.

In earlier generations, children were encouraged to use their right hands instead of their left, creating stressful situations for both parents and children. Studies of left-handedness in the population by age group show proportionally more young left-handers, probably an indication that parents and teachers are no longer trying to switch these children into using their right hands.

Probably the biggest stress factor facing individuals who are left-handed is that handwriting techniques, scissors, and other kitchen and household tools are not designed with them in mind. However, at the end of the 20th century, catalogs with special products made for left-handers abound.

Scientists are unsure of what neurological factors cause handedness. There is some evidence that, before birth, all humans are potentially right-handed. Changes occur as the fetus develops or in the birth process that create left-handedness. The male hormone testosterone, produced by both men and women, may have something to do with left-handedness. The hypothesis is that an unusually high amount of testosterone produced by the mother before birth may enable the right side of the brain, the area that controls the left side of the body, to dominate. Studies have linked left-handedness with pregnancy in older mothers, Cesarean deliveries, and difficult labor.

Studies also show that while there is a predominance of left-handers in the schizophrenic and retarded populations, left-handers statistically score higher than the general population on standardized tests. Research on college students showed that left-handers entered fields such as the graphic arts, architecture and the sciences, which tend to be nonverbal. This is probably a reflection of the fact that the right side of the brain controls spatial reasoning ability and other nonverbal skills.

Many famous criminals were left-handed. Evidence from the crimes of Jack the Ripper points to the fact that he was left-handed, as were Billy the Kid, John Dillinger, and Albert Henry DeSalvo, known as the Boston Strangler, and his lawyer F. Lee Bailey. However, not all left-handers are famous for their crimes. Other well known left-handers were Pablo Picasso, Leonardo da Vinci, Benjamin Franklin, Babe Ruth, Marilyn Monroe, and presidents Harry Truman and George Bush.

SOURCES:
Coren, Stanley. *The Left-Hander Syndrome: The Causes and Consequences of Left-Handedness*. New York: The Free Press, 1992.
Kahn, Ada P., and Jan Fawcett. *The Encyclopedia of Mental Health*. New York: Facts On File, 1993.

leisure   See HOBBIES; RECREATION; VACATIONS.

lesbianism   Defined as female HOMOSEXUAL-ITY, lesbianism is a term derived from the Greek poetess Sappho, who lived on the island of Lesbos. Women who practice lesbianism (lesbians) prefer women as sexual partners, although some lesbians have or have had heterosexual partners. Lesbians are part of the "gay community" along with homosexual men. In the late 1990s, lesbians still face some stresses of nonacceptance by their families, childhood friends, coworkers and bosses, and members of their community-at-large.

More and more lesbian couples have become parents (co-mothers) through artificial insemination and ADOPTION. While facing all the concerns and stresses of parenthood, they may encounter particular stressors because of their choice of living situation.

The "gay liberation" movement during the 1970s and 1980s encouraged homosexuals to meet and discuss their important issues and provided a political organization to work toward legal change and fight job discrimination. The National Gay Task Force is a clearinghouse for these groups and provides information on local organizations.

FOR FURTHER INFORMATION:
The National Gay Task Force
80 Fifth Avenue
New York, NY 10011
Phone: (212) 741-1010

SOURCES:
Harris, Mary B., and Pauline H. Turner. "Gay and Lesbian Parents." *Journal of Homosexuality* 12, no. 2 (Winter 1985-86): 101–13.
Jay, Karla, ed. *Dyke Life. From Growing Up to Growing Old, a Celebration of the Lesbian Experience*. New York: Basic Books, 1995.
McDaniel, Judith. *The Lesbian Couples Guide: Finding the Right Woman and Creating a Life Together*. New York: HarperPerennial, 1995.
Polikoff, Nancy. "Lesbian Mothers, Lesbian Families: Legal Obstacles, Legal Challenges." *Review of Law and Special Change* 14 (1986): 907–14.
Slater, Suzanne. *The Lesbian Family Life Cycle*. New York: Free Press, 1995.

life change events   See GENERAL ADAPTATION SYNDROME; LIFE CHANGE SELF-RATING SCALE; SELYE, HANS.

life change self-rating scale   The original life change rating scale was developed as a predictor of illness based on stressful life events by authors Holmes and Rahe and presented at the Royal Society of Medicine in 1968. In many variations, this type of rating scale has been used to help individuals determine their composite stress level within the last year.

To take this test, mark any of the changes listed below that have occurred in your life in the past 12 months. Your total score indicates the amount of stress you have been subjected to in the one-year period. Your score may be useful in predicting your chances of suffering

LIFE CHANGE SELF-RATING SCALE

Event	Value
Death of spouse	100
Divorce	73
Marital separation	65
Death of close family member	63
Personal injury or illness	53
Marriage	50
Fired from work	47
Marital reconciliation	45
Retirement	45
Change in family member's health	44
Pregnancy	40
Sex difficulties	39
Addition to family	39
Business readjustment	39
Change in financial status	38
Death of close friend	37
Change to different line of work	36
Foreclosure of mortgage or loan	30
Change in work responsibilities	29
Son or daughter leaving home	29
Trouble with in-laws	29
Outstanding personal achievement	28
Spouse begins or stops work	26
Starting or finishing school	26
Change in living conditions	25
Trouble with boss	23
Change in residence or school	20
Change in recreational habits	19
Change in church or social activities	19
Change in sleeping habits	16
Change in eating habits	15
Vacation	13
Christmas season	12
Minor violation of the law	11

Your total score: _____

Adapted from Holmes, Thomas and Richard Rahe. "The Social Readjustment Rating Scale." *Journal of Psychosomatic Research* (Oxford) 11 (1967):213–18.

illness in the next two years due to physiological effects of serious stressors.

What your score means

A total score less than 150 may mean you have only a 27% chance of becoming ill in the next year. If your score is between 150 and 300, you have a 51% chance of encountering poor health. If your score is more than 300, you are facing odds of 80% that you will become ill; and as the score increases, so do the odds that the problem will be serious. To avoid these consequences, attention to RELAX-ATION and STRESS relief can help.

SOURCE:
Adapted from Holmes, Thomas and Richard Rahe. "The Social Readjustment Rating Scale." *Journal of Psychosomatic Research* (Oxford) 11 (1967): 213–18.

light therapy   See PSORIASIS; SEASONAL AFFEC-TIVE DISORDERS.

listening   Hearing with thoughtful attention; a skill necessary for good COMMUNICATION between individuals. It is an active process in which one gives complete attention to what others are saying and how they are saying it. According to Deborah Tannen, author of *Talking from 9 to 5: How Women's and Men's Conversational Styles Affect Who Gets Heard, Who Get Credit and What Gets Done at Work*, "Listening taps two important areas, gathering information and developing relationships." Active listening can reduce the stress of communication not only in business but in personal life as well.

By using nonverbal gestures such as a nod of the head or a smile, active listeners can convey concern and reinforce or encourage the

REDUCE STRESS WITH BETTER LISTENING SKILLS

- Focus on the speaker; use eye contact. Keep interruptions, such as phone calls and other conversations, down to a minimum.
- It helps to question the speaker. You can gently guide a conversation, show that you are interested in what he/she is saying, and what you might want to learn.
- Don't judge the person speaking; concentrate on the information he/she is presenting.

other's verbalizations. Listeners contribute by asking good questions, providing FEEDBACK on what they hear, and seeking consensus or pointing out differences of opinion within a group. On the other hand, people feel listened to when more than just their ideas get heard; they feel valued, and they will contribute a lot more to the conversation.

See also BODY LANGUAGE.

SOURCES:
Nichols, Michael P. *The Lost Art of Listening* New York: Doubleday, 1995.
Tannen, Deborah. *Talking from 9 to 5: How Women's and Men's Conversational Styles Affect Who Gets Heard, Who Gets Credit and What Gets Done at Work.* New York: William Morrow, 1994.

lithium See MANIC-DEPRESSIVE DISORDER; PHARMACOLOGICAL APPROACH.

live-in Common term for members of the opposite sex who share a domicile without the benefit of marriage. In many cases, stresses arise when one individual decides he or she wants to get married and the other does not. Additionally, stresses arise if the couple decides to break up. Besides the hurt feelings and blows to the ego, there may be mutually owned property or equipment, and live-ins may face the same dilemmas as a couple going through a DIVORCE.

Live-in is a term that evolved during the last two decades of the 20th century when this practice became fairly common in the United States among men and women of all ages. The demographic term for this situation, used by the United States Census Department, is POSSLQ (person of the opposite sex sharing living quarters).

See also FRIENDS; INTIMACY; RELATIONSHIPS.

living will See END OF LIFE CARE.

loneliness State of mind relating to lack of companionship or separation from others. It is different from being alone, which is a ques-

tion of choice. It is this lack of choice that make loneliness so stressful.

When people feel lonely, they are most likely to react in one of two ways. The first is a sadness response indicated by too much time spent eating, sleeping, and crying. The other response is "creative solitude" where a person finds a way to deal with loneliness such as reading a "good book" or watching a movie, listening to or playing music, using artistic talents to paint, crochet, quilt, weave, or do ceramics, spending time in the garden, or pursuing other interests and HOBBIES. When people deal with loneliness creatively, they are in fact fighting BOREDOM and, in that process, they become happier, calmer, and less stressed.

Some lonely people fit the shy, retiring stereotype; others compensate for their feelings by trying to become the center of attraction whether it be in the classroom or at a party. Individuals who have spouses and families can be lonely even though they are surrounded by people. Adolescents and teenagers may become lonely when they long to be part of their peer group and are not. Many widowed or divorced people in their later years become lonely as their friends die and they find it increasingly difficult to make new friends.

Conditions such as mental and physical DISABILITIES or language or ethnic barriers, sometimes produces isolation that results in loneliness.

Research on loneliness
In some cases, loneliness results from a sense of loss, a feeling that the past was better than the present. A 1990 Gallup poll showed that loneliness is most common among the widowed, separated, and divorced. Over half of this group felt lonely "frequently" or "sometimes" compared with 29% of the married participants. Adults who had never married fell in between. According to the survey, women are more likely to be lonely than men,

possibly, not because they genuinely have less companionship but because they place more importance on friendship and are more willing to confess to being lonely.

Loneliness is often a factor in DEPRESSION, drug ADDICTION, and alcoholism. In recent years, many studies have shown that the more connected to life individuals are, the healthier—mentally and physically—they will be.

According to *The Complete Guide to Your Emotions and to Your Health,* results of a survey conducted by social researchers Rubenstein and Shaver indicate that loneliness has little to do with the number of people in a given living situation, but is more apt to be defined by people's expectations of life and reactions to their environment. Rubenstein and Shaver's questionnaire drew 22,000 respondents over the age of 18. The survey confirms that "feeling lonely"—regardless of living arrangement—is associated with greater health risks, including some psychological symptoms such as ANXIETY, depression, CRYING spells, and feeling worthless. Nearly one-quarter of the people who lived alone fell into the "least lonely" category. They had more FRIENDS on the average than people who lived with other people and were less troubled by symptoms of stress such as HEADACHES, ANGER and irritability.

By comparison, young people who continued to live with parents after college appeared to be the loneliest of all respondents. Rubenstein explains, "A young person in this situation has different expectations. If there's no girlfriend or boyfriend in the picture, they face a social-psychological conflict. For young adults, in particular being alone—especially on Saturday night—can be a stigma. This makes them feel rejected and lonely."

Key to combating loneliness is maintaining a feeling of self-worth and the ability to care not only for yourself but also for other people and other things. Altruistic people lose themselves in others. The process can block out depression, make us less aware of our own inadequacies, and help us surmount our personal problems. When you maintain a pattern of caring, whether for a house, a garden, pets, or other people, you are protecting yourself against despair. And in the process, you'll live a more happy and healthy existence—whether alone or in the company of others.

See also ALCOHOLISM AND ALCOHOL DEPENDENCE; COPING; GENERAL ADAPTATION SYNDROME; VOLUNTEERISM.

SOURCES:

Beck, Alan, and Aaron Katcher. *Between Pets and People. The Importance of Animal Companionship.* New York: Putnam, 1983.

Padus, Emrika. *The Complete Guide to Your Emotions and Your Health: Hundreds of Proven Techniques to Harmonize Mind and Body for Happy, Healthy Living.* Emmaus, Pa.: Rodale Press, 1992.

Wilson, Marlene. *You Can Make a Difference!* Boulder: Volunteer Management Associates, 1990.

loss   See GRIEF.

low back pain   See BACK PAIN.

lump in the throat   Many individuals experience a "lump in the throat," which is the feeling of a need to swallow but, upon swallowing, the sensation does not go away. The medical term for this unpleasant situation is *globus hystericus.* Some individuals have this feeling before a stressful event, such as a court appearance, a public speaking engagement, a role in a play, or a singing solo, and they are concerned that they will not be able to speak or sing. Dryness and muscular contraction play a causative role.

RELAXATION and BREATHING techniques can help overcome this feeling. For some, MEDITATION and GUIDED IMAGERY is also helpful.

See also ANXIETY; STRESS.

manic-depressive disorder Disorder characterized by mood disturbances and changes. It is a mental health disorder that puts stress on the individual as well as those around him or her because there may be moods of mania as well as DEPRESSION or a swing between the two states (bipolar disorder). In the manic state, the individual is excessively elated, agitated, hyperactive, and has accelerated thinking and speaking patterns; in the depressed state, the individual feels extremely sad, helpless, and hopeless.

An individual in a manic state will show an abnormal increase in activity and believe that he or she is capable of achieving any goal. There may be a grandiose sense of knowing more than others, extravagant spending of money, little need for sleep, increased appetite for food, alcohol, and sex, or inappropriate bursts of LAUGHTER or ANGER. Severe mania may result in violence and hospital admission is often required.

Relatively mild symptoms of the manic state are known as *hypomania.* First appearance of manic attacks is usually before age 30, and they may last for a few days or several months. When attacks begin after age 40, they may be more prolonged. Mania often runs in families and may be genetically transmitted.

Depression is more common than mania. Depression affects about one in 10 men and one in five women at some time in their lives. Mania (unipolar or bipolar) affects only about eight per 1,000 people, men and women equally. The recovery rate from manic-depressive disorder is about 80%.

Severe manic-depressive illness often requires hospitalization. Antidepressant medications and, in some cases, electroconvulsive therapy are used in treating depression. Antipsychotic drugs are prescribed to control the symptoms of mania. To prevent relapse, lithium is often used. Many people who have manic-depressive illness lead healthy, well-balanced lives when taking lithium under the guidance of their physician.

See also AFFECTIVE DISORDERS; PHARMACOLOGICAL APPROACH.

manic episode See MANIC-DEPRESSIVE DISORDER.

marijuana A drug derived from the plant *Cannabis sativa*, is used as a stress reliever by some people because it is said to intensify sensory experiences, including seeing, hearing, tasting, and touching. It may make the user feel relaxed, but in some cases it creates feelings of ANXIETY and distrustfulness.

There is no accepted medical use for smoking marijuana, although THC (delta-9 tetrahydrocannabinol) in capsule form is prescribed in certain carefully selected medical cases. The only marijuana currently approved for medical use is the synthetic form of its most active component, tetrahydrocannabinol, available as Marinol. It was developed as an antiemetic for chemotherapy patients.

Advocates of medicinal marijuana continue their efforts for easier access to the illicit drug. Proponents cite anecdotal evidence that smoked marijuana restores appetite in patients with AIDS wasting syndrome, controls chemotherapy-induced nausea and vomiting, reduces interocular pressure in glaucoma patients, and alleviates painful spasticity in multiple sclerosis. Most of mainstream medicine disagrees, however, and insists that the health risks far outweigh the potential benefits.

Marijuana, in the later 1990s, is federally designated as a Schedule I drug, like LSD and heroin, with high potential for abuse and no medical application. Advocates want marijuana downgraded to Schedule II, where it would be classified like cocaine and morphine as having a proven therapeutic value.

See also ADDICTIONS.

marital therapy   Many individuals who are stressed by a difficult or troubled MARRIAGE choose to engage in marital therapy. This may involve couples in therapy, or therapy for each individual alone. The therapy may be directed toward overcoming specific problems, such as COPING with the other's DEPRESSION, helping one partner manage MONEY better, helping one partner overcome an unwanted compulsion, such as GAMBLING, or toward saving a marriage that might end in DIVORCE. Psychological counseling or sexual therapy, or a combination of both, may be involved in marital therapy.

In some cases, just the suggestion of marital therapy is a source of stress to one or the other partners. For the therapy to have a chance at succeeding, it is essential that both partners participate.

See also BEHAVIOR THERAPY; INTIMACY; PSYCHOTHERAPIES; RELATIONSHIPS; REMARRIAGE; SEX THERAPY.

marriage   The marriage of one man with one woman, or monogamy, is the most common form of marriage in the Western world. As a personal arrangement, marriage means a lifelong emotional and legal commitment to another individual. For people unwilling to make a commitment, the thought of marriage is extremely stressful. In the 1990s, many young people developed a fear of commitment and avoided marriage until their late thirties. Marriage later in life brings with it the stress of the BIOLOGICAL CLOCK for women and increased anxieties about becoming parents before both the woman and the man are too old.

From a romantic commitment that was entered into for life and was almost a social requirement as recently as the 1950s, tradiational marriage became a subject that aroused feelings of rebellion and disdain in the late 1960s and 1970s. DIVORCE became more common and socially acceptable and premarital sex became more common. Many young people experimented with communal arrangements or simply lived together without benefit of the legalities of marriage.

Stresses involved in the marriage ceremony

Planning for the marriage ceremony may be stressful for one or both partners or for parents of the couple. Some weddings in the United States involve hundreds of guests, while other ceremonies take place in a judge's chambers or the study of a clergy person. Plans for large weddings may result in a yearlong period of stress for members of the wedding party. Ceremonies for marriage may be lengthy and complex or very simple, and ceremonies frequently contain elements of religious observance. In interfaith marriages, particularly, decisions must be made about who will perform the ceremony and in which tradition the wedding will be conducted. Good COMMUNICATION and mutual agreement between bride and groom are essential to avoid ongoing stress. Most marriage ceremonies are followed by the consumption of food, and planning this event can also be stressful for those involved who seek PERFECTION in the special day.

Marriage as a social construct

Most cultures and societies have included some form of marriage in their social structure. Romance and mutual selection and compatibility is generally considered less important in other cultures than in the modern Western world. In some societies, couples are promised to each other as children or even before birth. Family or tribal relationships and economic considerations quite often take precedence over individual wishes.

Some arranged marriages result in lifelong loving RELATIONSHIPS, while others lapse into marriages of convenience and for procreation, with one or more of the partners becoming involved with others. Polygyny, the union of one man and several wives, is practiced in some African tribes and in Islamic cultures. In Tibet, one woman may have several husbands who are brothers. The Catholic Church and other religious groups consider members of religious orders as being married to their divine being. Many religious groups have prohibitions against marrying outside the group. Most cultures prohibit INCEST to some degree.

Changing marriage patterns
Gloria Steinem, in *Outrageous Acts and Everyday Rebellions* (1980), issued a veiled warning that the reason that women are not attracted to GAMBLING is that the uncertainties and precariousness of marriage satisfy most women's gambling instincts. However, despite recent reports of the statistical difficulty of acquiring a husband and of career possibilities opened up by the WOMEN'S MOVEMENT, women still seem to favor marriage as a way of life. A Gallup poll in 1987 showed that only 8% of the women surveyed thought that being a single career woman was an ideal way of life, approximately the same percentage as when the question was asked in 1975.

Another Gallup poll indicated what may be a return to a more conservative approach to marriage and sexual relationships. Whether the conservatism is a product of a heightened interest in religion, an overall conservative trend, or fears about SEXUALLY TRANSMITTED DISEASES, the segment of the population who believe that premarital sex is wrong rose from 39% in 1985 to 46% in 1987.

Researchers say that while opposites may attract, they probably will not marry or stay married because of their differences and it is from the differences that stresses arise. People usually tend to marry within their own social and educational groups, although tendencies to marry within religious groups are declining. This tendency may be due in part to the fact that modern American life brings people of differing cultures and religions together, but still segregates somewhat by social and educational status.

Commuter marriages
A study by Barbara Bunker, State University of New York, noted that nearly one million American couples who work in different cities and see each other only on weekends feel no more stressed than dual-career couples who live in the same place. From previous research, Bunker knew that long-distance "commuter couples" experience specific strains different from those felt by dual-career couples living together full-time. Not surprisingly, the commuters were less pleased with their relationships, but more satisfied with their work lives and the time they had for themselves.

The researchers were surprised that the stay-at-home couples reported feeling just as much stress in their lives as did the commuters, and, in fact, felt more overloaded. Bunker and her colleagues speculated that people who see their spouses only on weekends are better able to focus fully on their work during the week and on their domestic lives when they are at home. This separation of work and family might make it easier to handle multiple roles, while stay-at-home couples must learn to manage all aspects of their lives simultaneously.

Alternative forms of marriage
Because so many traditional monogamous marriages have resulted in stress and divorce, many individuals have experimented with alternative marital-sexual relationships. While some of the stresses in traditional marriages are overcome by these alternative unions, many stressful situations also arise in them. At the latter part of the 20th century, the pos-

sibility of marriages between homosexual couples has become an issue for many individuals.

Open marriage. The concept of open marriage was espoused by Nena and George O'Neil in their book, *Open Marriage* (1972). Disadvantages of this system include possibilities for JEALOUSY and fear of losing one's spouse. Open marriage emphasizes equality and flexibility for both the male and female roles in the marriage and includes an agreement not to be emotionally, socially, or sexually exclusive. While this system attracted attention, it was largely discarded as generally unworkable for most couples.

Swinging. Sharing sexual activities between couples has been termed *swinging.* A couple may switch partners with another married couple, or a married couple may engage in sexual activities with a single female, single male, or an unmarried couple. Recreational swingers are primarily interested in sexual activities without close friendships or involvement with their sexual partners. Swinging first gained public attention during the 1950s (then known as "wife swapping"). Clubs and magazines devoted to swinging have existed. Major reasons for dropping out of the swinging scene include the stress of jealousy, the threat to marriage, and the threat of sexually transmitted diseases and the HIV virus.

See also COHABITATION; FATHERING, OLDER; LIVE-IN; MARITAL THERAPY; MOTHERS; REMARRIAGE; STEPFAMILIES.

FOR FURTHER INFORMATION:
American Association of Marriage and Family
 Therapy
1717 K Street NW (Suite 407)
Washington, DC 20006
Phone: (202) 429-1825

SOURCES:
Bunker, Barbara, et al. "Quality of Life in Dual-Career Families: Commuting Versus Single-Residence Couples." *Journal of Marriage and the Family,* May 1992.

Gottman, John Mordechai. *Why Marriages Succeed or Fail: What You Can Learn From the Breakthrough Research to Make Your Marriage Last.* New York: Simon & Schuster, 1994.

Roloff, Tamara L., and Mary E. Williams, eds. *Marriage and Divorce.* San Diego: Greenhaven Press, 1997.

Simpson, Eileen B. *Late Love. A Celebration of Marriage After Fifty.* Boston: Houghton Mifflin, 1994.

Steinem, Gloria. *Outrageous Acts and Everyday Rebellions.* New York: New American Library, 1983.

Stuart, R.B. "Spouse Selection," in Corsini, Raymond J. *Encyclopedia of Psychology,* vol. 3. New York: Wiley, 1984.

masked depression   Some people appear to be well but work hard at hiding DEPRESSION. For them, the hiding is a heavy source of stress. They outwardly do what they think is expected of them while inwardly they feel hopeless and even suicidal. They may have little facial animation, appear to have a fixed expression, and show little emotion. The terms "depressive equivalents," "affective equivalents," "hidden depression," and "missed depression" are other terms used for this situation. Some mental health professionals use the term "borderline depression" for such individuals.

See also AFFECTIVE DISORDERS; MANIC-DEPRESSIVE DISORDER; PHARMACOLOGICAL APPROACH.

massage therapy   A form of body therapy in which the practitioner applies manual techniques such as kneading, stroking, and manipulation of the soft tissues of the body, the skin, muscles, tendons, and ligaments with the intention of positively affecting the health and well-being of the client. Massage therapy helps many people relieve STRESS and body aches caused by tension and anxieties.

A professional massage increases blood flow and relaxes muscles. Massage therapy can provide anything from soothing RELAX-

ATION to deeper therapy for specific physical problems. It can aid in recovery from pulled muscles or sprained ligaments. Massage therapy can also ease many of the uncomfortable stresses of child bearing, the discomforts of BACK PAIN and exhaustion, as well as the pains of certain REPETITIVE STRESS INJURIES related to on-the-job activities.

According to the American Massage Therapy Association, once the massage is under way, many beneficial reactions are set in motion. Massage therapy can hasten the elimination of waste and toxic debris that are stored in muscles, increase the interchange of substances between the blood and tissue cells, and stimulate the relaxation response within the nervous system. Responses to massage therapy can help to strengthen the immune system, improve posture, increase joint flexibility and range of motion, and reduce blood pressure.

Types of massage
The most universally understood Western form of massage is Swedish, also called Esalen. It consists of many types of strokes: gliding the hand across the skin, kneading, lifting, squeezing and grasping the muscles, gentle pushing, friction, vibration, jostling and rocking, and percussion (hacking, chopping, and rapid pounding).

Oriental massage, sometimes referred to as SHIATSU or ACUPRESSURE, involves pressing at certain points along invisible energy meridians that run through the body; the practitioner looks for tight spots, knots, or anything that interferes with the flow of energy.

Deep tissue massage uses slow strokes and deep finger pressure to combat aching muscles, such as a stiff neck or bad back. Sports massage is a combination of stretching and Swedish or deep-tissue massage performed before or after strenuous exercise.

REFLEXOLOGY, the massage of the hands, feet, and ears, is based on the belief that spe-cific areas govern all parts of the body. For example, the tips of the toes correspond to the head, while the inside arch of the foot reflects the spine. The theory is that by stimulating the nerve endings of the different organs in the body, changes can be affected.

Choosing a massage therapist
According to the American Massage Therapy Association (AMTA), a qualified massage therapist should have a solid foundation in physiology and be knowledgeable about the inner workings of the body. Therapists from an accredited school have usually completed 500 hours of training, including classes in anatomy, first aid, and cardiopulmonary resuscitation.

The American Massage Therapy Association, founded in 1943, is the largest and oldest national organization representing the profession. Membership in the AMTA is limited to those who have demonstrated a level of skill and expertise through testing and/or education. All AMTA therapists must agree to abide by the AMTA Code of Ethics.

According to the AMTA, their number of members increased from under 5,000 in 1986 to over 20,000 in 1994.

Experiencing a massage
Most massage therapists work in small, semi-darkened rooms, where soft music of the client's choice will be playing. Some therapists offer a choice of scented candles. The massage therapist leaves the client alone to undress and lie down on a padded massage table. During the massage, the entire body is draped in a sheet; only the portion that is currently being worked on is exposed. Quiet is an essential feature of the massage experience. While conversation with the therapist may be limited, a person should speak up if experiencing discomfort, feeling hot or cold, or desiring more or less pressure, or wanting more attention paid to a certain area of the body, such as an aching back.

Massage is "productive down time." During the massage, the body becomes very heavy and sinks into the table. As the therapist's hands locate areas of tension, the individual consciously tries to let go and relax these areas. He or she lets go of a desire to control movement and allows the therapist to move limbs into whatever position is required.

Patricia Deer, a certified massage therapist and owner of Energy Breaks, Chicago, says that a good neck and shoulder massage may contribute toward better mental performance as well as relief of stress. One study reported that people who received 15-minute seated massages during their workday showed brain-wave patterns consistent with greater alertness. Those people were also able to complete arithmetic problems twice as fast and with half the errors, as they did before the massage. "Employers are increasingly recognizing the benefits of "mini-tune-ups" for people who sit at desks or computers much of the day," says Deer.

See also ALTERNATIVE THERAPIES; BODY THERAPIES; MIND-BODY CONNECTIONS; ROLFING.

FOR FURTHER INFORMATION:
American Massage Therapy Association
800 Davis Street (Suite 100)
Evanston, IL 60201
Phone: (847) 864-0123

masturbation   Usually refers to sexual self-stimulation for gratification and pleasure and usually to an experience of orgasm. The method is to massage the penis or clitoris with the hand. The subject of masturbation is stressful for many people because in previous generations, parents warned young people against masturbation, suggesting that doing so would lead to dire consequences such as acne, impotence, insanity, or worse. Thus many people who believed that they were going against cultural mores developed anxieties and GUILT about the practice. Now masturbation is considered normal behavior,

particularly among teenagers and adults without sexual partners.

The topic of masturbation has been the subject of several large-scale surveys. In one study, Alfred Kinsey (1884–1956), a sex researcher, found that more than 90% of men reported masturbatory experiences in their adolescence. In the 1980s, Shere Hite, a researcher on female sexuality, reported that 82% of American women masturbated.

Sex therapists during the latter part of the 20th century use masturbation as a technique to instruct clients in learning to know what pleases them so that they can later instruct a partner.

Compulsive masturbation is an obsessive urge to masturbate without sexual feeling or satisfaction. Such an individual may substitute masturbation for a lack of social satisfaction that arises from shyness, or an inability to establish relationships with the opposite sex, or to relieve anxieties.

See also SAFE SEX; SEX THERAPY.

SOURCE:
Kahn, Ada P., and Linda Hughey Holt. *The A–Z of Women's Sexuality.* Alameda, Calif.: Hunter House, 1992.

mathematics anxiety   Experiencing stress related to practical applications of mathematics in everyday life, such as counting small change or reading timetables. Additionally, math ANXIETY results because mathematics is an abstract science and many people have difficulties understanding abstractions.

As simple a chore as balancing a checkbook causes many individuals to perspire and experience a more rapid heartbeat. Many students who are good in all subjects experience feelings of discomfort in math classes. Why this happens isn't a clearcut issue. There are many factors involved in why this happens; the individual may be unsure of his or her abilities regarding adding and subtracting or there may be a fear of making a mistake. In a school setting, making a mistake when called upon would be embarrassing.

meditation   A learned technique to relieve STRESS and involves deep RELAXATION brought on by focusing attention on a particular sound or image and breathing deeply. One directs thoughts away from work, family, relationships, and the environment. During meditation, the heart rate, blood pressure, and oxygen-consumption rate decrease, temperature of the extremities rises and muscles relax.

Meditation also has been shown to reduce a number of medical symptoms and improve health-related attitudes and behaviors. For example, people with chronic obstructive pulmonary disease (COPD) who practiced meditation reduced the frequency and severity of episodes of shortness of breath and the number of visits to emergency rooms. People with heart disease, hypertension, CANCER, DIABETES, and chronic PAIN have reported feeling more self-confident, more in CONTROL of their lives and better able to manage stress after mastering the meditation technique. Meditation has been used successfully by individuals who have PANIC ATTACKS AND PANIC DISORDER.

Meditation may bring out increased efficiency by eliminating unnecessary expenditures of energy. Individuals who practice meditation sometimes report a beneficial surge of energy marked by increased physical stamina, increased productivity on the job, the end of writer or artist's "block," or the release of previously unsuspected creative potential.

Learning to meditate

Meditation is a very self-disciplined routine and a way to learn more about one's own thoughts and feelings. Simple procedures can be learned easily. The basics include sitting in a quiet room with eyes closed, breathing deeply and rhythmically with attention focused on the breath. Also, there may be a focus on either a special word or "mantra," such as "peace," which one repeats over and over again, or on steadily watching an object, such as a candle flame for a 20-minute period once or more daily.

Meditation relies on the close links between mind and body. When one meditates, the alpha brainwaves indicate that the body is relaxed and free from physical tension and mental strain. BIOFEEDBACK monitoring has indicated that meditation encourages the brain to produce an evenly balanced pattern of alpha and theta brain wave rhythms. This means that the body is relaxed and the mind calm, yet alert. The "relaxation response" sets in, which is the opposite of the physical tension that results from stress.

Individuals who meditate frequently report that they are more aware of their own opinions after beginning meditation. They are not as easily influenced by others as they were previously and can arrive at decisions more quickly and easily. They may be more self-assertive and more able to stand up for their own rights effectively. Additionally, researchers have shown that the meditating person may become less irritable in his or her interpersonal relationships within a relatively short period of time after beginning meditation.

Types of meditation vary

Modern meditation techniques are derived from spiritual practices in Eastern cultures dating back more than 2,000 years. Traditionally, the benefits of the techniques have been defined as spiritual in nature, and meditation has constituted a part of many religious practices. In the latter part of the 20th century, however, simple forms of meditation have been used for stress management with excellent results. Contributing to the rising interest is the fact that these meditation techniques are related to biofeedback (which

---

SITUATIONS IN WHICH MEDITATION MAY REDUCE STRESS

- Tension or anxiety
- Chronic fatigue
- Insomnia and hypersomnia
- Abuse of alcohol or tobacco
- Excessive self-blame
- Chronic sub-acute depression
- Irritability, low tolerance for frustration
- Strong tendencies to submissiveness
- Difficulties with self-assertion
- Prolonged bereavement reactions

---

also emphasizes a delicately attuned awareness of inner processes) and to muscle relaxation and visualization techniques used in BEHAVIOR THERAPY.

There are two basic types of meditation. One is *concentration* and the other, *insight*. Concentration types, such as TRANSCENDENTAL MEDITATION, often use a special sound or silently repeated phrase to focus attention and screen out extraneous thoughts or stimuli. *Insight-oriented meditations,* such as *mindfulness meditation,* accept thoughts and feelings that arise from moment to moment as objects of attention and acceptance. The goal of mindfulness is an increased awareness of what is happening in one's mind and body right now. Recognition and acceptance of present reality provide the basis for changes of attitudes and conditions.

See also ALTERNATIVE THERAPIES; BENSON, HERBERT; GUIDED IMAGERY; KABAT-ZINN, JON.

SOURCES:

Benson, Herbert. *The Relaxation Response.* New York: Morrow, 1975.

Chopra, Deepak. *Creating Affluence: Wealth Consciousness in the Field of All Possibilities.* San Rafael, Calif.: New World Library, 1993.

———. *Creating Health: How to Wake Up the Body's Intelligence.* Boston: Houghton Mifflin, 1991.

Kabat-Zinn, Jon. *Full Catastrophe Living: Using the Wisdom of Your Body and Mind to Face Stress, Pain and Illness.* New York: Delacorte, 1991.

———. *Wherever You Go, There You Are: Mindfulness Meditation in Everyday Life.* New York: Hyperion, 1993.

Kerman, D. Ariel. *The H.A.R.T. Program: Lower Your Blood Pressure Without Drugs.* New York: HarperCollins, 1992.

Mahesh Yogi, Maharishi. *Science of Being and Art of Living: Transcendental Meditation.* New York: Meridian, 1995.

memory   An ability to learn by observation and to retain, remember, and call up information presented through the senses. Many people feel stressed and anxious because of their poor memories and inability to recall things at will. Some people fear they are developing ALZHEIMER'S DISEASE when their memory fails them. During periods of extreme stress, many people experience memory difficulties.

The exact amount of retention depends on factors such as the thoroughness of the learning, on repetition, and on the nature of the content. The more thoroughly the person learns, the greater the duration and amount of retention. Many people retain visual images of what they have learned, such as people, objects, pictures, or the printed page. Children have superior visual imagery, but this ability usually declines after about the age of 15.

Individuals have recall in various steps. Immediate recall involves remembering from a few seconds to a few minutes; an example is remembering a phone number long enough to write it down. Short-term recall involves memory from a few minutes to a few days. Long-term memory refers to memory from a few days to a few years.

Verbalizing the memory involves finding the right words, which then calls into play the entire left side of the brain where words are stored. All parts of the brain are required for comprehension and storage of memory.

A poor memory may be due to poor learning, but sometimes there are psychological reasons for FORGETTING a fact, an event, or a person. This may be called motivated forgetting, as the person subconsciously tries to forget. Many people have a tendency to forget unpleasant things, but when forgetting becomes extreme it is called repression. When thoughts associated with GUILT, shame, or FEAR are pushed into the unconscious mind, tension and ANXIETY may result.

How memory works

There is ongoing research to determine just how the memory works. However, researchers agree that certain events occur in the central nervous system. It has been suggested that there are chemical and/or physical changes in brain cells and nerve pathways. Another theory is that memory is established in the cerebral cortex through a scanning process comparable to that of a computer. Memory is a cell-to-cell transmission of information across a synapse that has both electrical and chemical properties. This interaction and transmitting across cell walls takes place in a split second. Memories of smell, touch and taste are placed in several places in the brain, awaiting a similar stimulus, such as the smell of a familiar food, to reactive the memory.

Age-related memory impairment

Many individuals are less able to remember certain types of information as they get older. The term "age-associated memory impairment" (AAMI) is used to describe minor memory difficulties that come with age. AAMI is often most noticeable when the individual is under severe stress. When the person is relaxed, he or she will be able to remember the forgotten material with no difficulty. There is no treatment for AAMI, but written reminders, lists, the use of association to remember names, and allowing more time to remember may be helpful.

Amnesia and other forms of memory loss

Amnesia may be produced by physical or chemical changes in the brain. If the cause is psychological, the loss of memory is a defense against experiences that have been extremely painful and intolerable. Amnesia may be total or only for certain events or periods of time. Paramnesia is a false or distorted memory and serves as a protection against unbearable anxiety. The individual fills in the gaps in his memory by statements that are not true, although he believes they are. This condition occasionally occurs in senility and in alcoholic psychoses. Hyperamnesia is an extreme degree of retentiveness and recall. There is unusual clarity of memory images. It occasionally occurs in individuals faced with death and also in mental prodigies, but is more common in individuals during hypnosis and in a drug intoxication induced by amphetamines and hallucinogens. Impressions arising from emotionally colored events are registered with more than usual intensity and the result is that one has a vivid recollection of details.

Getting help

Individuals should seek professional help for memory difficulties if they feel extremely stressed, anxious, or fearful because of the loss; if they feel out of touch with reality because they cannot remember what day of the week it is or where they are; or if they feel that forgetting things is upsetting their work or home life. Local hospitals that have geriatric centers may be a helpful resource; additionally, local departments of health may be able to make referrals to centers that have facilities for memory evaluation.

SOURCES:
Kra, Siegfried J. *Aging Myths: Reversible Causes of Mind and Memory Loss.* New York: McGraw Hill, 1985.
Mark, Vernon H. *Reversing Memory Loss: Proven Methods for Regaining, Strengthening, and Preserving Your Memory.* Boston: Houghton-Mifflin, 1992.

menopause   Cessation of menses (menstrual periods). Menopause occurs at midlife (average age 50–51), when a woman's ovaries stop producing eggs (ovulating) and monthly bleeding from the uterus ceases. During the climacteric (a period of time when gradual hormonal changes occur before and after menopause itself), the ovaries gradually produce less estrogen and progesterone.

Menopause occurs at a time in women's lives when they have many psychosocial concerns as well as concerns about their changing bodies. Many women experience particular stresses, conflicts, and challenges at this time. In generations past, the "change of life" was considered to be a time when women would be naturally irritable and even irrational. Many of women's complaints around the time of menopause were written off by doctors as being "all in your head." Now, however, it is recognized that other issues in a woman's life at midlife contribute to her stress level in addition to changes in hormonal levels.

Women face many health care controversies around the time of menopause. A major one is the issue of hormone replacement therapy, which, in the latter 1990s, is still somewhat controversial. While some authorities say that hormone replacement therapy can help prevent osteoporosis, heart disease, and ALZHEIMER'S DISEASE, others caution that there may be cancer-related risks. However, advances in hormone replacement therapy have made the medications safer to use and with fewer side effects. Hormone replacement therapy helps many women who have hot flashes and vaginal dryness. However, differences of opinion regarding hormone replacement therapy by experts leave many women feeling stressed, confused, and in search of additional opinions.

Stress during menopause

Many women are affected by a variety of stressors around the time of menopause. One is a feeling that they are no longer attractive to men; another is a feeling of loss because they are no longer able to bear children. They may be divorced or widowed and facing a husband's retirement or their own. They may be dealing with grown children who have returned home, or may be anticipating financial difficulties due to an inflationary economy.

Physiological and sexual concerns

Physiological problems add to many women's stress level, too. They may be plagued by HOT FLASHES and they experience embarrassment when these occur. Hormone replacement therapy can help women who suffer from hot flashes, and so can HERBAL MEDICINE administered under the guidance of an herbal practitioner. Other aids to relieve some discomforts are layering clothing, avoiding wool fabrics close to the skin, and using a portable fan. When vaginal dryness occurs along with diminishing estrogen levels, these factors may contribute to DYSPAREUNIA and sexual difficulties. What a husband or lover may interpret as lack of interest may actually be fear of painful intercourse or serious discomfort during intercourse. A thorough physical examination by a gynecologist should be sought, with sex therapy useful in some cases.

Population trends

The number and popularity of educational programs featuring speakers on the topic of menopause and hormone replacement therapy is a testimony to the concern about menopause and ongoing confusion. At the end of the 1990s, there is also considerable interest in the subject of menopause by the popular media because of the population trend. By the year 2000, the number of women around age 50 will increase dramatically because the BABY BOOMER generation will enter midlife. Research on menopause will increase and women at midlife will continue to seek solutions to controversies about therapies. With more definitive information, some of the stress associated with menopause may be relieved.

See also ALTERNATIVE THERAPIES.

SOURCES:

Avis, Nancy E., ed. *Menopause: Myths & Realities.* Watertown, Mass.: New England Research Institutes, 1996.

Holt, Linda Hughey, and Ada P. Kahn. *50 Ways to Cope With Menopause.* Lincolnwood, Ill.: Publications International, 1994.

Kahn, Ada P., and Linda Hughey Holt. *Midlife Health: A Woman's Practical Guide to Feeling Good.* New York: Avon Books, 1989.

Merz, Beverly, ed. "The Evidence for Estrogen." *Harvard Women's Health Watch,* April 1997.

Wright, Karen. "Menopause Naturally." *Health,* January-February 1996.

menstruation   Term for the uterine bleeding that commonly occurs in WOMEN approximately once a month between PUBERTY and MENOPAUSE. Some young women in the United States begin menstruating as early as age nine and as late as age sixteen. Many have an irregular pattern of menstruation varying from one- to three-month intervals. Periodic flow varies from extremely light to moderate or very heavy. Blood loss during each period averages about one ounce but can vary from a third of an ounce to almost two ounces. Although the menstrual period usually lasts about four to five days, it can last fewer or more days and still be considered within the range of normal. The fact that there are so many individual differences between women's menstrual patterns is often a source of stress for women.

Historically, for many women, the onset of menstruation (menarche) has been filled with wonder, awe, and sometimes fear. Menstruation marks the beginning of physical adulthood for women, as bearing children becomes possible after menarche. Young women can become pregnant shortly after the onset of menstruation, and this can lead to unwanted children and the stresses of childraising.

Understanding menstruation

Menstruation is the removal of the lining of the uterus that is prepared each month to provide for a potential PREGNANCY. At the same time, the ovary ripens an egg (ovum) each month and releases it (ovulation) so that it can be fertilized and implanted in the uterus. When fertilization does not occur, the uterus empties and these cyclical preparations begin again. Menstruation usually begins two weeks after ovulation if the egg is not fertilized.

Menstruation is caused by cyclic fluctuation of the hormones estrogen and progesterone. During a "typical" menstrual cycle, ovarian estrogen is produced in response to stimulation from the pituitary hormones known as follicle stimulating hormone (FSH) and luteinizing hormone (LH). At midcycle, ovulation occurs in response to an "LH surge" and the ovary forms a small cyst (a corpus luteum) in the follicle that has surrounded the egg or ovum. Progesterone is produced, which causes structural changes in the uterine lining. If the ovum is fertilized and implants in the uterine lining, menstruation does NOT occur; hence a late menstrual period may be a signal of pregnancy or of some menstrual irregularity.

Stressful aspects surrounding menstruation

Premenstrual syndrome (PMS). Many women experience higher levels of stress, or are more irritable or depressed just before and during their menstrual periods. Some notice annoying bloating, fluid retention, breast tenderness, and HEADACHES. Some women who have migraine headaches find that the onset is associated with their menstrual periods. Most women cope successfully with their symptoms by getting a little extra rest, limiting or decreasing salt intake, and recognizing the temporary nature of the annoyances. Women who have excessive premenstrual symptoms should bring them to the attention of a physician.

Sexual intercourse during menstruation. In some cultures, menstruating women have been excluded from society during their periods. Over centuries, concerns regarding menstruation have included the notion that sexual intercourse during menstruation is harmful to both men and women's health, and that deformed children may result from intercourse during this time. Historically, some men have avoided contact with menstruating women out of fear of castration, or that menstrual blood was meant to form the body of a child and therefore is filled with potent and dangerous energy.

Menstrual cessation. When periods stop for an unexplained reason, great feelings of stress ensue as a woman may fear pregnancy or disease. Absence of menstruation is called *amenorrhea*. Amenorrhea is normal prior to puberty or after menopause; it occurs frequently as a response to extreme stress, weight loss, or to a wide range of hormonal, physical, or emotional causes. Anorexia nervosa, an EATING DISORDER, usually results in amenorrhea. Runner's or athlete's amenorrhea is a commonly observed syndrome in which women undergoing rigorous physical training temporarily cease having periods.

Pain. Painful menstruation is known as dysmenorrhea, and is a source of stress for the sufferer because the discomfort often leads to lost days from work, school, or social activities. Cramplike pain (cramps) may be associated with the passage of uterine clots and may start just before or during menstruation and may last only while the mass is passing out of the uterus, or may continue for hours or days. Many women feel cramps in their lower abdomen, lower back, and thighs. Medications may relieve discomfort.

Personal protection. Protecting clothing and hiding the fact that a woman is having her menstrual period has been a concern for generations. The most common ways of disposing of menstrual fluid are use of externally worn sanitary napkins (in Britain, known as sanitary towels) or internally worn tampons.

Internally worn tampons can be used by young women from the start of menstruation. Physicians say that virginity is intact until one's first act of sexual intercourse. The hymeneal ring, a tissue between the internal and external genital organs, is usually large enough to admit a tampon, which has been slightly lubricated for easier insertion. Many women of all ages find tampons a neater way to deal with menstruation, and a way to avoid external irritation of the genital area with a sanitary napkin.

During the 1980s, concern about a condition called toxic shock syndrome, a serious infectious disease linked to tampon usage, caused many women to stop using tampons. However, with proper attention to hygiene and frequent replacement of tampons, women need not fear toxic shock syndrome. Also, some of the materials used in tampons have been changed by the manufacturers, making them safer to use.

Relief for menstrual stress

The stresses brought about by menstrual irregularities can be somewhat ameliorated with medical help and self-helps. Women who have menstrual irregularities should discuss them with their physicians, as there are many individual variations contributing to irregularities. In some cases, menstrual dysfunction is accompanied or caused by failure of the ovaries to ovulate, and the menstrual dysfunction may be associated with infertility. Treatment may consist of various female sex hormones, such as estrogen, progesterone, or thyroid. In some cases, menstrual difficulties are cleared up by a dilatation and curettage (D and C), a surgical scraping of the lining of the uterus.

Many women learn to prevent normal menstrual discomforts by practicing general good health measures, such as exercise, a nutritious diet, adequate rest, and improving and maintaining good posture.

See also UNWED MOTHERS.

SOURCES:

Allen, Patricia. *Cycles: Every Woman's Guide to Menstruation.* New York: Pinnacle, 1983.

Delaney, Janice, et al. *The Curse, a Cultural History of Menstruation.* New York: E.P. Dutton, 1976.

Holt, Linda Hughey, and Melva Weber. *Guide to WomanCare.* New York: Random House, 1984.

Kahn, Ada P., and Linda Hughey Holt. *The A–Z of Women's Sexuality.* Alameda, Calif.: Hunter House, 1989.

Marzollo, Jean. *Getting Your Period. A Book About Menstruation.* New York: Dial Books for Young Readers, 1989.

mental retardation Impaired intellectual function that results in an inability to cope with the normal responsibilities of life. To be classified as mentally retarded, a person must have an IQ below 70 and impairment must be present before the age of 18. For families, stress results from COPING with the responsibilities of raising a retarded child. Early diagnosis is extremely important so that special education and training programs can be started and the child given every opportunity to learn.

It is crucial that families then seek professional help to define the retardation problem honestly and clearly. Next, they must gather information on community resources in order to make informed decisions about their child's future. While every state and most urban areas now have special governmental departments concerned with retardation where advice and consultation are available, accessing these agencies is not always easy and they are often bureaucratic.

Faced with the sadness and difficult problems of raising a retarded child, one of the first decisions families must make concerns institutionalization. Unless the child has debilitating physical problems as well as severe retardation, most families will opt to keep the child at home.

While the mentally retarded child remains a child all his or her life, they can experience feelings, concerns, emotions, fears, wonder, discovery, love, and laughter, as do all children. A retarded child does learn when given good training and support. If they are well cared for in a responsible and loving home, they will thrive and some may become reasonably independent and self-supporting.

FOR FURTHER INFORMATION:

American Association on Mental Deficiency (AAMD)
1719 Kalorama Road NW
Washington, DC 20009
Phone: (202) 387-1968

Association for Retarded Citizens (ARC)
P.O. Box 6109
Arlington, TX 76005
Phone: (817) 640-0204

National Down's Syndrome Society
141 5th Avenue
New York, NY 10010
Phone: (212) 460-9330

SOURCES:

Dolce, Laura. *Mental Retardation.* New York: Chelsea House, 1994.

Dunbar, Robert E. *Mental Retardation.* New York: Franklin Watts, 1991.

Grossman, Herbert J., et al., ed. *AMA Handbook on Mental Retardation.* Chicago: American Medical Association, 1987.

McNey, Martha. *Leslie's Story: A Book About a Girl with Mental Retardation.* Minneapolis: Lerner Publications, 1996.

mergers The transformation of two or more corporations into one organizational structure for reasons of growth, economy of scale, diversification or vertical integration. They are becoming increasingly common in the late 1990s.

In their book *The Human Side of Mergers and Acquisitions*, Buono and Bowditch state, "mergers and acquisitions can sufficiently transform the organizational structures, systems, processes; in one or both of the firms involved people often feel stressed, disoriented, frustrated, confused, and even frightened."

Emotions felt by employees during mergers may arise in stages and can be conflicting. These emotions range from shock, disbelief, ANGER, and hopelessness to excitement and high expectations for the future. When the merger is completed, employees move slowly toward acceptance, often experiencing a period of mourning and GRIEF. When a proposed merger does not go through, it usually means that one of the companies is seeking change and sometime down the road the change will occur. This outlook compounds the stress for employees, particularly at the management level where there is bound to be job redundancy.

An analysis of LAYOFF announcements in the summer months of 1995 by the outplacement firm of Challenger, Gray & Christmas showed that one out of three jobs cut was a result of mergers. Such job cuts could be attributed to corporate restructuring and plant and office closings.

Staff reductions that occur due to mergers create less dissatisfaction and bitterness when they are handled with sensitivity and concern. Where possible, staff redundancies can be managed through attrition, early RETIREMENT, and attractive severance packages. When involuntary termination is necessary, decisions should be made objectively and supported by outplacement assistance and related job search services.

Most of those who lose their jobs through mergers may have little financial loss, as they are usually white-collar employees who are given generous severance packages. However, they often experience the stress of having to rethink their careers and relocate to obtain new employment.

See also DOWNSIZING; WORKPLACE.

SOURCE:
Buono, Anthony F., and James L. Bowditch. *The Human Side of Mergers and Acquisitions: Managing Collisions Between People Cultures and Organizations.* San Francisco: Jossey-Bass, 1989.

midlife crisis Certain stressful situations that occur at or around middle age are often referred to as "midlife crisis." Men and women both experience these stressors. For some, stresses occur as individuals realize that they have reached the prime of their lives and so begin to question whether or not they have achieved their goals. Others reset goals and, in some cases, turn their lives in new directions.

Specific stressors that occur at midlife include children growing up and leaving home, job loss, forced RETIREMENT, DIVORCE, widowhood, loss of a sex life because of lack of a partner, seeking a new partner, REMARRIAGE, stepchildren, and care of ELDERLY PARENTS.

Men and women at midlife realize that they no longer have the physical strength and stamina that they had when they were younger. For women, MENOPAUSE marks the end of their fear of having unwanted children. Many men and women begin to fear that they are losing their attractiveness and sex appeal and so turn to COSMETIC SURGERY for such procedures as relieving age lines or removing excess body fat. They may embark on strenuous courses of exercise at health clubs and gyms in an effort to retard effects of aging. Some resort to purchasing of sports cars to make themselves feel younger. Divorces occur as one of the spouses becomes involved with another younger partner.

See also EMPTY NEST SYNDROME; MENOPAUSE; SELF-ESTEEM; STRESS.

SOURCE:
Kahn, Ada P., and Linda Hughey Holt. *Midlife Health. A Woman's Practical Guide to Feeling Good.* New York: Avon Books, 1989.

migraine See BIOFEEDBACK; GENERAL ADAPTATION SYNDROME; HEADACHES; MENSTRUATION; PAIN.

migration Leaving one's country to settle in another. Doing so can set in motion a stressful mourning process similar to that which occurs after losing a loved one. The country one is leaving appears as an object, a nonhuman object, with which one develops a relationship.

At first, loss of country might appear more stressful for the involuntary emigrant; however, it is no less difficult for the voluntary one. Some relatives and friends might feel abandoned and resent the person leaving. Although the emigrant adjusts to a new life in the new country, at the same time he or she may long for the old country.

Some may prolong their stress by holding on to a fantasy of transience in the new country for as long as 30 years. For example, by not learning the language of the new country or, more subtly, by not becoming a citizen.

Culture shock

Another stressful aspect of migration is culture shock, which is the result of a sudden change from a known environment to a strange, unknown one. The impact can be violent and, combined with the mourning process set in motion by the loss of that which is familiar, can cause a threat to the newcomer's identity. The sense of the continuity of the self and the sense of self-sameness, is threatened. At the same time, the consistency of one's own interpersonal interactions is disrupted. No longer is there the same confirmation of one's identity in interaction with the environment. As an example, an American living in a hostile country would be acutely aware of his nationality. Whether in a hostile country or not, environmental clues that normally confirm the emigrant's identity are absent and are replaced by unfamiliar phenomena, including language, architecture, housing, manner of dress, food, music, and smells.

One means of COPING with the stress of a new environment is to try to translate the unfamiliar into the familiar. For example, an individual from a forested country may look at tall buildings in a city and say that tall buildings look like the forest. There may have been a similar mechanism at work when the early American settlers chose an area that was physically like the one they left, thus reducing the psychologically "unsettling" effect of beginning a new life in a strange environment.

See also ACCULTURATION; HOMESICKNESS; MOVING.

SOURCE:
De Vryer, Miepje A. "Leaving, Longing, and Loving: A Developmental Perspective of Migration." *Journal of American College Health,* 38 (September 1989).

mind-body connections Health philosophers in the late 20th century emphasize the mind-body connections or links between the mind, brain, and other organ systems. Research studies have demonstrated that psychological as well as physical stress has effects on health. Increasingly, physicians are recognizing that BEHAVIOR THERAPY and ALTERNATIVE THERAPIES such as GUIDED IMAGERY, RELAXATION, BIOFEED-BACK, and HYPNOSIS are useful adjuncts in the comprehensive care of many patients, many of whom have stress-related disorders.

The term "mind-body" medicine relates to many treatments and approaches, ranging from MEDITATION and relaxation training to social SUPPORT GROUPS planned to engage the mind in improving physical as well as emotional well-being.

According to Herbert Benson, M.D., author of *The Relaxation Response,* "Too often in the practice of modern medicine, the mind and body are considered to be separate and distinct, which is not in our best interests. Because of specialization, patients are no longer treated as whole persons. Instead, we are separated into groups of organs and specific symptoms are not considered in context."

ADVANTAGES OF MIND-BODY CONNECTIONS FOR STRESS RELIEF

- Can be used along with standard medical practices.
- Financial cost of procedures is low.
- Physical and emotional risk is minimal; potential benefit is great.
- Many can be taught by paraprofessionals.
- No high-tech interventions.
- May improve quality of life by reducing pain and symptoms for people with chronic diseases.
- May help control or reverse certain underlying disease processes.
- May help prevent disease from developing.

In *The Mind/Body Effect,* Dr. Benson emphasized the need for practicing behavioral medicine, which incorporates the principles of medicine, physiology, psychiatry, and psychology. Patients are viewed in their entirety, with the realization that what happens in their mind has direct bearing on the state of their physical health.

In *The Mind/Body Effect,* Dr. Benson makes it clear that psychological factors often induce physical ailments. He indicates that, in extreme cases, fear and a sense of hopelessness can even induce death.

Many conditions have been found to respond to such techniques when they are used alone or in combination with standard medical and surgical treatments. These include HIGH BLOOD PRESSURE, coronary artery disease, CANCER, chronic PAIN, TMJ syndrome, HEADACHES, eczema, PSORIASIS, IRRITABLE BOWEL SYNDROME, ARTHRITIS, rheumatic diseases, ASTHMA, and DIABETES.

The Mind/Body Group at Boston's Beth Israel Hospital

The Mind/Body Group is part of a program of the Division of Behavioral Medicine at Beth Israel Hospital and is headed by Herbert Benson, M.D., a cardiologist. It is one of many programs across the country to help individuals suffering from a variety of medical disorders, including cancer, arthritis, and diabetes.

The program uses a variation of the relaxation response, the meditation method pioneered by Dr. Benson. Since the early 1980s, the group has taught people to use the power of their minds to help themselves bring about the relaxation response, learn how to change their own physiology, and finally have some sense of CONTROL over themselves and their lives.

An example of mind-body connection: diabetes control

Dr. Joan Borysenko, one of the group and an instructor at Harvard Medical School who is trained in cell biology and psychology and is an innovative researcher in PSYCHONEUROIMMUNOLOGY (PNI), has developed a program for diabetics. These sessions are attended only by diabetics, creating a therapeutic dynamic group identity. Members of the group give each other social support in their relaxation procedures and encourage each other to follow the regimen. Results indicate that in those who practiced the relaxation response and exercised, blood sugar was lowered. Thus, diabetics had a drug-free technique in controlling levels of blood sugar that could help minimize damage from the disease and help them live longer and with better quality of life.

See also KABAT-ZINN, JON; OFFICE OF ALTERNATIVE MEDICINE; PRAYER; RELIGION; SIEGEL, BERNIE; SOCIAL SUPPORT SYSTEM; WEIL, ANDREW.

SOURCES:

Benson, Herbert. *Beyond the Relaxation Response.* New York: Berkeley Press, 1985.

———. *The Mind/Body Effect: How Behavioral Medicine Can Show You the Way to Better Health.* New York: Simon & Schuster, 1979.

———. *The Relaxation Response.* New York: Avon Books, 1975.

Borysenko, Joan. *Minding the Body, Mending the Mind.* New York: Bantam, 1988.

Goleman, Daniel, and Joel Gurin, eds. *Mind Body Medicine: How to Use Your Mind for Better Health.* Yonkers, N.Y.: Consumer Reports Books, 1993.

Kerns, Lawrence L. "A clinician's guide to mind-body treatments." *Chicago Medicine* 97, no. 22 (November 21, 1994).

Locke, Steven, and Douglas Colligan. *The Healer Within.* New York: New American Library, 1984.

mindfulness meditation See ALTERNATIVE THERAPIES; KABAT-ZINN, JON; MEDITATION; MIND-BODY CONNECTIONS.

miscarriage The spontaneous loss of a PREG-NANCY before the fetus is capable of surviving outside the uterus. Many women who experience miscarriage also experience symptoms of extreme STRESS, GRIEF, and DEPRESSION for a period of time after the event. They feel the loss, even though the child was never born and they never saw the child.

Family and friends sometimes may seem less sympathetic toward women who have suffered miscarriages than toward those whose babies are stillborn or die in early infancy. Many are encouraged to try to achieve another pregnancy very soon. Those who do try often overcome their depressed feelings, but for those who have difficulty in achieving another pregnancy, mourning over the lost pregnancy may continue.

Miscarriage: what is it?

Understanding the physiology involved in the process may help women who experience miscarriage to mentally adjust to the situation. Early miscarriages are usually the result of defects in the fetus. Later miscarriages, which occur in the middle trimester, are more likely to be caused by an incompetent cervix, uterine abnormalities, toxemias, or preexisting chronic disease.

Women who miscarry after some strenuous activity may feel GUILTY and some even believe that they induced the miscarriage. Usually this is not the case. Normal exercise does not usually induce miscarriage. Most women who have been tennis players, hikers, or swimmers usually are advised by their obstetricians to continue exercising throughout their pregnancy (or until the last two months).

The first sign of the possibility of miscarriage is vaginal bleeding, with or without cramping; however, not all vaginal bleeding indicates miscarriage. Some bleeding may be associated with implantation, or it may come from the vagina, vulva, or cervix. If bleeding occurs from the uterus without any dilation of the cervix, and usually without pain, the situation is termed *threatened abortion*. With appropriate medical care, cases of threatened abortion can be salvaged, and many women have healthy babies who were in the "threatened" stage during pregnancy. Treatment includes rest.

Late miscarriage may be the most stressful and difficult for a woman (and the infant's father) to accept. If she has had good medical care and followed her obstetrician's advice, she should not feel that anything she did or did not do induced the miscarriage. In a later miscarriage, when the placenta and embryo are totally evacuated, the term used is *complete abortion*. When placental tissue remains in the uterus, the term is *incomplete abortion*, and the tissue must be removed by curettage.

Miscarriage is also known as *spontaneous abortion*; the term "miscarriage" is more commonly used because it is more socially acceptable. Both terms refer to the loss of an embryo or fetus before maturity.

See also POSTPARTUM DEPRESSION.

mitral valve prolapse See PANIC ATTACKS AND PANIC DISORDER.

modeling A BEHAVIOR THERAPY technique in which a person learns by observation without reinforcement from a therapist. The troubled individual watches someone else perform a particular action such as giving a speech in public (in the case of one who is fearful about speaking in front of others) and then gradually become able to perform the action without fear. In a traditional learning sense, modeling is a form of social learning; children learn appropriate culturally-acceptable behaviors in this way from parents and elders.

See also PUBLIC SPEAKING.

money   A cause of stress in one way or another for most people. Lack of money is stressful, and having money to invest or spend, wisely or unwisely, is also a source of stress. Money is involved in every aspect of life, from housing to education to social life.

For some, money arouses stressful feelings of ENVY—possibly one reason that those who have it may be reluctant to discuss it and those who lack it may pretend that they are well off. Parents may be reluctant to reveal their financial matters to their children, which may lead them to fantasize that they are quite well off, in serious financial straits, or simply lead them to think that money is a TABOO subject.

For practical purposes, many households have no disposable assets to respond to emergencies and absorb shocks. There are more stresses on those in this situation. There are effects on one's sense of CONTROL, optimism, happiness, security, and SELF-ESTEEM.

Western tradition offers two conflicting messages regarding money: that of self-denial, generosity, and spirituality, and that of capitalism and materialism. The most practical attitude seems to be that it is good to have money, but not to flaunt it or even discuss it.

Sigmund Freud wrote that "Money questions will be treated by cultured people in the same manner as sexual matters, with the same inconsistency, prudishness, and hypocrisy." Approaching the end of the 20th century, society has lost a good deal of reluctance to discuss sex openly and honestly, but issues involving money are still handled carefully. For example, knowing the price of a friend's dress or furniture might really be of some interest other than idle curiosity, but usually the question is asked indirectly or with elaborate apologies.

As a group, the very rich are a minority and may experience the same stressful feelings of isolation and alienation that other minorities experience. Middle- and upper-middle-class children sense that both rich and poor children are different and may reject them for that reason. Marriage among the wealthy is often riddled with divorce and extramarital affairs, possibly because the marriages are frequently entered into for financial or social rather than emotional reasons. If both spouses are well-to-do, each may go his or her own way and never have to form the cooperative couple of the middle class. When wealthy men or women "marry down" they may acquire a more attractive and personable spouse than they deserve. However, day-to-day living may make some of the stresses of this type of relationship difficult.

Children of the wealthy may experience a stressful type of upbringing in which one or both parents may be traveling or preoccupied with social or business events much of the time. The child may have to live up to the larger-than-life achievements and reputation of his family. At the same time, he may be indulged in ways that reduce the possibilities of his ever developing the characteristics and talents to meet his family's expectations.

See also PERFECTION; SHOPAHOLISM.

SOURCES:
Kahn, Ada P., and Jan Fawcett. *The Encyclopedia of Mental Health.* New York, Facts On File, 1993.
Krueger, David, ed. *The Last Taboo.* New York: Brunner/Mazel, 1986.

monoamine oxidase inhibitors (MAOIs)   See PHARMACOLOGICAL APPROACH.

moods   A mood is an emotion that determines how a person feels and often relates to his or her stress level. Examples of moods include sad or glad and angry or happy.

According to the American Psychiatric Association (in *Diagnostic and Statistical Manual of Mental Disorders,* 4th ed.), for diagnostic purposes, moods are characterized as follows:

Dysphoric: An unhappy or sad mood, such as depressed, anxious, or irritable.

Elevated: A more cheerful than usual mood.

Euphoric: A feeling of extreme well-being; also occurs in MANIC-DEPRESSIVE DISORDER. This type of mood is beyond what most people rate as simply "feeling good."

Euthymic: Feeling good; absence of depressed or elated mood, and feeling able to cope with life.

Irritable: A feeling of internal tension and being easily annoyed and provoked to anger.

See also AFFECTIVE DISORDERS; DEPRESSION.

SOURCES:

American Psychiatric Association. *Diagnostic and Statistical Manual of Mental Disorders,* 4th ed. Washington, D.C.: American Psychiatric Association, 1994.

Justice, Blair. *Who Gets Sick: How Beliefs, Moods and Thoughts Affect Your Health.* Los Angeles: J.P. Tarcher, 1988.

Kals, W.S. *Your Health, Your Moods and the Weather.* Garden City, N.Y.: Doubleday, 1982.

mothers Traditionally, they protect and nurture offspring. They give their infants and children emotional warmth as well as sensory stimulation, both of which are necessary for them to develop a sense of self-worth and an ability to deal effectively with stresses of the environment.

For many women, motherhood may serve purposes other than the simple desire for a child. For example, children may seem to be the solution for a stressful or troubled MARRIAGE. Women may expect their children to succeed where they have failed and may live vicariously through their offspring. Faced with her older children maturing and the threat of no longer being needed, some women will have another child rather than explore the next phase of life.

Changing images of mothers

The media at the end of the 20th century reflect the fact that mothers have changed, or possibly the audience has grown more realistic and tolerant, even admiring, of different types of mothers. For example, in the 1950s and early 1960s television mothers were always homemakers, dispensing wisdom and charm, while dressed appropriately. Title roles in the later 1990s include unmarried mothers and WORKING MOTHERS.

Today, many mothers undertake the double role of having a career and family, sometimes out of economic necessity. However, a Gallup poll measured a growing tendency to perceive this as desirable in spite of the conflicts. Between 1975 and 1987 the percentage of women polled who felt that marriage, children, and a full-time job were not only possible, but also a preferable way of life, rose from 32% to 43%. However, even though women work they still tend to be saddled with home, family, and social responsibilities. While men may be willing to stay home with a sick child or leave work punctually because of a family obligation, they may not be met with the understanding they need from their employers.

Working mothers' responsibilities include getting themselves to work and quite often getting their child to a DAY CARE facility. Some mothers of school-age children may have to deal with the worries of having "latch key" children. Careers may have to be adapted to eliminate travel or situations where the mothers are inaccessible to a telephone. HOBBIES, interests, or just having time for oneself are almost nonexistent on such a mother's schedule. Faced with these pressures, more women are expressing an interest in limiting their family to one child or staying home with their children and/or trying to work from their home. Many women who completed their education in the late 1970s, began careers, married, and had children, tried HAVING IT ALL—meaning marriage, family, and career—and feel constantly stressed by all factors. During the 1990s, women who work outside the house are opting for less aggressive career tracks so that they can spend more time with their families and have less stress in their lives.

See also ADOPTION; MOTHERS-IN-LAW; REMARRIAGE; STEPFAMILIES; UNWED MOTHERS.

SOURCES:
Jetter, Alexis, Annelise Orleck, and Diana Taylor, eds. *The Politics of Motherhood: Activist Voices From Left to Right.* Hanover, N.Y.: University Press of New England, 1997.
"U.S. Women Endorse Jobs, Marriage and Children." *The Gallup Report,* December 1987, 24–25.

mothers-in-law   The butt of many jokes, which comedians find good for a laugh. While jokes may reflect some underlying social truths, in practice, many spouses have excellent RELATIONSHIPS with their in-laws; many don't.

Sometimes stresses and conflicts arise between a daughter-in-law and her husband's MOTHER or the husband and the wife's mother. The source of these conflicts may be the children's repressed resentments of their own parents being projected toward in-laws; ethnic, social, and religious differences; or the mother-in-law's own stress in adjusting to the departure of her children and the aging process. Open lines of COMMUNICATION may improve the situation.

See also LISTENING; PARENTING.

SOURCE:
Kahn, Ada P., and Linda Hughey Holt. *The A–Z of Women's Sexuality.* Alameda, Calif.: Hunter House, 1992.

motion sickness   Uncomfortable feeling of queasiness, NAUSEA, and DIZZINESS. It occurs because of constant motion, along with conflicting signals from the eyes, inner ears, and sensors in muscles and joints. Anticipating motion sickness is a source of stress for many people, and some even avoid certain situations because of their fears.

Motion sickness occurs when in a moving vehicle, such as a car, boat, or airplane. Many people develop motion sickness during a car trip on a bumpy road. Other people require more unstable conditions, such as a ride aboard a pitching boat to become upset. Still others do not experience motion sickness, and their doubts about a sufferer's discomfort lead to further stress for the unfortunate ones.

Understanding motion sickness and using self-help techniques
Understanding how motion sickness occurs may help relieve its attendant stress. On a ship, for example, the eyes record movement, the inner ears detect rolling motion, yet the body is stationary. One technique that helps many people is focusing on the horizon or on a fixed, distant object instead of looking at swirling waves or roadside trees that seem to be moving. Preventive measures and natural remedies also may prevent, or at least relieve, the dizziness, nausea, vomiting, and clamminess symptomatic of motion sickness. Over-the-counter medications work by depressing signals from the inner ear and by quieting the gastrointestinal tract and decreasing nausea. Most of these preparations should be taken an hour or so before departure.

In an airplane, motion is less pronounced in an aisle seat over a wing, preferably on the right side where there is less swaying, because most flight patterns call for left turns. In a car, ride in the front seat and, unless driving, lean back against a stable headrest to minimize inner-ear reaction to movement. Looking down or reading while riding can produce motion sickness because of the apparent movement outside the windows. Being the driver also helps as drivers seldom suffer from motion sickness. At sea, reserve a midship cabin near the waterline where motion is minimal and, as much as possible, stay topside in the middle of the deck.

Eat lightly before a trip and eat small amounts at frequent intervals while traveling. It is easier to become queasy on an empty stomach. Sucking on a lemon or eating olives at the first sign of nausea are folk remedies that work for some people. They may work because motion sickness creates superfluous saliva, which trickles down to the stomach and contributes to nausea. Lemons and olives contain mouth-drying agents that diminish the queasiness.

Fortunately, most sufferers from motion sickness find relief as soon as they get off the airplane, out of the car, or off the ship. Symptoms and their stress usually disappear quickly.

mourning   See GRIEF.

moving   Moving involves relocating to another place of residence, or possibly to another place of work or business. Moving is a source of stress for many people because it removes them and their families from familiar surroundings, families, friends, neighbors, schools, and sports and other activities. Moving may be the third most stressful event, after the death of a loved one and divorce. The length of the distance moved may increase the level of stress, as visiting the old familiar territory becomes more difficult.

However, moving should become less of a national source of stress because fewer Americans are moving. According to the U.S. Census Bureau, one in six Americans moved between March 1993 and March 1994. That was down from one in five who moved over a similar period nearly a decade earlier. More than 26 million of the 1993–94 movers stayed within the same county. Eight million moved between counties in the same state, seven million moved to another state and 1.2 million left the United States.

As people age, they become less likely to move, according to the U.S. Census report. The group least likely to move in 1993–94 were persons 75 to 84 years old, of whom only 4.9% moved. That rate is not significantly different, however, from the 5.8% of persons 85 and over who moved.

Work-related moving
Despite these statistics, many people move because of their jobs. According to a survey of 503 companies by Runzheimer International, a relocation data collection company in Rochester, Wisconsin, the companies surveyed reported an average of 155 relocations during 1994. The average cost to relocate a homeowning employee domestically was $34,700. Relocation to a high-cost-of-living city such as New York or Los Angeles can add as much as 15% to the expense of a move.

One of the stressors people find in moving is "sticker shock." Home prices in the new location could be a pleasant surprise, and they find they can buy more house than they had before for less money. Unfortunately, that is not always the case, and some couples are faced with "downsizing" their living accommodations in the new more costly setting.

Many companies turn to specialized providers of relocation services who range from small, often geographically specialized concerns, to real estate conglomerates that handle thousands of relocations each year and are responsible for orchestrating all details of a move. When a company decides to transfer an employee to another city, sometimes on short notice, it should do so with as little stress as possible for the employee and the employee's family. From the employee's viewpoint, the key question concerns what level of support the employer will provide in the move. According to Stephen C. Roney, president of Coldwell Banker Relocation Services in Mission Viejo, California, "from the employer's viewpoint, the key issue is ultimately one of productivity."

Migration from one country to another carries with it all the stresses of moving as well as adapting to new culture.

See also ACCULTURATION; MIGRATION.

muscle relaxants Pharmacological agents that act on the central nervous system or its associated structures to reduce muscle tone and spontaneous activity. Many people experience tense, tight, or strained muscles as a result of stress or injury and some resort to these prescription medications instead of or in addition to using mind-body techniques for RELAXATION. Many skeletal muscle relaxants also function as minor tranquilizers.

See also MIND-BODY CONNECTIONS; PHARMACOLOGICAL APPROACH.

music A basic social and cultural activity of mankind, involving sounds produced by the voice or by instruments. Music is often used a therapy to reduce stress and help people relax. It is a way to connect with people and a way of getting through to people who are otherwise unreachable. Some songs embody life experiences and may bring back memories of courtship, a wedding or even wartime. For example, in many nursing homes, individuals who have been very untalkative and unresponsive may start to tap their feet to music, particularly live music that they watch as it is performed, or will begin to hum or even sing.

According to Oliver Sacks, American neurologist, author of *The Man Who Mistook His Wife for a Hat* and a pioneer in developing therapies, music organizes motor functions, thus smoothing out, for example, the uncontrolled movements that afflict patients with Parkinson's disease and enabling people with speech losses to sing the words to familiar melodies.

Historical background: music and healing
Using music as a relief of stress and as a healer is not a new concept. In Greek mythology, Apollo was god of both music and medi-

---

STRESS-RELIEVING RESPONSES TO MUSIC

- Heart rate acceleration is correlated with loudness, tempo, and musical complexity; heart rate deceleration is correlated with resolution of musical conflict, decreasing loudness, and slowing tempo.
- Stimulative music increases heart rate; sedative music decreases heart rate.
- Rock music leads to heart deceleration.
- Tachycardia (fast heartbeat) is associated with driving rhythms and increasing dynamics; bradycardia (slow heartbeat) is associated with changes in rhythm, texture, and dynamics.
- Sedative music significantly increases finger temperature.
- Blood pressure is affected by music listening, but the type of music that effects these changes is unknown; music is effective in reducing blood pressure in essential hypertensives.
- Music that is enjoyed increases respiration.
- Music decreases stomach acid production.
- Popular music produces more electroencephalograph (EEG) changes than classical music, particularly in middle-aged subjects. Popular music causes a decrease in blood flow to the brain in young adults; classical music promotes brain blood flow enhancement in middle-aged subjects.

---

cine. His son Aesculapius became god of medicine and cured mental diseases with song and music. Plato, a Greek philosopher, believed that music influenced a person's EMOTIONS and character. According to the Bible, David's harp-playing relieved King Saul's melancholy (DEPRESSION).

In his plays, Shakespeare referred to the healing powers of music. The first English-language book on music as therapy, *Medicina Musica*, was written in the early 1700s by Richard Browne, an apothecary. Browne said music could "soothe turbulent affections" and calm "maniacal patients who did not respond to other remedies."

Music therapy was used in the early part of the 19th century in the form of brass bands for patients with the then-identified mental disorders, including ANXIETY. In the 20th century, particularly during World War II, many American psychiatric hospitals began active music therapy programs. In 1950, the National Association for Music Therapy (NAMT) was organized; in 1954, NAMT recommended a curriculum for preparation of music therapists. Subsequent organizations of music therapists were formed in England, Europe, South America, and Australia. Since the 1980s there has been a growing focus on medical/physiological applications of music therapy.

Music and stress management

Music therapy may be effective in reducing stress because it addresses the whole person concurrently and simultaneously on physical, affective, cognitive, and social levels. Music is a noninvasive technique with few if any side effects, with relative ease of administration and with increasing therapeutic promise as indicated by studies in many fields.

Researchers have looked at the influences of music in managing stress in many anxiety-provoking situations. One example is test taking: Anxiety levels appear to rise in the absence of music, while they are held constant with music. Music may have more effect on highly anxious subjects. Stimulative music may increase worry and emotionality; more sedative music decreases these feelings.

The effects of music in reducing stress and anxiety associated with various medical procedures has been studied. For example, music appears to improve mood and to comfort adult patients in general hospitals and to reduce anxiety significantly in chronically ill patients. Several studies have reported successful applications of music to reduce anxiety during PREGNANCY. Additionally, music is reported to decrease PAIN responses during labor and to elicit positive psychological responses.

A number of studies have examined the effects of music in dental procedures. Listening to music causes significant reductions in heart rate, blood pressure, and stress hormones, and significantly decreases the need for pain relieving medications. There is also an improvement in the patient's feeling of CONTROL, as he/she has a choice of music. The pain threshold and tolerance during dental procedures increase with music.

In a study of chronic pain, patients playing self-selected tape-recorded music reported not only a reduction in the emotional experience of suffering but also a reduction in the actual sensation of pain. In addition to reducing pain, particularly in pain clinics, music has been offered during chemotherapy as a form of relaxation and distraction to bring overall relief and to reduce nausea and vomiting.

Surgeons and music

A study reported in the *Journal of the American Medical Association* (1994) offered data to support the belief of many surgeons that music calms them and aids their performances. Researchers at State University of New York, Buffalo, devised a controlled laboratory experiment in which 50 male surgeons, aged 31 to 61—all reporting that they typically listen to music during surgery—performed a complex math task under three separate conditions: while listening to music of their own choosing, while listening to music selected by the researchers, and with no music.

Changes in skin conductance, pulse rate, and blood pressure, all responses associated with stress, were dramatically lower with the physicians' music, somewhat lower with the researchers' music, and highest with no music at all. Music also appeared to improve speed and accuracy.

Researchers selected Pachelbel's *Canon in D*, an orchestral piece often used in commercially prepared stress reduction tapes. Participants' selections covered a range of musical styles, including classical, jazz, and Irish folk. Category of music, regardless of tempo or instrumentation, seemed to have no significant impact on results, as long as the music was of the surgeon's own choosing.

Researchers pointed out that since all participants were already enthusiastic believers in the benefits of music and eager to participate in this study, they did not speculate about the effects on surgeons who customarily choose not to listen during surgery.

Music and worker productivity
According to a report by Greg Oldham, professor of organizational behavior at the University of Illinois at Urbana-Champaign, allowing employees to listen to personal stereo headsets can improve productivity. Among 75 employees who wore headsets an average of 20 hours during the work week, productivity increased by 10% over a four-week period. Among 181 employees who did not wear headsets during the same period, there was no change in productivity. According to Oldham, the headset wearers were less nervous, less fatigued, more enthusiastic and more relaxed at work than were the employees in the control group. The most popular types of music were oldies and country music.

See also ALTERNATIVE THERAPIES; ARTHRITIS; STRESS MANAGEMENT.

SOURCES:
Aldridge, David. "The Music of the Body: Music Therapy in Medical Settings." *ADVANCES, The Journal of Mind-Body Health* 9, no. 1 (Winter 1993).
Allen, K., and J. Blascovich. "Effects of Music on Cardiovascular Reactivity among Surgeons." *Journal of the American Medical Association* 272 (1994): 882–84.
Crowley, Susan L. "The Amazing Power of Music." *Bulletin* (American Association of Retired Persons), February 1992.
Hodges, D.A., ed. *Handbook of Music Psychology.* Lawrence, Ks.: National Association for Music Therapy, 1980.
Lehrer, Paul M. and Robert L. Woolfolk. *Principles and Practice of Stress Management.* New York: Guilford Press, 1993.

music therapy See MUSIC.

myocardial infarction See HEART ATTACK.

nail biting A difficult habit to break. In spite of the stereotype of the nervous nail biter, nail biting does not correlate with specific personality qualities. However, many children as well as adults bite their nails when affected by stress. Situations that cause ANXIETY, FEAR, BOREDOM, PAIN, or tension relate to nail biting.

With some people, nail biting continues because it is a routine and unconscious HABIT without an obvious underlying cause. Many people are embarrassed and bite their nails only when no one is around to see them. A somewhat universal habit, nail biting has no relationship to sex, race, or intelligence. It is estimated that over 50% of the population has had the nail biting habit at some point in life. Nail biting usually starts in childhood after the age of three and frequently ends in adolescence when peer pressure and personal grooming become important. About 20 to 25% of adults remain nail biters. More women than men seek help to break the habit.

There seems to be a slight hereditary tendency to nail biting, but, because family members are prone to mimic each others' habits, this is hard to establish. It seems, however, that a nail-biting parent is likely to have trouble correcting a nail-biting child.

See also NERVOUS HABITS; OBSESSIVE-COMPULSIVE DISORDER.

SOURCE:
Smith, Frederick Henry. *Nail Biting: The Beatable Habit.* Provo, Ut.: Brigham Young University Press, 1980.

naturopathy A form of alternative medicine. It is based on two principles: the accumulation of waste products and toxins in the body causes disease; symptoms of disease are the body's way of trying to get rid of these substances. Proponents believe that nature heals itself by strengthening the healing powers within, and that individuals can do the same by dealing with factors that potentially hinder wellness. In addition to the accumulation of waste products and toxins, these hindrances include bodily structural imbalances, emotional stressors, and detrimental lifestyles.

The goal of naturopathy therapy is to free the body to heal itself by enhancing its self-healing power. Practitioners agree that it is the ultimate goal of any type of wellness practitioner to encourage the body's own life force to operate more efficiently within the individual. He/she may encourage the individual to use many techniques for controlling STRESS and promoting wellness, including nutritional and herbal supplements, BREATHING and EXERCISE programs, and MEDITATION.

See also ALTERNATIVE THERAPIES; HERBAL MEDICINE; NUTRITION.

FOR FURTHER INFORMATION:
American Association of Naturopathic Physicians
P.O. Box 20386
Seattle, WA 98102
Phone: (206) 323-7610

nausea A feeling of sickness in the stomach that causes a loathing for food and an urge to vomit. Some people experience nausea when under stress or recalling an anxiety-producing experience from the past. Others experience stress from the DIZZINESS, light-headedness, or sweating that accompanies nausea.

When individuals become nauseated before certain events, such as a public speaking appearance or a dramatic performance, playing in a sports event or taking an examination, BEHAVIOR THERAPY techniques can help. However, in all cases of repeated nausea, physical causes should be ruled out before undergoing psychotherapy for the condition. Some medications may produce nausea as a side effect in susceptible individuals.

See also PERFORMANCE ANXIETY; SOCIAL PHOBIA.

nervous habits   Habits that include involuntary twitches and facial tics and voluntary behaviors such as nose picking, thumb sucking, and nail biting. These habits may be a reaction to STRESS or a means of relieving stress and anxieties for some people. If the individual has a strong desire to overcome these nervous HABITS, in some cases BEHAVIORAL THERAPY techniques will help.

See also ANXIETY; IRRITABLE BOWEL SYNDROME; NAIL BITING; OBSESSIVE-COMPULSIVE DISORDER.

networking   Using one's contacts in business and in personal life to acquire information, to achieve some professional advantage, or to expand one's circle of friends. It is a useful technique in finding out about marketing and industry trends and is unsurpassed for generating job leads and interviews. The stress involved in networking is that the individual may be bothering his friends, casual acquaintances, or complete strangers; the individual may fear rejection in these efforts. Despite the stress, networking has become an important part of finding work.

One of the important rules of networking is that people should never call anyone with whom they don't have a connection or referral. According to Marilyn Moats Kennedy, managing partner of Career Strategies, Chicago, the goal in networking is to amass a list of 400 people with similar interests and skills in your target industry who will remember your name and answer your calls. To gain that network, Kennedy recommends forming concentric circles starting with coworkers, past employers, friends, relatives, and other people with whom you have contact within your community and personal life. Not to be overlooked is an immediate former boss. A survey by Lee Hecht Harrison, an outplacement firm based in New York, indicated that as many as one in three job seekers get help in their networking efforts from their former boss.

Kennedy calls the people in the first concentric circle the individual's inner sanctum. Having asked each inner sanctum person for contacts, these contacts become a second concentric circle. The third concentric circle consists of people referred by the second circle.

Keeping a log of the networking calls you make each day is an important part of the process. Through contacts, certain employers or job descriptions are identified for follow up. Other information coming from referrals should be collected and filed for future use.

See also JOB CHANGE; JOB SECURITY.

SOURCE:
Burg, Bob. *Endless Referrals. Networking Your Everyday Contacts Into Sales.* New York: McGraw Hill, 1994.

neurotransmitters   Chemicals that carry messages from one nerve cell to another or to muscle cells; these messages are transmitted within a fraction of a second.

Norepinephrine (a neurotransmitter) is released by the adrenal gland in response to signals triggered by STRESS, exercise, or by an emotion such as fear. Norepinephrine helps maintain a constant blood pressure by stimulating certain blood vessels to constrict when the blood pressure falls below normal. Serotonin (a neurotransmitter) is thought to be involved in controlling states of consciousness and MOOD.

See also ANXIETY; DEPRESSION; PHARMACOLOGICAL APPROACH.

nightmare   A frightening DREAM characterized by a sense of oppression or suffocation that usually wakes people up during sleep. It occurs, most frequently, during REM (rapid eye movement) sleep and during the later part of the nighttime sleep period. Immediately after a nightmare, people feel very stressed. They have a clear recollection of the dream accompanied by intense uneasiness.

Children often have nightmares after a day filled with great excitement, such as a first day of school or seeing a frightening movie or TV show. When they grow older and can distinguish a dream from reality, they are less frightened when nightmares occur.

Some individuals suffer nightmares as part of POST-TRAUMATIC STRESS DISORDER (PTSD), particularly those who have witnessed a crime, been a victim of a crime, or served in a battle. They may relive their experience in the nightmare and wake up just as frightened as they felt when the event first happened.

See also BEHAVIOR THERAPY.

SOURCE:
Krakow, Barry. *Conquering Bad Dreams & Nightmares: A Guide to Understanding, Interpretation and Cure.* New York: Berkeley, 1992.

night shift   See SHIFT WORK.

noise   See ENVIRONMENT; RANDOM NUISANCES.

norepinephrine   A hormone secreted by nerve endings in the sympathetic nervous system and by the adrenal glands. Its primary function is to help maintain a constant blood pressure by stimulating certain blood vessels to constrict when the blood pressure falls below normal.

In some cases, an injection of the hormone may be given in the emergency treatment of shock or severe bleeding. Excessive levels of norepinephrine in the brain have been associated with manic states.

Norepinephrine is also sometimes called noradrenaline.

nostalgia   A longing to return to a place where one may have emotional ties or a yearning to return to some past period or irrecoverable condition.

When nostalgia is characterized by excessive or abnormal sentimentality, it becomes stressful because it is related to feelings of isolation. According to Miepje DeVryer, in the *Journal of American College Health,* nostalgia should be distinguished from the stress of experiencing HOMESICKNESS, which tends to be resolved by returning "home."

In contrast, when the individual longs or yearns for a lost past, and does so without desire to actually return, he is merely experiencing a normal response to nostalgia. His memories are usually of experiences with places and things rather than people. He is encompassed by a bittersweet feeling, painful and stressful on the one hand, pleasurable and soothing on the other.

See also ACCULTURATION; LONELINESS; MIGRATION; MOVING.

SOURCE:
DeVryer, Miepje A. "Leaving, Longing and Loving: A Developmental Perspective of Migration." *Journal of American College Health* 38 (September 1989).

nursing homes   Homes that provide care at various levels for individuals who cannot care for themselves. Older persons today are faced with stressful choices in determining how they will spend their final years. Adult children, as well, feel the tremendous stress of helping their parents make the right choice. In some cases, they must make the choice for the parents when the parents are unable to do it themselves.

For some older adults, the preference will be to remain in their own home; others may choose to move in with their children. However, the latter option may not be as viable as it was in years past. Space could be at a premium in their children's homes, and both husband and wife may be tied down to a job. Even more likely, these adult children may be at the beginning of their RETIREMENT years, having only recently shed the responsibility of their own sons and daughters.

Some older adults will find comfort and safety in housing complexes built specifically to meet the needs of senior citizens. In these complexes, they will have all the conveniences of independent living combined with meal service and planned social, cultural, and recreational activities.

Any of these options work as long as the older persons involved remain independent and healthy. However, when illness and physical limitations related to living longer occur, the need for full-time care becomes a priority. It is that priority that often is best met in a nursing home environment.

In the United States in the later 1990s, over 1.5 million people live in nursing homes and the number is increasing every year. According to a report in *Today's Chicago Woman* (November 1995), "Today's housing choices for the elderly are modern, clean, sun-filled environments, designed for the comfort, enjoyment, freedom, and security of their residents." The article describes levels of care that are offered, ranging from 24-hour skilled nursing and rehabilitative facilities to residential care facilities providing room and board and social activities and sometimes, but not always, health care services as well. The article singled out the most important feature of a long-term care facility as the quality of care delivered, which can only be as good as the staff who delivers it.

See also ELDERLY PARENTS; HOSPITALIZATION.

SOURCE:
Yeh, Elizabeth. *How to Achieve Quality of Life and Care in a Nursing Home.* Houston: Rosenwasser Publishing, 1996.

nutrition   The study and science of the food people eat and drink and the way food and drink are digested and assimilated in the body. STRESS plays an important role in nutritional aspects of life. At times of certain mental or physical illnesses, an individual's nutrition may be less than optimal. For exam-

---

TAKE THE STRESS OUT OF CHOOSING A NURSING HOME

- Tour the facility for cleanliness, safety and security.
- Check the activity calendar.
- Ask to see its annual report/financial statement.
- Observe and talk with residents or drop in unannounced.
- Look for conveniences such as handrails, call buttons, and other devices designed specifically to assist older people.
- Observe how personal privacy is respected.
- Determine what help is available in making the transition.

---

ple, a severely depressed person may have little interest in eating, and lose weight, or a patient with a chronic illness, such as cancer, may have little appetite because of chemotherapy. ALCOHOLISM and substance abuse can suppress the appetite, leading to a decrease in food intake.

In Western societies today, many people feel stressed over the relationship between diet and health. The focus is on the danger of too much fat in the diet, and on the effects of food additives, coloring, and preservatives. Inadequate intake of protein and calories may occur in people who restrict their diet and try to lose weight. This can lead to EATING DISORDERS such as anorexia nervosa. It can also occur because of mistaken beliefs about diet and health. Emphasis on thinness in our society has led many to poor nutritional habits in an effort to lose weight. Hence one's perception of BODY IMAGE may interfere with proper nutritional intake.

Psychotropic medications can contribute to inadequate nutrition for some individuals. For example, dry mouth, a side effect of some medications, may make eating less pleasurable than usual. Other side effects that interfere with one's ability to maintain good nutrition include glossitis, nausea, abdominal pain, vomiting, and diarrhea.

Mental impairment, caused by organic mental disorders and MENTAL RETARDATION or alcoholism and drug abuse, can result in an inability to make decisions about eating. The lack of judgment may be reflected in inappropriate selection or preparation of meals. MEMORY impairment associated with some of these disorders may cause one to forget to eat, even after frequent reminders, or forget that one has already eaten, and eat a second meal.

See also OBESITY; WEIGHT GAIN AND LOSS.

SOURCES:

Bland, Jeffrey S. "Psychoneuro-Nutritional Medicine: An Advancing Paradigm." *Alternative Therapies* 1, no. 2 (May 1995).

Napier, Kristine. "Nutrition: Fat Is Everyone's Issue." *Harvard Health Letter* 21, no. 3 (June 1996).

Thomas, Patricia, ed. "Nutrition: High-Protein Diets: Where's the Beef?" *Harvard Health Letter* 22, no. 3 (January 1997).

O

obesity Obese refers a person's body fat. While the words "obese" and "overweight" are usually used synonymously, they are actually measured differently. Scientists use a scale called the body measurement index (BMI) to measure obesity. BMI is computed by multiplying weight in pounds by 700 and dividing the result by the square of a person's height in inches. Overweight refers to an excess of total fat, bone, muscle, and water.

Obesity is a source of STRESS and ANXIETY for many of the one-third of all Americans who meet the criteria of being "20 percent or more above their ideal weight" and are fast realizing that crash diets alone will not solve their problems. Obesity can affect a person's SELF-ESTEEM, feeling of attractiveness, and mental well-being. It can lead to social withdrawal and have debilitating effects on the body.

The public image of obesity is changing; once obesity was considered the look of the lazy and the gluttonous. However, news of recent breakthroughs in the genetics of obesity, and drugs under development to fight obesity, are giving the general public a view long shared by researchers and many overweight Americans, that obesity is a long-term disease.

Estimates indicate that about 25% of the American population is obese. About 5% to 10% of children and 13% to 23% of all adolescents, especially girls, suffer from obesity. Obese teenagers are more likely to turn into obese adults.

Causes

There are no clear reasons why people become obese. Although obesity occurs when the calories absorbed by the body exceed those that are being used, obese people do not necessarily eat more than those who are not obese.

It is thought that obese people have a lower metabolic rate, which is the amount of energy needed to maintain the body's functions, because they are less physically active.

Since children of obese parents are much more likely to be obese than children of thin parents, genetics may play a role in obesity. Psychologist Kelly D. Brownell, director of the Yale Center for Eating and Weight Disorders, has said that "genetics may cause obesity to occur, but our environment makes it happen." By environment he means, "A world in which we are inundated with media images of thinness that few of us could attain; filled with labor-saving devices that keep us physically inactive; and full of cheap, seductive food that is rich and fat in calories."

Treatment

Researchers agree that a healthy diet and exercise can fight obesity. The diet should be one that provides the obese person 500 to 1,000 calories less than his or her energy requirements. Regular exercise, which burns extra calories, particularly aerobics, is considered a must. However, in children and adolescents, increasing physical activity can be complicated by interference with growth. For adults, increasing physical activity not only controls weight, but also protects against a list of illnesses, including DIABETES, heart disease, and CANCER.

When obesity is threatening the life of the individual, various radical procedures have been used. These include wiring the jaw so that only reduced-calorie liquids can be consumed, and stapling the stomach to reduce its size, causing the person to feel full after eating a small amount.

In sum, nothing is more effective than psychological motivation to help obese people to lose weight by dieting and exercise and to keep it off.

See also BODY IMAGE; DIETING; EATING DISORDERS; NUTRITION; WEIGHT GAIN AND LOSS.

FOR FURTHER INFORMATION:
American Society of Bariatric Physicians
5600 S. Quebec (Suite 1600)
Englewood, CO 80111
Phone: (303) 779-4833

National Association to Aid Fat Americans
P.O. Box 188620
Sacramento, CA 95818
Phone: (916) 443-0303

SOURCE:
Merz, Beverly, ed. "Obesity Drugs Redux." *Harvard Women's Health Watch* 4, no. 6 (February 1997).

obsessive-compulsive disorder (OCD) An ANXIETY DISORDER characterized by a person's obsessions, which are repeated intrusive, unwanted thoughts that may lead to carrying out ritualized, compulsive acts. This disorder affects 2.4 million Americans and is a cause for stress for the sufferer as well as family members, coworkers, and friends.

OCD may come on suddenly, often beginning in early childhood, around age eight to 10. The disorder is twice as prevalent in the general population as panic disorder or schizophrenia. OCD is partly inherited and partly the result of environmental factors. Personality traits of orderliness and cleanliness are said to be related to OCD and certain brain disorders can result in compulsive behavior.

Obsessions
Obsessions come into the mind involuntarily and recur. Sufferers are not able to ignore them; they consider these thoughts, such as fear of being infected by germs or dirt and constant doubt about such things as turning the coffeepot off or locking the front door, senseless and somewhat unpleasant, but unrelenting.

Compulsions
A normal lifestyle routine is impossible for many OCD sufferers because they constantly repeat rituals that take up considerable time. People who have OCD are aware that their compulsions and rituals are irrational, but they cannot help themselves. Some are ashamed of their actions and hide them from family and friends, often delaying treatment for years.

Hand washing, checking, and counting are the most common compulsions among people with this disorder. Other types of rituals relate to fastidiousness and PERFECTION, such as cleaning the house, showering, repeating names or phrases, hoarding, avoiding objects, and performing tasks extremely slowly and repeatedly.

OCD and links with depression
Researchers speculate that OCD may be closely associated with DEPRESSION. Some individuals experience only OCD while others suffer from both OCD and depression. The link between OCD and depression is borne out by laboratory tests on patients who have the two illnesses. For example, obsessive-compulsives, like some people who have depression, do not stop producing dexamethasone, a steroid naturally produced in the body, during a dexamethasone suppression test. When the steroid is injected into the body, the body should stop producing dexamethasone on its own. OCD patients continue to make the steroid. Also, obsessive-compulsives, like depressed people, show an abnormal lapse in the time it takes between first falling asleep and the first dream, normally from one to two hours. When researchers looked at the immediate family members of people suffering from OCD, they found a high percentage had depression or manic-depressive disorder. Many OCD sufferers have symptoms associated with depression, such as GUILT, indecisiveness, low self-esteem, ANXIETY, and exhaustion.

BEHAVIOR THERAPY FOR OCD

Technique	Action experienced	Anticipated effect
Prevention of response	Individual gradually delays performing ritual for longer intervals.	Helps reduce compulsion.
Thought stopping	Individual tries to voluntarily interrupt obsessive thoughts.	Helps decrease obsessions.
Imagery	Individual is encouraged to imagine being exposed to feared situation and prevent an unwanted response.	Help decrease obsessions and anxiety.
Modeling	Therapist actively models response.	Alters patient's unwanted behaviors to more acceptable ones.
Exposure	Individual is gradually exposed to the feared thought or object.	Reduces anxiety; decreases obsessions and compulsions.

Pharmacological and behavior therapies

PHARMACOLOGICAL APPROACHES include use of prescription medications for some individuals. Researchers have learned that medications that affect the serotonergic system (such as clomipramine and fluoxetine) can be useful in relieving symptoms in some patients.

BEHAVIOR THERAPY is one of the most effective treatments for OCD. During therapy sessions, the person is exposed to situations that cause extreme stress and anxiety and provoke compulsive behaviors. The individual is not allowed to go through the usually performed rituals, such as excessive hand washing after handling money. This technique works well for people whose compulsions focus on situations that can be easily recreated. For those who follow compulsive rituals because they fear catastrophic events that cannot be recreated, individuals must rely more on imagination.

FOR FURTHER INFORMATION:
Obsessive-Compulsive Disorder Foundation
P.O. Box 70
Milford, CT 06460-0070
Phone: (800) 639-7462

Anxiety Disorders Association of America
11900 Parklawn Drive (Suite 100)
Rockville, MD 20852
Phone: (301) 231-9350

SOURCES:
American Psychiatric Association. *Obsessive-Compulsive Disorder.* Washington, D.C.: American Psychiatric Association. 1988.
Kahn, Ada P., and Jan Fawcett. *The Encyclopedia of Mental Health.* New York: Facts On File, 1993.
Reyes, Karen. "Obsessive-Compulsive Disorder: There Is Help." *Modern Maturity,* November–December 1995, 78.

occupational stress See JOB CHANGE; JOB SECURITY; WORKPLACE.

Office of Alternative Medicine (OAM) An increasing number of people in the United States are turning to ALTERNATIVE THERAPIES for stress reduction and improvement of wellness. This trend encouraged the United States medical establishment not only to take notice but also to establish the Office of Alternative Medicine within the National Institutes of Health in 1992.

One of OAM's primary mandates from Congress is to award research grants to scientists studying the effects of alternative therapies on stress as well as various illnesses. The OAM strives to fund research projects and to establish an information clearinghouse on alternative medicine so that the public, policy makers, and public health experts can make informed decisions about health care options.

Many of the grants awarded by the OAM focus on strategies to reduce stress and related disorders. For example, research grants awarded by the OAM have included studies on ACUPUNCTURE for unipolar depression, MASSAGE THERAPY for HIV, HYPNOSIS for chronic lower back pain, massage therapy for post-surgical outcomes, MUSIC therapy for psychosocial adjustment after brain injury, classical HOMEOPATHY for health status, T'AI CHI for mild balance disorders, GUIDED IMAGERY for ASTHMA, imagery and RELAXATION for breast cancer, Ayurvedic herbals for Parkinson's disease, BIOFEEDBACK and relaxation for DIABETES, and YOGA for OBSESSIVE-COMPULSIVE DISORDER.

Since its inception, hundreds of awards have been granted. For example, in 1995, the NIH designated eight specialty research centers to study the effectiveness and safety of such treatments as acupuncture, herbs, massage/body work, and chiropractic and vitamin therapy. The grants provide a proving ground to determine if it is the alternative therapy that works or if it is the patients' belief in the therapy that helps them get better. Alternative practitioners are encouraged about the potential for scientific evidence confirming the value of therapies that do not involve drugs, surgery, or other invasive procedures. Such evidence may prove to physicians that alternative therapy has credibility.

The Office of Alternative Medicine provides a directory of alternative health care associations relating to holistic health care, diet/nutrition/lifestyle changes, MIND-BODY CONNECTIONS, art, music, dance and humor therapy, traditional and ethnomedicine, structural and energetic therapies, pharmacological and biological treatments, bioelectromagnetic applications, and more.

See also AYURVEDA; CHIROPRACTIC MEDICINE; MEDITATION; NATUROPATHY.

FOR FURTHER INFORMATION:
Office of Alternative Medicine
National Institutes of Health
6120 Executive Blvd. (Suite 450)
Rockville, MD 20892-9904
Phone: (301) 402-4741

SOURCE:
Burton Goldberg Group, eds. *Alternative Medicine: The Definitive Guide.* Puyallup, Wash.: Future Medicine Publishing, 1993.

Ohashiatsu Based on the same system of Oriental medicine as ACUPUNCTURE; a form of therapy useful for relief of stress in some people. Ohashiatsu addresses the body's energy meridians and points along those meridians called *tsubos.* Instead of using needles, however, the practitioner of Ohashiatsu uses hands, elbows, and sometimes even knees as tools. The goal is to achieve a feeling of deep RELAXATION, harmony, and peace.

Ohashiatsu adds psychological and spiritual dimensions to traditional SHIATSU by incorporating Zen philosophy, movement, and MEDITATION to balance the energy of body, mind, and spirit.

See also ALTERNATIVE THERAPIES; BODY-THERAPIES; MIND-BODY CONNECTIONS.

orgasm See SEXUAL RESPONSE CYCLE.

overeating See OBESITY; NUTRITION; WEIGHT GAIN AND LOSS.

P

pain   A feeling that can range from mild distress to unbearable, acute suffering. It occurs following injury or as a result of disease when the body's sensory nerve endings are stimulated.

Pain is not restricted to a specific type of stimulus; it can be aroused by extreme stimulation of any sense. Loud noise and bright lights can be painful, as can be HEADACHES, toothaches, cancer, inflammation of tissue and muscles, and bone breakage.

In his book *Painstoppers*, author Norman D. Ford identifies stress as the genesis of pain. Ford says, "Stress occurs only when we perceive life through a filter of fear-based, negative beliefs. Stress is the underlying cause of some 70 percent of all chronic pain. Virtually all pain in the neck, upper and lower back, and shoulders is stress-related and so are most headaches. Such pain-provoking diseases as ulcers, irritable bowels, rheumatoid ARTHRITIS, cancer, and heart disease are also stress related. Overeating because of emotional stress also leads to OBESITY, which worsens the pain of osteoarthritis."

Psychiatrist Lawrence S. Schoenfeld, Ph.D., of the Pain Clinic, University of Texas Health Science Center, San Antonio, states, "People usually think of the physical aspects, but in chronic pain, that's only one component." Also to be considered, he continues, is the patient's emotional state, beliefs, and prior conditioning. An individual's EMOTIONS—for example, ANXIETY, DEPRESSION, or ANGER—can add to or magnify the perception of pain. According to Schoenfeld, "We often can't fix or significantly alter the body, but we can alter the mood and thought processes, and change reinforcements that affect a patient's motivation."

REDUCE STRESS: PARTICIPATE IN PAIN CONTROL

- Identify small steps toward independence from pain, such as accepting the pain and not blaming others for your problems.
- Track pain levels and activities with awareness of the difference between physical pain sensations and emotional pain distress.
- Check the "costs/benefits" in relation to participation in family activities, work and play, and relationships with people.
- Express feelings and anxieties; learn ways to decrease anger responses.
- Block negative thoughts; use relaxation techniques to fight the chronic stress of sleep disturbance, fatigue, poor concentration, increased muscle tension, anxiety, depression, and loss of self-control—all of which amplify pain.
- Distract yourself by focusing on the environment, singing or using imagery to concentrate on pleasant, dramatic, and healing thoughts.
- Indulge in healthy pleasures and fun.
- Focus on the pain and the thoughts and feelings that accompany the pain.
- Reclaim an active life by setting short- and long-term goals.
- Exercise on a regular basis; increase the amount gradually. Modify how you use your body, such as during lifting, bending, and sitting, and what you use for physical support—chairs, desks and counters, wrist bands and other methods.
- Prepare for flareups by knowing the specific pain relievers that work best for you.

Treatment

Course of treatmellt at the Texas pain clinic is based on how patients are categorized: somatic, those whose pain is primarily of physical origin, with some psychological issues possible; psychogenic, those who experience pain but have nothing physically wrong; malingering, those who are either faking or greatly exaggerating their pain. Treatments include RELAXATION training, HYPNOSIS, BIOFEEDBACK, behavior modification, and family, marital, and sexual counseling.

In *Mental Medicine Update*, Robert Ornstein, Ph.D., and David S. Sobel, M.D. stated that 10% to 30% of Americans suffer from chronic or recurrent pain, which extracts a heavy toll on health, ability to work, and sense of well-being. While feelings of anxiety, frustration, and loss of control and confidence can amplify the experience of pain, it does not mean that the pain is not "real." It just means that emotions make it worse. In addition to physical treatment of pain, the authors suggest behavioral self-management that includes mind-body strategies such as relaxation techniques, SUPPORT GROUP therapy, and biofeedback training. To those suffering chronic pain, Ornstein and Sobel suggest that when they become partners in pain treatment, they become part of the solution.

See also ALTERNATIVE THERAPIES; CHRONIC ILLNESS; GUIDED IMAGERY.

FOR FURTHER INFORMATION:
American Academy of Pain Medicine
5700 Old Orchard Road
Skokie, IL 60077
Phone: (847) 966-9510

American Pain Society
P.O. Box 186
Skokie, IL 60076
Phone: (847) 475-7300

Pain Management Guidelines
Agency for Healthcare Policy Research
P.O. Box 8547
Silver Spring, MD 20907
Phone: (800) 358-9295

SOURCES:
Ford, Norman D. *Painstoppers: The Magic of All-Natural Pain Relief.* West Nyack, N.Y.: Parker Publishing, 1994.
Ornstein, Robert, and David Sobel. "RX: Managing Chronic Pain." *Mental Medicine Update* 4, no. 1 (1995).

palpitations A conscious sensation of the heart's beating harder and faster than normal or skipping beats. Whereas normally people are not aware of how their hearts beat, many of them experience palpitations when they participate in strenuous exercise or have stress-producing experiences.

Thumping or fluttering feelings in the chest do not normally indicate heart disease and may be a result of heavy use of caffeine, alcohol, or smoking. An arrhythmia (irregular beat) may cause a palpitation. Individuals may feel faint and breathless and their pulse may be as high as 200 beats per minute but remain regular. Hyperthyroidism, overactive thyroid glands, may also cause palpitation by speeding up the heartbeat.

Many individuals experience palpitations during panic attacks or as a phobic reaction to a stimulus they fear. For example, a person who is phobic about dogs may experience palpitations just at the sight of a dog walking on the sidewalk. Although the dog is on a leash and does not pose any threat, the phobic individual may experience palpitations along with sweaty palms, weak knees, and DIZZINESS.

Those who experience palpitations may fear that they are having a heart attack or that they are going to die. For many people, just thinking these thoughts and becoming afraid of imagined consequences can cause palpitations to increase. Symptoms of ANXIETY, such as palpitations, are treated with BEHAVIOR THERAPY and, in some cases, drug therapy.

If an individual experiences palpitations for several hours or the feeling recurs over several days, or if they cause chest pain, breathlessness, or dizziness, a family physician, general internist, or specialist in cardiology should be consulted as soon as possible. If palpitation episodes are brief, they are probably within the range of normal. Some medications may produce palpitations in individuals.

See also ANXIETY DISORDERS; PANIC ATTACKS AND PANIC DISORDER; PHARMACOLOGICAL APPROACH; PHOBIAS.

panic attacks and panic disorder   A panic attack is a short period (five to 10 minutes) of suddenly occurring, intense fear or discomfort, usually for no apparent reason. The feeling may be caused by stress but it also causes extreme stress in the affected individual because it is usually accompanied by a fear of dying, a sense of imminent danger or impending doom, and an urge to escape.

Panic attacks are considered one of several ANXIETY DISORDERS. They can occur in a variety of anxiety disorders, such as panic disorder, AGORAPHOBIA, SOCIAL PHOBIAS, and POST-TRAUMATIC STRESS DISORDER.

The word "panic" is derived from the name Pan, whom Greeks worshiped as their god of flocks, herds, pastures, and fields. Pan loved to scare people and make eerie noises to frighten passersby. The fright he aroused was known as "panic."

Criteria for diagnosis

To be diagnosed as a panic attack, organic factors have to be ruled out as the cause of the disturbance. The panic incident must include at least four or more of the characteristic symptoms, which are a sense of breathing difficulty, PALPITATIONS or rapid heartbeat, sweating, trembling, shaking, feelings of smothering or choking, chest pains, nausea or abdominal distress, DIZZINESS or light-headedness, paresthesia, and chills or hot flushes.

HYPERVENTILATION (fast, shallow breathing) worsens the symptoms and leads to a pins and needles sensation and to a feeling of derealization or depersonalization. These symptoms are usually the result of underlying emotional conflicts such as fear of being trapped or loss of emotional support.

According to the *Diagnostic and Statistical Manual of Mental Disorders,* 4th ed. (DSM-IV), typically the first attack occurs in individuals in the late teens. Initially, attacks are unexpected and do not occur immediately before or on exposure to a stressful situation, such as a simple phobia or social PHOBIAS. Subsequently, certain situations may be identified with having a panic attack, such as crossing a bridge or being on an escalator. Once a panic attack has occurred in a particular setting, the individual may become fearful that it will happen again and tend to avoid that situation.

The context of panic attacks

When a health professional assesses the significance of the problem, it is important to determine the context in which it occurs. According to DSM-IV, three characteristic types of panic attack relate in different ways to the onset of the attack and the presence or absence of situational triggers:

Unexpected panic attack: The onset of the attack is not associated with any situational trigger.

Situationally bound attack: The attack almost invariably occurs immediately on exposure to, or in anticipation of, the stressful situational trigger.

Situationally predisposed panic attack: More likely to occur on exposure to the situational cue or trigger, but is not invariably associated with the cue and does not necessarily occur immediately after exposure to the stressful factor.

Panic disorder

When panic attacks recur frequently and disrupt an individual's life, the condition is known as panic disorder. Sufferers (1% to 2% of the population) may have attacks ranging from two or three a day to two to four times a week. This type of disorder tends to run a fluctuating course and becomes worse when the individual comes under stress. Panic disorder usually begins during periods of choices, transitions, separation, and added responsibilities. There is often a family history of panic disorder. For example, first-degree relatives of patients with panic disorder are at a markedly higher risk of developing the disorder (15% to 20% compared to 1% in the general population).

In diagnosing panic disorder, the essential feature is the presence of recurrent, unexpected panic attacks followed by at least one month of persistent concern about having another panic attack, worry about the possible implications or consequence of the attacks, or a significant behavioral changed related to the attacks.

Personality characteristics

Personality characteristics of those who have panic disorder vary considerably. However, H. Michael Zal, a clinical professor of psychiatry at the Philadelphia College of Osteopathic Medicine, has observed some common factors. Additionally, cross-sectional studies of persons with panic disorder or agoraphobia have demonstrated personality traits of dependency, avoidance, low SELF-ESTEEM, and interpersonal sensitivity. One common attribute shared by panic-prone people may include placing a great value on CONTROL. Any loss or threatened loss of control, particularly changes in their life-styles, causes them to feel anxious and stressed. According to Dr. Zal, panic-prone people overvalue their independence and feel great discomfort in acknowledging their dependency needs. They are often reluctant to accept help and prefer helping others. Known to repress feelings, they feel anxious when their EMOTIONS surface. As perfectionists and compulsive individuals, they have high expectations of themselves and others.

It is difficult to estimate how many men suffer from panic disorder because men may attempt to mask their symptoms by drinking alcohol or by other means. This type of self-medication can develop into a secondary problem. Many men go to family physicians, see multiple specialist, or end up in emergency rooms, thinking they have physical dis-

orders. They complain of lower gastrointestinal problems, which are sometimes a symptom of panic disorder. When the panic disorder is treated, these gastrointestinal symptoms disappear.

Treatment for panic disorder

Treatment for the stresses that come with panic disorder may involve COGNITIVE THERAPY, BEHAVIOR THERAPY, or medical therapy. Often a combination of treatments is specifically chosen for each patient. Treatment begins with education about the illness and encouragement to reenter situations the person has come to avoid. Help for some individuals is in cognitive therapy (changing how they think and dealing with their feeling of anxiety). For others, behavior therapy (changing how they act in response to certain situations and using desensitization techniques to gradually expose sufferers to the situations they have avoided) is useful.

During the late 1990s, ALPRAZOLAM (trade name, Xanax) was the first and only medication approved in the United States for panic disorder. Previously, various studies indicated that tricyclic antidepressant drugs (such as imipramine) provided an effective, safe treatment for panic disorder. However, these medications typically take three to six weeks for noticeable improvement, and side effects including anxiety symptoms occur in up to one-third of the patients.

Three-quarters of patients who have to take drugs will need long-term drug therapy, while another 25% will not be helped regardless of how long they take drugs. Overall, a quarter of the patients who do take drugs are helped permanently and will not have to continue them.

Help for panic disorder sufferers

Treatment for panic disorder is not limited to medical or psychotherapeutic intervention. Family members can help in recognizing panic disorders by being alert to the individual's level of anxiety. Because symptoms can be hidden, repeated avoidance of situations is often the best clue. Family members can give the sufferer support, be good listeners, and talk openly and constructively among each other. Instead of enabling the person to avoid a situation, family members can help him or her make a small step forward by finding something positive in that effort. Most important, family members should be patient and accepting and not sacrifice their own lives nor build resentment toward the sufferer.

See also PHARMACOLOGICAL APPROACH; TACHYCARDIA.

FOR FURTHER INFORMATION:
Anxiety Disorders Association of America
11900 Parklawn Drive (Suite 100)
Rockville, MD 20852
Phone: (301) 231-9350

National Mental Health Association
1021 Prince Street
Alexandria, VA 22314
Phone: (800) 969-NMHA; (800) 969-6642

SOURCES:
American Psychiatric Association. *Diagnostic and Statistical Manual*, 4th ed. Washington, D.C.: American Psychiatric Association, 1994.
Kahn, Ada P. "Panic Attacks" and "Family Members Can Help Sufferers Cope with Attacks." *Chicago Tribune*, June 23, 1991.
Zal, H. Michael. *Panic Disorder: The Great Pretender.* New York: Insight Books, Plenum Press, 1990.

parenting   Caring for and nurturing children. The term may also apply to the situation when grandparents take over the care of their grandchildren because their sons or daughters are no longer able to fulfill their responsibilities.

Of all the roles in life, parenting is one of the most important; it is one for which there is the least preparation and which therefore brings with it a great deal of STRESS. For those with little instruction and no experience, the stress of parenting begins with the basics of feeding, bathing, and caring for the baby. As role models, parents provide moral and ethi-

cal values; as disciplinarians, they reward good conduct and withhold reward when conduct is bad. They deal with family disputes including sibling rivalry and, at the same time, try to avoid playing favorites, recognizing the needs of all their children. Keeping children safe throughout their lifetime is a constant concern.

Parenting involves responding to problems and concerns of children, both physical and mental. As children grow, parents watchfully wait to step in when there is trouble while recognizing their own capacities and respecting their children's need to do things for themselves.

Parenting adult children
When children become adults, the parenting role often becomes one of friend and companion. Many adult children and their parents enjoy the same sports activities, traveling together, and sharing hobbies. Characteristics of a good relationship while the children were growing up, such as open and honest communications, carry over into later life.

Eventually the young people leave home and some parents are faced with the EMPTY NEST SYNDROME and no longer feel needed. While this may be a time of stress and loneliness, it is a time when parents can explore their own interests and enjoy the intimacy they shared as newlyweds.

DIVORCE carries with it special stresses for the parents as well as children. Another stressful dimension of parenting is when grandparents take over the role of parents. A growing number nationwide have assumed the financial, physical, and emotional responsibility for their grandchildren. Grandparents Raising Grandchildren was founded in 1988 to provide the information and resources needed for those facing this stressful challenge. Current census figures indicate 4.7 million children living with grandparents and 1.1 million being raised by grandparents alone; however, this may be an understatement because the figures do not cover informal living arrangements.

See also BIRTH ORDER; ELDERLY PARENTS; SIBLING RELATIONSHIPS; STEPFAMILIES; WORKING MOTHERS; UNWED MOTHERS.

FOR FURTHER INFORMATION:
Grandparents Raising Grandchildren
P.O. Box 104
Colleyville, TX 76034
Phone: (817) 577-0435

SOURCES:
Johnson, John, D.W. Johnson, and R.T. Johnson. "Peer Influences," in Corsini, Raymond J., ed. *Encyclopedia of Psychology*, vol. 2. New York: Wiley, 1984.
Leach, Penelope. *The Child Care Encyclopedia*. New York: Alfred A. Knopf, 1984.
Rogers, Fred. "Parenting: A Lifelong Commitment." *The Rotarian*, September 1995, 12–14.

Peck, M(organ) Scott   American psychiatrist, author and lecturer (1936–   ) and author of several best-selling books, including *The Road Less Traveled: A New Psychology of Love, Traditional Values and Spiritual Growth* and *The Road Less Traveled and Beyond.* Peck postulates that when an individual accepts the inherent stresses in life, he can transfer weakness into strength through self-discipline and love. This "real love" is "an act of the will to extend oneself for the purpose of nurturing one's own or another's spiritual growth."

For many years, Peck has had an interest in the growing interface between RELIGION and science. He received his M.D. from Case Western Reserve University and his A.B. from Harvard University.

See also GENERAL ADAPTATION SYNDROME; HARDINESS; PRAYER.

SOURCE:
Peck, M. Scott. *The Road Less Traveled and Beyond.* New York: Simon and Schuster, 1997.

peer group   A group whose members are of "equal" standing with each other. This refers to people who are of the same age, educational level or have the same job or profession. A peer group can cause stress for the individual because it can influence feelings of self-concept, SELF-ESTEEM, attitudes, and behaviors.

Peer group relationships are important to children as well as adults. While children look to each other for acceptance and approval, so do adults who are seeking new friends and acceptance in a group.

Peers are crucial to psychological development of the individual throughout life. Children learn to cooperate, work together, handle aggressive impulses in non-destructive ways, and explore differences between themselves and their friends. Throughout the school years, children rely on their peers as important sources of information and may use peers as standards by which to measure themselves. Many look to their peers as models of behavior and for social reinforcement as often as they look to their own families.

Some children who do not learn to combat LONELINESS by fitting into a peer group may develop emotional problems later in life. These children who feel "different" from their peers may endure particular stresses as they work toward "fitting in." Such children may be those who are in recently divorced families, recently "merged" families with two sets of parents, or adopted children of single parents. However, there are children, when there are no extenuating circumstances, who are born "loners" and shun the values of their peers.

For adults, the increasing mobility that often cuts them off from family and longtime friends has made the development of peer relationships at work and in other social and community activities extremely important.

Peer pressure
Peer pressure is the influence of the peer group on the individual. It begins in adolescence, because teenagers want to belong to a

group. Teenagers react to the physical changes they are going through, as well as their changing responsibilities and experiences by close bonding with those in their own age group. Music, language, and clothing are held extremely important by the peer group. The rallying cry of teenagers often is "everybody's doing it, or everyone has it." Parents frequently become stressed by this peer pressure on their youngsters. They may also fear that the influence of friends may lead their children to genuinely damaging activities such as experimenting with drugs, irresponsible sexual activity, criminal behavior, or dropping out of school.

Peer pressure doesn't end with the teens but becomes more subtle in the ways it affects adults. It may be caused by ADVERTISING that brings the "keeping up with the Jones" philosophy that every one else on the block has one; it may arise from the COMPETITION generated by the BABY BOOMERS who influenced their generation by placing a high value on possessions, or it may be human nature that among peers there will always be leaders who have the power to influence.

See also PARENTING; PUBERTY.

peptic ulcer   Ulcers in the part of the digestive tract where gastric (stomach) secretions are present are known as peptic ulcers. They may occur in the esophagus, stomach, or duodenum. STRESS may create an opportunity for peptic ulcers to develop because it can cause people's stomachs to churn out excess gastric acid. However, there is no proof that stress actually causes ulcers, and many people in pressure-related jobs never develop them.

The symptoms of peptic ulcers sometime disappear for periods of days, weeks, or months, only to reappear, often after a person has become emotionally tense or nervous, or has picked up an infection that disturbs the chemical balance of the system. Other symptoms are loss of appetite, belching, feeling bloated, weight loss, nausea, and vomiting.

Every day, an estimated 4,000 Americans develop a peptic ulcer. Heredity can be a factor. If a person's blood relatives have had ulcers, his or her chance of getting one is increased two or three times. Two additional risk factors are involved in getting ulcers: smoking and overuse of aspirin. Smoking cessation improves the odds against getting an ulcer. Aspirin can adversely affect the protective lining of the stomach and duodenum.

Types of ulcers
There are two common types, *duodenal* and *gastric*. A duodenal ulcer is a sore that occurs in the duodenum, the first part of the intestine into which the stomach empties. More than 80% of all peptic ulcers are found in this area in young or middle-aged people. A sharp, gnawing pain may occur one to three hours after meals and will usually go away when a little food is eaten. Pain may also occur in the middle of the night when food has left the stomach and the ulcer is being bathed in acid. Individuals may often feel extremely hungry, but eating sweets and foods that stimulate the secretion of the acid will probably start or intensify the pain.

Gastric ulcers are sores in the lining of stomach. Increasingly, they have become a disease of older people, most often occurring between the ages of 55 and 65; men and women are equally affected. The pain may begin with a meal or soon after and feels relatively constant. It is not likely to be relieved by eating food and may even be made worse with eating. Antacids may not provide any relief.

Advice about diet and medication
Bland diets were once recommended for ulcer patients, but that is rarely the case anymore. A physician may suggest that the sufferer avoid any foods that irritate the stomach, but will probably write a prescription for an ulcer medication. Several pharmaceutical products now are available that are quite successful at eliminating ulcer pain and healing the ulcer itself.

TIPS TO AVOID THE STRESS OF LIVING WITH AN ULCER

- Avoid foods that cause you to experience ulcer pain.
- Avoid alcohol, juice, and caffeinated drinks such as coffee, tea, and cola beverages.
- Eat three nutritionally balanced meals each day.
- Milk may relieve some pain at first but actually causes the stomach to produce even more acid. Ask your doctor if you should avoid milk.
- Take medication exactly as your doctor prescribes it.

Even when symptoms vanish, taking medication as prescribed is necessary. This is extremely important since the ulcer may not quite be healed, even if the pain has been relieved. Most ulcers generally heal within four to six weeks of treatment, but they can rapidly recur if the medication is stopped too soon. Duodenal ulcer can be a chronic condition and there is a good chance that the ulcer will recur. Some physicians recommend that certain people take, on an ongoing basis, a reduced dosage of ulcer medication to prevent recurrence.

See also RELAXATION.

FOR FURTHER INFORMATION:
National Digestive Disease Education and
   Information Clearinghouse
Box NODIC
Bethesda, MD 20892
Phone: (301) 468-6344

perfection   The state of being expert, proficient, flawless, without fault or defect. It is an unrealistic goal, a drive toward the impossible and unattainable and is a source of stress for many people. Perfectionists are very achievement-oriented. They are unable to select what is important and have the faulty idea that perfectionism equals quality.

The perfectionist faces stress and frustration with failure of any kind, imagined, real, large, or small. The obsession with perfection ultimately results in fragmentation of self, loss of efficiency, sleep deprivation, less time for exercise, rest and quiet meals, increased use of alcohol and drugs and, ultimately, exhaustion. The perfectionist ideal leaves out the important fact that people are only human, and have limitations of body, mind, and spirit.

Many people believe the myth that overachieving will bring recognition and perhaps even love. Today's society measures individuals in terms of productivity and accomplishment. However, there is a delicate balance between the amount of work the human body and mind can do and the amount of time required for rest and regeneration. That balance point differs for each person and is affected by feelings of stress, emotional overload, illness, and fatigue.

Overcoming perfectionism
People who are plagued by the need to be perfect and the stresses that are incurred should realize their own limitations and reevaluate personal priorities. They must decide what is important and what is not and set realistic deadlines and short- and long-term goals, and choose values that matter.

CONQUER PERFECTIONISM: AVOID STRESS

- Look for sources of satisfaction in simple pleasures.
- Pursue special interests such as painting, music, gardening, reading, or handicrafts.
- Take better care of the personal self with improved diet, rest, and exercise.
- Concentrate on the process of achieving a goal instead of the goal itself.
- Establish friendships outside work and family.
- Set personal priorities and stay with them.
- Find time to be alone and become better acquainted with yourself.

See also OBSESSIVE-COMPULSIVE DISORDER; SELF-ESTEEM.

SOURCES:
Riess, Dorothy Young. "The Perils of Perfection." *Better Health Newsletter,* March 1989.
Shaw, Jean, ed. "Perfectionism: Internal Source of Stress Has High Emotional and Physical Costs." *Women's Health Advocate Newsletter* 4, no. 5 (July 1977).

performance anxiety　Many people experience extreme stress over any kind of performance because they fear failure, CRITICISM, or not measuring up to real or imaginary standards. Issues of SELF-ESTEEM are involved. Time and energy spent in thinking about their fears may interfere with concentration on preparation and on the performance.

For some individuals, performance anxiety may cause loss of sleep, indigestion, DIZZINESS, or even faintness. However, if properly directed, the nervous energy generated by stress before a performance can become an advantage. When focused on the best possible outcome, for example, that there will be a standing ovation, the individual will be challenged to do a good job.

Performance anxiety is a common stressor to people who speak publicly before large or small audiences, as well as musicians, actors, and other on- and off-stage performers. Anyone who is the central focus of other people's attention can experience performance anxiety.

Coping with performance anxiety

Many individuals use MEDITATION and deep BREATHING exercises to reduce stress before performances. Others carry a good luck charm, which provides their anxieties with a placebo-like effect. Some follow certain rituals before every performance: establishing a routine way of getting dressed, avoiding certain foods or beverages (caffeine and alcohol particularly) or taking a walk. For severe cases of performance anxiety, physicians may pre-scribe medication; however, medications may have side effects.

See also PUBLIC SPEAKING; SOCIAL PHOBIA; STAGE FRIGHT.

performance review　Reviews that are held separately from salary reviews and are annual (sometimes bi-annual) management evaluations of how well employees are doing their jobs. The evaluations, held face-to-face, are a source of stress for both the managers and the employees. According to Dr. Susan E. Brodt, assistant professor of business administration, Duke University, "The process of job evaluations often is so stressful because most companies do not do them correctly." Brodt researched how some 100 firms do employee reviews and concluded that they may be a waste of time because the important topics were often not discussed. Brodt added that appraisals "generally are conducted too late to change performance, often long after problems occur. They're anxiety-filled and people tend to avoid sensitive subjects." Finally and tragically, Brodt continues, they can lead to misunderstandings in which talented employees are fired or forced to leave the company.

Chris B. Bardwell, a Chicago-based human resource consultant, argues in favor of performance reviews "because employees need to know areas in which they should improve and also areas where they are having success."

However, it has been reported that when layoffs occur, employees often feel that performance evaluations are either not used at all or are purposely downgraded to justify terminations. One study on termination showed that 75% of the survey respondents had received "excellent" or "outstanding" in their last reviews and were still let go. As a management tool, performance reviews are often seen as political devices—inflated to assure maximum merit raises and deflated to speed up the termination procedure—according to which way the wind is blowing.

See also JOB SECURITY; LAYOFFS; MERGERS; WORKPLACE.

personality   The sum of all of an individual's behavioral and emotional tendencies. Personality develops from the interaction of many complex factors, including heredity and environment. Many theorists hold that genetics is more important than environment, while others take the opposite view.

Personality characteristics may be predictors of how well an individual copes with the stresses of life. According to studies by psychologist Suzanne O. Kobasa and associates at the University of Chicago, survivors, or people with "HARDINESS," share three specific personality traits that appear to afford them a high degree of stress resistance: they are committed to what they do, they feel in CONTROL of their lives, and they see change as a challenge rather than a threat.

Personality disorders

For some individuals, personality traits and patterns are severe enough to cause them extreme stress and interfere with normal functioning. Such individuals are said to have a personality disorder. Personality disorders usually are recognizable by adolescence or earlier, continue through adulthood, and become less obvious in middle or old age. They involve behaviors or traits that affect recent and long-term functioning. Individuals may have more than one personality disorder at a time. Their patterns of perceiving and thinking are usually not limited to isolated episodes, but are deeply ingrained, inflexible, maladaptive, and severe enough to cause mental stress or anxieties, or interfere with interpersonal relationships and normal functioning.

Personality tests

Personality tests are questionnaires designed to determine various traits, assist in psychological research and, at times, determine the suitability of an individual for a particular field of work or job assignment. Personality tests measure many aspects of an individual's being, such as how easily she is disturbed by stressors, how she relates to people and her degree of extroversion or INTROVERSION.

See also HOSTILITY; TYPE A PERSONALITY; TYPE B PERSONALITY; TYPE C PERSONALITY.

personal space   The invisible zone of privacy that individuals unconsciously put between themselves and other people. Although personal space is something rarely noticed, when it is invaded by someone approaching too closely, people may feel stressed and become anxious, irritated, and even hostile.

According to Lisa Davis, in *In Health,* "we invite others in to our personal space by how closely we approach them, the angle at which we face them, and the speed with which we break a gaze. It's a subtle code but one we use and interpret easily and automatically, having absorbed the vocabulary since infancy."

Anthropologists have reported that people follow fairly established rules regarding how far apart they stand, depending largely on their relationship to each other. For example, friends, spouses, lovers, parents, and children tend to stand inside a "zone of intimacy," or within arm's reach, while a personal zone (about four feet) is comfortable for conversation with strangers and acquaintances.

The size needed for personal space depends on many variables, including the individual's cultural background, gender, and the nature of the occasion. Individuals from North European or British ancestry usually want about a square yard of space for conversation in uncrowded situations. However, people from more tropical climates choose a smaller personal area and are more likely to reach out and touch the occupant of another space. In Mediterranean and South American societies, social conversations include much eye contact, touching, and smiling, typically while standing at a distance of about a foot. In the United States, however, people usually stand about 18 inches apart for a social conversation; while they will shake hands, they tend to talk at arm's length.

Understanding cultural and gender differences in interpretations of personal space is becoming more important as intercultural trade and business transactions escalate. The interpretation of personal space leaves much room for misinterpretation. Consultants have developed businesses interpreting for people of all nationalities the meaning and use of personal space to relieve the possibilities for occurrences of stressful situations. It is possible that a culture's use of space is evidence of a reliance on one sense over another. For example, Middle Easterners get much of their information through their senses of smell and touch, which require a close approach, while Americans rely primarily on visual information, backing up in order to see an intelligible picture.

See also ACCULTURATION; CROWDING; MIGRATION.

SOURCES:

Davis, Lisa. "Where Do We Stand?" In *Health*, September/October 1990.

Freedman, Jonathan L. *Crowding and Behavior*. New York: Viking Press, 1975.

Padus, Emrika, ed. *The Complete Guide to Your Emotions & Your Health*, rev. Emmaus, Pa.; Rodale Press, 1994.

pets   Pets reduce the stress of LONELINESS, provide companionship, and give owners a sense of order in their lives. No matter what, the routine of caring for pets provides a distraction from life's stressful problems and draws the owners out of themselves. According to *Health* (November-December 1994), 60% of American households have a pet.

Researchers have found that pets can be important factors in reducing stress and providing positive effects on human health. James Serpell, a zoologist at the University of Pennsylvania says: "People who acquire pets report fewer minor health problems such as colds, flus, and backaches. They tend to think less about their problems and are happier with their lives."

According to a University of Pennsylvania study, blood pressure drops sharply when people simply stroke a cat or dog. A study of 5,741 Australians reported that those who owned pets had cholesterol and triglyceride levels markedly lower than those who did not. Some nursing homes and other institutions may have pets in residence or programs through which pets visit residents or patients.

A UCLA study reported that older adults who had pets made fewer visits to doctors than those without. Caring for an animal seemed to make them feel less anxious about their own health. Many dentists keep aquariums in their offices because it seems that dental patients suffer less anxiety if they watch fish in an aquarium before oral surgery.

In an effort to learn more about the symbiotic relationship between humans and pets, the American Animal Hospital Association asked pet owners questions about day-to-day interactions with their pet in a pet owner survey. Results from the survey show that: 75% of dog owners and 69% of cat owners spend 45 to 60-plus minutes each day engaged in activities with their pets; 69% of dog owners and 60% of cat owners said they give their pets as much attention as they would to their children; 59% of the dog owners and 57% of the cat owners admitted to having their pet sleep with them or next to or under the bed; and 54% of survey respondents claimed that they feel an emotional dependence on their pets. The survey was conducted by AAHA drawn from its membership. Respondents were pet owners from 39 states, the provinces of Canada, and the District of Columbia, who take their pets to AAHA veterinarians.

Choosing the right pet

It is said that the world is divided into "dog people" and "cat people." Cat owners admire their pets' independence, graceful shape and movements, and wild instincts. Since cats tend to require less human companionship than dogs, they are ideal for busy people who must be away from home for long periods of time. Dogs, on the other hand, have been called the "yes men of the animal world." They have an affectionate, emotional nature and an appetite for food, regardless of whether they are really hungry or if it is good for them. Most important, dogs offer unconditional love and act out human behavior, which their more inhibited masters can enjoy vicariously.

Stress of pet loss

The death of a pet can be a devastating and stressful experience. The child who has lost a pet is inconsolable for a time; however, this brush with genuine loss may lead to maturity. Adults who lose pets often are reluctant to express themselves freely about their sorrow because they fear that others will think their behavior is childlike and self-indulgent. The fact that veterinary hospitals now send a sympathy card or letter of condolence on the death of a pet shows the awareness of the stressful effect of a pet owner's loss.

See also GRIEF.

SOURCES:

American Veterinary Medical Association. *Animal Health News and Feature Tips.* Summer 1995.

Dossey, Larry. "The Healing Power of Pets: A Look at Animal-Assisted Therapy." *Alternative Therapies* 3, no. 4 (July 1977).

Laskas, Jeanne Marie. "When the Nine Lives Are Over." *Health,* March 1997.

pharmacological approach   Therapy for disorders caused or worsened by stress are often treated with a pharmacological approach. In many cases, prescription medications are used in combination with psychotherapy, BEHAVIOR THERAPY, or some of many ALTERNATIVE THERAPIES. Prescription medication is often helpful for individuals who have ANXIETY DISORDERS, DEPRESSION, AGORAPHOBIA,

PANIC ATTACK AND PANIC DISORDER, OBSESSIVE-COMPULSIVE DISORDER, POST-TRAUMATIC STRESS DISORDER, as well as other disorders. In many cases, use of MEDITATION, BIOFEEDBACK, GUIDED IMAGERY, and RELAXATION therapy continue to be helpful after prescription medication is stopped.

While there are many effective techniques for managing stress without medications, the pharmacological approach may be helpful, sometimes just for the short term. Anxiety disorders, like some medical conditions, can be controlled but not cured; chronic conditions require long-term management, often with a combination of alternative therapies as well as pharmacological therapies.

The best principle with pharmacological therapy is to use the lowest effective dose for the shortest possible period of time. However, before any medication is taken, an individual should have a thorough medical and psychiatric examination.

Categories of medications

There are three major classes of medications used for the disorders discussed in this book: *benzodiazepines* (BZDs), *cyclic antidepressants,* and *noncyclic antidepressants.* Additionally, a number of pharmacological agents are categorized as "other antianxiety medications."

Alcohol is the oldest antistress drug and remains the most frequently used (and misused) nonspecific tranquilizer. BARBITURATE DRUGS have been available since 1903; they are respiratory depressants and are contraindicated in people with respiratory insufficiency. In the 1930s, a series of "nonbarbiturate, non-BZD" hypnotic drugs were developed. Many of them carried the same problems as the barbiturates and most are no longer available. In 1957 the first BZD, chlordiazepoxide (Librium) was introduced for the safe management of anxiety.

Benzodiazepine drugs (BZDs)

BZDs are popular choices in the late 1990s for the pharmacological management of anxiety.

Other indications for BZDs include insomnia, seizures, muscle spasms, and the induction of anesthesia. All BZDs have similar anxiolytic, sedative, and anticonvulsant properties.

The length of BZD treatment varies between individuals. Some individuals continue medications for several years. Generally, long-term anxiolytic treatment should continue for at least two weeks after complete remission of symptoms. The dose should then be tapered off, and, if possible, the medication should be discontinued. Should the symptoms return, the medication can be used again but, upon remission, tapered off.

Antidepressant medications

Antidepressants usually are not recommended for treating episodic anxiety or even excessive anxiety. However, in cases of depression for which they are prescribed, doses will vary between individuals.

Most drugs used to treat depression either mimic certain NEUROTRANSMITTERS (biochemicals that allow brain cells to communicate with each another) or alter their activity. Antidepressants are thought to decrease the activity or concentration of these neurotransmitters, which occurs during depression. The major neurotransmitters involved appear to be NOREPINEPHINE, SEROTONIN, and dopamine. The precise pharmacologic mechanisms of antidepressant drugs, as well as the balances of neurotransmitters in individuals who have depression, still are not entirely understood. As newer, more specific antidepressants are developed, understanding of antidepressants and depression evolves and improves.

Historical development of antidepressants

Antidepressant medications were developed during the 1950s after physicians noted that tuberculosis patients treated with iproniazid sometimes became extremely cheerful. The notion that this elevated mood might be a side effect of the drug led to the development of a class of antidepressants known as monoamine oxidase inhibitors (MAOIs). They were followed by the tricyclic antidepressants and lithium.

The three major categories of antidepressants are *tricyclic antidepressants* (TCAs), *monoamine oxidase inhibitors* (MAOIs), and *lithium*. There are also "novel" antidepressants.

Commonly, antidepressant medications take up to two to three weeks before having a full effect (although side effects may begin immediately). The time elapsing before the drug becomes therapeutic varies with the drug. Antidepressants may have to be taken regularly for months, even years, if their gains are to continue. For some individuals, relapse often occurs upon stopping the drug.

Tricyclic antidepressants

Tricyclic antidepressants are referred to as "tricyclic" because the chemical diagrams for these drugs resemble three rings connected together. An example of a tricyclic antidepressant is imipramine, which has been used since the late 1950s. Tricyclics elevate mood, alertness, and mental and physical activity, and improve appetite and sleep patterns in depressed individuals. When given to a nondepressed person, tricyclics do not elevate

---

BENZODIAZEPINE DRUGS

Trade name	Generic name
Long Acting	
Librium	chlordiazepoxide
Klonopin	clonazepam
Tranxene	clorazepate
Valium	diazepam
Dalmane	flurazepam
Paxipam	halazepam
Centrax	prazepam
Doral	Quazepam
Short Acting	
Xanax	alprazolam
Ativan	lorazepam
Serax	oxazepam
Restoril	temazepam
Halcion	triazolam

ANTIDEPRESSANT MEDICATIONS

Trade name	Generic name
Cyclic antidepressants	
Anafranil	clomipramine
Asendin	amoxapine
Aventyl, Pamelor	nortriptyline
Elavil, Endep	amitriptyline
Ludiomil	maprotiline
Norpramin, Pertofrane	desipramine
Sinequan, Adapin	doxepin
Surmontil	trimipramine
Tofranil, Janimine	imipramine
Vivactil	protriptyline
Monoamine oxidase inhibitors (MAOIs)	
Eldepryl	selegiline/deprenyl
Eutonyl	pargyline
Marplan	isocarboxazid
Nardil	phenelzine
Parnate	tranylcypromine
Examples of "Novel" antidepressants	
Desyrel	trazodone
Prozac	fluoxetine
Wellbutrin	bupropion

COMMONLY USED TRICYCLIC ANTIDEPRESSANTS

Trade name*	Generic name
Anafranil	climipramine
Asendin	amoxapine
Aventyl	nortriptyline
Elavil	amitriptyline
Emitrip	
Endep	
Enovil	
Janimine	imipramine
Norfranil	
Norpramin	desipramine
Pamelor	
Sinequan	doxepin
Surmontil	trimipramine
Tipramine	
Tofranil	
Tofranil-PM	
Vivactil	protriptyline

* Trade names as used in the United States.

mood or stimulate the person; instead, the effects are likely to increase anxiety and arouse feelings of unhappiness.

Tricyclic antidepressants are generally well tolerated, relatively safe, and cause minimal side effects. Their antidepressant effects, however, often take several weeks to appear; because of this lag, tricyclics are not prescribed on an "as-needed" basis.

Some depressed individuals may respond well to one tricyclic, but not at all to another. Due to the time lag of several weeks before any beneficial effects show up, a physician will try first one drug for the time needed, and then, if results are not noticeable, prescribe another tricyclic, and give it several weeks. Such trials, with their waiting and uncertainty, may lead to some anxiety and stress for both the individual and physician.

Some of the more well-known tricyclic antidepressants (and their trade names) are shown in the accompanying chart.

Side effects of tricyclic antidepressants. Side effects of tricyclic antidepressants include excessive dry mouth, sweating, blurred vision, HEADACHE, urinary hesitation, and constipation. Drowsiness and DIZZINESS, as well as vertigo, weakness, rapid heart rate, and reduced blood pressure upon standing upright are likely to occur early on, but usually disappear within the first several weeks. Tricyclics should be used cautiously in persons with heart problems.

Drug interactions and cautions. Tricyclic antidepressants and MAO inhibitors are not recommended to be combined except under unusual circumstances. A common drug interaction involves the combination of tricyclics and alcohol, and possibly other sedatives, as tricyclics enhance effects of these substances. In large doses, use of other anticholinergic drugs (those that block effects of acetylcholine, a chemical released from nerve endings in the parasympathetic division of the autonomic nervous system) may interfere with actions of histamine, serotonin, and norepinephrine. Side effects may include slurred speech, confusion, hallucinations, and memory deficits, particularly short-term memory impairment.

Monoamine oxidase inhibitors (MAOIs)

MAO inhibitors (MAOIs) are primarily used for individuals who have not responded adequately to tricyclic antidepressants. These drugs are generally considered somewhat less effective than the tricyclics, and, due to a wider range of potential and often unpredictable complications, use is limited. However, MAOIs may be prescribed for certain types of depressions and generalized anxiety disorders and are used to help individuals who have panic attacks.

When a tricyclic antidepressant is tried and discontinued because of ineffectiveness, a gap of several days is recommended before the monoamine oxidase inhibitor is tried. In the reverse case, where the MAOI is ineffective and is to be replaced by a tricyclic, a much longer period of two weeks between medications is recommended.

Interactive effects. A drawback of the MAOIs, as a group, is that they may lead to unpredictable and occasionally serious interactions with some foods and drugs. For example, combining MAOIs with a class of drugs called sympathomimetic drugs may lead to serious complications; common nasal decongestant sprays often include phenylpropanolamine or phenylephrine, both sympathomimetics. Also, cough and cold preparations or any preparation not specifically recommended by a physician should be avoided. The pain drug Demerol should not be given with MAOIs, but other pain relieving drugs, for example, morphine, can safely be used.

Individuals taking MAOIs must avoid the amino acid tyramine or they may experience a dangerous rise in blood pressure. Tyramine is present in many foods, including alcoholic beverages, cheese, liver, lima beans, and beverages containing caffeine and chocolate.

A side effect of MAOIs is that they lower blood pressure, an effect not well understood by researchers; one MAOI, pargyline, is used to treat hypertension.

Lithium

Lithium is effective in individuals who have both depression and mania and in preventing future episodes. It acts without causing sedation, but, like the tricyclics and MAO inhibitors, requires a period of use before its actions take effect. Side effects of lithium may rule it out for use as an antidepressant; there may be nausea and vomiting, muscular weakness, and confusion.

Other treatments for depression

ALPRAZOLAM (Xanax) may lift depression, although it is primarily a drug used to treat anxiety and panic disorder. In some individuals, alprazolam has shortened or interfered with panic attacks and also induced sleep. In depressed individuals with a high level of anxiety, alprazolam may be added to tricyclic antidepressants.

Development of "novel" antidepressant medications

In the last several decades, while conventional antidepressants have been helpful for many individuals, limitations of these antidepressants have been noted, namely their lack of specificity of action, delayed onset of action, side-effect profile, and potential for lethality in overdose. Approximately 20% to 30% of depressed persons do not respond to traditional antidepressants.

During the late 1980s and 1990s, the emergence of newer antidepressants, such as fluoxetine and bupropion, offered the advantages of antidepressants with fewer side effects and less potential for lethality in overdose. However, research has shown that both of these agents have unique side effects. Their overall efficacy appears to be no greater than conventional antidepressant treatments, and they also have a delayed onset of action.

The goal of recently developed antidepressants is to act faster and more powerfully than previously used antidepressants, with less frequent and less severe side effects and with more ability to target an individual's specific type of depression. Newer antidepressants are *unicyclic, bicyclic,* or of other molecular configurations. Where tricyclics and MAOIs are understood to influence chemicals known as neurotransmitters, the newer antidepressants are technically classified by their preferential influence over individual neurotransmitters—norepinephrine, serotonin, or dopamine.

Fluoxetine. Fluoxetine (Prozac), one of the "novel" antidepressants, was introduced in the United States in 1988. Fluoxetine is part of a class of selective serotonin reuptake inhibitors (SSRIs) with low toxicity and free of many side effects attributed to tricyclic antidepressants. Fluoxetine is not sedative, has no anticholinergic side effects, and does not promote weight gain. Another SSRI, Sertaline, has similar advantages.

Like other antidepressant drugs, fluoxetine does not help everyone with depression. It has its own unique side effects, including possible nausea and weight loss, both usually time limited, insomnia, and anxious agitation that occurs rarely and is dose-related. Most people adjust to these side effects.

Other antianxiety medications
Beta-blockers. Beta blockers (beta-adrenergic receptor antagonists) are frequently used in treating hypertension, angina, and migraine headaches. They are occasionally used to help individuals with symptoms of anxiety such as rapid heartbeat, tremor, tingling, perspiration, blushing, and chest constriction. A number of beta blockers are effective in treating both generalized anxiety and situationally produced anxiety, such as SOCIAL PHOBIA and PERFORMANCE ANXIETY.

Buspirone. Buspirone (trade name: BuSpar), is considered a "novelty" anti-anxiety agent and is pharmacologically unrelated to BZDs or other anxiolytics. It is popular because it causes less sedation and has less potential for dependence than other anxiolytics. However, there is a four-week lag in efficacy; with BZDs individuals notice a rapid onset of improvement.

See also AFFECTIVE DISORDERS; BENZODI-AZEPINE DRUGS; EXOGENOUS DEPRESSION; HERBAL MEDICINE; IMMUNE SYSTEM; MANIC-DEPRESSIVE DISORDER; MIND-BODY CONNECTIONS; PSYCHOTHERAPIES; VALIUM.

SOURCES:
Appleton, William S. *Prozac and the New Antidepressants: What You Need to Know About Prozac, Zoloft, Paxil, Luvox, Wellbutrin, Effexor, Serzone, and More.* New York: Plume, 1997.
Carlin, Peter. "Treat the Body, Heal the Mind." *Health.* January/February 1997.
Kahn, Ada P., and Jan Fawcett. *The Encyclopedia of Mental Health.* New York: Facts On File, 1993.
Sachs, Judith. *Nature's Prozac: Natural Therapies and Techniques to Rid Yourself of Anxiety, Depression, Panic Attacks and Stress.* Englewood Cliffs, N.J.: Prentice-Hall, 1997.
Turkington, Carol. *Making the Prozac Decision: A Guide to Antidepressants.* Los Angeles; Lowell House, 1994.
Wilkinson, Beth. *Drugs and Depression.* New York: Rosen Publishing Group, 1994.

phobia   An irrational, intense fear of an object or situation and a strong desire to avoid the feared object or situation. Most people have minor fears, for example, experiencing some ANXIETY when unable to avoid contact with bugs, bees, and other undesirable encounters. However, when a fear interferes with normal social function, causes significant distress, and is out of proportion to any real or apparent danger, it is considered a phobia.

Phobia sufferers are subject to a great deal of stress because they cannot explain or understand their fear. Nor can they voluntarily control their anxiety response and their need to avoid the dreaded stimulus or situation.

Phobic reactions that occur when the phobic stimulus appears include: *persistent and irrational panic, dread, horror or terror; rapid heartbeat, shortness of breath, trembling and overwhelming desire to flee the situation; and avoidance of the situation*

Phobias are classified by the American Psychiatric Association (*Diagnostic and Statistical Manual of Mental Disorders,* 4th ed.) as the most common form of ANXIETY DISORDER. People of all ages, at all income levels, and in all geographic locations suffer from phobias. Between 5.1% and 12.5% of Americans suffer from phobias. Broken down by age and gender, phobias are the most common mental health concern among women in all age groups and the second most common illness among men over age 25.

Categorizing phobias

Phobias cannot be neatly classified because fear of almost any situation can occur and may be associated with any other psychological symptoms. However, in a general way, phobias can be classified as:

Specific phobias, also known as *simple phobias.* Specific phobias are characterized by a persistent, irrational fear of, and compelling desire to avoid, *specific* situations or objects. The category of specific phobias contains an endless list of fears, as almost any object or situation can be phobic for any given individual.

Commonly recognized specific phobias relate to particular animals (dogs, rats, mice, birds, spiders, and snakes); enclosed spaces (claustrophobia), such as being in an elevator or sitting in the middle of a theater row; darkness; heights; or thunderstorms. Some specific phobias have to do with transportation, such as driving across bridges, riding in trains, or flying in airplanes.

Phobias related to the sight of blood or injury are unique types of specific phobias. Unlike other specific phobias, which cause increased pulse and other physiological signs of arousal, blood and injury phobias produce lower pulse and blood pressure, and bring on fainting spells.

A person who has a specific phobia experiences stressful physiological symptoms and behavior typical of many phobic disorders. However, because these fears are so specific, the individual can usually manage to avoid contact with the object of their phobia. On the other hand, individuals who fear common situations, such as riding in elevators or going over bridges, may not easily avoid these stressful stimuli.

How simple phobias start is not well understood. Researchers differ in their explanations; some report that direct conditioning—for example, a traumatic event—is an important factor, while others say that indirect learning experiences or exposure to negative instructions and vicarious experiences are also influential. Opinions vary regarding effects of family influences on specific fears. While some experts say that the majority of simple phobics come from families in which no other member of the family shares the same fear, some studies have found relatively strong associations between the fears of mothers and children. Many simple phobics are dependent or anxious individuals, and their family backgrounds may have contributed to these characteristics. Individuals who have simple phobias may not recall the origin of their fear. Treatment of the phobic symptom, however, does not have to wait until the origin is uncovered.

Specific phobias can begin at any age. However, certain phobias are more common among certain age groups. For example, infants often fear loud noises and strangers. Fear of animals, which is prevalent in children between the ages of nine to 11, stays with many girls after age 11 but disappears in most boys. Fear of aging occurs most commonly in people over age 50.

SOCIAL PHOBIA involves fear of being scrutinized by others. People with social phobias may fear making mistakes, being criticized, and making fools of themselves. They also may fear eating or making a speech in public, using public toilets, writing in public, and making complaints. Because of the fear of interacting with the opposite sex, strangers, or aggressive individuals, social phobics are stressed when they are in social or business situations such as parties, meetings, and interviews. Some individuals will participate in a particular activity only when they cannot be seen—for example, swimming in the dark. Social phobias develop over many months or years, but sometimes a precipitating event can be determined.

Social phobics have ongoing problems with excessive stress, generalized anxiety, dependence, and DEPRESSION. Sweating, fainting, blushing, and vomiting may all be symptoms of social phobia.

Usually social phobias begin in a range from 15 to 30 years of age. They tend to persist throughout adulthood, unlike specific or simple phobias, which tend to diminish as the individual enters young adulthood. Many such individuals have traits that interfere with social and marital adjustment.

Some social phobics attribute their fears to direct conditioning, some to vicarious factors, and some to instructional and informational factors; direct negative learning experience may play an important role. Development of social phobias may be influenced somewhat by parental behavior. For example, parents who have few friends and are socially anxious in the presence of others may influence their children to react in similar ways. Also, the presence of anxiety in children is often associated with criticism and verbal punishment.

AGORAPHOBIA. Possibly the most stressful and serious of the phobias. Agoraphobics are afraid to leave a safe place such as their home or be apart from a safe person such as a spouse or close relative. Such separations cause intense anxiety and panic. A small percentage of agoraphobics remain housebound, sometimes for many years.

Symptoms of agoraphobia include a wide range of avoidance behaviors, including a fear of entering public places or open spaces, traveling, social interaction, and even being alone. Agoraphobics often have physiological symptoms such as palpitations, lightness in the head, weakness, atypical chest pain, and difficulty in breathing. Some agoraphobics have panic attacks. Agoraphobics express fears of losing CONTROL, going insane, embarrassing themselves, and dying.

Phobias of internal stimuli. These are fears that develop within the individual without reason. As an example, fear of dying from an illness, such as cancer, heart disease, or venereal disease, for which there are no physical symptoms. Some of these fears, which occur in both sexes, may be regarded as an extreme form of hypochondria. Often characteristic of depressive illnesses, these phobias improve when the depression improves.

Obsessive phobias. Examples of obsessive phobias are fear of harming people or babies, fear of swearing, or a fear of contamination that leads to obsessive hand washing and cleaning. Such phobias usually occur along with other obsessive-compulsive symptoms.

Treatment of phobias
Many forms of therapy, ranging from BEHAVIOR THERAPY to psychoanalysis, are used by qualified psychiatrists, psychologists, social workers, and other mental health professional to treat phobias.

In behavior therapy, the therapist focuses on the symptoms and attempts to change the physiological reactions. There are phobic people who have good results with exposure therapy. They are able to face their feared object or situation and, as a result, are desensitized. Many others are helped with BIOFEEDBACK, RELAXATION, GUIDED IMAGERY, and MEDITATION therapies.

Sometimes antianxiety drugs and a variety of other medications can help people face their phobic situations and overcome them.

Pharmacological treatment for phobias varies with individuals and should be used only with supervision by a physician or mental health professional.

See also ALTERNATIVE THERAPIES; OBSESSIVE-COMPULSIVE DISORDER; PANIC ATTACKS AND PANIC DISORDER; PERFORMANCE ANXIETY; PHARMACOLOGICAL APPROACH; PSYCHOTHERAPIES; PUBLIC SPEAKING.

FOR FURTHER INFORMATION:
American Psychiatric Association
1400 K Street NW
Washington, DC 20005
Phone: (202) 682-6000

Anxiety Disorders Association of America
11900 Parklawn Drive (Suite 100)
Rockville, MD 20852
Phone: (301) 231-9350

National Mental Health Association
1021 Prince Street
Alexandria, VA 22314-2971
Phone: (703) 684-7722

SOURCES:
American Psychiatric Association. *Diagnostic and Statistical Manual of Mental Disorders,* 4th ed. Washington, D.C.: American Psychiatric Association, 1994.
Bourne, Edmund J. *The Anxiety & Phobia Workbook.* Oakland: New Harbinger Publications, 1995.
Kahn, Ada P., and Jan Fawcett. *The Encyclopedia of Mental Health.* New York: Facts On File, 1993.
Monroe, Judy. *Phobias: Everything You Wanted to Know, But Were Afraid to Ask.* Springfield, N.J.: Enslow Publishers, 1996.
Nardo, Don. *Anxieties and Phobias.* New York: Chelsea House, 1992.

physician-assisted suicide See END-OF-LIFE CARE.

physicians   Stress affects physicians, just as it does members of any other occupational group. An increasing number of American physicians are becoming employees in managed care systems, and this possibly means that they will have less AUTONOMY and less CONTROL over their time management. Some physicians will change their profession entirely or will find other work in the health care field, such as medical administrators, government analysts, or health journal editors.

According to Peter Orton, in *Canadian Family Physician,* among family physicians, stressors predicting job dissatisfaction and lack of mental well-being have included the demands of the job and patient expectations, interference with family life, constant interruptions at work and home, practice administration, and greater external management of the profession.

Stress has effects on physicians, staff, family, and patients. Among physicians, stress is a leading cause for SUICIDE, accidental poisoning, alcoholism, liver disease, substance abuse, and ANXIETY and DEPRESSION; marital problems and accidents increase because of these factors.

The effect on physicians' families often goes unnoticed until it is too late. While spouses believe their partners are emotionally drained, physicians deny it. Spouses often comment on physicians' inability to discuss emotional problems and complain that they are essentially left to bring up their children as single parents. This has an effect on marital relationships, particularly when it is a relationship between two doctors.

Staff and patients also suffer from physicians' stress. Staff may be blamed for the physicians' mistakes and be the butt of their short tempers. Patients complain of being kept waiting for doctors' appointments and hurried through their examinations.

Still, there are many benefits in being a physician, particularly a family physician. Historically, they have had autonomy, job security, and career opportunities. Their work allows for a regular sharing of experiences with colleagues.

Preventing stress
Once a stress-related problem is recognized by physicians, they can try to reduce demands on

their time. Stressors should be identified at an early stage and practical steps taken to reduce them. In some cases, physicians need to improve their organizational skills, become proactive, and take control. This involves using tools of human resource management, time management, delegation, COMMUNICATION, and teamwork.

COPING mechanisms can be improved by seeking support in the WORKPLACE and at home. Time should be allocated for family, exercise and relaxation.

SOURCES:

Chambers, R. "Health and Lifestyle of General Practitioners and Teachers." *Occupational Medicine* 42, no. 2 (1992): 69-78.

McCue, J. "The Effects of Stress on Physicians and Their Medical Practice." *New England Journal of Medicine* 306 (1982): 458–63.

Orton, Peter. "Stress and Family Physicians." *Canadian Family Physician* 41 (February 1995).

placebo effect   The therapeutic benefit of a chemically inactive substance that has no medicinal effect but that superficially resembles an active pharmacological effect or therapy. The word "placebo" Latin and means "I shall please." Patients believe that taking a placebo will have positive effects on their health, and this can be an important factor in relieving the stresses involved in many illnesses and conditions.

Usually the word "placebo" refers to a pill or capsule that has no pharmacologically active substance; however, the term "placebo effect" is not restricted to therapy with an inert pill. It applies also to therapeutic results, both psychological and physiological, that occur by any method that has no demonstrable specific action on the disorder being treated.

Sometimes placebos induce reactions because of the power of suggestion. For example, individuals enrolled in a "double-blind" study do not know if they are taking a placebo or the real drug, and many improve because they think they are taking an active substance. The placebo effect was described in *The Healing Mind,* by Irving Oyle. "Whatever you put your trust in can be the precipitating agent for your cure."

According to Alan H. Roberts, in *Mind/Body MEDICINE*, patients improve after treatment because of specific effects or placebo effects, or a combination of the two. A full evaluation of any treatment includes a determination of whether the treatment is effective and the degree to which improvements are a consequence of understanding specific and nonspecific factors and how they work. Although it is commonly understood that placebo effects account for approximately 33% of treatment effectiveness, recent reviews and studies indicate that placebo effects in clinical situations may be as high as 70% when both doctors and patients believe that a treatment will be efficacious.

See also ALTERNATIVE THERAPIES; MIND-BODY CONNECTIONS; PRAYER.

SOURCES:

Oyle, Irving. *The Healing Mind: You Can Cure Yourself Without Drugs.* Millbrae, Calif.: Celestial Arts, 1975.

Roberts, Alan H. "The Power Placebo Revisited: Magnitude of Nonspecific Effects." *Mind/Body MEDICINE* 1, no. 1 (March 1995).

plant closings   See CORPORATE BUYOUT; COST-CUTTING; DOWNSIZING; LAYOFFS; MERGERS.

plastic surgery   Any operation carried out to repair or reconstruct skin and underlying tissues that have been damaged or lost by injury or disease, malformed since birth, or changed with aging. Plastic surgery techniques enable an injured or diseased person to regain some sense of SELF-ESTEEM and remove the stress of coping with the deformity. Operations performed mainly to improve appearance in a healthy person are known as COSMETIC SURGERY.

The scope of plastic surgery improved dramatically during the 1990s by the use of microsurgical techniques to join blood vessels, allowing transfer of blocks of skin and muscle from one part of the body to another.

See also BODY IMAGE.

play therapy Used in psychotherapy as a treatment for stress-related problems in children. It is based on the theory that all play in children has some symbolic significance.

Children choose from toys, such as dolls and puppets, and drawing and art materials, such as clay and finger paint, and games. These activities mirror children's emotional life and fantasies, enabling them to act out feelings and thoughts that cause anxiety and stress. Observing them at play helps the therapist diagnose the source of the child's stresses. Play therapy is also referred to as analytical play therapy and ludotherapy.

See also PSYCHOTHERAPIES.

poison ivy Poison ivy (including sumac and oak) can cause severe skin rashes and is the most common cause of allergic reactions in the United States. It affects 10–50 million Americans every year and can be a very stressful experience.

Itching, burning and blistering cause stress for poison ivy sufferers; they also experience stress from knowing that they can get poison ivy without coming in contact with the plant. The colorless or slightly yellow oil (urushiol) that oozes from any cut or crushed part of the plant, including the stem and the leaves, is easily spread. Sticky, and virtually invisible, it can be carried on the fur of animals, on garden tools and sports equipment, or on any objects that have come into contact with a crushed or broken plant. The effect on the skin can be neutralized to an inactive state by water.

Once the urushiol touches the skin, it penetrates in a few minutes. In those who are sensitive, a reaction appears in the form of a line or streak of rash, sometimes resembling insect bites, within 12 to 48 hours. Redness and

swelling will be followed by blisters and severe itching. It is additionally stressful because the rash can affect almost any part of the body, especially areas where the skin is thin; the soles of the feet and palms of the hands are thicker and less susceptible.

First-aid treatment includes thorough cleansing of the infected area, sponging with alcohol, and applying calamine lotion. Severe reactions should be reported to a physician, who may prescribe corticosteroid drugs to be taken by mouth or injection.

Prevention is the best cure. One should be watchful for the plants whenever out of doors. If going to areas where poison oak or ivy is likely to grow, wear protective clothing.

See also ALLERGIES.

FOR FURTHER INFORMATION:
American Academy of Dermatology
930 Meacham
Schaumburg, IL 60172-4965
Phone: (708) 330-0230

politically correct Term coined in the early 1990s that refers to a sensitivity about many causes, including the needs and problems of minorities and disabled people, avoidance of sexist and racist terms and attitudes, and respect for animals and the environment. In an effort to be "politically correct," politicians, government officials, and organizational leaders are adding an additional stressor to their own activities as well as those of their constituents who must use an additional caution in their actions.

SOURCE:
Kahn, Ada P., and Jan Fawcett. *The Encyclopedia of Mental Health.* New York: Facts On File, 1993.

postpartum depression DEPRESSION immediately following the delivery of a baby. It is probably caused by hormonal changes after the birth as well as stressful psychological factors. Postpartum depression ranges from extremely common and short-lived "maternity blues" or "baby blues" to a state of serious depression in which the mother may have to be hospitalized.

Some women become depressed after CHILDBIRTH because they fear being a parent or being a failure as a parent. They feel less loving toward the baby than they think they should and feel sexually unattractive to their mates because their bodies have not regained normal shape. Women may be overwhelmed with chores of a new baby, and sleep deprivation, caused by the baby's frequent waking during the night, can lead to additional stresses of irritability and chronic fatigue. If women go from careers outside the home into full-time motherhood, they may also suffer a loss of SELF-ESTEEM. With reassurance and support from family and friends, this type of "blues" lasts only two or three days. However, in about 10% to 15% of women the depression is more marked and lasts for weeks. There is a constant feeling of tiredness, difficulty sleeping, restlessness and loss of appetite. These symptoms are more likely to happen when there is a strained relationship with the father, financial or other concerns, no family support or a personality disorder. First-time mothers, single mothers, or women who suffered from depression during PREGNANCY are likely sufferers. The condition may clear up on its own or may be treated with antidepressant drugs.

Persistent, severe depressions may become major depressions or bipolar (manic-depressive disorders) and require psychiatric treatment.

post-traumatic stress disorder (PTSD) ANXIETY DISORDER produced by an unusual and extremely stressful event, such as assault, an act of violence, rape, natural disaster, or physical injury. PTSD has been referred to as battle fatigue or shell shock when it occurred from military combat.

Often PTSD surfaces several months or even years later, although its symptoms can occur soon after the event. Sufferers characteristically reexperience the trauma in painful recollections or recurrent DREAMS or nightmares. Some have diminished emotional responsiveness ("numbing"), feelings of estrangement from others, insomnia, disturbed sleep, difficulty in concentrating or remembering, GUILT about surviving when others did not, avoidance of activities that cause recollection of the traumatic event, and intensive thoughts related to the event. Avoidance behavior also affects sufferers' relationships with others because they often avoid close emotional ties with family, colleagues, and friends.

Sometimes the re-experience comes as a sudden, painful rush of EMOTIONS that seem to have no cause. These emotions may be anger or intense fear. Some PTSD sufferers endure anxiety and panic attacks as a result. During panic attacks, their throats tighten, BREATHING and heart rate increase, and they may feel dizzy and nauseated.

Overcoming PTSD
Individuals who have PTSD can learn to work through the trauma and pain and resolve their anxieties. Individual psychotherapy is one of many useful therapies. PTSD results, in part, from the difference between the individual's personal values and the reality of what he/she witnessed or experienced during the traumatic event. Psychotherapy helps the individual examine his/her values and behavior with the goal of resolving the conscious and unconscious conflicts that were created. Additionally, the individual works to build SELF-ESTEEM and self-control, develops a reasonable sense of personal accountability, and renews a sense of integrity and personal pride.

In many cases, family therapy is recommended because members of the family may affect and be affected by the PTSD sufferer. Some spouses and children report that their loved one does not communicate, show affection, or share in family life. The therapist can help members of the family recognize and cope with the range of emotions they feel and, when needed, help them improve their communication skills and learn techniques for parenting and stress management.

A newer technique for PTSD involves "rap" groups, in which survivors of similar traumatic events are encouraged to share their experiences and reactions. Group members help each other realize that many people have gone through the same thing and experienced the same emotions. Over time, the members will experience an improved self-image and self esteem. Antidepressant medications have also been reported to reverse symptoms of PTSD.

See also COMMUNICATION; CONTROL; COPING; LISTENING; PSYCHOTHERAPIES.

FOR FURTHER INFORMATION:
Anxiety Disorders Association of America
11900 Parklawn Drive (Suite 100)
Rockville, MD 20852
Phone: (301) 231-9350

National Association of Veterans Administration
  Chiefs of Psychiatry
54th Street and 48th Avenue
Minneapolis, MN 55417
Phone: (612) 725-6767

National Institutes of Mental Health
5600 Fishers Lane
Rockville, MD 20857
Phone: (301) 443-2403

U.S. Veterans Administration
Mental Health and Behavioral Sciences Services
810 Vermont Avenue, NW (Room 915)
Washington, DC 20410
Phone: (202) 389-3416

SOURCES:
Catherall, Donald Roy. *Back From the Brink: A Family Guide to Overcoming Traumatic Stress.* New York: Bantam Books, 1992.
Kahn, Ada P., and Jan Fawcett. *The Encyclopedia of Mental Health.* New York: Facts On File, 1993.
Porterfield, Kay Marie. *Straight Talk About Post-Traumatic Stress Disorder: Coping with the Aftermath of Trauma.* New York: Facts On File, 1996.

powerlessness   Lacking the authority or capacity to act. It is a stressful situation for most people because they feel that they lack CONTROL and know that they cannot significantly affect the outcome of a situation.

For some people, feelings of powerlessness underlie DEPRESSION, suspiciousness, and aggressive behavior. Powerlessness is also associated with withdrawal, passivity, submissiveness, apathy, increased frustration, agitation, ANXIETY, AGGRESSION, acting-out behavior, and even violence.

A person who feels powerless may be unable to set goals or follow through on activities relating to school, work, or family life. This feeling can be induced by illness and hospitalization, because such events compromise a sense of self. Strategies to help people who feel powerless include teaching them to gain control of a situation and helping them to develop better means of COPING with the stressors in life.

See also AUTONOMY; SELF-ESTEEM.

SOURCE:
McFarland, Gertrude K., and Mary Durand Thomas. *Psychiatric Mental Health Nursing.* Philadelphia: J.B. Lippincott, 1991.

prayer   Act of the individual speaking to God in adoration, confession, supplication, or thanksgiving. According to researchers, repeating a prayer can help reduce stress and improve physical ailments by lowering the heart rate, breathing rate, and brain wave activity.

At a national conference on faith in Boston in 1995, experts said that the idea of prayer is gaining support among cost-conscious health organizations. "The supposed gulf between science and spirituality in healing does not always exist," said Herbert BENSON, M.D., a Harvard Medical School professor. Benson explained that scientific studies have demonstrated that, by repeating prayers, words, or sounds and passively disregarding other thoughts, many people are able to trigger a specific set of beneficial physiological changes. Studies show that this RELAXATION response decreased visits to health maintenance organizations by 36%.

Another internationally known authority in the field of mind-body medicine, Larry DOSSEY, M.D., said that the power of prayer to heal should no longer be regarded as just a matter of faith. Dossey is a physician who has practiced medicine for more than 20 years. He has become a believer, not in RELIGION, but in a growing body of research suggesting that prayer is an important scientifically verifiable factor in healing. "I have come to regard it as one of the best-kept secrets in medical science," he says in his book, *Healing Words: The Power and the Practice of Medicine.*

See also ALTERNATIVE THERAPIES.

SOURCES:
Dossey, Larry. *Healing Words (The Power of Prayer and the Practice of Medicine),* San Francisco: Harper, 1993.
———.*Meaning and Medicine (Lessons from a Doctor's Tales of Breakthrough and Healing).* New York: Bantam/Doubleday, 1991.

pregnancy The period while a woman is carrying an embryo/fetus from conception to birth; it is marked by a cessation of menses. Many women may find that their MOODS are more changeable and that they are subject to mental, emotional, and physiological stresses at this time. They may experience bouts of DEPRESSION, become easily annoyed or angered, feel more lethargic than usual, and be subject to periods of CRYING. Emotional changes are due to hormonal as well as emotional adjustments involved in pregnancy.

An important influence in reducing the natural stressors of pregnancy is a supportive emotional environment during and after the pregnancy. While most couples have a positive attitude, others have children to please the grandparents or because "everybody's doing it." In some cases, conception occurs in an attempt to save a marriage that is dysfunctional or to deal with anxiety about sterility. There are also anxieties relating to such questions as: Was the child wanted, was an abortion attempted or considered, or are there hereditary disorders in the family. However, these anxieties usually are replaced by positive feelings as signs of life are experienced and the pregnancy progresses.

For many women, an early symptom of pregnancy is morning sickness, which is sometimes considered "imaginary" but is a very real problem for sufferers. Nausea during the first months of pregnancy may be due to a low level of vitamin B^6, or may occur because of the natural slowing down of a pregnant woman's digestive process. When food remains undigested in the stomach for longer periods than normal, nausea and the urge to vomit occurs. Morning sickness usually diminishes or disappears by the time the pregnancy is in the fourth month. Other symptoms of pregnancy that can be troublesome are CONSTIPATION, HEMORRHOIDS, HEARTBURN, urinary tact infections, swollen ankles, BACK PAINS, varicose veins, leg cramps, and breathlessness.

Women may cope with the psychological stresses of pregnancy better when they begin participating in "prepared CHILDBIRTH" classes, offered by many hospitals, which teach prospective parents about the physiological changes that occur during pregnancy and labor. These classes provide exercises to help the prospective mothers learn to relax and reduce tension. An example is the popular Lamaze method, named for a French obstetrician, which involves breathing and relaxing methods and massage routines for the expectant mother and her coaching partner right through the birth itself.

Men and pregnancy
Couvade (the French word for *hatching*) is the term applied to the range of sympathetic

physical changes men go through during their wives' pregnancy. Some men actually experience such symptoms as nausea, fatigue, back pain, and weight gain as a result of the stresses of anticipated fatherhood. In Western cultures, however, men have a role in pregnancy and often participate in prenatal education classes and the birth event itself.

Baby blues

Endocrine changes after childbirth as well as fatigue from being awakened during the night to feed the newborn often lead to POST-PARTUM DEPRESSION, or "baby blues." Some women become weepy a few days after giving birth. Some who experience clinical depressive symptoms may partially reject the infant and feel withdrawn. This response becomes evident in difficulties in feeding and patterns of mother-child interaction. In most cases, postpartum depression does not last more than two weeks. However, if it persists longer or if a woman develops irrational fears, despair, hopelessness, and violent anger toward the new baby, professional help should be sought.

Fears lead to stress in pregnancy

Fears of pregnancy stem from both psychological and physical sources. For example, unmarried women fear conceiving and bearing a child out of wedlock, while some married women do not want a child; some fear the pain of childbirth, while others are frightened of dying during childbirth; some fear that their pregnancy makes them unattractive to their husbands, while others are concerned about returning to their original physical appearance.

Many women become anxious and embarrassed by the physical symptoms associated with pregnancy. Morning sickness, food cravings, frequent urination, water retention, bloating, and swollen breasts are some of their complaints. First-time mothers may not understand the movements of the fetus and

fear that their baby is abnormal or dead. Recent findings about effects on the fetus of the mother's smoking and alcohol consumption have caused many pregnant women to abstain out of fear that they will have an unhealthy baby.

Pregnancy and sexual intercourse

Marital stress arises for many couples during pregnancy when they become concerned about the advisability of continuing sexual intercourse during pregnancy. In many relationships, partners may fear hurting the fetus or the man may fear hurting the woman. Depending on the course of the pregnancy, gynecologists usually allow women who have no unusual vaginal discharges, pain, or other symptoms, to continue sexual relations until the seventh month. In later months, modifications of coital position are suggested to assure that intercourse will not harm the baby or cause a miscarriage.

Teenage pregnancy

Twenty percent of all live births in the United States are to adolescent mothers. The adolescent pregnancy rate in the United States is greater than in any other Western country. Infants of teenage mothers are at significantly higher risk for "failure to thrive" syndrome, physical abuse, school failure, and behavior disturbances. Many teenage mothers are unmarried and will face difficulties in continuing with their own education and finding employment. Unfortunately, many adolescent fathers do not provide assistance or maintain contact with their young families.

Some adolescent girls who become pregnant may have had the fantasy of becoming autonomous and independent from their families. These ideas quickly disappear as the young women face the reality of the need for dependence. Many such young women, both before and after the pregnancy, have persistent low moods and poor SELF-ESTEEM. Usual developmental landmarks, including separation and disengagement from her family, pursuit of academic and career goals, and the experience of individuation, may be missed as the adolescent girl must continue to rely on her family throughout the pregnancy and often beyond.

Pregnancy loss

Experts say that 20% to 30% of expectant couples will face the emotional pain and stress of prenatal loss. When a miscarriage occurs very early in a pregnancy, some people think it's "nature's way," and that the couple should put the miscarriage behind them and go on with their lives. Jane Summers, M.D., director, Women's Mental Health Program, Pennsylvania Hospital, disagrees. "You cannot predict the level of attachment based on the length of pregnancy." According to Dr. Summers, parents-to-be develop a fantasy of their baby. When pregnancy loss occurs, they lose their fantasy baby: Even though they never got to see their baby smile or hear the baby coo, the child is real to them in many ways.

Dr. Summers added: "Pregnancy loss has much in common with other losses and, in some ways, can be more painful. When an adult dies, mourners have memories of the deceased that can be shared. The parents of an unborn infant have only their private hopes and dreams. There are no tangible memories to laugh and cry about with others."

While women may have a harder time dealing with the loss, some men have a particularly hard time, too. Says Martin Rosenzweig, M.D., director, Mood Disorder Programs, Pennsylvania Hospital, "People extend sympathy to a woman in a way that may not be extended to a man." Although not as obvious, men also may have dreams for their unborn child. Often his spousal role may prevent a man from sharing his feelings, because he must be strong for his wife. At the same time, the wife may interpret his silence as not caring. That's why it is so important for

---

HELPING OVERCOME THE STRESS OF PREGNANCY LOSS

- For parents who have experienced a loss: After several weeks have passed, don't hesitate to seek medical facts to help clarify misconceptions and facilitate your grieving process.
- Join a support group and share your experience with others.
- Plan how you will spend anniversary dates.
- Accept the help and support of family and friends.
- Give yourself time to heal.
- For friends and relatives of the grieving parents: don't trivialize the parents' GRIEF with clichés such as "Don't worry, you'll have another."
- Don't turn away from the grieving couple; try to provide a sympathetic ear and support, except when the couple doesn't want to talk.
- Help with tasks such as minding the grieving couple's other children, shopping, or preparing meals.
- If the baby was named, refer to the name and recognize anniversary dates.

---

couples to talk to each other about how they feel about the loss.

Typically, reaction of couples to the initial loss follows a continuum. First, couples feel numb, empty, and shocked and are often in a state of disbelief. Denial, which may turn to anger or rage, can follow. Next comes a series of "what ifs." What if the wife hadn't gone dancing; what if the husband hadn't taken the wife camping? Would the baby be alive? Though these reactions are unrealistic, they are typical feelings of self-blame.

Emotions can be accompanied by physical reactions as well. Couples may notice changes in sleeping and eating habits, or feel anxious or tired. With time most people come to terms with their loss. However, if symptoms continue for too long, professional support can help. A therapist can help people to come to terms with guilt and anger, and separate reality from perception.

Assisted reproduction techniques
Pregnancy and motherhood without marriage has become more culturally acceptable in some Western countries. Today, couples who cannot conceive can become parents with use of "assisted reproduction" techniques including *in vitro* fertilization and artificial insemination. Surrogate motherhood is also gaining some degree of acceptance, despite legal complications. Women who delay motherhood into their late thirties or early forties, because of their own or their husbands' careers or because of the attraction of the single life, face diminished fertility and greater anxiety about possibility of birth defects, which increase with maternal age. However, amniocentesis (testing the amniotic fluid to detect abnormalities in the fetus) can allay some fears of women who postpone motherhood.

See also INFERTILITY; UNWED MOTHERS.

FOR FURTHER INFORMATION:
American College of Obstetricians and
   Gynecologists
409 12th St. SW
Washington, DC 20024-2188
Phone: (202) 638-5577

American College of Nurse-Midwives
1522 K St. NW (Suite 1000)
Washington, DC 20005
Phone: (202) 289-0171

Planned Parenthood Federation of America
810 Seventh Avenue
New York, NY 10019
Phone: (212) 541-7800

SOURCES:
Eisenberg, Arlene, Heidi Eisenberg Murkoff, and Sandee Hathaway. *What to Expect When You're Expecting.* New York: Workman Publishing, 1984.
Kahn, Ada P., and Jan Fawcett. *The Encyclopedia of Mental Health.* New York: Facts On File, 1993.
Rockwell, Beverly. "Expectant Fathers: Changes and Concerns." *Canadian Family Physician* 35 (May 1989): 663–65.

premenstrual syndrome (PMS)   See MENSTRUATION.

pro-choice and pro-life   Pro-life is the term used for those in favor of upholding the right to life for the developing fetus and who are therefore against abortion; pro-choice is the term used for those in favor of a woman's right to choose whether or not to have an ABORTION.

These terms arose in the United States in the 1970s and by the early 1980s had become central to political debate and an important election issue. Pro-life advocates, along with pro-family advocates who want a return to values based on the family unit, oppose legalizing abortion. Pro-choice advocates believe their position supports the civil rights of all women. The controversy between these groups continued throughout the 1990s, erupting in shootings and bombings by pro-lifers and causing emotional stress for individuals on both sides of the issue.

progressive muscle relaxation   Also known as progressive RELAXATION; a stress management procedure in which individuals learn to make heightened observations of what goes on under their skin. They learn to control all of the skeletal muscles so that any portion can be systematically relaxed or tensed by choice.

First, there is recognition of subtle states of tension. When a muscle contracts (tenses), waves of neural impulses are generated and carried to the brain along neural pathways. This muscle-neural phenomenon is an observable sign of tension.

Next, having learned to identify the tension sensation, the individual learns to relax it. Relaxation is the elongation (lengthening) of skeletal muscle fibers, which then eliminates the tension sensation. This general procedure of identifying a local state of tension, relaxing it away, and making the contrast between the tension and ensuing relaxation is then applied to all of the major muscle groups.

As a stress management technique, progressive relaxation is effective only when individuals have the ability to selectively elongate their muscle fibers on command. They can then exercise the self-control required for progressive relaxation and more rationally deal with the stressful situation.

See also ALTERNATIVE THERAPIES; BIOFEEDBACK.

SOURCES:

Jacobsen, E. "The Origins and Development of Progressive Relaxation." *Journal of Behavior Therapy and Experimental Psychiatry* 8 (1977): 119–23.
————*Progressive Relaxation,* 2nd ed. Chicago: University of Chicago Press, 1983.
Lehrer, Paul M., and Robert L. Woolfolk, eds. *Principles and Practice of Stress Management,* 2nd ed. New York: Guilford Press, 1993.

prostate cancer   The prostate is a walnut-sized gland located at the base of the bladder in males. It surrounds a part of the urethra, the tube that carries urine from the bladder through the penis. Prostate cancer is a malignant growth in the outer zone of the prostate gland. It is the second most common CANCER in men; particularly during the latter part of the 20th century, the threat of prostate cancer, which seems to be on the rise, has become a stressful issue. However, the increase in incidence may be partially attributed to early examinations for the disease. When prostate cancer is discovered at an early stage, the outlook for recovery is very good.

This disease is especially common in African-American men and may run in families. The fathers and brothers of men who have prostate cancer appear to have three times the risk of dying from the disease.

Symptoms are caused by enlargement of the prostate and include difficulty in starting urination, poor flow of urine, and increased frequency of urination. Eventually the flow of urine may cease because the urethra is blocked or because cancer has spread to the bladder and ureters. In advanced cases, pain may be in the nerves of the pelvis or be spread by cancer to anywhere in the body.

Cancer of the prostate is diagnosed when the physician feels the prostate through the rectum and it is hard and knobby. This is verified by ultrasound scanning, pyelography, and prostatic biopsy. Also, a simple, painless blood test is available to detect prostate cancer. Treatment may be surgical removal of the prostate, radiation, or hormonal therapy.

SOURCES:

Goldfinger, Stephen E. "The Big Chill: Prostate Cancer." *Harvard Health Letter* 20, no. 11 (September 1995).
————. "Carnal Knowledge: Diet and the Prostate." *Harvard Health Letter* 19, no. 9 (July 1994).
————. "Radioactive Seeds: Prostate Cancer." *Harvard Health Letter.* 21, no. 3 (January 1996).
Jacobsen, S.J., et al. "Incidence of Prostatic Cancer Diagnosis in the Era Before and After Serum Prostate-Specific Antigen Testing." *Journal of the American Medical Association* 274, no. 18 (November 8, 1995): 1445–49.

prozac   See PHARMACOLOGICAL APPROACH.

psoriasis   A common and persistent skin disease characterized by thickened patches of inflamed, red skin covered by silvery scales. It causes physical discomfort as well as social embarrassment. The diagnosis of psoriasis is a source of stress to affected individuals because there is no treatment that permanently cures the disease.

In the United States, two out of every hundred people between the ages of 10 and 30, have psoriasis (four to five million people). Approximately 150,000 new cases occur each year. Psoriasis cannot be passed from one person to another, although it is more likely to occur in individuals whose family members have it. The name of the disease comes from the Greek word meaning "itch."

Causes of psoriasis

Dermatologists say that specific causes are unknown; however, there may be an abnormality in the functioning of certain white cells in the bloodstream, which triggers inflammation in the skin, causing the skin to shed itself too rapidly, every three to four days. New spots may be noticed 10 to 14 days after the skin is cut, scratched, or severely sunburned. Psoriasis also can be activated by infections, such as strep throat, and by certain medications. Dry skin and lack of sunlight sometimes bring about flareups of the disease.

Forms of psoriasis

Forms of psoriasis differ in the shape and pattern of the scales, how long they last, and where they are. The most common form begins with little red bumps, which gradually grow larger and form scales. Although the top scales flake off easily and often, scales below the surface stick together. When they are removed, the tender, exposed skin bleeds; these small red areas grow, sometimes becoming quite large. The most common sites affected by psoriasis are the elbows, knees, groin and genitals, arms, legs, scalp, and nails. It often appears in the same sites on both sides of the body.

Psoriasis affects nails by pitting them, and causing them to loosen, thicken, or crumble. Inverse psoriasis occurs in the armpit, under the breast, and in skin folds around the groin, buttocks, and genitals. Guttate psoriasis usually affects children and young adults. It often shows up after a sore throat, with many small, red, drop-like, scaly spots appearing on the skin. It often clears up without treatment in a few months or less.

Diagnosis and treatment of psoriasis

Dermatologists make a diagnosis of psoriasis by examining the skin, nails, and scalp, and may take a skin biopsy for microscopic examination. The goal of treatment is to reduce inflammation and slow down rapid skin cell division.

Psoriasis attacks may improve with moderate exposure to sunlight or an ultraviolet lamp and use of a smoothing, emollient cream. Moderate attacks are treated with an ointment containing coal tar or anthralin. Other methods of treating psoriasis include corticosteroid drugs, PUVA (a type of phototherapy) and some types of anticancer drugs, such as methotrexate.

Some patients with severe psoriasis are treated with the Goeckerman treatment, named for a Mayo Clinic dermatologist who first reported the treatment in 1925. The treatment combines coal tar dressings and ultraviolet light and is performed in specialized centers.

Dermatologists and researchers are continually testing new drugs and treatments. Currently, there is considerable interest in investigating other medications, such as cyclosporin, a drug used in patients who receive organ transplants.

See also PAIN.

SOURCE:
Goldfinger, Stephen E. "Scales of Injustice: Psoriasis." *Harvard Health Letter,* 20, no. 2 (December 1994).

psychiatrist A physician (medical doctor with an M.D. degree) who specializes in the diagnosis and treatment of mental, emotional, or behavioral problems; some psychiatrists do research in the field of mental health. Many people who cannot cope with the stresses in their lives seek help from psychiatrists. Psychiatrists trace the patient's personal and family history to seek possible causes of a problem. A psychiatrist can prescribe counseling, individually or in groups, and medications and, if necessary, can admit patients to hospitals.

Psychiatrists are trained in a variety of diagnostic techniques and therapies. There is a strong medical emphasis because of the rapid development of techniques of psycho-pharmacology which require a knowledge of pharmacology, physiology, cardiology, and endocrinology, all subjects taught in medical training. Recent advances in neuroscience, as it relates to behavior, have provided a strong medical and psychosocial focus for psychiatry.

In addition to providing direct patient care, many general, child, and adolescent psychiatrists devote time to other professional activities, such as administration, medical teaching, and research, and many work in more than one setting. Psychiatrists today are likely to devote at least part of their practice hours to salaried and managed care settings, including health maintenance organizations, preferred provider organizations and large hospital systems.

Cooperation and consultation between psychiatrists, primary care physicians, and other health care practitioners continues to be important for the provision of comprehensive care to patients. Especially in rural areas, primary care providers are critical gatekeepers for the diagnosis and treatment of mental health problems. The detection of mental disorders and the treatment of the less severe disorders, including the prescription of medications, often take place in a primary medical setting. Primary care physicians, however, are less likely than psychiatrists to treat patients with serious or complex mental disorders, such as patients with dual diagnoses or comorbidity of psychiatric and medical illnesses. Primary care physicians are more likely to prescribe medications for anxiety, while psychiatrists are more likely to prescribe drugs for DEPRESSION.

See also PHARMACOLOGICAL APPROACH; PSYCHOTHERAPIES.

SOURCES:
"The Future of Psychiatry." *Journal of the American Medical Association* 264, no. 19 (November 21, 1990).

Manderscheid, R.W., and M.A. Sonnenschein, eds. *Mental Health, United States, 1990.* DHHS Pub. No. (ADM) 90–1708. Washington, D.C.: Government Printing Office, 1990.

psychoanalysis   The mode of treatment for mental health disorders developed by Sigmund Freud and his followers at the beginning of the 20th century. He believed that mental disorders were a result of the failure of normal emotional development during childhood.

Some individuals who suffer from extreme stresses in their lives, with which they cannot cope, seek psychoanalysis. The therapy aims to help the patient understand his or her emotional development and to make appropriate adjustments in particular situations.

Psychoanalysis is practiced by clinicians who have undergone specialized training after residency training. Individuals who practice psychoanalysis are usually medical doctors, but not necessarily so. Those who are not must pass certain examinations given by an accredited institute of psychoanalysis. Psychoanalysts must undergo psychoanalysis themselves to resolve their own emotional problems before they start their practice. The American Psychoanalytic Association has more than 3,000 members, and the International Psychoanalytical Association numbers over 7,500.

Analysts use features of free association, dream analysis, and the development and working through of transference or distortions in the individual's relationship with the analyst. Sessions are usually held four or five times a week and a completed analysis may take three to five years, but length of treatment varies considerably with the nature of the problems being treated.

Changes in the field
According to *Psychiatric News* (September 6, 1991), the nature of psychoanalysis is changing to include multiple theoretical viewpoints

that work synergistically. There is a proliferation of psychoanalytic publications dealing with clinical and theoretical issues, as well as the application of psychoanalytic study to other fields such as history, literature, anthropology, and art.

See also PSYCHOTHERAPIES; SELF-PSYCHOLOGY.

psychodrama An adjunct to psychotherapy in which the patient acts out certain roles or incidents; this is sometimes useful for individuals trying to overcome the serious effects of stresses in their lives. The roles or incidents may or may not be related to people closely involved with the individual or may concern situations that they find particularly stressful.

The purpose of psychodrama is to bring out hidden concerns and to allow expression of a person's disturbed feelings. Therapeutic value comes from the release of pent-up emotions and from insights into the way other people feel and behave. Psychodrama is often carried out with a partner or in a group. In many cases, use of music, dance, and pantomime may be included.

The technique was developed by J.L. Moreno, a Viennese psychiatrist, in 1921. Psychodrama is considered an early form of group therapy or group psychotherapy.

See also ALTERNATIVE THERAPIES; DANCE THERAPY; PSYCHOTHERAPIES.

psycho-imagination therapy (PIT) A technique that uses waking imagery and imagination to effect personality changes and alter the ways in which an individual copes with stress. The basic proposition of psycho-imagination therapy is recognizing people's needs to become aware of how they define themselves in relation to others and how they think others define them.

See also ALTERNATIVE THERAPIES; PSYCHOTHERAPIES.

psychologist A non-medical specialist in diagnosing and treating mental health concerns such as difficulties in coping with stress. In most states, a psychologist has a Ph.D. degree from a graduate program in PSYCHOLOGY. Licensed psychologists receive insurance reimbursement, have hospital privileges, and act as expert witnesses in court cases.

Prior to World War II, psychologists were primarily involved in academic institutions, with only a few individuals employed outside universities and actively engaged in mental health services. After 1977, with the passage of the Missouri psychology licensure act, all 50 states and the District of Columbia granted statutory recognition to the profession.

Along with dramatic growth in the number of practitioners, there has been a significant expansion in the psychologist's role as provider of mental health care. For example, today psychologists are involved in almost every type of mental health setting, including institutional or community based, research or treatment oriented, or general health or mental health focused. Within these environments, psychologists' roles have also expanded beyond traditional activities of diagnostic assessment and psychotherapy to include primary prevention, community-level intervention strategies, assessment of service delivery systems, and client advocacy.

Psychology has many subspecialties, which include child, developmental, school, clinical, social, and industrial; some psychologists have private practices, are employed by health care facilities, or teach in universities.

Psychologists cannot prescribe medications; they refer patients requiring medication to a physician.

See also BEHAVIOR THERAPY; PSYCHIATRIST; PSYCHOTHERAPIES.

psychology The study of the processes of the mind, such as memory, feelings, thought, and perception, as well as intelligence, behavior, and learning. Within this field, there are many different approaches. For example, behavioral psychology studies the way people react to events and adapt to stress; neuropsychology relates human behavior to brain and body functions; and psychoanalytic psychology emphasizes the role of the unconscious and the experiences of childhood.

Clinical psychology

Clinical psychology is a branch of psychology specializing in the study, diagnosis, and treatment of behavior disorders. This branch of psychology became popular in the United States during the late 1940s and 1950s. Much of the research in clinical methods, diagnosis, and therapy has taken place within departments of clinical psychology.

In most states, clinical psychologists must be licensed to treat clients and, in some states, they must have a Ph.D. degree. Training for the Ph.D. in clinical psychology includes course work, development of research skills, and clinical practice.

See also BEHAVIOR THERAPY; PSYCHO-THERAPIES.

SOURCE:

Manderscheid, R.W., and M.A. Sonnenschein eds. *Mental Health, United States, 1990.* DHHS Pub. No. (ADM) 90–1708. Washington, D.C.: Government Printing Office, 1990.

psychoneuroimmunology (PNI) Relatively new branch of science that studies the interrelationships among the mind (psycho), the nervous system (neuro), and the IMMUNE SYSTEM (immunology). The aim of this field is to investigate and document interrelationships between psychological factors and the immune and neuroendocrine systems. Research efforts include looking at effects of emotional STRESS on the immune system and health. In a general way, PNI seeks to understand the scientific basis of the MIND-BODY CONNECTION.

Authors Locke and Colligan, in *The Healer Within,* explain that a premise of PNI is that the immune system does not operate in a biological vacuum but is sensitive to outside influences. PNI researchers speculate that there is a line of communication between the mind and the cells that are the immune system. Tendrils of the brain's nerve tissues run through important sectors of the immune system, including the thymus gland, bone marrow, lymph nodes, and spleen. Hormones and NEUROTRANSMITTERS secreted by the brain have an affinity for immune cells. Also, certain states of mind and feelings can have strong biochemical results.

The field began in 1981 with the publication of a book edited by Robert Ader (*Psychoneuro-immunology*). While most of the research presented was primarily based on animal models of stress and illness, the collection paved the way for clinical research with humans.

During the later 1980s and 1990s, researchers from various backgrounds were drawn to this new discipline. Social psychologists, experimental psychologists, psychiatrists, immunologists, neuroendocrinologists, neuroanatomists, biologists, oncologists, and epidemiologists, among other specialists, have all made contributions to PNI research. Together, they seek to explain the way in which the brain and mind contribute to illness or keep people healthy.

PNI and cancer

Considerable research has been done with PNI and cancer patients. Work has progressed beyond looking at cell activity and now evaluates the role of ALTERNATIVE THERAPIES, such as group therapy, in inducing immune response in cancer patients, allowing identification of potentially helpful support modalities, and evaluation of possible mechanisms of action. In 1995, a pilot study was conducted to differentiate the effect of support from that of imagery/RELAXATION on immune function, and to explore the relationship of emotional well-being and quality-of-life measures to the immune function.

Arthritis and the PNI link

A research study evaluating personality traits of people who have rheumatoid arthritis was undertaken by Robert Fathman, Ph.D., a Dublin, Ohio, clinical psychologist, and Norman Rothermich, M.D., professor emeritus, Ohio State University, Columbus. "We found that rheumatoid arthritis sufferers have a personality that leads them to try overly hard to be nice to other people, not to lean on others for emotional support, and to stow things inside, especially anger," they concluded. Many rheumatoid arthritis sufferers also had a situation of long-term tension or anger in their lives. "These traits seemed to precede the disease, not result from it. The end result is that repressed anger 'eats them up'." Rheumatoid arthritis is considered an autoimmune disease, in which the immune system mutinies against the body.

In a well-known study in the field of psychoneuroimmunology, psychiatrist George Solomon, M.D., and Rudolf H. Moos, Ph.D., both then at the Stanford University School of Medicine, discovered that the difference between people who develop rheumatoid arthritis and those who do not lies in their psychological profile. People who have the rheumatoid factor in their blood but stay in good psychological condition will not get arthritis. On the other hand, those who are genetically predisposed and endure long periods of stressful anxiety and/or DEPRESSION or suffer some major emotional upset are at a higher risk for arthritis.

See also HUMOR; LAUGHTER; PLACEBO EFFECT; STRESS MANAGEMENT.

SOURCES:

Locke, Steven, and Douglas Colligan *The Healer Within*. New York: New American Library, 1984.

Moye, Lemuel A. "Research Methodology in Psychoneuroimmunology: Rationale and Design of the Images-P Clinical Trial." *Alternatives Therapies* 1, no. 2 (May 1995).

Padus, Emrika, ed. *The Complete Guide to Your Emotions and Your Health*, rev. Emmaus, PA.: Rodale Press, 1994.

Schwartz, Carolyn E. "Introduction: Old Methodological Challenges and New Mind-Body Links in Psychoneuroimmunology." *Advances: The Journal of Mind-Body Health* 10, no. 4 (Fall 1994).

psychotherapies   The treatment of mental and emotional concerns by psychological methods. In a psychotherapy, a therapeutic relationship between the patient and a therapist (psychotherapist) is established. The relationship is focused on the patient's symptoms. Patterns of behavior—mood swings, low SELF-ESTEEM, and not being able to deal with stress—can benefit from this interaction between patient and therapist.

There are many types of psychotherapist who can be recommended by friends, family physicians, or local community mental health centers. There are several rules to follow when choosing a therapist. Check out credentials. Know whether the therapist is a PSYCHIATRIST, PSYCHOLOGIST, or psychiatric social worker. Determine where the person received training, and check with that institution. Also, because there are professional societies for many specialties, check with the appropriate organization to see that the therapist has appropriate accreditation.

Choosing a psychotherapist

People seeking help may be faced with the question of who to choose. If they recognize what their problems are and there are just occasional periods of feeling moody, a psychiatrist may not be needed. Guidelines for selecting psychotherapist rather than a psychiatrist include:

The end of the stressful problem is in sight, but the individual just can't get there by him/herself.

The individual realizes that symptoms are of short duration and that the stress that brought them on can be identified.

However, a person who has tried going to a therapist and has not found relief, may need a psychiatrist because of the following reasons:

MDs are the only mental health therapists who can prescribe medications.

For certain emotional illnesses, medications may be helpful.

The individual has incapacitating or debilitating symptoms.

The individual has other concurrent medical problems for which care and medications are being received.

There is a history of mental illness in the family; other family members have ever been hospitalized for mental illness; or the individual requires hospitalization for a mental problem.

Group therapy

Group therapy is treatment of emotional or psychological problems in groups of patients or in self-help support groups led by a mental health professional. These groups attract individuals with similar concerns. For example, such groups may be for recently widowed persons (GRIEF), divorced people (self-esteem), parents who have lost a child to SUDDEN INFANT DEATH SYNDROME, people suffering from DEPRESSION, or those concerned with OBESITY.

Therapy groups include from three to 40 people but work best with 10 to 12 participants who meet for an hour or more, once or twice a week. There is therapeutic interaction among the individuals in the group; members find that others share their feelings and experiences and this helps them feel less alone and less helpless.

Group therapy is useful for people who have personality problems, ALCOHOLISM, drug dependency, EATING DISORDERS, and ANXIETY DISORDERS.

Co-therapy

This is a form of psychotherapy in which more than one therapist works with an individual or group. Co-therapy is also known as combined therapy, cooperative therapy, dual leadership, multiple therapy, and three-cornered therapy. Co-therapists work in various areas. For example, in SEX THERAPY one therapist is a male and the other is female to encourage both viewpoints in sexuality problems concerning a married couple.

Geropsychiatry

This is a specialized form of mental health care that addresses the complexities involved between mental and physical illness in the elderly. For example, an elderly patient who might appear to have psychotic symptoms may be experiencing symptoms of toxicity resulting from taking two or more incompatible drugs. Many psychosomatic disorders and chronic conditions manifest themselves with symptoms of depression. Physicians specializing in geropsychiatry are located in community hospitals where they can provide a safe and secure environment and offer psychological evaluation in conjunction with medical testing and liaison services for elderly patients being treated for medical or surgical conditions.

An increasing number of hospitals are adding this component to their mental health programs. Some hospitals contract with various managed care organizations which provide these services.

Family therapy

Family therapy is a form of psychotherapy that focuses on the family unit, or at least the parent and child (in single-parent families), rather than separate treatment of one or more family members. It is based on the theory that an individual who is troubled or is mentally ill should not be seen in isolation from the family unit. Family members become aware of how they deal with each other and are encouraged to communicate more openly with each other. The discussions and confrontations lead to understanding.

Family therapy usually focuses on here-and-now stresses and their practical solutions. It can be helpful when at least one member has a relatively serious problem, such as recurrent depression, or needs ongoing assistance in coping with outbursts of anger and emotional withdrawal.

Family therapy has become increasingly popular for dealing with problems of children and adolescents. Typically, the therapy group will consist of both parents, or a parent and stepparent, two separated parents, or other parental pairings depending on the environment in which the child lives. In many cases, the child is brought to a mental health professional because of difficulties in school, such as exhibiting aggressive behavior or cutting classes.

See also COMMUNICATION; LISTENING; MARITAL THERAPY; SUPPORT GROUPS.

puberty The developmental stage between childhood and adulthood. It is the term used for the physical and emotional changes of adolescence: It usually occurs between the ages of 10 to 15 in boys and girls. This is a stressful period for many young people, as when they enter puberty they are no longer children but are not accepted by society as adults. Tensions exist between children's dependence on their parents and their increasing desire for independence from their parents.

Many young people feel stressed by the emotional ups and downs they experience. They may laugh, cry, or explode in anger without any apparent reason. Parents, teachers, and others need to be understanding, patient, tolerant, and sympathetic to help the adolescents weather this transition successfully.

Sexual and physical changes

Puberty, also defined as the period at which maturation of the sexual organs occurs, begins at about age 11 or 12 for girls and 13 or 14 for boys. However, there are wide variations; some girls begin to menstruate as early as age 8 or 9 and others as late as age 16. In Western cultures, the average age at which adolescents reach sexual maturity has been steadily decreasing over the last century, possibly as a result of better nutrition and medical care.

Many physical changes occur during puberty. In boys, this includes an increase in the secretion of male hormones and in testicular functions, and enlargement of the external sex organs. Nocturnal emissions or WET DREAMS are a normal, automatic release at night for secretions that accumulate in the boy's sexual organs. Hair increases on the boy's legs, pubic area, chest, underarms, and face. Later his voice deepens. A spurt of growth in height and general filling-out usually occurs shortly before the start of this period.

Adolescents, particularly boys, often feel stressed by comparisons with their peers concerning physical development. Early-maturing boys seem to have advantages on later-maturing boys; they do better in athletics, are generally more popular, and have a positive sense of SELF-ESTEEM.

In girls, female hormone production and ovarian activity increase, the uterus matures and nearly doubles in size, the breasts develop, and mammary glands mature. The pelvis also widens and rounds, and hair begins to show on the legs, pubic area, and underarms. MENSTRUATION and ovulation begin, often irregularly at first.

Body weight may double during puberty, due to muscle growth in boys and increased fat in girls.

Communications between generations

Adolescents need guidance and reinforcement along the way; it is important that they and their parents keep the lines of COMMUNICATION open. They may have questions about the physical, sexual, and personality changes that they are experiencing as well as concerns about making appropriate choices and decisions. Today's teenagers face many external sources of stress, such as peer pressure, drugs and alcohol, and the possibility of teenage pregnancy. For some, internal sources of stress may lead to EATING DISORDERS and SCHOOL problems.

See also INTERGENERATIONAL CONFLICTS; LISTENING; PARENTING.

public speaking The art of making speeches to an audience. Individuals can experience stress related to public speaking ranging from mild apprehension to true phobic reactions. The anticipation of giving a speech in public may arouse feelings ranging from only a mild form of ANXIETY, which might be considered normal, to feelings of rapid heartbeat, faintness, DIZZINESS, nausea, or other symptoms of a phobia.

An individual may suffer a mild degree of stress as a common reaction to being asked to give the speech, preparing it, and, finally, getting up in front of people to give it. There may be apprehension about how one looks or sounds and what people will think about the speech. All these apprehensions, however, could spur the individual to making the best possible presentation.

A truly social phobic person who is phobic about public speaking probably would not accept such an invitation, nor would an individual who has an extreme fear of failure.

People who manage to give a speech in public but are extremely uneasy often exhibit behaviors such as shuffling the feet, pacing, no eye contact, facial tics or grimaces, moistening the lips and clearing the throat frequently, and noticeably perspiring.

Issues of self-confidence and SELF-ESTEEM are involved in the stress of public speaking. People who have given many speeches and feel confident about the subject matter, as well as their appearance, will probably experience only a mild degree of stress.

See also PERFORMANCE ANXIETY; SOCIAL PHOBIA; STAGE FRIGHT.

public transportation See RANDOM NUISANCES.

R

random nuisances Annoying or unpleasant situations with which individuals cope. They may include difficult things such as commuting in traffic, finding a parking spot, depending on public transportation when the weather is bad; or annoying things like construction noise outside your office window, phone calls from telemarketers at dinnertime, last-minute dinner guests, or zippers that get stuck at a critical moment. Such nuisances differ for each person, but if they are perceived as stressful, they take their toll.

Successful people regard random nuisances as "small stuff." There is a saying, "Don't sweat the small stuff; it's all small stuff." As stressors, random nuisances may seem small. However, the response to some of life's "small stressors" may escalate into physical responses, such as ANGER and rage, that are similar to responses to major stressors.

Hans SELYE explained the concept of STRESS with two basic ideas: The body has a similar set of responses to many of life's stressors; this he called the GENERAL ADAPTATION SYN-DROME (G.A.S.). Also, stressors can make an individual ill. To prevent illness induced by stressors, keeping a positive perspective on life and everyday occurrences is essential. The individual should endeavor to cope with the small stressors and keep them from escalating into more serious consequences.

Many individuals find that MEDITATION at the end of a day helps them meet challenges of home, children, and paying bills. Others find that participating in regular EXERCISE helps them forget about the random nuisances of each day.

See also HARDINESS; RELAXATION.

rape Forcible sexual intercourse against the will of the partner. There is some variation among states as to the actual definition. In many states, sexual assault need not involve either force, actual penetration, or ejaculation; in others, genital contact under the threat of force or even implied threat of force meets the legal definition.

Rape is an extremely stressful situation for the victim and her/his family members. The psychological effects of rape are severe. Many victims suffer significant ANXIETY, DEPRESSION, and post traumatic stress reactions that last for years and can adversely affect their professional, personal and sexual lives.

While rape has traditionally been an offense between a man and woman, there has been an attempt to remove gender identification and to include homosexual rape and other offenses, such as sexual contact between an adult and an underage child or adolescent and INCEST.

Traditionally, women have feared violent sexual assault by a stranger. However, society now recognizes that forced intercourse can occur with perpetrators known to the victim, even the husband. The incidence of "date rape" (rape by a person with whom one has had a social engagement) is increasingly reported.

Rape is now recognized as more a crime of violence than one of sexuality; rapists often have a history of other types of violent crime. As courts and law enforcement agencies have been more sympathetic toward victims, the number of reported rapes in the United States has increased dramatically.

Rape victims may be physically injured at the time of the assault. They may be shot, knifed, or beaten, and immediate medical attention is usually given to injuries. The rape itself can cause perineal bruising or lacerations, particularly if the victim is very young, anal penetration occurs, and/or dangerous objects are used in the assault. Cultures are taken for gonorrhea and other SEXUALLY TRANSMITTED DISEASES and appropriate antibiotics may be recommended. If a victim is exposed to HERPES or AIDS, there is, at present, no effective way of preventing these diseases.

After reporting a rape and being examined at a medical facility, the rape victim's body and clothing will be examined for traces of blood, semen, hair, or clothing of the rapist. Recent development of DNA "fingerprints" from semen and blood permit accurate identification of the person responsible.

Women at risk for pregnancy may be offered "morning after" contraception. Unfortunately, many victims fail to press charges either out of fear of having to relive the incident in court or out of fear of shame or reprisal.

Prevention of rape will depend on major restructuring of the way society views violence against women and prevention of the drug, alcohol, and poverty problems that lead to violent crimes. To a lesser extent, self-defense and ASSERTIVENESS TRAINING for women can decrease the risk to those women but fail to address the underlying psychopathology of the rapist.

SOURCES:
Clark, Stephanie. "Perspectives on Sexual Assault." *Canadian Family Physician* 35 (January 1989): 77–80.
Harrison, Maureen, and Steve Gilbert, eds. *The Rape Reference: A Resource for People at Risk.* San Diego: Excellent Books, 1996.
Miller, Maryann. *Drugs and Date Rape.* New York: Rosen Publishing Group, 1995.

recreation   The activities people do as a means of diversion or refreshment. For many people, these activities restore health and offset the effects of stress in everyday life.

Recreation comes in many forms. Sports activities such as tennis, golf, bowling, ice skating, rollerblading, and bike riding are activities many people enjoy. Others play cards, sing in choirs, act in plays, keep a journal, or go to movies, plays, and concerts. Most forms of recreation help individuals cope with stressors in their lives because they divert attention from them.

At times, recreation itself can be stressful. Examples are games in which individuals are highly competitive or participation in community theater, when individuals may experience STAGE FRIGHT or fear of forgetting their lines. It is important to choose a balance of recreational activities that meet the need for personal satisfaction and achievement, as well as to bring healing to the spirit, mind, and body.

See also EXERCISE; HOBBIES; MIND-BODY CONNECTIONS; RELAXATION; VOLUNTEERISM.

SOURCES:
Austin, David R. *Therapeutic Recreation. An Introduction.* Englewood Cliffs, N.J.: Prentice-Hall, 1991.
Miller, Thomas Ross. *Taking Time Out. Recreation and Play.* Woodbridge, Conn.: Blackbirch Press, 1996.

reflexology   A form of body therapy based on the theory that every part of the body has a direct line of communication to a reference point on the foot, hand, and ear. By massaging these reference points, professional reflexologists say they can help the corresponding body parts to heal. Through improved circulation, elimination of toxic by-products, and overall reduction of stress, the body responds and functions better because it is more relaxed.

See also ALTERNATIVE THERAPIES; BODY THERAPIES.

SOURCE:
Feltman, John, ed. *Reflexology. Hands on Healing.* Emmaus, PA.: Rodale Press, 1989.

USING REFLEXOLOGY TO REDUCE STRESS

- Choose a quiet place.
- Apply a few drops of a light, absorbent, greaseless lotion to your feet and massage them, continuing until the lotion is totally absorbed.
- Grasp the ankle, heel, or toes of one foot firmly in one hand, place the thumb of your other hand on the sole of your foot at the heel and apply steady, even pressure with the edge of your whole thumb.
- Keep your thumb slightly bent at the joint and use a forward, caterpillar-like motion. This is called thumbwalking; press one spot, move forward a little, press again, and so on.
- When you reach the toes, start again at a new spot on the heel. Continue until the entire bottom of the foot has been worked. Then fingerwalk the top of the foot. Work your entire foot twice this way.

---

relationships Relationships are formed between individuals connected by affinity. These relationships include the individual's FAMILY, spouse, lovers, friends, and business or professional associates. Good relationships are healthy and nurturing and act as a buffer against outside stressors. However, even the most meaningful relationships can at times be nonsupportive and sources of stress.

Relationships and health

Best friends fit this category: He or she is on the same wave length with you and understands your personal situations, such as dealing with a difficult boss or overbearing parent; appreciates and admires who you are, even if there isn't always agreement on what is being done or said; gives you compliments and makes you feel important in his or her life.

According to S. Leonard Syme, Ph.D., University of California at Berkeley, people who have a close-knit network of intimate personal ties with other people seem to be able to avoid disease, maintain higher levels of health and, in general, deal more successfully with life's difficulties. Dr. Syme and his research team found that people with many social contacts had the lowest death rate, and people with the fewest contacts had the highest rates. Single, divorced, and widowed people have higher rates of many diseases. Widows, particularly in the first year after their husbands' deaths, have many more symptoms of physical and mental disease as well as death rates that are four times higher than average. "One can guard against the ill effect of being single through a solid network of friends and associates," says Dr. Syme.

Socially isolated people may be more likely to adopt self-destructive health habits and may get depressed and become suicidal or accident-prone. "All diseases are 'social diseases,'" says Dennis Jaffe, author of *Healing from Within*. "It's as though a breakdown in the social support structure precipitates a breakdown in the body's immune system."

This breakdown in the body's immune system resembles the body's stress response. People who lack outlets for stress release are susceptible to a list of stress-related illnesses. Having one or two close friends with whom they feel free to say anything is invaluable. When they are overwhelmed, they don't trust

---

COMPONENTS OF A HEALTHY RELATIONSHIP

- Realism: openness and honesty with each other
- Trust: allowing the individuals to share their feelings
- True friendship: having no hidden motives
- Forgiveness: accepting the individual as he or she is
- Security: knowing that individuals can count on one another
- Vulnerability: exposing weaknesses that allow the relationship to grow

their own judgment, and an objective view from a friend can help.

Romantic relationships

Romantic relationships are far riskier and potentially more stressful to the individual's emotional and physical well-being than people realize. Not only are feelings likely to be hurt, SELF-ESTEEM damaged, and trust betrayed, but there can be physical and mental battery by an outraged spouse. America's high DIVORCE rate suggests that INTIMACY has painful consequences.

According to Geraldine K. Piorkowski, author of *Too Close for Comfort: Exploring the Risks of Intimacy,* romantic relationships can be stressful because they are related to the process of getting close to another person. As we become more intimate (both emotionally and sexually), we reveal our deepest secrets, hopes, inadequacies, and even fantasies. We become more vulnerable, and thus easily cut to the core by a hostile comment, act of betrayal, or moment of rejection.

Further, Piorkowski says, stress arises in relationships when our emotional needs and expectations are unrealistic. Also, we may lose our AUTONOMY and wind up feeling suffocated by the other's demands; their neediness may drain energy needed to pursue our own desires and interests. We may be blamed for all the problems in the relationship and suffer GUILT and loss of self-confidence as a result

Relationships and support groups

A lack of connections with other people can be detrimental to health, says Dr. Andrew Weil, author of *Spontaneous Healing.* "Surrounding yourself with supportive people is an important step for any healing you need to do. Whenever I take a family history from a patient, I always ask about people who are helping or hindering someone's illness. For example, sometimes a friend or family member who means well only make matters worse, maybe by not wanting the patient to express sadness about being sick or show discomfort from pain."

In terms of building relationships through support groups, Dr. Weil urges patients to find and develop relationships with people who have the same conditions and who have improved rather than simply to join a SUPPORT GROUP. "I find that some support groups can be counterproductive and cause more stress for the individual," he says. "For example, some patients with cancer are horrified and extremely stressed when they see another person with a more advanced form of the disease. There is a similar phenomenon with chronic fatigue syndrome."

Some people are more fatalistic about their illness while others tend to be positive thinkers. This should be factored into any relationships developed through a support group, and especially with the regular people in your life, suggests Dr. Weil.

See also COMMUNICATION; DATING; INTERGENERATIONAL CONFLICTS; LISTENING; LIVE-IN; MARRIAGE; PARENTING.

SOURCES:
Gilbert, Roberta M. *Extraordinary Relationships. A New Way of Thinking About Human Interactions.* Minneapolis: Chronimed Publishing, 1992.
Jaffe, Dennis T. *Healing From Within.* New York: Knopf, 1980.
Padus, Emrika, ed. *The Complete Guide to Your Emotions and Your Health.* Emmaus, PA.: Rodale Press, 1992.
Piorkowski, Geraldine K. *Too Close for Comfort: Exploring the Risks of Intimacy.* New York: Insight Books, 1994.
Weil, Andrew. *Spontaneous Healing: How to Discover and Enhance Your Body's Natural Ability to Maintain and Heal Itself.* New York: Knopf, 1995.

relaxation A feeling of freedom from anxiety and tension. Internal conflicts and disturbing feelings of STRESS are absent. Relaxation also refers to the return of a muscle to its normal state after a period of contraction.

People who are very tense and anxious can learn to relax using relaxation training, a form of BEHAVIOR THERAPY or ALTERNATIVE THERAPY. Relaxation techniques are methods used to consciously release muscular tension and achieve a sense of mental calm. Historically, relaxation techniques have included MEDITATION, T'AI CHI, MASSAGE THERAPY, YOGA, MUSIC, and AROMATHERAPY. More modern developments include AUTOGENIC TRAINING, PROGRESSIVE MUSCLE RELAXATION, HYPNOSIS, BIOFEEDBACK, and aerobic EXERCISE.

Many of these techniques were developed to help people cope with stresses brought on by the challenges of life. They are different approaches to relieving stress by bringing about generalized physical as well as mental relaxation. Relaxation techniques have in common the production of the relaxation response as one of their stress-relieving actions. Additionally, relaxation may counter some of the immunosuppressing effects of stress and may actually enhance the activity of the IMMUNE SYSTEM.

Relaxation training programs are commonly used in conjunction with more standard forms of therapy for many chronic diseases. The MIND-BODY CONNECTION between relaxation and ill health has been demonstrated in many conditions. Some of the physiological changes that occur during relaxation include decreased oxygen consumption, decreased heart and respiratory rates, diminished muscle tension, and a shift toward slower brain wave patterns.

The "relaxation response"

In the 1970s, Herbert BENSON, M.D., a cardiologist at Harvard Medical School, studied the relationship between stress and hypertension. In stressful situations, the body undergoes several changes, including rise in blood pressure and pulse and faster breathing. Dr. Benson reasoned that if stress could bring about this reaction, another factor might be able to turn it off. He studied practitioners of TRANSCENDENTAL MEDITATION (TM) and found that once into their meditative states, some individuals could willfully reduce their pulse, blood pressure, and breathing rate. Dr. Benson named this "the relaxation response." He explained this procedure in his book (written with Miriam Z. Klipper) *The Relaxation Response* (1976).

Relaxation applications

Relaxation training can be particularly useful for individuals who have "white coat hypertension," which means that their blood pressure is high only when facing certain specifically stressful situations, such as having a medical examination or visiting a dentist. It can also help reduce hostility and anger, which in turn affect the body and the individual's physical responses to stress. Anxieties can lead to panic attacks, nausea, or gastrointestinal problems.

There are many applications of relaxation training to help individuals learn CONTROL over their mental state and body and in treating conditions as diverse as high blood pressure, cardiac arrhythmia, chronic pain, insomnia, premenstrual syndrome, and side effects of cancer treatments. Relaxation training is an important part of childbirth classes to help women cope with the pain of labor.

In a training program, individuals are instructed to move through the muscle groups of the body, making them tense and then completely relaxed. Through repetitions of this procedure, individuals learn how to be in voluntary control of their feelings of tension and relaxation. Some therapists provide individuals with instructional audio tapes for use during practice, while other therapists go through the procedure repeatedly with their clients.

To determine the effectiveness of relaxation training, some therapists use biofeedback as an indicator of an individual's degree of relaxation and absence of ANXIETY.

See also GUIDED IMAGERY; HOBBIES; KABAT-ZINN, JON; RECREATION.

SOURCES:

Benson, Herbert. *Beyond the Relaxation Response.* New York: Berkeley Press 1985.

———. *The Relaxation Response.* New York: Avon Books, 1975.

Goleman, Daniel, and Joel Gurin, eds. *Mind Body Medicine. How to Use Your Mind for Better Health.* Yonkers, N.Y.: Consumer Reports Books, 1993.

Lehrer, Paul M., and Robert L. Woolfolk, eds. *Principles and Practice of Stress Management,* New York: Guilford Press, 1993.

Locke, Steven, and Douglas Colligan. *The Healer Within.* New York: New American Library, 1984.

religion   The service and worship of God. It is a commitment to a personal set or institutionalized system of attitudes, beliefs, and practices. Religion helps many people cope with stresses of life because it gives them a sense of security, meaning, order, and an ethical pattern for living.

Faith in God

Belief and trust in and loyalty to God or belief in the doctrines of religion historically have been an avenue for relieving stress and increasing an individual's physical and mental health. Studies regarding benefits of religion indicate that religious beliefs offer some protection from hypertension, death from heart disease, and cancer. While a physician cannot recommend a patient participate in religion, asking about such behavior and positively reinforcing it may improve the patient's quality of life. In some cases, it may prove to be a useful piece of evidence that patients will use to alter their survival behaviors.

Involvement with religion very often increases in older adults, an observation that led researchers headed by psychiatrist Thomas Oxman at Dartmouth Medical School to investigate the role religion might play in the health of the elderly. They found that those who derive at least some strength and comfort from religion are more likely to survive longer after cardiac surgery than those who do not. Researchers looked at the effect on survival of a number of biomedical, psychological, and social factors as well as religious feeling and activity. Those who said they found at least some strength and comfort from their religious feelings were three times more likely to survive than those who had no comfort from religious faith. Those who participated in social and community activities, such as church suppers, senior centers, or historical societies, had three times the survival rate of those who did not participate in any organized activity. Those who had both protective factors—religious and social support—showed a tenfold increase in survival.

However, while religion contains elements that are supportive, it also contains elements that may be damaging to a person's management of stress. For example, the promise of reward in the afterlife has inspired and comforted many, but has also been held responsible for making believers passive or accepting of hardships and inequities, which they could overcome through their own efforts, because they hope for a better life in the beyond.

Religion in wartime

A survey of World War II veterans offered interesting insights into the religious state of mind of men who experienced the stresses of warfare. About 26% said that the war made them more religious; 19% that war made them less religious. Fifty-eight percent of those surveyed said that even though their religious conviction may have increased, decreased, or remained the same, their war experiences made them more interested in the subject of religion. The veterans exhibited an even stronger tendency when describing their religious attitude during battle. Most were of the opinion that everyone prays in combat. An interesting variation was the comment, "There were atheists in fox holes, but most of them were in love," implying that the thought of a loved one might carry a man through danger almost as well as an appeal to a higher power.

The influence of religion on mental health

Between 1930 and 1960, theologian Paul Tillich (1886–1965), philosopher Martin Buber (1878–1965) and psychoanalyst Rollo May (1909–94) published important works attempting to synthesize religion, psychology, and modern philosophical movements. An interest in combining the mental health disciplines with the influence of religion has encouraged the development of training in pastoral counseling in recent years. In the early 1970s, priest-sociologist Andrew Greeley (1928–), in his book *Unsecular Man: the Persistence of Religion,* described a conservative, religious social trend that recently has become more obvious in movements such as the creationist opposition to secular humanism in education and the political influence of religious leaders and celebrities publicizing their "born again" experiences.

Religion in America

Two surveys, one in 1991 for *Time* and one by the Gallup poll, indicated that while religion is a strong influence in the United States, there seems to be a lack of confidence or awareness of its importance. For example, the *Time* survey showed that 78% of those surveyed felt that children should be allowed to say PRAYERS in public schools. Sixty-three percent said that they would not vote for a presidential candidate who did not believe in God. Fifty-five percent said that there was too little religious influence in American life, and 65% felt that religious influence was decreasing. The latter opinion can be both supported and contradicted by the Gallup Poll, depending on one's point of reference. The percent of those surveyed by Gallup who felt that religion was "very important" or "fairly important" to them personally, was about 85%, and has remained fairly constant since the 1970s. Attendance at church or synagogue during

the previous week had actually risen slightly from a low of 40% in the 1970s to 43% in 1989, while actual membership had dropped from 73% in 1965 to 68% in 1989. If contrasted with figures from the 1950s, which were 49% church or synagogue attendance and 95% feeling that religion was very or fairly important to them personally, American life does appear to be less religious than in the past, although not on a strong downward trend.

The Gallup survey further defined the religious people in the population. Women, non-whites, adults over the age of 50, southerners, and those with annual incomes under $20,000 are most likely to place importance on religion. On the other hand, the wealthy have a high rate of church attendance and membership.

See also ALTERNATIVE THERAPIES; MEDITATION; MIND-BODY CONNECTIONS.

SOURCE:

Koenig, Harold George. *Is Religion Good for Your Health: The Effects of Religion on Physical and Mental Health.* New York: Haworth Pastoral Press, 1997.

relocation The need to transfer to a new company location as part of a promotion or lateral career move. Transfers may also become necessary due to reorganizations and MERGERS. A fact of life and a stressor for most workers and their families today, relocation means losing a SUPPORT GROUP (FRIENDS and/or relatives), finding a new residence and new community resources (places to worship, schools, doctors, dentists, etc.), handling the move (packing and unpacking), and, in the case of dual careers, the need for one spouse to find new employment and the possible financial impact of that.

Children probably suffer the most stress during relocations. New schools can mean new methods of teaching and new textbooks, and, most important, new friends. Research has shown that adults who as children moved frequently due to parent job transfers may find it difficult to form lasting friendships and have not learned the necessary skills to form intimate relationships.

Frequent transfers can be hard on all members of the family. They have been known to trigger a group of stress reactions called the mobility syndrome, which can include DEPRESSION, deterioration of health, dependency on one's own family for emotional satisfaction, reclusiveness, a high rate of alcoholism and drug dependency, and marital discord that often leads to divorce. There is an increase of acting out behavior on the part of children and teenagers. Many of these stress reactions require professional help.

For the first time, many people are assessing the viability of a transfer not only in terms of careers and the financial and housing implications of the move, but also in terms of the quality of life for themselves and their families. Since relocation often becomes a primary part of a promotion, it is important to see if it matches family values and priorities as well as the individual's career plan. Whatever the decision, applying COPING techniques and strategies is necessary to handle the resulting stress.

See also ACCULTURATION; GENERAL ADAPTATION SYNDROME; MIGRATION; MOVING; NOSTALGIA.

remarriage Entering into a MARRIAGE contract between a couple when one or both of them has been left a widow or widower or when there has been a DIVORCE. Bride and groom bring with them remembrances, some good and some bad, of previous marriages. If there are children, establishing new family RELATIONSHIPS as well as maintaining old family ties are major concerns. Widows or widowers who experienced "good marriages" are less likely to have fears and apprehensions than those who are divorced.

Many people do find their second marriage, particularly after a divorce, a source of stress. For example, some divorced men and women marry a person very similar to their first spouse and encounter similar difficulties. Others try very hard to find a quality that was lacking in their first spouse. As a consequence, they may marry a person who has that particular quality but may be blinded to other ways in which they are actually incompatible.

Divorced or widowed persons may remarry out of emotional and financial need without understanding themselves first or resolving their feelings about their previous marriage. Ex-mates may interfere when one or the other remarries and family members may make it obvious that they preferred the previous spouse. In some cases, men and women are stressed by feelings of GUILT about how the second marriage has affected their children or previous spouse.

In remarriages, the husband is frequently several years older than the wife and may not want more children, while she may be eager for a family. The financial strain on a man called upon to support two families is very often disruptive and is also a source of stress.

Being accepted into the family, a stressor for many, may relate to the circumstances of the courtship. For example, if a woman was the "other woman" while the new husband was still married, his relatives may regard the wife as a "home wrecker." If a recently widowed woman marries too soon, her relatives may think the marriage was disrespectful to the deceased.

Statistics on remarriage
According to a 1987 report, 46% of all marriages were remarriages for the bride or groom or both. More widows than widowers remarry, but divorced men are more likely to remarry than divorced women. Nineteen percent of divorced men remarry within a calendar year of their divorce; 8% of widowed men marry within a year of the death of their wives. Divorced men have good reason to remarry. Death rates for divorced men who

remain single are far higher than for divorced women who do not remarry.

While divorced and widowed people remarry at a high rate, the divorce rate for these unions is higher than for first marriages. Responses to a survey concerning the failure rate of second marriages consistently listed two leading causes: children and money. Friction between stepparents and stepchildren is common.

In American contemporary society, some couples choose not to marry for a variety of reasons, ranging from not wanting to lose alimony payments, to waiting for vesting in a pension plan, to fear of making a mistake. Many older individuals who are past childbearing and child rearing years opt for a LIVE-IN arrangement instead of remarriage.

See also INTIMACY; STEPFAMILIES.

SOURCES:

Kahn, Ada P., and Jan Fawcett. *Encyclopedia of Mental Health,* Facts On File, 1993.

Statistical Abstract of the United States, 1991. Washington, D.C.: U.S. Department of Commerce, 1991.

Wilson, Barbara Foley. "The Marry-Go-Round," *American Demographics,* October 1991, 52–54.

repetitive stress injuries (RSI) Injuries that result from repetitive motions, such as using a computer or certain types of factory work. As people spend more time at computers, sitting at a desk, looking at a screen, and typing information, they become more and more open to repetitive stress injuries. Human beings are not meant to do repetitive motions all day in work spaces not set up to accommodate either the equipment or their bodies. The result is damage to muscles in the fingers, wrists, hands, arms, neck, head, and back.

The rate of RSIs is increasing as more Americans turn to computers at work and at home. RSIs are affected by the individual's work pacing, work stress, environment conditions and personality traits.

The kinds of problems computer users report include shooting pains in the arms,

---

AVOIDING REPETITIVE STRESS OF COMPUTER USE

- Select chairs and desks that can be adjusted for maximum work comfort. The desk should be high enough and feet should be on the floor.
- Support your back with a pillow to keep posture correct and relieve strain.
- Be sure your keyboard and mouse are at a comfortable level; raise or lower if necessary.
- Avoid flexing wrists; use a contoured wrist-support device.
- Take work breaks—stretch, roll the neck, and use hand squeezing exercises; stand up and walk about.
- Keep monitor at arm's length (24 inches) from face.
- If pain persists, see a doctor. Work space or work habit changes, physical therapy, special exercises, medication, braces, or surgery may be recommended.

---

acute pain or stiffness in the arms, neck, shoulders, and/or back, acute wrist or finger pain, numbness or tingling in the fingers, hands, arms, or shoulders, and chronic pain in the neck, shoulders, or back.

A specific type of repetitive stress injury relating to wrist-and-hand disorders is CARPAL TUNNEL SYNDROME, and it has been identified as one of the fastest growing occupational illnesses. Carpal tunnel syndrome is the result of inflamed tendons in the wrist.

FOR FURTHER INFORMATION:

Association for Repetitive Motion Syndromes
P.O. Box 514
Santa Rosa, CA 95402
Phone: (707) 571-0397

repression See MEMORY.

resolutions Statements of will or intent. Many people make resolutions at the beginning of the new year, and later in the year are stressed by the fact that they cannot live up to their own hopes and expectations. Commonly, people determine to change their negative behaviors and HABITS into positive ones, such as losing weight, stopping SMOKING, exercising more, and working hard to improve themselves.

Often people are earnestly trying to change their habits, but find that doing so becomes increasingly hard. Other responsibilities get in the way and often the time is used for other tasks. They feel frustrated and finally abandon the resolution with the thought that it might become a resolution the next year. To avoid the stress and FRUSTRATION of unkept resolutions, Mark Groder, author of *Business Games: How to Recognize the Players and Deal with Them*, suggests:

Know your own limits; don't make resolutions that are too ambitious.

Consider the obstacles in keeping your resolution; set your priorities.

Use breaking a resolution as an opportunity for self-understanding; perhaps you were overly optimistic in making it.

See also PERFECTION; SELF-ESTEEM; WEIGHT GAIN AND LOSS.

SOURCE:
Groder, Martin. *Business Games. How to Recognize the Players and Deal with Them.* Des Moines: Boardroom Classics, 1995.

retirement Retirement usually means that the individual is withdrawing from the work force of his or her own free will. It generally occurs when people are around age 65 or older, but in times of economic problems due to DOWNSIZING, LAYOFFS, and MERGERS, it can occur earlier.

Retirement, highly desired by some, produces stresses including ANXIETIES, BOREDOM, and feelings of lack of productivity and loss of SELF-ESTEEM for others. Some retired people feel that they are not contributing members of society and become depressed and withdrawn. Some miss the identity and the prestige they formerly received from their position at work.

Those who adjust the best to retirement and experience the least stress seem to be the people who participate in new activities and make new acquaintances. Most retired people enjoy having more time for family and FRIENDS, for travel, for continuing their education, and for pursuing HOBBIES.

People who have planned ahead for their retirement generally start an interest or hobby before stopping work. For example, some individuals start to learn a musical instrument while others pursue a woodworking or sewing hobby. Many do volunteer work to help others who are in need of assistance. In most of the big cities in the United States, there is a "job corps" of senior citizens willing to donate their time and use their knowledge in business and industry.

Continuing education classes at local colleges and universities are targeted to retired people who enjoy learning. A great many of these people participate in Elderhostel activities, where they travel to college campuses all over the world to study and tour.

Retirement and second careers
Retirement is no longer a once-in-a-lifetime happening. Some individuals who retire go back to paid positions in an area in which they already have an expertise; some go to an entirely different area. Researchers at the University of Southern California tracked 2,816 American men who turned 55 between 1966 and 1976. Approximately one-third went back to work for an average of two more years after they retired. Other significant findings indicated that the average American male retires between ages 61 and 62, that white-collar workers stay on the job about two years longer than blue-collar workers, and that blue-collar workers spend an average of 10 years in retirement; white-collar workers, 12.

Wives of retired men are sometimes affected by their mates' retirement. A study reported in *Modern Maturity* (December 1991–

January 1992) indicated that most women polled reported satisfaction with their husbands' retirement. Effects of retirement on 413 upper-middle-class women married to men retired an average of 16 years were examined. More than one-third of the women had no problems with their husbands' retirement, and two-thirds said they were fully prepared for it. Only 12% said they felt stressed by some loss of personal freedom, and 5% to 6% reported an increase in household chores. Among those who said they would have done things differently, the majority mentioned the need to be better prepared financially for their later years.

Planning ahead relieves stress

Relieving some of the stresses of retirement depends largely on pre-retirement planning and the retirement process itself. A variable in life satisfaction during retirement is socioeconomic status. According to the College of Family Physicians of Canada, those with middle and upper incomes report a higher degree of adaptation. Household income drops drastically (one-half to one-third). Many retirees experience poverty for the first time. Financial problems are the major reasons for stress and dissatisfaction with retirement.

Actual financial hardship may differ from perceived financial hardship. Strategies to cope with the stress of reduced income include expenditure reduction, rearrangement of assets, or continued activity in the labor force. Education is the most influential factor related to successful coping with reduced income.

See also AGING; HARDINESS; RECREATION; VOLUNTEERISM.

SOURCES:

Dennis, Helen, and John Migliaccio. "Redefining Retirement: The Baby Boomer Challenge." *Generations: Journal of the American Society on Aging* 21, no. 2 (Summer 1997): 45.

Godin, Seth. *If You're Clueless About Retirement and Want to Know More.* Chicago: Dearborn Financial, 1997.

Manchester, Joyce. "Aging Boomers and Retirement: Who is at Risk?" *Generations: Journal of the American Society on Aging* 21, no. 2 (Summer 1997): 19.

right sizing   See DOWNSIZING; LAYOFFS; MERGERS; WORKPLACE.

risk   See DECISION-MAKING.

rolfing   One of many contemporary BODY THERAPIES used to relieve stress and improve emotional and physical health. It is a form of deep tissue massage and is a combination of the disciplines of Eastern philosophical systems and practices and Western knowledge of muscular and skeletal structure.

The technique, which is often combined with other body therapy techniques, was developed by Ida Rolf (1896–1979), an American biochemist. As a young woman, she had an accident and was successfully treated by both an osteopathic physician and a yoga instructor. She combined these two techniques with the medical system of homeopathy, a practice that calls upon the patient's own healing powers rather than merely treating symptoms. The therapy gained recognition through Rolf's work at the Esalen Institute in California during the 1960s. From what had been considered the fringe or one of many ALTERNATIVE THERAPIES, Rolfing and other body therapies entered the mainstream of mental and physical treatments in the mid-1900s.

Rolfing focuses on the network of connective tissue—fascia, tendons, and ligaments—that contains the muscles and links them to the bones. Whenever connective tissue fails to work effectively, pain can result. For many, Rolfing helps to heal the body by bringing it into proper alignment and proper relationship to the forces of gravity. A Rolfing practitioner puts pressure on certain areas of the patient's connective tissue to improve the structure of the body. Certified Rolfers have had training in human anatomy, physiology, kinesiology, and various massage techniques.

Locating a Rolfing therapist

The Rolf Institute, headquartered in Boulder, Colorado, has produced Rolfers since 1972. There are more than 600 practitioners across the United States and in 23 other countries. The institute provides a complete listing of its graduates, their addresses, and telephone numbers. The institute also has a free pamphlet that lists books, videotapes, and audiovisual information currently available about Rolfing.

See also MASSAGE THERAPY.

FOR FURTHER INFORMATION:
The Rolf Institute
P.O. Box 1868
Boulder, Colorado 80306
Phone: (303) 449-5903

SOURCE:
Rolf, Ida P. *Rolfing: Reestablishing the Natural Alignment and Structural Integration of the Human Body for Vitality and Well Being.* Rochester, VT.: Healing Arts Press, 1989.

runner's high   A certain feeling of physical and mental well-being and a relief of stress is often reported by individuals who run or jog. This may occur during or after a period of EXERCISE, when the cardiovascular system works harder and longer than it usually does. For example, about 30 to 40 minutes of jogging may produce the feeling of "runner's high" in many individuals.

There is a common misconception that runner's high is caused exclusively by the release of ENDORPHINS, brain chemicals that can reduce pain and elevate mood in a manner similar to opiate drugs. In addition to the release of endorphins, exercise causes the body to discharge many neurochemicals that trigger physiological reactions. For example, stimulation of the sympathetic nervous system along with activation of the endocrine system's adrenal medulla causes an increased heart rate and delivery of more oxygen to the brain, contributing to the relief of stress.

See also RECREATION.

S

"safe sex" Avoiding behaviors that may lead to SEXUALLY TRANSMITTED DISEASES, AIDS, or PREGNANCY. Safe sex involves being in a monogamous relationship, knowing one's partner, avoiding sexual relationships with known drug users, and using CONDOMS and spermicidal agents properly. The need for practicing safe sex causes stress for many individuals who fear contracting a disease or find preparations and precautions annoying. For some couples, use of a condom becomes a stressful issue.

See also BIRTH CONTROL; SEXUAL REVOLUTION.

"sandwich" generation This so-called generation includes people in midlife who have responsibilities for taking care of ELDERLY PARENTS as well as their own almost adult or adult children. Stresses abound because of the multiple and sometimes conflicting roles. Stressors include living arrangements, financial constraints, and time constraints, as in many cases both individuals in a midlife couple are still working.

To improve such stressful situations, open COMMUNICATION between all parties involved is essential. Young people need to realize that their concerns must be balanced with the concerns of the elderly, to reduce some of the stress on the middle generation. Those caught in the middle need to take time for themselves and their own interests. RELAXATION techniques can also be helpful.

See also INTERGENERATIONAL CONFLICTS; LISTENING; PARENTING.

school This term refers to learning institutions, including nursery schools and preschools. The stress caused by fear of going to school may cause a child to be absent, tardy, or simply refuse to attend school. Fear of going to school may begin as early as kindergarten, but usually develops during elementary or junior high school. In many cases, the child begins to devise reasons for staying home. Some develop symptoms, such as nausea, stomachaches, or HEADACHES; others leave home for school, then return without their parents knowing that they are absent from school, or spend their day elsewhere. Cases of extreme refusal to attend school may be considered school PHOBIA. (Fear of school, or school phobia, is known as didaskaleinophobia.)

School avoidance (also known as school refusal or school absenteeism) is one of the most common ANXIETY DISORDERS in children. Avoidance may result from many aspects, such as anxiety over separation from the parents or getting along with teachers, a discipline issue, a complication of a mood disorder, or a fear of failure.

Overcoming the stresses of school

Helping a child who feels stressed by school attendance should begin with discussions with the child and the teacher or teachers involved, and investigating possible causes of the child's problem within the school or school transportation situation.

Reasons may include low SELF-ESTEEM; being bullied, teased, or criticized; or feeling inferior to others. Situations surrounding actual school issues should be considered, such as riding on the school bus, eating in the school lunchroom, using the public washrooms, and undressing in the gym locker rooms. Issues of BODY IMAGE may be involved.

With appropriate counseling and conferences with teachers or other school officials, all concerned can develop a new understanding of the children's stresses regarding school.

Treatment of a child who avoids school should be regarded as crisis intervention. The goal should be to get the child back in school as soon as possible and attending regularly with less fear and more confidence to meet the daily challenges.

Stresses on school teachers
In today's urban societies, teachers face more stresses than just in the classroom. Some neighborhoods in inner cities are populated by gang members, gun carriers, and drug dealers. From the time teachers leave their car in the parking lot, enter through a metal detecting machine, and arrive in their classrooms, there can be considerable uneasiness. Dealing with young people who are concerned only with getting through school and who nearly dare teachers to teach them something, is stressful for even the most dedicated of teachers. Counseling services within the school can be helpful.

See also COPING; CRITICISM; PARENTING; PERFECTION; UNDERACHIEVEMENT.

seasonal affective disorder (SADS)   A form of mild DEPRESSION resulting from the stress of not seeing much sunshine or daylight for months at a time. It is characterized by severe mood swings corresponding to the change of seasons. Depression usually becomes more prevalent during the winter months, while the mood improves with the coming of spring.

The incidence of SADS, which an estimated 35 million Americans suffer from, rises with geographic latitude, affecting 1.4% of Floridians but almost 10% of the population of New Hampshire.

Role of genetics
People who eat more, sleep more, and are more depressed during the winter months may have family members experiencing similar changes, according to an article in the *Archives of General Psychiatry.* Researchers from Washington University School of Medi-

cine surveyed 4,639 adult twins from Australia to determine if there is a biological predisposition to seasonal rhythms in mood and behavior (seasonality). Two types of seasonality were described: one characterized by a winter pattern and a second by a summer pattern of depressive mood disturbance. The researchers found that winter was much more likely than summer to lead to changes in mood, energy, social activity, sleep, appetite, and weight. They also found a "significant genetic influence" on those changes; 17% reported that they felt worse during the winter and 8% reported that they experienced a summer pattern of worsening in mood.

The researchers concluded, "There is a tendency for seasonality to run in families, and this is largely due to a biological predisposition. These findings support continuing efforts to understand the role of the stress of seasonality in the development of mood disorders."

Role of light therapy
Therapy for SADS includes use of specially made bright lights that extend the hours of illumination during short winter days and help reset the body's CIRCADIAN RHYTHMS. In some cases, a PHARMACOLOGICAL APPROACH and PSYCHOTHERAPY are useful.

See also CLIMATE.

SOURCES:
Anderson, Janis L., and Gabrielle I. Weiner. "Seasonal Depression." *Harvard Health Letter* 21, no. 4 (February 1996).
Madden, Pamela A.F. "Seasonal Changes in Mood and Behavior." *Archives of General Psychiatry,* January 1996.
Rae, Stephen. "Bright Light, Big Therapy." *Modern Maturity,* February-March 1994.

secondary depression   A DEPRESSION occurring in an individual who has another illness, either mental or physical, preceding the depression. For example, depression may accompany psychiatric disorders such as

OBSESSIVE-COMPULSIVE DISORDER, ALCOHOLISM AND ALCOHOL DEPENDENCE (most common); depression may occur after or together with a medical illness. Careful evaluation of secondary depression by a physician is essential to determine the cause and course of treatment to reduce the stress the individual is experiencing.

See also PHARMACOLOGICAL APPROACH.

secrets Bits of information people hide or are afraid to tell. Some feel stressed about keeping their secrets or learning the secrets of others. The word "secret" is derived from the Latin *secretus,* meaning "separate" or "out of the way." The current definition, according to the *American Heritage Dictionary of the English Language* includes: "Something kept hidden from others or known only to oneself or to a few. Concealed from general knowledge or view. Dependably close-mouthed; discreet. Not visibly expressed; private; inward."

Most people know something that fits the above definition of secrets. However, the definition does not include many people who are uncomfortable and stressed. They think that there is something wrong in having a secret, don't know what to do about it, and feel scared and threatened. Many people struggle lifelong with the keeping of secrets. A person's own secrets become all-consuming, such as having committed a crime, attempted suicide, having mental illness in the family, or his or her own sexual orientation. There are women and men who are secret alcoholics, agoraphobics afraid to venture out of their homes, women who have had abortions or, after giving birth, gave babies away, and people who know they are adopted and never told their spouses. Some people keep prior marriages secret; others are or were victims of abuse by their husbands or wives. Hiding these secrets, as well as non-visible disabilities, such as vision or hearing impairment, diabetes or cancer, produces stresses that can lead to ANXIETY DISORDERS.

Many people who hide secrets CATASTROPHIZE (constantly asking "what if"). Catastrophizing is predicting in the imagination the actuality of a negative event. They project the "worst case" scenario into the future and act on it as if it were true. As individuals continue worrying about hiding a secret, or worrying about what might happen if they tell, the stress produced leads to body tension, causing psychophysiological illnesses such as HEADACHES and stomachaches, and behavior symptoms such as irritability, short temper, difficulty concentrating, anxieties, DEPRESSION, and frustration.

Sharing secrets

Divulging secrets at the wrong time to the wrong people can be embarrassing, shameful, and may interfere with one's life and lifestyle. On the other hand, telling a secret at an appropriate time to an appropriate person, may help one feel freer, unburdened, and able to let go of real or imagined fears. According to Kahn and Kimmel, authors of *Empower Yourself,* secrets can be divided into those to keep, those to let go of and those to share. Many couples share secrets—the intimacies of their RELATIONSHIP. Family members and business associates share secrets. For many the sharing of secrets helps bond their loving and supportive relationships.

See also COMMUNICATION; INTIMACY.

SOURCES:
Kahn, Ada P., and Sheila Kimmel. *Empower Yourself: Every Woman's Guide to Self-Esteem.* New York: Avon Books 1997.
Pennebaker, James W. *Opening Up. The Healing Power of Confiding in Others.* New York: William Morrow, 1990.

security object A special object, such as a favorite toy or blanket, that gives a child comfort and reassurance. If the object is taken away or lost, even temporarily, the child will experience great stress and probably cry inconsolably. Loss of a child's security object also causes stress for parents, as they must find ways to help the child deal with the loss.

See also GRIEF; PARENTING.

self-confidence See SELF-ESTEEM.

self-esteem Accepting oneself, liking oneself and appreciating one's self-worth. A high degree of self-esteem is a major characteristic of successful COPING with stress. Low self-esteem can lead to mental and physical disorders, such as DEPRESSION, poor appetite, HEADACHES, insomnia and, in extreme cases, SUICIDE.

Many people become stressed when they compare themselves with others or use unrealistic standards set for them by others. Those who think they do not measure up, have low levels of self-esteem and may feel inferior, either intellectually or physically. In contrast, individuals with high self-esteem feel confident and capable. People with low self-esteem often become workaholics and depend on approval from others.

Lack of self-esteem has been indicated as one possible causative role for social ills, including juvenile delinquency, crime, and substance abuse. Lack of self-esteem can be life threatening, particularly in young people, where it is a major factor in depression and suicide.

Causes of low self-esteem

While causes of low self-esteem vary between individuals, there are many common themes. Some have low self-esteem because of physical appearance, for example, individuals who are overweight. This can be overcome by seeking counseling regarding a diet and exercise program. Some have prominent facial features, such as a misshapen nose or ear; with counseling and possibly cosmetic surgery, improvements can be made in both appearance and outlook.

Abuse is another common cause. Having been abused as a child, either sexually or psy-chologically, or having been an abused spouse or in a codependent relationship can have a lasting effect on a person's self-esteem.

Some children lose their self-esteem on the athletic field because they do not compete well or do not have the physical ability to keep up or are bullied by team members. Other children lose self-esteem in the classroom when they are stressed by doing subjects they find hard. Simple comments and CRITICISM by teachers can be stressful to a child and can lower self-esteem. For example, a child told that he or she cannot sing well and should just mouth the words, may lose his confidence in ever trying to sing again. A high school student criticized because of a tendency to stutter may become afraid to stand up and speak in front of a crowd. In many cases, low self-esteem can lead to the stresses of social fears and phobias.

In a Gallup poll in 1992, 612 adults were interviewed and asked about situations that would make them feel very bad about themselves. Situations included not being able to pay bills, being tempted into doing something immoral, having an abortion, getting a divorce, losing a job, feeling they had disobeyed God, being noticeably overweight, doing something embarrassing in public, and being criticized by someone they admired. People over 50 or more years old were more likely to feel bad about these situations than younger people.

See also BODY IMAGE; CODEPENDENCY; DATING; DOMESTIC VIOLENCE; INFERIORITY COMPLEX; INTIMACY; OBESITY; RELATIONSHIPS; SCHOOL; SOCIAL PHOBIAS; UNDERACHIEVEMENT.

SOURCES:
Hazelton, Deborah M. *Solving the Self-Esteem Puzzle.* Deerfield Beach, Fla. Health Communications, 1991.
Hillman, Carolynn. *Recovery of Your Self-Esteem.* New York: Simon & Schuster, 1992.
Kahn, Ada P., and Sheila Kimmel. *Empower Yourself: Every Woman's Guide to Self-Esteem.* New York: Avon Books, 1997.

self-help groups The concept behind self-help groups is sharing feelings, perceptions, and concerns with others who have had or still have the same experience. According to the American Medical Association, self-help groups typically exhibit the following characteristics and benefits:

Common problem: Members immediately identify with one another.
*Mutual aid/helper therapy:*Members benefit as much from giving help as from receiving it.
Network for support: Members provide a network of emotional and social support through regular and special gatherings, telephone calls, newsletters, visits, and computers.
Unconditional acceptance: Members are usually encouraged to share their personal situations in a nonjudgmental, caring environment.
Shared information: Through the group process and written material, members capture and share their successful techniques for COPING.
Low cost: Expenses are shared through collections at meetings, minimal membership dues, or fundraising projects.

The self-help movement, with growing strength and visibility, has led to increased openness and understanding of many disorders, such as ANXIETY DISORDERS and CHRONIC ILLNESS. Such groups help many people develop better coping skills to meet the challenges they face.

Self-help techniques

Self-help groups utilize group discussions as well as audio and videotapes. Self-help can work if the individual is motivated to make it work. In fact, even with psychotherapy under the guidance of a professional, much of the improvement in a person's ability to cope with STRESS actually comes from self-help.

Many individuals join SUPPORT GROUPS to learn self-help techniques for particular situations. These include MEDITATION and PROGRESSIVE MUSCLE RELAXATION. Both are skills that

can be learned and applied to relieve stress, ANXIETY, and PHOBIAS.

See ALTERNATIVE THERAPIES.

FOR FURTHER INFORMATION:
National Self-Help Clearinghouse
22 West 42nd Street
New York, NY 10036
Phone: (212) 642-2944

SOURCE:
American Medical Association. *Healthcare Resource and Reference Guide.* Chicago: American Medical Association, 1993.

self-hypnosis See HYPNOSIS.

self-psychology Term for the psychological system propounded by Heinz Kohut (1913–81), an Austrian-born American psychoanalyst. His theory holds that all behavior as well as stresses can be interpreted in reference to the self. He proposed that even a young child has tendencies toward assertiveness and ambition, idealization of parents, and the beginnings of values. All these tendencies contribute to strong ties between the infant and parent.

Kohut believed that the real mover of psychic development is the self, rather than sexual and aggressive drives, as Sigmund Freud suggested. Kohut used the term self-object to describe an object in an infant's surrounding that the infant regards as part of himself or herself. People with narcissistic personality disorder cannot separate adequately from the self-object and thus cannot perceive or respond to the individuality of others. Kohut believed that the lack of empathic response between parent and infant is the cause of later stresses and psychological disorders in the growing child.

Kohut explained his major theories in several publications, including *The Analysis of the Self* (1971), *The Restoration of the Self* (1977) and *The Search for the Self* (1978).

See also PSYCHOTHERAPIES.

FOR FURTHER INFORMATION:
Kohut Archives
Institute for Psychoanalysis
180 North Michigan Avenue
Chicago, IL 60601
Phone: (312) 726-6300

SOURCES:
Kohut, Heinz. *The Analysis of the Self.* New York:
    International Universities Press, 1971.
———. *The Psychology of the Self.* New York:
    International Universities Press, 1978.
———. *The Restoration of the Self.* New York:
    International Universities Press, 1977.

self-talk   Messages one gives to oneself, often stemming from comments heard during childhood or earlier negative experiences. Negative self-talk may include such statements as "I can't do this; this will never work out; I'm no good at this." On the other hand, positive self-talk may include such messages as "I've done this before; everything will work out; I'll find a way."

Negative self-talk is a source of stress for many people because it discourages them from taking any risks or making desired changes in their lives. Negative self-talk interferes with SELF-ESTEEM. Positive self-talk can help relieve stress because it reinforces confidence in one's own abilities.

SOURCE:
Kahn, Ada P., and Sheila Kimmel. *Empower Yourself: Every Woman's Guide to Self-Esteem.* New York: Avon Books, 1997.

Selye, Hans (1907–82)   An Austrian-born Canadian endocrinologist and psychologist, well known for his work in STRESS research. He introduced the concept of stress during the early 1940s. He is the author of *The Stress of Life* (1956) and *Stress without Distress* (1974).

He defined stress as "the nonspecific response of the body to any demand made upon it. It is more than merely nervous tension." He categorized over 1,000 physiological occurrences related to stress and adaptation. His theory is a description of what one may expect with chronic exposure to stressors, and with the body's attempts to adapt and return to "normality."

In 1950, Selye coined the term "GENERAL ADAPTATION SYNDROME" (G.A.S.). Selye borrowed the term "stress" from physics, and applied it to the mutual actions of forces that take place across any section of the body to threaten HOMEOSTASIS. Although not all states of stress were harmful, according to Selye, he held that the more severe, protracted, and uncontrollable situations of psychological and physical distress led to disease states. His concept of G.A.S. focused on the reaction of the body to illness or foreign substances as opposed to concentrating on specific illnesses and their treatment.

Although his work was controversial during his time, mental health disciplines profited from his ground-breaking work in stress research. His concept of stress opened new avenues of treatment through the discovery that hormones participate in the development of many degenerative diseases, including coronary thrombosis, hardening of the arteries, high blood pressure, arthritis, peptic ulcers, and even cancer.

Selye received his medical training in Europe; he did most of his innovative research on the effects of stress in Montreal at McGill University and the Institut de Medicine et de Chirurgie Experimentales de l'Universite de Montreal, of which he was director for many years. He received his medical degree and his Ph.D. from the German University in Prague. Selye earned doctorates in medicine, philosophy, and science, as well as at least 19 honorary degrees from universities around the world. He authored more than 32 books and more than 1,500 technical articles.

See also DIS-STRESS; EUSTRESS; STRESS MANAGEMENT.

SOURCES:

Selye, Hans. *The Stress of Life.* New York: McGraw-Hill, 1956.

———. *Stress without Distress.* Philadelphia: J.B. Lippincott, 1974.

sense of humor   See LAUGHTER.

separation anxiety   A stressful feeling one experiences when separated from parents or individuals with whom one has an attachment. Infants and toddlers normally experience stress and anxiety when separated from parents or caregivers, but the intensity usually diminishes by the time the child is four to five years old. Children who fear separation cry, cling to the parent, and demand to be held and cuddled.

Symptoms of separation anxiety in childhood may be HEADACHES, stomachaches, and other vague complaints in an effort to keep the parent from leaving or to keep the child home from SCHOOL. School phobia, or school avoidance, is sometimes a case of separation anxiety. What some children fear is that something dreadful will happen to their parent(s) if they are away, or that the parent will not be there when the child returns.

Sometimes the parent (usually the mother) has a fear of danger when her child is away from her, which is transmitted to the child and augments the child's own fears. The mother of a child with separation anxiety may need supportive psychotherapy to help relieve her own stresses as well as those of the child.

See also AGORAPHOBIA; GRIEF; SECURITY OBJECT.

serotonin   A NEUROTRANSMITTER found in the central nervous system, in many tissues, in the lining of digestive tract, and in the brain, serotonin influences SLEEP and emotional arousal and is indirectly involved in the psychobiology of DEPRESSION. Low levels of serotonin may contribute to development of depression. Some antidepressant medications increase the levels of serotonin and norepinephrine, another neurotransmitter.

See also PHARMACOLOGICAL APPROACH.

serotonin reuptake inhibitors (SRIs)   See DEPRESSION; PHARMACOLOGICAL APPROACH.

sex appeal   Usually refers to personal appeal or physical attractiveness for members of the opposite sex. A healthy, good-looking face, attractive hair, and an attractive body shape are generally the embodiment of sex appeal in the United States today. Individuals with these characteristics are featured in advertisements and in films. People may find these advertisements a source of stress as they seem to feel that these models are a threat to their SELF-ESTEEM.

A person who has sex appeal may be said to be "sexy" based on cultural patterns and personal tastes. For example, men who are muscular and athletic are considered sexy, as are women who are relatively slim but have large breasts. At other periods in history, women who were plump were considered attractive, as shown in paintings of Peter Paul Rubens, a Flemish painter (1577–1640) whose nudes gave our vocabulary the term "Rubenesque," to refer to the well-developed and heavier body shapes.

See also ADVERTISING; BODY IMAGE; EATING DISORDERS.

sex drive   A level of desire to have sexual activity. This level varies in strength and is different for women and men and at different ages and stages of their lives. Differences may be due to stress or to inhibitions influenced by parental, religious, and peer group attitudes about sex.

People's expression of sexual desire may differ also, according to whether or not they have a partner. For example, sex researchers have found that some widowed postmenopausal women who have no partner believe that their sex drive is not very strong, while women in the same peer group who date and have male companions feel a strong sex drive.

While some researchers believe that sex drive decreases with age, many older adults will attest to the fact that sex drive can persist throughout all stages of life. Good health, freedom from chronic disease, and companionship with others of the opposite sex stimulates the sex drive to continue until older age.

If individuals feel that they are lacking in sex drive, medical consultation may be helpful.

See also SEX THERAPY; SEXUAL DIFFICULTIES.

sexism An attitude or belief that one sex is superior to the other in certain situations. The attitude seems to cause stress for all concerned. The term often refers to male attitudes about women, such as "women in public office might cry if they are upset," or "a woman shouldn't be trained for a high-paying job because she will leave to have children." To a large extent the WOMEN'S MOVEMENT during the latter half of the 20th century fought and overcame sexism.

See also SEXUAL HARASSMENT.

sex therapy Includes counseling and treatment for SEXUAL DIFFICULTIES that are not due to medical or physical causes. People may encounter sexual difficulties because of stress, while at the same time sexual difficulties are a cause of stress for them. The purpose of sex therapy is to address the anxieties that a couple has about sexual activity by learning what normal sexual behavior is and by increasing their enjoyment of sex by gradually engaging in intimate activities. Couples learn to communicate better with each other regarding sexual matters and preferences, retrain their approaches and response patterns, and thus reduce their feeling of stress.

Sex therapy techniques

Sex therapists use several techniques. One is sensate focus therapy, in which the couple explores pleasurable activities in a relaxed manner without sexual sensations. The couple might start with massage of non-erogenous areas of the body. Gradually, as anxieties diminish, the couple progresses to stimulation of sexual areas and finally to sexual intercourse.

Other techniques sex therapists use are directed toward reducing premature EJACULATION, relieving vaginismus (muscle spasm of the vagina), and helping both partners reach orgasm.

For sexual difficulties related to physical causes or illness, individuals should consult a physician, particularly specialists in gynecology or urology.

See also ANORGASMIA; COMMUNICATION; DYSPAREUNIA; INTIMACY; LISTENING; SEXUAL PREFERENCES; SEXUAL RESPONSE CYCLE.

SOURCE:

Kahn, Ada P., and Linda Hughey Holt. *The A–Z of Women's Sexuality.* Alameda, Calif.: Hunter House, 1992.

sexual difficulties Any conditions that interfere with the process leading to and including enjoyment of sexual intercourse (coitus). Sexual difficulties are extremely stressful for the individuals involved. Indeed, many marriages and relationships break up because of sexual stress.

The opposite of sexual difficulties are feelings of contentment after a pleasurable and satisfying sexual encounter. An individual has a feeling of intense fulfillment in the orgasmic and resolution phases of the SEXUAL RESPONSE CYCLE. This is accompanied by a feeling of extreme RELAXATION, sometimes a "high" feeling and emotional closeness with the partner.

There are temporary sexual difficulties and there are dysfunctions or situations that persist lifelong. Use of some prescription drugs may cause sexual dysfunction for some individuals; it may be possible that other similar drugs can be substituted by a physician that do not have these unpleasant side effects.

Examples of female sexual difficulties include ANORGASMIA, DYSPAREUNIA (painful sexual intercourse), and VAGINISMUS. Examples of male sexual dysfunctions include IMPOTENCE, difficulty in maintaining erection, premature EJACULATION, and retarded ejaculation.

Sexual fears

Many people are under stress and that stress tends to impair or weaken their sexual responses to partners. For example, some women fear experiencing pain during intercourse or fear that they will not experience ORGASM. Some men fear that they will not be able to achieve or maintain an erection long enough for a satisfying experience for their partners.

The stress of CHRONIC ILLNESS can cause people to fear that they will not be able to enjoy sexually fulfilling experiences. For example, some husbands after heart surgery fear the sexual act itself; their wives fear that sexual activity will harm their husbands.

The threat of acquiring a SEXUALLY TRANSMITTED DISEASE (STD) or the HIV virus (known as the cause of AIDS) is a contemporary fear of many people who are not in monogamous relationships. These fears can largely be overcome by the use of SAFE SEX practices.

See also BEHAVIOR THERAPY; COMMUNICATION; HUMAN IMMUNODEFICIENCY VIRUS; SEX THERAPY.

sexual harassment Unwelcome and unwanted sexual attention, usually on the job; it is particularly stressful for the person experiencing it. The harassment may involve men toward women, women toward men, or the same-sex individuals; it may include jokes, remarks, and questions about the other's sexual behavior, "accidental" touching, and repeated and unwanted invitations for a date or for a sexual relationship. It can be verbal, visual, physical, or written.

Sexual harassment is defined in terms of its effect on the recipient. This means that behavior meant to be humorous or well-intentioned is sexual harassment if it is offensive to the individual at the receiving end. It is not the intent of the sender of the behavior that counts because what one person may view as harmless can be objectionable to others.

According to the Human Resource Department, Rush North Shore Medical Center, Skokie, Illinois, 90% of harassment is stopped by a request from the victim. In 76% of cases where victims ignored the harassment, it continued. When propositioned, 67% of men are flattered and 83% of women are not. Equally important, 63% of women and 15% of men are insulted.

Of all incidents of sexual harassment reported to the Equal Employment Opportunities Commission in fiscal year 1990, 92% were reported by women. Women in lower positions are far less likely to tell a harasser who holds a higher organizational position that his/her conduct is unwelcome. However, in a research study of female medical students, 61% reported having been sexually harassed by residents or interns and 48% claimed to be harassed by patients.

A United States Supreme Court decision (*Meritor* v. *Vinson*) in 1980 declared that sexual harassment is a form of sex discrimination and, therefore, a violation of Title VII of the 1964 Civil Rights Act. During the 1980s, American society became increasingly aware of sexual harassment. For example, in the study by the U.S. Merit Systems Protection Board reported in 1988, federal workers were more inclined to define certain types of behavior as sexual harassment than in 1980.

In 1987, 42% of women and 14% of men employed by the federal government said they experienced some form of uninvited and unwanted sexual attention. Federal workers in the survey believed that sexual harassment was not worse in the federal government than in the private sector. The workers reported that the most frequently experienced type of uninvited sexual attention was "unwanted

EXAMPLES OF SEXUAL HARASSMENT

- Dirty jokes or sexually oriented language
- Nude or semi-nude photos, posters, calendars, or cartoons
- Obscene gestures, lewd actions, or leering
- Introduction of sexual topics into business conversations
- Requests for dates or sexual favors that are not mutually acceptable
- Unwelcome hugging, patting, or touching

sexual teasing, jokes, remarks, or questions." The least frequently experienced type of harassment reported was "actual or attempted rape or assault." When victims of sexual harassment took positive action in response to unwanted sexual attention, it was largely informal action, and in many cases, was effective. For both sexes, simply asking or telling the offender to stop improved the situation most frequently. Threatening to tell others or telling others was the second most effective action for women, while avoiding the person(s) was the second most effective action for men.

Sexual harassment during the survey period of May 1985 through May 1987 cost

SEXUAL HARASSMENT: WHAT TO DO

- Tell the offender promptly and clearly that the conduct is unwelcome and unacceptable. Do this verbally or in writing, or both.
- Document in writing every incident, with specific details of the offensive behavior and your response.
- Do not feel guilty. Sexual harassment is not your fault. By clearly voicing your expectations, you force the offender to choose whether to change the unwelcome behavior or to purposely continue it.
- If the problem continues, tell your supervisor. If your supervisor is the harasser, talk to another executive or report it to the department of human resources.

the federal government an estimated $267 million, which involved job turnover, sick leave, individual productivity, and work group productivity.

In the late 1990s, cases of sexual harassment in the military services were uncovered. Stresses arose when enlisted men and women felt obligated to follow requests of their superiors. Disciplinary charges occurred in many cases and led to discharge, which will probably serve as a deterrent to ongoing sexual harassment in the military.

Sources:
Sexual Harassment in the Federal Government: An Update. Washington, D.C.: U.S. Merit Systems Protection Board, June 1988.
"Sexual Harassment: What Am I Supposed to Do?" Skokie: Rush North Shore Medical Center, 1995.

sexuality   The ability to think and behave as a sexual being; also, any aspect of human thought or behavior that has sexual meaning. It implies a self-concept of oneself as a sexual being as well as having the capacity to respond to erotic stimuli and sexual activity. Sexuality encompasses being comfortable with sexual fantasies and erotic zones of the body as well as with one's own gender identity. However, no specific set of behavior or SEXUAL PREFERENCE is necessary to have a good sense of one's own sexuality. Social, psychological, and biological dimensions to human sexuality lead to stress for many people.

See also SEXUAL DIFFICULTIES.

sexually transmitted diseases (STDs)   Diseases that affect both men and women and are generally transmitted during sexual intercourse. STDs cause individuals considerable stress because of physical discomforts, psychological pain, possible INFERTILITY, and the potential that they may be life-threatening, as in the case of AIDS.

STDs cause psychological distress for many reasons, including a need to communicate the problem to one's partner and a need to disclose information about past sexual activities and partners. The term SAFE SEX relates to sexual practices that aid in the prevention of STDs as well as AIDS.

The stresses and long-term effects caused by two STDs, syphilis and gonorrhea, have been with human beings for centuries. Those two diseases were commonly referred to as venereal diseases long before the term STD was coined. Syphilis and gonorrhea are still prevalent, and on the increase due to the upswing in other concurrent STDs. These other STDs became notably widespread during the latter decades of the 20th century. They include chlamydia, herpes, hepatitis B, as well as genital warts, and other vaginal infections.

Individuals who are widowed or divorced and who begin dating and seeking new partners after their loss, as well as never-married individuals, are concerned about STDs. Fear of acquiring STDs has led many formerly sexually active people to seek fewer sexual partners. Such concerns have also increased the use of condoms, which, when appropriately used, are thought to reduce the likelihood of spreading most STDs (as well as AIDS).

Differentiating sexually transmitted diseases

Chlamydia is two or three times more common than gonorrhea (see below) but less well known. The disease affects men and women, but women are less likely to notice symptoms in early stages. The signs in women are unusual vaginal discharge, irregular bleeding, bleeding after intercourse, or deep pain during and after intercourse. Untreated infections in women can lead to infections in the Fallopian tubes and uterus (pelvic inflammatory disease). Men may notice clear, mucous-like discharge from the penis and burning during urination. Chlamydia is treated with antibiotics, and sexual partners must be treated to avoid a ping-pong effect of reinfection. Thus, when one individual discovers

that he or she has it, psychological concerns arise regarding telling the partner(s) and encouraging treatment.

Herpes (technically known as HERPES SIMPLEX or herpes virus hominus; HSV) outbreaks cause either single or multiple blisters, which occur on mucous membranes such as lips or vagina. Herpes simplex I causes most oral "cold sores"; herpes simplex II causes most genital herpes. Transmission can occur when a herpes blister comes in contact with any mucous membrane or open cut or sore. Herpes is most often transmitted through sexual intercourse and can also be transmitted during mouth-genital contact, or with manual contact during heterosexual or homosexual relations.

Attacks of herpes occur or recur when the individual is under stress, fatigued, or has another illness. Women who know that they have the herpes infection are concerned about giving birth, as the infection can be transmitted to the baby during the birth process. Women who have active vaginal herpes blisters are routinely given Cesarean sections.

Hepatitis B may develop about two months after sexual activity. It usually is acquired during sexual intercourse with an infected individual. Hepatitis B is common among intravenous drug users in the United States as well as those who travel in underdeveloped countries. People who are concerned about getting Hepatitis B can obtain an immunization against it; the immunization is recommended for health care workers, for household workers, and for sexual partners of individuals already infected by Hepatitis B.

Genital warts. Warts, or small bumps on the mucous membrane of the vulva, the clitoral hood, in the perineum, inside the vagina, in the anus, on the penis, or in the urinary tract, may be genital warts; they are caused by a sexually transmitted virus. Genital warts cause discomfort and stress to the sufferer and may be particularly painful during sexual intercourse or when the sufferer wears tight clothing. Certain strains of the wart virus have been implicated as a cause of cervical cancer. If either partner has a history of genital warts, a condom should be used during sexual intercourse to avoid transmission. Genital warts can be removed by a physician.

Gonorrhea and syphilis. Gonorrhea (also known as the "dose," "clap," or "drip") is caused by a bacteria that can infect the genital organs and spread to other parts of the body; complications include pelvic inflammatory disease, joint pains, heart disease, liver disease, meningitis, and blindness. Because there are fewer symptoms in women than men, gonorrhea usually is detected later in women. In a woman, the gonorrhea germs travel to the uterus, Fallopian tubes, and ovaries. As the disease advances, she may feel abdominal pain. Males may notice painful urination and pus discharging from the penis.

Gonorrhea is treated with large doses of penicillin, usually injected, with follow-up doses of oral antibiotics. In recent years, many cases of penicillin-resistant gonorrhea have appeared. This makes the disease even more fearsome than in the past, when penicillin was hailed as the "magic bullet" against gonorrhea.

Syphilis, though less common than gonorrhea, can result in serious complications when untreated. Syphilis has been known as "lues," "syph," "pox," and "bad blood" and is caused by a microorganism from the spirochete family. An initial outbreak ("primary syphilis") causes a large punched out lesion called a chancre. After this initial outbreak, symptoms may not recur for several months, after which a skin rash or secondary syphilis occurs. Years later, central nervous system symptoms in the form of mental aberrations and a stumbling gait may occur ("tertiary" syphilis). Treatment with penicillin or other antibiotics is usually effective during the early stages of the disease and will prevent complications.

Unlike infections with herpes, chlamydia, and gonorrhea, which can be transmitted at

---

HOW TO REDUCE RISKS OF ACQUIRING AN STD

- Have sexual contact with only one partner who limits contact to you only. Have a monogamous relationship.
- Ask your partner about any suspicious looking discharges, sores, or rashes. Look your partner over.
- Use condoms. Condoms provide some (though not complete) protection against STDs. However, the condom must be put on before sexual activity begins and not removed until the end of the activity.
- Use foam, a diaphragm with spermicides, or sponge spermicides, which kill many infectious agents; these should be used in addition to the condom.
- If one partner has a STD, the other partner must be informed and treated at the same time to avoid reinfection. Avoid the "ping-pong" effect of infection.

---

birth, congenital syphilis is a prenatal infection. Fetal infection may occur at any time during pregnancy. It is more likely to occur if the mother has primary, secondary, or early latent syphilis, as many organisms are present in the circulation during these stages.

ACQUIRED IMMUNODEFICIENCY SYNDROME (AIDS) has become a widely known disease during the latter part of the 20th century. The AIDS virus is known to be transmitted by direct exchange of body fluid, such as semen or blood, and thus is considered a sexually transmitted disease.

FOR FURTHER INFORMATION:
National VD Hotline
American Social Health Association
Phone: (800) 227-8922; CA: (800) 982-5883

American Social Health Association
P.O. Box 13827
Research Triangle Park, NC 27709
Phone: (919) 361-2742

SIECUS (Sex Information and Education Council of the U.S.)

130 W. 42nd Street (Suite 2500)
New York, NY 10036
Phone: (212) 819-9770

SOURCES:
Kahn, Ada P., and Linda Hughey Holt. *The A–Z of Women's Sexuality.* Alameda, Calif.: Hunter House, 1992.
Sack, Fleur. *Romance to Die For: The Startling Truth About Women, Sex and AIDS.* Deerfield Beach, Fla.: Health Communications, 1992.

sexual preferences   The choices women and men make when experiencing attraction to and participating in sexual activities with other men, women, or both genders. These may be influenced by environment, early childhood experiences, possibly genetic makeup, and early hormonal exposure effects on central nervous system development.

HOMOSEXUALITY refers to sexual attraction to members of the same sex. Bisexuality refers to sexual attraction to members of the opposite sex and members of the same sex. Stresses involve perceiving oneself as different from most people and at times not understanding one's attractions.

See also LESBIANISM.

sexual response   A physiological reaction to sexual stimulation and arousal. In women, vaginal lubrication is an early sign in the SEXUAL RESPONSE CYCLE. In men, erection of the penis occurs. Responsiveness is a highly individual matter, largely determined by mutual feelings of love and affection between the partners and a wide variety of emotional and physical circumstances. Levels of responsiveness vary between individuals, and vary within the same individual at different times. Many people experience stress about their responses, not realizing that a wide range of differences are considered normal.

See also SEX THERAPY.

sexual response cycle   The physiological processes and events that occur during sexual intercourse. Many people experience stress in their sexual relationships because of lack of understanding of what this cycle should be. An explanation as proposed by Masters and Johnson in their landmark work, *Human Sexual Response* (1966), may relieve some of this stress.

They describe four phases in the cycle: *excitement, plateau, orgasm,* and *resolution.* In reality, sexual activity usually proceeds in a smooth-flowing, continuous manner with various phases overlapping and imperceptibly merging into one another.

Excitement phase. Arousal begins; excitement may result from kissing, being caressed or touched in erogenous areas by one's partner. This excitement may occur quickly or more slowly due to stress, fatigue, intake of alcohol, or age. Vasocongestion in women results in vaginal lubrication; in men, erection of the penis. In women, the glans (tip) and shaft of the clitoris enlarge; the nipples may become erect. Some males have nipple erection during the excitement phase. A woman's inner labia (labia minora) swell and open up (a vasocongestion response); and the outer lips (labia majora) move apart and flatten out. The upper two-thirds of the vagina expands to accommodate the entrance of the penis. The uterus and cervix also pull up during excitement, resulting in a "tent effect" within the vaginal walls and creating a larger cervical opening. Both women and men show an increase in pulse rate and blood pressure. In men, the skin of the scrotum becomes thicker, the scrotal sac tenses, the scrotum is pulled up and closer to the body, and the spermatic cords shorten, elevating the testes.

Plateau phase. Vasocongestion reaches its peak. In women, an "orgasmic platform" forms; this is a swelling or thickening of the tissues surrounding the outer third of the vagina, making the size of the vaginal entrance somewhat smaller; there may be an increased gripping of the penis. The clitoris retracts or draws up into the body, making the shaft about half as long as before. Excitement builds until there is enough tension for orgasm. In men, the penis is completely erect during the plateau phase even though there may be some variations in the firmness of the erection. The coronal ridge at the edge of the glans swells, the testes become engorged with blood and may be double their unaroused size. They pull up higher and closer to the body. A few drops of liquid, secreted by the Cowper's glands, appear at the tip of the penis. This liquid is not ejaculate but may contain active sperm; thus intercourse without any means of contraception may result in pregnancy even though the man believes he is withdrawing before EJACULATION.

Both women and men experience further increase in breathing rate, pulse rate, and blood pressure during this phase.

Orgasm. Orgasms vary within the same man or woman at different times, depending on many factors, which may include their level of arousal, physical condition, or the mood of the moment. In women, the process of orgasm includes a series of rhythmic muscular contractions of the orgasmic platform; they may also feel some degree of contraction around the opening of the vagina. Some women describe a feeling of very comfortable warmth and sudden relaxation of their entire body accompanying orgasm. A woman's partner cannot always tell when she has reached orgasm; COMMUNICATION between partners enhances enjoyment for both. Women usually do not reach orgasm as quickly as men; partners usually develop a pace in their sexual cycle to accommodate to each other's responses. According to researchers, some women never consciously experience orgasm. An inability to achieve orgasm is not abnormal nor does it necessarily make a woman's experience unsatisfying.

In men, orgasm consists of a series of rapid rhythmic contractions of the pelvic organs. First, the vas, seminal vesicles, and prostate contract, forcing the ejaculate into a bulb at the base of the urethra, which Masters and Johnson describe as "ejaculatory inevitability." In the next stage, the urethral bulb and the penis itself contact rhythmically, forcing semen outward.

Resolution. After orgasm, the body returns to a relaxed and unaroused state. Usually a feeling of deep relaxation occurs in both women and men who experience a return to normal breathing, pulse rate, and blood pressure. They may be covered with a thin glow of perspiration, not from the physical exertion but as a response of the resolution phase.

See also ANORGASMIA; EJACULATION; IMPOTENCE; LISTENING; SEXUAL DIFFICULTIES.

SOURCES:
Hite, Shere. *The Hite Report: A Nationwide Study of Female Sexuality.* New York: Macmillan, 1976.
Kahn, Ada P., and Linda Hughey Holt. *The A–Z of Women's Sexuality,* Alameda, Calif.: Hunter House, 1992.
Kinsey, Alfred C., Wardell B. Pomeroy, Clyde E. Martin, and Paul H. Gebhard. *Sexual Behavior in the Human Female.* Philadelphia: W.B. Saunders, 1953.
Masters, William H., and Virginia Johnson. *Human Sexual Response.* Boston: Little, Brown, 1966.

sexual revolution The term "sexual revolution" refers to changes in sexual attitudes and behaviors in the United States during the 1960s, 1970s, and early 1980s. With the changes came increased stresses for many people as more choices of life-style became socially acceptable. Generally, there were more liberal attitudes toward premarital sexual activity, changes in the double standard in which sexual activity had previously been seen as more acceptable for men than for women, and more open discussion of women's sexual needs. Increases in premarital activity evolved in part as a result of development of better and easier means of BIRTH CONTROL, including oral contraceptives during the late 1950s.

For many young people, DATING habits during the sexual revolution included sexual intercourse early in the relationship. However, with the increase of SEXUALLY TRANSMITTED DISEASES and ACQUIRED IMMUNODEFICIENCY SYNDROME (AIDS) in the heterosexual population since the 1980s, people have become more cautious and selective about their sexual partners and monogamy has regained favor.

The sexual revolution was closely tied with the WOMEN'S MOVEMENT. Many college dormitories became coeducational, and there was wider acceptance of unmarried adults "living together." While this arrangement was acceptable to many, for others it was a source of stress.

shell shock   See POST-TRAUMATIC STRESS DISORDER.

shiatsu   Considered an ALTERNATIVE THERAPY that may be useful for some individuals to prevent or relieve the effects of stress. Shiatsu is a specific method for manipulating *tsubos* (points along the meridians where the flow of energy may become blocked). The manipulation may occur through pressing with the fingers and hands, or through the use of elbows, knees, and feet. The points that are manipulated are known as ACUPRESSURE or ACUPUNCTURE points. Manipulation of the body's approximately 360 *tsubos* is thought to release the flow of energy (*chi*). There are many forms of shiatsu.

See also BODY THERAPIES.

SOURCE:
McCarty, Patrick. *A Beginner's Guide to Shiatsu: Using Finger Pressure for the Relief of Headaches, Back Pain, and Hypertension.* Garden City Park, N.Y.: Avery Publishing Group, 1995.

shift work   Usually refers to working a series of hours earlier or later in the day than the more usual 9 to 5 routine. Some work an afternoon shift, from 4 to 11 P.M.; others work the night shift, from 11 P.M. to 7 A.M. People who do shift work experience many unique stresses. How well one adapts to shift work depends on how well one handles the interruption of the body's CIRCADIAN RHYTHMS. The break in circadian rhythm can affect mental ability, alertness, and temperament. Thus some night shift workers experience anxiety and lapses in memory as a result of SLEEP deprivation.

Individuals who do shift work also suffer social stresses. For example, many people function on a 9 to 5 schedule, with most socialization occurring after work and on weekends. For night-shift people to have a family or social life, they must schedule creatively. Spouses and children of shift workers also experience stress because of this schedule.

A study of 79,000 nurses published in *Circulation* (December 1, 1995) indicated that those who worked irregular shifts for more than six years had a moderately higher risk of suffering a heart attack than coworkers on regular shifts.

How night shift workers can avoid stress
"The best strategy is to stay on one shift as long as possible. You'll have the best chance of getting restful sleep that way; you'll be more alert and potentially safer," says Rebecca Smith-Coggins, M.D., a Stanford University emergency medicine physician who studies what happens when people's sleep habits change.

"People who work random shifts in a 24-hour work environment suffer in their ability to perform specific physical tasks and to make decisions. Other studies have shown that when workers are shifted forward rather than randomly, they perform better and have fewer sick days. However, it still takes two weeks to get used to a night shift after a day shift," according to Smith-Coggins.

Workers new to the night shift can help themselves adjust by knowing that they won't get a full six to eight hours' sleep in one stretch immediately. To help make the change,

Smith-Coggins advises that new night workers take a three-hour nap before starting work, then sleep again after their shift. "Studies as well as our own experience among emergency department workers point to this double sleep pattern as the easiest way to switch over," she says.

Eventually most shift workers will find themselves sleeping longer after they get home and napping less before they start work. Ultimately, a full "night's" sleep is possible in the morning, after working the night shift.

Changing work shifts

For people who must change shifts, the healthiest approach seems to be to start the new shift later in the day. For example, it's easier on sleep and rest patterns to change from an eight-hour shift starting at 7 A.M. to one starting at 3 P.M. rather than the reverse. Moving forward is better because most humans operate on a 25-hour sleep-wake cycle. "Our body temperature and other natural functions rotate as if the day were 25 hours long. You can see how that works by studies that place people in a darkened setting with no clues about time. They develop a natural tendency to get up one hour later every day, a clear indication that we are on a forward rather than back or static cycle," Smith-Coggins explained.

Other ways for night workers to get more efficient rest include darkening the bedroom as much as possible or using a sleep mask. Ear plugs or so-called white noise, such as a humming sound from a fan or air conditioner, can help. It is also helpful to maintain the same bedtime rituals, such as relaxing with a book or television show, particularly if the material is not unsettling.

SOURCES:
Hurley, Margaret, and Elizabeth A. Neidlinger. "To Shift or Not to Shift." *Schumpert Medical Quarterly* 9, no. 2 (October 1991).
Smith-Coggins, Rebecca. "Night Shifts Can Be Easier." *Circulation*, December 1, 1995.

shopaholism   A compulsion to shop. While some people view shopping as recreation and a way to reduce stress, for others, shopping can lead to a compulsive syndrome. Excessive shopping shares some characteristics with OBSESSIVE-COMPULSIVE DISORDER, in which people perform certain rituals to relieve tension. In this way, compulsive shopping is similar to the problems of alcoholics or gamblers who exhibit obsessive behavior.

Compulsive shoppers buy things in order to forget the stresses of their lives and make themselves feel good. However, over time it takes more and more spending and buying to improve their moods.

Probably 2% of Americans can be described as compulsive buyers, and another 2% to 3% are on the verge. In a 1991 symposium on compulsive buying during a conference of the American Psychological Association in San Francisco, advertisers, store owners and credit card companies drew some blame for encouraging irresponsible spending. After studying hundreds of compulsive buyers, researchers concluded that such buyers have a knack for deluding them-

---

COPING WITH THE STRESS OF SHOPAHOLISM

- Shop with a list and buy only what is on the list.
- Shop with a partner who will help you resist
- Avoid browsing and avoid sales. The excitement can trigger a shopping spree.
- Develop new social outlets. Cultivate groups of friends with whom you can share activities as a healthful alternative to shopping.
- Learn alternatives for COPING with stress. People with addictive illnesses usually do not cope well with stress.
- Physical exercise is a good stress reliever and will clear your mind for better concentration later on.
- Avoid using credit cards. Use them only for business, if you need to.

selves when they want to buy something. They believe that they will have the money to pay for the items when the bills come, but in reality they will not.

Many people who are normally good about balancing their budgets overbuy around holidays, so for individuals who are compulsive shoppers, the problem will be magnified. Excessive shopping can be attributed in part to an attempt to promote a better self-image through buying multiple or expensive gifts, to change people's perceptions about the giver, to make an economic statement, or to serve as a substitute for weaker aspects of the giver's relationship with others.

Support group for shopaholics

Debtors Anonymous is a support group for overspenders based on the 12-step recovery program of Alcoholics Anonymous. DA members work toward financial solvency the way AA members work toward abstinence. Experienced DA members review new members' finances and help them formulate an action plan for resolving debts and a spending plan for the future. DA members look to one another for support, hope, and strength in dealing with the stresses of indebtedness.

FOR FURTHER INFORMATION:
Debtors Anonymous
P.O. Box 400
Grand Central Station
New York, NY 10163-0400
Phone: (212) 642-8220

SOURCES:
Kahn, Ada P., and Jan Fawcett. *The Encyclopedia of Mental Health.* New York: Facts On File, 1993.
O'Connor, Karen. *When Spending Takes the Place of Feeling.* Nashville: Thomas Nelson, 1992.

shyness   Generally refers to excessive discomfort, embarrassment, and INHIBITION in the presence of others, which can lead to avoidance. Shyness is a source of stress for many individuals who recognize their shyness.

Shy people generally would like to be more dynamic, outgoing, and outspoken. They may be eager to meet new people and learn new activities, but are often reluctant to do so because of discomfort and anxiety about what to say or do. Excessive shyness sometimes becomes a SOCIAL PHOBIA.

Shyness is fairly common in children and adolescents. However, as the young person develops an increasing sense of SELF-ESTEEM, shyness often disappears.

See also PHOBIAS; PUBERTY.

sibling relationships   Relationships between brothers and sisters; stresses include COMPETITION between siblings who often vie for parental attention. The situation first occurs after the birth of a new baby, when an older sibling feels "displaced." The feelings of rivalry may persist among siblings throughout life. One child may be continuously compared with another, and the parents may further the feeling of rivalry by appointing one child as the better example. Throughout school, brothers and sisters may strive to outdo one another.

PERSONALITY differences may account for sibling rivalry. For example, while one sibling may be extroverted, have an outgoing personality, and make friends easily, another sibling may be more introspective, find it difficult to mingle but excels in school. The introspective sibling may be jealous of the extroverted sibling's sociability, while the extrovert may be jealous of the other sibling's academic achievements.

Sibling rivalry may persist even after the death of parents, when brothers and sisters become jealous over uneven distribution of their parents' possessions.

See also BIRTH ORDER; JEALOUSY.

sick building syndrome   Refers to illnesses caused by working or living in modern buildings. Symptoms may be caused by air-conditioning systems, fluorescent lighting systems, and not enough ventilation. Modern buildings are tighter in construction and depend on air circulators, as opposed to outside air from windows, for ventilation. A contemporary personal and societal source of stress, sick building syndrome was once known as "building-related illness." Symptoms may include HEADACHES, itchy eyes, nose and throat, dry cough, diminished mental acuity, sensitivity to odor, and tiredness.

Additionally, stressful symptoms may be caused by the FRUSTRATION of feeling closed in and not being able to control the amount of heat or light in the immediate ENVIRONMENT. Thus the stress of the syndrome is also related to feelings of lack of personal CONTROL.

A ripple effect sometimes occurs when one employee in such a building begins complaining of illness. Soon others believe that they too have headaches as a result of the WORKPLACE. An outbreak of Legionnaire's disease, a form of pneumonia, from bacteria in an air-conditioning system was first identified among American Legion conventioneers in a Philadelphia hotel during the 1970s; outbreaks of Legionnaire's disease occurred as recently as 1995. Organisms responsible for the disease as a contaminant of water systems were responsible for earlier epidemics of pneumonia, although the cause had not been known.

The influence of sick building syndrome as a source of employee stress was recognized on a large scale when complaints of sick building syndrome to the U.S. Department of Occupational Safety and Health (OSHA) doubled between 1980 and 1981. Recognized by the insurance industry under the name "tight building syndrome," Fireman's Fund Insurance Company established its own "tight building syndrome" laboratory in late 1983, after investigating 48 buildings in the United States and discovering that about one-third presented health hazards from indoor air pollution.

Relief of stress caused by sick building syndrome

Individuals who believe they are being made ill by their building should consult their company psychologist, if there is one, or department of human resources. Reports should be filed in a timely way so that investigations can be made. Removal of the pollutant, if possible, is essential. There may be possibilities to improve air balance and adjustment, including percentage of outside air being circulated. All humidifiers, filters, and drip pans must be checked. Overall maintenance of the building should be evaluated, and cleaning materials, air fresheners, and moth repellents should be selected carefully. New carpeting should be installed on a Friday, allowing ventilation of the building over the weekend.

Additionally, individuals should determine if there are any possible steps they can take to relieve their personal stress. These may include requesting being moved to another part of the building, or bringing a small electric fan or heater to work. If necessary, a short vacation away from the pollutants may be helpful.

FOR FURTHER INFORMATION:
National Safe Workplace Institute
1121 Spring Lake Drive
Itasca, IL 60143-3201
Phone: (630) 285-1121

SOURCE:
Griffin, Katherine. "When Your Office Calls in Sick." *Health,* January-February 1993.

SIDS See SUDDEN INFANT DEATH SYNDROME.

Siegel, Bernie S(hepard), M.D. (1921–) Surgeon, lecturer, and author of the best-selling book, *Love, Medicine and Miracles.* Through his leadership of Exceptional CANCER Patients (ECaP), a California SUPPORT GROUP that he founded, Dr. Siegel encourages members try to help heal themselves. By sharing their FEAR and ANGER with each other, ECaP members undergo a form of stress reduction and alternative therapy that, according to Siegel, aids in the healing process. They utilize the concept of "carefrontation," a loving, safe, therapeutic confrontation, which facilitates personal change and healing and helps relieve the stress of chronic illness.

Siegel believes that getting well is not the only goal; learning to live without fear and to be at peace with life and ultimately death is also important. He utilizes group therapy involving patients' dreams, drawings, and images. Dr. Siegel travels extensively to speak, facilitate workshops, and share his techniques and experiences.

Dr. Siegel completed his surgical training at Yale New Haven Hospital and the Children's' Hospital of Pittsburgh. He received his M.D. from Cornell University and his B.A. from Colgate University. He has been a practitioner of pediatric and general surgery.

See also SELF-HELP GROUPS; PSYCHO-THERAPIES.

SOURCE:
Siegel, Bernie S. *Love, Medicine & Miracles.* New York: Harper & Row, 1986.

simple phobia (single or specific phobia) A simple PHOBIA is an intense, irrational fear that persists and compels a person to avoid one specific situation or object. Almost any situation or object such as heights, bridges, dogs, or cats can become a specific phobia for an individual. This kind of fear is an intense source of stress for the suffering individual. Help can be obtained with BEHAVIOR THERAPY.

See also ANXIETY DISORDERS.

single women and conception See UNWED MOTHERS.

skin cancer See SUNLIGHT.

sleep The natural state of lowered consciousness and reduced metabolism. Lack of sleep and inability to sleep are sources of stress for many people, while for others, sleep difficulties are symptoms of stress. Difficulties related to sleep are among the commonest problems patients complain about when they visit physicians.

Age, state of health, medication, and psychological state affects sleep. DEPRESSION is a major factor that interferes with sleep, causing some individuals to sleep too much and preventing others from getting to sleep or sleeping through the night. Individuals who have a CHRONIC ILLNESS or PAIN often experience interrupted sleep. Sleeping habits affect most people's MOODS and their ability to cope with stress. Many feel somewhat irritable and short tempered without adequate sleep.

Men and women show some differences in sleep patterns. For example, as they age, men lose their ability for deep sleep (delta sleep) sooner than women, even though more women complain about insomnia and light sleeping. Men begin to lose their deep sleep in their late 40s and 50s, while women continue to have deep sleep later in life.

The old adage "early to bed and early to rise" is too generalized a plan for most people, says Rosalind Cartwright, M.D., of Rush-Presbyterian-St. Luke's Medical Center, Chicago. "There are many individual patterns of sleep that work well. Some elderly people don't go to bed until 4 A.M. They stay awake until then, reading, knitting, or doing some creative work. They wake up at 8 A.M. when everyone else does and they feel good. Such individuals once went to bed at midnight and worried about staying awake for hours; now they turn those hours into doing something constructive."

Sleep disorders
There are two basic categories of sleep disorders. One is known as *DIMS,* or *disorders of initiating or maintaining sleep.* These include getting to sleep, staying asleep, or waking too early.

The other is known as *DOES,* or *disorders of excessive sleep.* Characteristics may include falling asleep inappropriately and a difficulty in awakening. Such individuals are known as *hypersomniacs.*

Sleep apnea is another common and more serious disorder of sleep. It involves brief periods of ceasing to breathe. There may be at least 250,000 people in the United States who cease breathing so often or for such long periods of time at night that they are tired all day and are likely to drift off into sleep at any moment. They must walk around often to fight off sleep and cannot drive safely.

Sleep apnea is marked by loud SNORING, prolonged periods between breaths (apnea), weight gain, and elevated blood pressure. Diagnosis of sleep apnea can be made from a tape recording at the bedside of the snorer. If there are repeated pauses of more than 10 seconds between snores, it may mean that the oxygen level in the brain is going down. The person must wake himself/herself to restart the brain. There is treatment for sleep apnea, and it is important that such people be treated because this disorder causes a strain on the heart.

Repetitive nocturnal myoclonus involves involuntary jerky motions of the legs or episodes of twitching that disturb sleep. This is an uncomfortable sensation that occurs just before falling asleep. The individual feels an urge to get up and walk around. This sensation may increase with age and frequently runs in families; it is more common in individuals age 50 to 60 than in younger people.

Sleep difficulties of menopausal women. Many midlife women experience stress because of changes in their sleep patterns around MENOPAUSE. Some changes may be due to HOT FLASHES or to other factors involving individual psychosocial stresses. According to Dudley Dinner, M.D., director, Sleep Disorders Center, Cleveland Clinic Foundation, while women may sleep seven to eight hours at age 20, they may decrease to six or six-and-a-half hours between ages 55 and 60. Also, sleep tends to become more "fragmented." Women in this age group may awaken oftener and spend more time awake during the night, although their total time in bed may increase.

Sleep disturbance related to medication. A side effect of medications can be sleepiness; all medications should be taken only under a physician's supervision. Some medications may make sleep apnea worse.

Medications used for inducing sleep. Individuals who are stressed by an inability to fall asleep or stay asleep sometimes have sleeping medications prescribed for them. Often at a time of great bereavement, such as after the death of a spouse or parent, an individual will have difficulty sleeping and can be helped with the assistance of an appropriately prescribed medication for short-term use.

Dreaming. Most dreaming takes place during the REM stage. Nightmares of being unable to move have a real basis during this phase of sleep because of the limpness of the muscles. People will probably forget DREAMS unless they awaken during a REM period or within 10 minutes afterward (see below).

Sleepwalking (somnambulism) may occur while asleep during NREM (nonrapid eye movement) sleep; this affects about 5% of adults and many more children. For unknown reasons, boys are more likely to sleepwalk than girls. A child may sleepwalk after awakening from a nightmare or night terror, and may scream, talk, or even urinate in an inappropriate place. It is difficult to awaken a sleepwalker; the best approach is to calmly lead him or her back to bed. However, in a household where an individual is known to sleepwalk, it is best to close off stairwells and remove objects in possible pathways to prevent injury.

Sleep research

Evaluation of sleep disturbances is carried out in many sleep laboratories across the United States. Sessions for a troubled sleeper in a sleep laboratory depend on the diagnosis and how complex the problem is. For example, some tests for narcolepsy, a disorder of excessive daytime sleepiness, are done during the day, with a series of five short naps. However, most sleep lab evaluations are done during the night. Patients are monitored for many things, including naso-oral air flow and heart rate. Insomniacs are tested to determine how much they really sleep. Typically, many physiological parameters are measured. There is an intercom from the control room, and researchers can talk to the patient's room or tape record what is going on in any room.

Stages of sleep

With use of an electroencephalogram (EEG), a graphic depiction of the brain's electrical potentials recorded by scalp electrodes, sleep is divisible into two categories: non-rapid eye movement (NREM) sleep and rapid eye movement (REM) sleep. Dreaming sleep is another term for REM sleep. There are four stages of NREM sleep. Stage I occurs immediately after sleep begins, with a pattern of low amplitude and fast frequency. Stage II has characteristic waves of 12–16 cycles per second known as sleep spindles. Stages III and IV have progressive further slowing of frequency and an increase in amplitude of the wave forms. After the beginning of sleep, over a period of 90 minutes, a person goes through the four stages of NREM sleep and goes from them into the first period of REM sleep. Dreaming usually occurs during REM sleep and short cycles (20–30 minutes) of REM sleep recur about every 90 minutes throughout the night. This type of sleep is so named because of the coordinated rapid eye movements that occur.

FOR FURTHER INFORMATION:
American Sleep Disorders Association
604 Second St. SW
Rochester, MN 55902
Phone: (507) 287-6006

HOW TO GET A GOOD NIGHT'S SLEEP

- Avoid stressful situations before bedtime. Postpone discussions of problems until morning, whenever possible. Avoid lengthy telephone conversations that may upset you before bedtime.
- If you have an argument or tension-filled discussion late at night, don't go to bed mad.
- If you are alone and feel hostile, call a friend and talk. Venting may help you unload and you will sleep better.
- Drink a cup of warm milk before bedtime. Eat a light snack. Avoid stimulating beverages containing CAFFEINE, such as coffee, cola beverages, and chocolate.
- Take a warm, relaxing bath before going to bed.
- Relax in bed and read something you enjoy. As your mind becomes engrossed, your muscles will relax. When your body is relaxed, you are likelier to become sleepy and ready for sleep. Watching television may have the same effect.
- Read something you find very dull. When your mind cannot handle what you present, your internal coping mechanism of falling asleep may take over. Watching television may have the same effect.
- Experiment by changing your environment. Make the room warmer or colder. Use different combinations of covers. Some people like the feeling of the "weight" of blankets, while others do not. If you like warmth without weight, use an electric blanket. Some have dual controls so that each bed partner can have individual arrangements.
- Avoid using sleeping pills. People build up a tolerance to them and some have daytime hypnotic effects. Some pills induce sleep apnea.
- If you must take a sleeping pill during times of extreme stress, such as after the death of a loved one, after surgery, or during extreme jet lag, take short-acting sleeping medications (see above).
- Nightly use of a sleeping medication may not be effective after a while. If you have to use them at all, use them only every other night or every third night.
- Avoid taking naps during the day; go to bed a little later each night.

SOURCES:

Borbely, Alexander. *Secrets of Sleep.* New York: Basic Books, 1984.

Carey, Benedict. "The Slumber Solution." *Health,* July-August 1996.

Hales, Dianne. *The Compete Book of Sleep.* Reading, Mass.: Addison-Wesley Company, 1981.

Kahn, Ada P., and Jan Fawcett. *The Encyclopedia of Mental Health.* New York: Facts On File, 1993.

sleep apnea   See SLEEP.

slips of the tongue   Saying one thing but meaning another. Such slips may be stressful for the person who speaks them as well as a source of embarrassment, or even CRITICISM and ridicule by listeners.

Sigmund Freud theorized that these acts have a subconscious basis with some motivation that is not recognized by the person who commits them. This type of behavior is temporary and correctable. Although undesirable, it tends to fall within normal limits and is not considered a disorder. Slips of the tongue are also known as "lapsus lingae."

SOURCE:

Campbell, Robert Jean. *Psychiatric Dictionary.* New York: Oxford University Press, 1981.

smoking   The inhaling and exhaling of tobacco by using cigarettes. A major public health problem in the United States, smoking is a source of stress for non-smokers as well as smokers. It is only in the late 1990s that cigarette companies have reluctantly admitted that the nicotine contained in cigarettes is habit-forming and addictive. Many smokers say they want to quit but cannot; expressing and following through with the desire to quit smoking becomes a source of stress for them.

Effects of smoking

Nicotine affects the central nervous system through routes that differ from other drugs, but it produces very similar results, such as pleasurable euphoria, dependency, and with- drawal symptoms when stopped suddenly. Smokers who quit may experience genuine physical discomfort and cravings. With- drawal symptoms from nicotine include HEADACHES, irritability, upset stomach, BREATHING and circulation problems, trouble sleeping, DIZZINESS, and numbness.

The actual physiological effects of smoking are somewhat at odds with the sensations that smokers report. When nicotine enters the bloodstream, it raises the heart rate and blood pressure and dilates the arteries. It also raises the level of glucose in the blood. However, smokers report a sense of relief from stress despite the stimulating effects of nicotine. Smokers claim it improves short- term memory, intellectual performance, and concentration.

While most smokers do not resort to devi- ate behaviors to maintain their habit, partici- pants in the Stop Smoking Clinics at Rush North Shore Medical Center, Skokie, Illinois, admitted going through ashtrays, garbage cans, and gutters, looking for butts that might still have a salvageable few puffs, if their own supplies were depleted. These recovered smokers are repulsed to think that they ever performed such acts.

Stresses between smokers and non-smokers

While scientists have documented the harm- ful effects of smoking, many smokers still believe that it is their "right" to smoke when and where they want to. Since anti-smoking laws were enacted in the United States during the 1980s and early 1990s, there have been fre- quent incidents of anger and hostility between smokers and non-smokers. Non- smokers maintain the "right" to clean air. Increasingly, workplaces are changing over to non-smoking and setting up outdoor smoking areas for smokers. In the large cities of America, most restaurants have non-smoking areas. Those that don't will not attract non- smokers. For asthmatics and those with other respiratory disorders, smoke in the air is more than an annoyance; being forced to breathe in secondhand smoke can make them feel physically ill.

Eventually the United States may become a smokeless society. However, in Third World countries, the numbers of smokers is unfortunately increasing and cigarette consumption is rising.

Consequences of smoking

The main harmful components of cigarette smoke are tar, nicotine, and carbon monoxide. The lungs retain 70% to 90% of these chemicals when one inhales. Tarry substances clog the lungs and affect breathing. Carbon monoxide decreases the ability of red blood cells to carry oxygen throughout the body.

Smoking lowers one's resistance to infection and ulcerative diseases. It also increases one's risk for bad breath, severe gum diseases, tooth loss, and premature aging of the skin, which many people find sources of stress. Pregnant women who smoke have higher rates of miscarriage, stillbirth, premature birth, low birth weight, and complications of PREGNANCY. Infants of mothers who smoke during pregnancy also have more of a chance of SUDDEN INFANT DEATH SYNDROME (SIDS) than do infants whose mothers did not smoke. Smoking is credited as a factor in nearly 500,000 deaths per year, representing more Americans than die from accidents, infectious diseases, murders, suicides, diabetes, and cirrhosis combined.

The disease most often associated with cigarette smoking is lung CANCER. One hundred years ago, if a doctor ever saw a case of lung cancer, he or she would have written it up in a medical journal. This disease, which only 50 years ago was almost unheard of, is now the leading cause of cancer deaths in men and women. Lung cancer, once believed to be predominantly a disease of males, in the mid-1980s overtook breast cancer to become the number one cause of cancer deaths for women. Over 85% of the people who die of lung cancer could have avoided the disease completely if they did not smoke. For this reason, coping with their deaths is doubly stressful for their family members.

Who smokes?

Many people experience smoking as a negative experience the first time they try. Some people may stop with the first cigarette, but for many, smoking becomes a habit that is difficult to break despite its link with disease. When adolescents begin smoking, it usually is the result of peer pressure. A desire to relieve stress, an attitude of rebellion, and a pattern of family smoking also seem to be factors that contribute to teenage smoking.

More teenage girls (14%) smoke than teenage boys (11%), according to a Gallup survey in 1989. In the general population, men have traditionally smoked more than women, although these figures are now somewhat even at 28% of men and 26% of women. Although their numbers have decreased, men are still heavier smokers than women. In a Gallup survey, one-fourth of men smoke more than a pack of cigarettes a day, while only 14% of the women in the survey exceed a pack a day. Smoking of less than a pack a day is common among the population in the 18- to 29-year-old age bracket.

Stop smoking programs

Almost all health risks decrease when one gives up smoking. As withdrawal symptoms subside, one is likely to notice "good" symptoms such as improved senses of taste and smell, increased energy, and enhanced SELF-ESTEEM and self-control. Regular exercise will enable one to avoid or minimize weight gain and keep the body in good physical shape.

Quitting smoking is not easy. Many stop-smoking programs exist to help cigarette addicts. However, for programs to be helpful, the individual must attend regularly and follow the rules set forth. For many, unfortunately, this is easier said than done. When one

---

STRESS RELIEVERS FOR THOSE WHO ARE QUITTING SMOKING

- List your reasons for wanting to stop and wanting to continue smoking.
- Note when and where you smoke the most.
- Set a date for quitting; tell your family and friends.
- Remove cigarettes, ashtrays, and matches from your home, car, and office.
- Minimize stressful situations and other occasions when you previously craved a cigarette.
- Spend time where smoking is prohibited.
- Reach for high-fiber, low-calorie snacks, such as vegetables or fruits when you have the urge to smoke.
- Talk to someone who is supportive until the urge to smoke passes.
- Increase aerobic exercise (walking, biking).
- Use relaxation techniques (such as meditation, guided imagery).
- Reward yourself for quitting smoking.

---

stops smoking, nicotine dependency may cause some stressful and unpleasant sensations. For example, one may temporarily experience withdrawal symptoms such as DEPRESSION, irritability, anxiety restlessness, trouble concentrating, headache, drowsiness, gastrointestinal disturbances, increased coughing, or difficulty sleeping.

Inhaling nicotine also seems to control weight in some smokers by lowering circulating insulin levels and thus decreasing their craving for sweets and tendency to store fat. This particular aspect of nicotine makes smoking appeal to those who are afraid of gaining weight when they stop smoking. However, a study reported in 1992 shows that the weight one gains after stopping smoking may be only temporary. Epidemiologist Yue Chen and colleagues at the University of Saskatchewan weighed 1,202 locals residents in 1977, and asked them whether they smoked. Six years later, they followed up on their survey with 709 of the residents. Of the 138 people who had stopped smoking, those who had quit recently had gained weight. The men had put on an average of 6.2 pounds, the women, 5.5. Those who had stayed away from cigarettes, however, gradually lost what they had gained, taking into account the normal amount of weight people add as they age. The smokers who had stopped the habit for more than two years had not gained any more than those who had never smoked, according to the researchers.

Many national organizations can help one affiliate with a stop-smoking program; check for a local chapter.

See also ADDICTION; EMPHYSEMA; HABITS.

FOR FURTHER INFORMATION:
American Cancer Society
1599 Clifton Road NE
Atlanta, GA 30329
Phone: (800) ACS-2345

American Heart Association
7320 Greenville Avenue
Dallas, TX 75231
Phone: (214) 373-6300

American Lung Association
1740 Broadway
New York, NY 10019
Phone: (212) 315-8700

Centers for Disease Control
Office of Smoking and Health
1600 Clifton Road, NEW (Mail Stop K-50)
Atlanta, GA 30333
Phone: (404) 639-3311

National Cancer Institute
9000 Rockville Pike
Building 31, 4A-21
Bethesda, MD 20892
Phone: (800) 4-CANCER

SOURCES:
Hammond, S. Katharine. "Environmental Tobacco Smoke Presents Substantial Risk in Workplaces." *The Journal of the American Medical Association,* September 26, 1995.
Spitzer, Joel. "Medical Implications of Smoking." Skokie, Illinois: Good Health Program, Rush North Shore Medical Center, 1995.

snoring   Noisy BREATHING through the open mouth during SLEEP; produced by vibrations of the soft palate. Snoring is stressful because it may deprive both the snorer as well as the bed partner of necessary sleep, resulting in irritability and tension for both the next day.

Frequently, snoring occurs as people sleep on their backs; their tongues slide back into a position that partially blocks the nasal passage, forcing mouth breathing, particularly in a deep sleep. It is more common in overweight people, partly because they are more likely to sleep on their backs and also because fatty tissue in their throats may cause blockage. Snoring also may be caused by enlarged tonsils, nasal problems, heavy drinking, smoking, or eating just before sleep.

Measurements of snoring volume have recorded decibel levels as high as the sound of a jack hammer or pneumatic drill. Robert W. Hart, M.D., writing in *Chicago Medicine* (Dec. 21, 1991), characterized snoring as "mild, moderate, severe, or heroic." According to Hart, the incidence of habitual snoring in an unselected population is estimated near 20%. However, in overweight males between the ages of 30 and 59, that incidence reaches 60%.

Snoring, sleep apnea, and stress

Many stressed individuals who report chronic fatigue and irritability are victims of sleep apnea, known as obstructive sleep apnea syndrome (OSAS). If untreated, OSAS can have lethal consequences when daytime sleepiness leads to automobile and industrial accidents, as well as consequences for interpersonal relationships because of short tempers due to tiredness.

OSAS is characterized by repetitive episodes of complete apnea or incomplete obstruction of the upper airways during sleep. OSAS is more common in males and postmenopausal females, with its frequency increasing with age and weight. The OSAS sufferer may complain of feelings of choking or suffocating during the night or feel panicky because of an inability to take in enough air. All these feelings are extremely stressful for the sufferer as well as his or her sleep partner.

Treatment options for OSAS include general measures, such as weight loss, abstinence from alcohol, pharmacological approaches for limited periods of time, oral and orthodontic devices, and surgical procedures, such as nasal surgery or uvulopalatopharyngoplasty (repair of the uvula, the small, fleshy protuberance that hangs from the middle of the lower edge of the soft palate, which is part of the mouth).

See also CHRONIC FATIGUE SYNDROME.

FOR FURTHER INFORMATION:
American Sleep Disorders Association
604 Second St. SW
Rochester, MN 55902
Phone: (507) 287-6006

SOURCES:
Borbely, Alexander. *Secrets of Sleep.* New York: Basic Books, 1984.
Lipman, Derek S. *Snoring From A to ZZZZ: Proven Cures for the Night's Worst Nuisance.* Portland, Or.: Spencer Press, 1996.
Pascualy, Ralph A. *Snoring and Sleep Apnea: Personal and Family Guide to Diagnosis and Treatment.* New York: Demos Vermande, 1996.

social phobia   The irrational fear and avoidance of being in a situation in which one's activities can be observed by others. It involves a fear of being embarrassed, humiliated, criticized, censured, or in some way evaluated in social settings by the reactions of others. The most common social phobia is fear of speaking in public, whether in front of a large audience or in front of a small group such as during a party. Other common social PHOBIAS include blushing, eating, drinking, writing, urinating, or vomiting in the presence of others. Some social phobics fear that their hands will tremble or shake as they eat or write and tend to avoid restaurants, banks, and other public places. They often avert their eyes when talking to another person. Some social phobics have been known to cross the street to avoid greeting people they know, and social phobics are fearful of attending parties, particularly with people they do not know.

Usually social phobias begin after puberty and peak after the age of 30, but social phobics have had lifelong SHYNESS and introverted habits. Both men and women suffer from social phobias and may have more than one at a time. Also, many agoraphobics have social phobias, and many social phobics have some agoraphobic symptoms.

See also AGORAPHOBIA; ANXIETY DISORDERS.

FOR FURTHER INFORMATION:
Anxiety Disorders Association of America
11900 Parklawn Drive (Suite 100)
Rockville, MD 20852
Phone: (301) 231-9350

SOURCES:
American Psychiatric Association. *Let's Talk About Phobias.* Washington, D.C.: American Psychiatric Association, 1988.
Marshall, John R. *Social Phobia: From Shyness to Stage Fright.* New York: Basic Books, 1994.

social support system A social support system involves an individual's relationships with others, including significant others, friends, people on the job, in the community and religious groups, as well as material resources. An individual with a stress concern may have an inadequate social support system because family members do not understand his/her circumstances and thus may not offer the assistance or encouragement that could be helpful.

Individuals with good social support systems seem to have better recoveries from illnesses and surgeries than those without such support.

See also SELF-HELP GROUPS; SUPPORT GROUPS.

social workers Workers trained to have expertise in counseling people regarding available community resources for various types of support and therapy; many of them provide counseling for individuals with concerns about stress. Social workers work in the public and private sector; they may work in publicly funded health and mental health clinics and in schools, family agencies, clinics, hospitals, and private practice. Some work in EMPLOYEE ASSISTANCE PROGRAMS (EAPs), alcohol and chemical dependency programs, and in religious settings.

In the 1960s and 1970s, with the establishment of comprehensive community mental health centers, clinical social workers provided a major proportion of outpatient mental health treatment services. In the 1980s, an increasing number of clinical social workers moved into full- or part-time private practice and these practices continue to grow.

In 1997, there were 150,000 members of the National Association of Social Workers (NASW), an organization limited to those persons who have a bachelor's, master's, or doctoral degree from a university program accredited by the Council on Social Work Education.

See also PSYCHOTHERAPIES.

FOR FURTHER INFORMATION:
National Association of Social Workers (NASW)
750 First Street NE (suite 700)
Washington, DC 20002–4241
Phone: (202) 408-8600

Council on Social Work Education
1600 Duke Street (Suite 300)
Alexandria, VA 22314
Phone: (703) 683-8080

SOURCE:
Manderscheid, R.W., and M.A. Sonnenschein, eds. *Mental Health, United States, 1990.* Washington, D.C.: Govt. Printing Office; DHHS Pub. No. (ADM) 90–1708, 1990.

somatization An individual experiencing physical symptoms as a response to psychological stress, in the absence of disease or out of proportion to a given ailment. For example, people experience physical symptoms such as fatigue, shortness of breath, or even pain as a response to stress.

Somatization can be hazardous to health because people who have ongoing complaints may undergo uncomfortable and invasive procedures that are not needed and can cause complications. Individuals who repeatedly report chest pains might eventually undergo coronary angiography to rule out serious arterial narrowing. Also, these individuals may be taking medications needlessly, some with serious side effects.

Individuals who "somatize" are said to have *somatoform disorders.* Treatment of somatization may include use of various PSYCHOTHERAPIES, RELAXATION exercises, MEDITATION, MASSAGE THERAPY, taking VACATIONS or dealing more effectively with stresses at home or in the WORKPLACE.

See also COPING; GENERAL ADAPTATION SYNDROME.

SOURCE:
Kahn, Ada P., and Jan Fawcett. *The Encyclopedia of Mental Health.* New York: Facts On File, 1993.

specific phobia   See SIMPLE PHOBIA; PHOBIAS.

spirituality   Spirituality has been described as experiencing the presence of a power, a force, an energy, or of God. This definition is from the writings of Herbert BENSON, M.D., president, The Mind/Body Medical Institute, and chief, Division of Behavioral Medicine, Deaconess Hospital, Boston. Spirituality, for many, is directly connected to PRAYER, faith, and RELIGION; belief systems help many individuals cope with symptoms of STRESS.

Dr. Benson's work at the Harvard Medical School considered the healing effects of spirituality; research later confirmed that some people experienced increased spirituality as a result of RELAXATION therapy whether or not they used a religious repetitive focus. This notion came about after Harvard researchers had systematically studied the benefits of mind/body interactions for more than 25 years. The research confirmed that when a person engages in a repetitive prayer, word, sound, or phrase and when intrusive thoughts are passively disregarded, a specific set of physiological changes ensues. There is decreased metabolism, heart rate and rate of breathing, and distinctly slower brain waves.

These changes are the opposite of those induced by stress and are an effective therapy in a number of diseases including HIGH BLOOD PRESSURE, cardiac rhythm irregularities, many forms of chronic PAIN, INSOMNIA, symptoms of CANCER and AIDS, premenstrual syndrome, ANXIETY, and mild and moderate DEPRESSION. To the extent that any disease is caused or made worse by stress, increased spirituality brought about by relaxation is an effective therapy.

See also ALTERNATIVE THERAPIES.

spouse abuse   See DOMESTIC VIOLENCE.

stage fright   An intense feeling of nervous anticipation that many people experience before giving a public speech or making an appearance on a stage. For some, the feeling occurs before they go on stage, while others experience it just as they enter the stage. Those who have been in theatrical productions, play a musical instrument or sing publicly, or have been videotaped, probably have experienced this feeling at some time. People who experience a high level of STRESS because of stage fright may view the audience as an adversary ready to judge them personally without regard to the content or message of their presentation.

Because of the stress caused by intense stage fright, some people go out of their way to avoid PUBLIC SPEAKING and public appearances; and some may actually develop a phobia. Symptoms of this phobia have many common characteristics; people may become dizzy and nauseated, have sweaty palms and weak knees, feel a rapid heartbeat, and experience difficulty breathing. While most people feel these symptoms in a very mild manner, phobics momentarily fear that they will die due to their rapid heartbeat and difficulty in getting enough air to breathe, even though they may be over-breathing. These symptoms may occur for only a few moments before going onstage, but as soon as they are onstage their nervousness disappears and they focus all of their attention and energy on their performance.

Many successful public figures have overcome stage fright. Some lose their fear by systematically becoming accustomed to appearing in front of people. BEHAVIOR THERAPY and RELAXATION techniques can help people overcome stage fright. Physical relaxation involves exercises to eliminate nervousness and ANXIETY and leads to physical ease and calmness. Mental and psychological relaxation involves exercises to develop objectivity, awareness, mental clarity, and a positive mental attitude.

Overcoming the stress of stage fright depends on the individual's developing confidence in his or her ability to speak or perform. Knowing the material well, whether it is a musical performance or a public speech, helps relieve stress. Confident individuals learn to convert their stress into positive energy.

See also ALTERNATIVE THERAPIES; ANXIETY DISORDERS; PERFORMANCE ANXIETY; SOCIAL PHOBIA.

SOURCE:
Desberg, Peter. *Controlling Stage Fright: Presenting Yourself to Audiences From One to One Thousand.* Oakland: New Harbinger, 1988.

stammering   See STUTTERING.

STDs   See SEXUALLY TRANSMITTED DISEASES.

stepfamilies   Families formed when a divorced or widowed parent remarries. Stresses in stepfamilies are more complex than in traditional nuclear families, possibly because society has not defined the role of the stepparent as it has of the natural parent. As a result, everyone may have different ideas regarding how stepparent and stepchild should get along. Frequently, stepparents feel that they should assume the role of an actual parent. This may be very uncomfortable and objectionable to their stepchildren, specially when the children continue to have a strong relationship with their own natural parent.

Children who live with a single parent may have had some sense of being the center of attention in the household and may have difficulty giving up that role with the arrival of a stepparent.

The living arrangements that are set up when two families merge may cause stresses and challenges to all involved. For example, some children may be in residence, some may visit. A child who had been living with one parent may suddenly decide he wishes to leave that parent, possibly because of a new stepparent in that household. If conflicts erupt between stepsiblings, parents may side with their own child, rather than making peace as they would in a traditional family.

Stresses may also arise in the stepparented household because there may be a highly charged sexual atmosphere in the home; the couple actually are newlyweds with children present. This may arouse real or potential relationships between stepsiblings, which are technically, although not biologically, incestuous. There is also a potential for technical incest between stepparent and stepchild, particularly if the stepparent is young, even close to the age of the child. In an attempt to be warm and friendly, some stepparents may unwittingly encourage these feelings in children.

In situations involving older couples and adult children, children may feel that their inheritance rights are threatened by the arrival of a stepfather or mother.

Many people help relieve the stresses brought about by the formation of a stepfamily with family counseling services and SUP-PORT GROUPS for stepparents and children.

See also DIVORCE; REMARRIAGE; SELF-HELP GROUPS.

FOR FURTHER INFORMATION:
Stepfamily Association of America
215 Centennial Mall (Suite 212)
Lincoln, NE 68508
Phone: (800) 735-0329

SOURCES:
Belovitch, Jeanne. *Making Re-marriage Work.* Lexington, Mass.: Lexington Books, 1987.
Wald, Esther. *The Remarried Family.* New York: Family Service Association of America, 1981.

stillbirth The death of a fetus between the 20th week of gestation and delivery. A still-birth causes a special kind of GRIEF and stress for the parents. Although they have never seen their child, they have imagined how he or she would look, what they would use for a name, and how the child would interact with others in the family.

After the stillbirth, there are no "real" memories, such as photographs or items the child actually used or touched. Friends and others in the family do not share the loss with the parents in the way that they might in the case of an older infant who died, making grief even more stressful for the parents.

Even though another child may arrive a year or more later, many parents of a stillborn never fully recover from their loss. Some remember the "due date" for years, and observe it with sadness, reviving the feeling of loss and sadness.

Major causes of stillbirth appear to be loss of oxygen to the baby, either because of a problem with the placenta or an umbilical cord accident before or during labor. However, for more than half of stillbirths, there is no known cause, and the lack of an explanation is also a source of stress for the grieving parents.

See also MISCARRIAGE.

stress The response of the body and mind to strains or burdens that demand adaptation; it is any hindrance that disturbs an individual's mental and physical well-being. These inter-ferences may range from RANDOM NUISANCES to life-threatening situations. From a scientific perspective, stress causes an imbalance in an individual's equilibrium (HOMEOSTASIS). Controlling stress is essential for wellness because continued exposure can lead to symptoms, such as HEADACHES or more seri-ous conditions such as HIGH BLOOD PRESSURE and DEPRESSION. Research has shown that stress also affects the IMMUNE SYSTEM and causes it to be less efficient in fighting off dis-eases. Coping well with stress also can improve an individual's chances of living with CHRONIC ILLNESS.

Understanding stress
Stress is an internal response to circumstances known as *stressors*. Stressors may be internal situations, such as feelings of insecurity or frustration, or external events, such as a bad review at work, or cancellation of an airplane flight.

Stressors can also be reactions to happy events as well as to bad news and unhappy events; there are good stressors derived from satisfying personal and professional events as well as unpleasant ones. For example, happy personal stressors may include get-ting married, having a baby, or moving to a new house; happy work stressors may include landing a new job or getting a pro-motion at work. Unpleasant stressors may include marital difficulties, illness, or being fired. Hans SELYE, pioneer in stress research and author of *Stress Without Distress* and *The Stress of Life,* termed the good events that cause stress as EUSTRESS and those that caused unpleasant effects as DIS-STRESS. Both types of stress cause physiological responses, including activation of the nervous system and of the FIGHT OR FLIGHT RESPONSE. That is why during stressful times, people may notice that they have a faster heartbeat and a sick feeling in their stomach; it is difficult to work or function efficiently at such times.

Stressors often represent significant changes in one's life or habits. How individuals accommodate to change influences the extent of stress they experience. Selye used the term GENERAL ADAPTATION SYNDROME to explain how individuals cope with stressors. He suggested that individuals experience events in different ways; what results in emotional strain and ANXIETY for one person may not bring about those reactions in others. Also, in the same individual, adaptations that are tolerated well at one time may not be handled so well at another.

Chronic stress results in ongoing wear and tear on the body's organs and systems, making them more susceptible to illness. When symptoms show up, many individuals begin to seek medical or psychological help. According to Herbert BENSON, M.D., Harvard cardiologist and author of *The Relaxation Response,* more than 80% of visits to physicians' offices may result from stress in patients' lives. "Physicians are aware of stress as a factor in diagnosing and treating many common health concerns." For example, many people seek help for gastrointestinal symptoms, an inability to SLEEP, headaches, depression, and chronic fatigue. They may have high blood pressure. "The best treatment is to get at the cause of the stress," recommends Catherine R. Landers, M.D., a member of the Department of Medicine at Rush North Shore Medical Center, Skokie, Illinois. "We know that physical problems, even if induced by stress, can interfere with the quality of one's work and ability to meet the needs of family members. Medications won't provide any long-lasting results. There are strong MIND-BODY CONNECTIONS. Helping the individual change his or her COPING styles usually works better than anything we can prescribe as medication."

Sources of stress

Stress can come from an individual's family, WORKPLACE or community connections. Stress within a family causes tension and difficulties in communicating effectively. There may be INTERGENERATIONAL CONFLICTS or situations arising from assisting ELDERLY PARENTS. In some cases, interpersonal stresses develop when an adolescent has two simultaneous feelings, such as wanting to be independent during PUBERTY and yet feeling dependent on parents. In a family, several people may be trying to cope with their own stress as well as the stress of others about whom they care. For example, when a father dies, the son tries to console his mother, even when struggling with his own sadness.

Stress that starts within the family can affect one's work and the reverse is also true. Family problems can make a person irritable on the job, distrustful of coworkers, and prone to mistakes and accidents. Likewise, a difficult day at the office can make a person short-tempered and hostile at home. Workplace factors that contribute to stress include lack of autonomy, lack of satisfaction, and feeling bored, underpaid, or overworked.

Many people feel stressed by demands made upon them from their community or religious activities. While these activities add to a person's SOCIAL SUPPORT SYSTEM, they may have taken on too many responsibilities, and are asked to take on more, and feel that there is not enough time to complete all of them adequately. Already feeling overwhelmed, but wishing to maintain their reputation as a "doer," they agree. Learning when to say "no" is an important skill to practice.

While stress can be physiologically devastating to many people, others find that stress actually raises their energy level and helps them focus their mind better on their work, family, or social activities. Some thrive on many kinds of stressors, such as COMPETITION and comparison with others. People who do so are often attracted to high-stress occupations and professions, or do well at competitive games and sports.

Learning to manage stress

"Stressors cannot be eliminated, so our goal should be to control and manage stress," says Elaine Shepp, LCSW, a psychotherapist on the staff at Rush North Shore Medical Center, Skokie, Illinois. She goes on to say, "It is possible to 'neutralize' the toxic effects of unrelenting stress. People who cope well with stress put their personal and professional lives into perspective. They may experience a constantly high level of pressure and unrealistic demands at work but develop their own ideals of conduct and test themselves by their own standards. They are able to prioritize their work and enjoy family life as well as their chosen recreational activities."

Experiencing stress is part of human nature. In his book, *Why Zebras Don't Get Ulcers*, Robert M. Sapolsky looks at how wild animals process stress and explains what humans can learn from them. "The key thing with humans is, we're all going to have a bit of stress response. It's part of life." Sapolsky goes on, "Three minutes or three hours (of stress response) is no problem, but do it chronically, and you're up a creek. The stress response increases blood pressure, which can led to a stroke. It also shuts down digestion, which can lead to ulcers."

In explaining why zebras don't get ulcers, Sapolsky said: "Because they don't have computers, they don't worry about mortgages, blind dates, or Social Security. They worry about lions, and with lions, it's all taken care of in three minutes, or it's all over in three minutes. No stress."

Relieving stress: an individual matter

Avenues toward relieving stress are personal matters. Many people find that regular physical workouts involving running, walking, or exercising in a gym or health club, or using equipment at home, helps them overcome their reactions to today's events and get ready to effectively face tomorrow's challenges. Using muscles is a way to use up some of the "fight or flight" readiness in the body.

A healthy diet with three meals a day is a basic for wellness and can also help prevent and relieve stress. Well-balanced meals provide a slow release of necessary nutrients throughout the day. For some people, too much CAFFEINE causes additional stress by bringing on symptoms of anxiety. "Crash diets" or "fad diets" can lead to anxiety, depression, and an inability to maintain an appropriate weight. Acceptance of one's BODY IMAGE and a good sense of SELF-ESTEEM will encourage people to maintain good NUTRITION as well as good health.

People use many ALTERNATIVE THERAPIES to relieve stress. These include ACUPUNCTURE, GUIDED IMAGERY, MEDITATION, PROGRESSIVE MUSCLE RELAXATION, and YOGA. Some use MASSAGE THERAPY or listen to MUSIC as stress relievers. However, what allows one person to relax may actually cause stress for another. An example is noise level in the workplace or at home. Each individual should try to create an environment in which to work and live that is the least stressful in order to focus on reaching his or her peak performance and a feeling of well-being.

HOBBIES help many people combat stress. Participating in an activity simply for the enjoyment of it, makes their stress level go down. Such hobbies may include dancing, art and painting, sewing, building model trains or planes, bird watching, or playing a musical instrument. Choices of hobbies are as diverse as human nature.

A social support system is important, too. Many people find relief from stress in talking with their support groups. When they are able to talk about their issues, problems, and concerns and get FEEDBACK from trusted, objective family and friends, people get an enlightened perspective that often helps them to lighten their stress load.

When professional help may be necessary

There are times when reactions to stress detract from a person's energy necessary for productive work and effective personal functioning. At these times, when talking to a friend just isn't enough, professional assistance is available. Those who seek professional help to overcome effects of extreme stress should not consider themselves "weak," says Shepp. "Seeking help is an intelligent way of using available tools to increase one's level of functioning. Counseling can help prevent BURNOUT and assist in dealing with life situations requiring the input of a non-involved, knowledgeable person."

Death of a close relative or friend, divorce or remarriage, marital difficulties, sexual problems, or illness of one's own or a family member are common stressful occurrences. Financial problems, such as facing a large mortgage or accumulated bills, can happen to anyone. Individuals faced with these and other serious life stressors may feel out of CONTROL and that their worlds are caving in around them.

If you find yourself feeling totally overwhelmed and decide to seek professional help, how should you select a psychotherapist and choose from a myriad of PSYCHOTHERAPIES? You may want to talk with a close relative, colleague, or friend who has experienced psychotherapy. However, if the issue of confidentiality is important to you, find a mental health professional or social worker in a hospital or community agency who can help direct you. The psychotherapist should be one with whom you have a sense of comfort, who also understands your particular stressors, and who can suggest practical ways for you to handle your stress. Find a therapist who is multifaceted in his or her approach to problems and knowledgeable about many options available to treat particular problems. Look for one who is open to consulting with other professionals who have additional expertise.

RECOGNIZE YOUR PERSONAL SIGNALS OF STRESS

Each person has unique sources of stress as well as personal signals of stress. Sources of stress come from within oneself (personal), from family life, from the workplace, and from community activities. Some common sources of stress and personal signals are listed below.

SOURCES OF STRESS

Individual stressors
- Aging
- Feeling unattractive or insecure
- Achievement or success problems
- Change in habits
- Relationship concerns
- Inability to pay bills; mortgage worries

Family stressors
- Death, illness, or injury of a family member
- Divorce; remarriage
- Marital difficulties; sexual difficulties
- Holidays, vacations
- Problems with children
- Young adult leaving home or returning home
- Lack of privacy
- Not enough time

Workplace/community stressors
- Difficulties with boss or coworkers
- Threatened layoffs
- Boredom; not enough work
- Overwork; underpayment
- Lack of autonomy
- Automation in the workplace

PERSONAL SIGNALS OF STRESS
- Irritability or bad temper
- Headaches; stomachaches; digestive problems
- Inability to sleep
- Grinding teeth
- High blood pressure
- Lethargy; inability to work; finger-tapping
- Depression; panic, or anxiety
- Fatigue; restlessness; accident proneness
- Sexual difficulties

See also ANGER; ANXIETY DISORDERS; BEHAVIOR THERAPY; CATASTROPHIZE; CORONARY ARTERY DISEASE; EXERCISE; KABAT-ZINN, JON; POST-TRAU-

---

CHECKLIST: COPING WITH STRESS

- Identify external stress-producing factors over which you have little or no control, such as on your job.
- Identify internal factors such as perfectionism and unrealistic self-expectations.
- Recognize your personal signs of stress, such as: Increased irritability with family members or coworkers
  Headaches; stomachaches; digestive disorders
  Overeating; increased alcohol consumption
  Sleeplessness; chronic fatigue
  Depression; feelings of hopelessness
- Separate your problems at home from your work concerns, and vice-versa.
- Be realistic in your daily outlook; don't expect too much of yourself or others.
- Prioritize your responsibilities; learn to occasionally say "no" to requests you consider unreasonable or undoable.
- Pay attention to a healthy life-style, such as eating a well-balanced diet and exercising.
- Reduce your consumption of caffeinated beverages, cut down on coffee, tea, and cola, which can increase your heart rate and your irritability level.
- Develop a regular habit of exercising; a 20-minute walk each day can be effective in fighting muscle tension.
- Develop a sense of humor; increase your ability to see humor in sometimes intolerable situations.
- Learn some RELAXATION techniques that work for you, such as deep breathing or listening to your favorite music.
- Seek professional help if you feel overwhelmed.

MATIC STRESS SYNDROME; PSYCHONEUROIMMUNOLOGY; RELATIONSHIPS; SUPPORT GROUPS; VOLUNTEERISM; WEIL, ANDREW.

SOURCES:

Benson, Herbert. *Beyond the Relaxation Response.* New York: Berkeley Press, 1985.

———. *The Relaxation Response.* New York: Avon Books, 1975.

Benson, Herbert, and Eileen M. Stuart. *The Wellness Book: The Comprehensive Guide to Maintaining Health and Treating Stress-Related Illness.* New York: Carol, 1992.

Carey, Benedict. "Don't Face Stress Alone." *Health,* April 1997.

Field, Tiffany, Olga Quintino, et al. "Job Stress Reduction Therapies." *Alternative Therapies* 3, no. 4 (July 1997).

Hornig-Rohan, Mady. "Stress, Immune Mediators, and Immune-Mediated Disease." *Advances: The Journal of Mind-Body Health* 11, no. 2 (Spring 1995).

Kahn, Ada P. "Stress" (pamphlet), Chicago: Mental Health Association of Greater Chicago, 1989.

———. "Win the Case Against Stress." Chicago Bar Association *Record,* May 1994.

———. "Women and Stress." *Sacramento Medicine,* September 1995.

Pelletier, Kenneth R. *Sound Mind, Sound Body: A Model for Lifelong Health.* New York: Simon and Schuster, 1994.

Sapolsky, Robert M. *Why Zebras Don't Get Ulcers.* New York: W.H. Freeman, 1994.

Selye, Hans. *The Stress of Life,* rev. New York: McGraw Hill, 1978.

———. *Stress Without Distress.* Philadelphia: J. B. Lippincott, 1974.

stress management   Refers to an individual's personal COPING skills for dealing with STRESS. It also refers to a multibillion-dollar industry that includes programs, products, services, and techniques to help people reduce stress on an individual or group basis. For example, stress management programs offer help to people interested in overcoming stress-related disorders ranging from EATING DISORDERS to issues of SELF-ESTEEM. Programs may include use of many ALTERNATIVE THERAPIES.

Many stress management programs are offered in the WORKPLACE and address such problems as ALCOHOLISM and other ADDICTIONS, finances, nutrition, and other employee concerns.

See also EMPLOYEE ASSISTANCE PROGRAMS; PSYCHOTHERAPIES.

SOURCE:

Murphy, Lawrence R. "Stress Management in Work Settings: A Critical Review of the Health

Effects." *American Journal of Health Promotion* 11, no. 2 (November/December): 112–35.

stressors See STRESS.

stroke An interruption to the blood supply of the brain, or leakage of blood outside vessel walls, that causes damage to a part of the brain. Sensation, movement, or function controlled by the damaged area may be impaired. Paralysis or some speech impairment may occur. Strokes are fatal in about one-third of cases and are a leading cause of death in developed countries. A stroke is a very stressful event in the life of the sufferer as well as the caregiver.

See also ATHEROSCLEROSIS; CORONARY ARTERY DISEASE; HEART ATTACK; HIGH BLOOD PRESSURE.

FOR FURTHER INFORMATION:
National Institute of Neurological Disorders and
    Stroke
9000 Rockville Pike
Bethesda, MD 20892
Phone: (301) 762-9922

National Stroke Association
300 E. Hampden Avenue
Englewood, CO 80110
Phone: (303) 762-9922

The Stroke Foundation
898 Park Avenue
New York, NY 10021
Phone: (212) 734-3461

stuttering A speech disorder involving repeated hesitation and delay in saying words or in which certain sounds are unusually prolonged. Stuttering is also known as stammering. Stuttering is stressful because it causes the sufferer embarrassment and ANXIETY. Some stutterers become socially withdrawn because they fear ridicule from others.

Stuttering usually starts in early childhood and may be a temporary situation. However, about half of the children whose stuttering persists after age five continue to do so throughout adulthood. Causes of stuttering

are not understood; theories say that it may be due to a subtle form of brain damage or may be related to a psychological problem.

When people who have a stammer become anxious or fearful, their stuttering becomes worse. For example, some children who are fearful of getting up and speaking in the classroom have difficulty getting words out. Interestingly, these same children feel no particular stress and have no difficulty in reading aloud or singing in unison.

Speech therapy helps some individuals improve their speech pattern; training may include learning to give equal weight to each syllable.

See also SOCIAL PHOBIA.

FOR FURTHER INFORMATION:
National Center for Stuttering
200 E. 33rd Street
New York, NY 10016
Phone: (212) 532-1460; (800) 221-2483

Stuttering Resource Foundation
123 Oxford
New Rochelle, NY 10804
Phone: (800) 232-4773

substance abuse See ADDICTION.

success A favorable outcome or attainment of wealth or stature, success can be a source of stress when it happens as well as when it does not happen. Some who view success as a source of stress, fear that they will not be able to reach a higher plateau or that they will not be able to fulfill other people's expectations. Others may fear that by achieving success they will have to move to a better neighborhood, bigger house, or send children to a better school. All these expectations may lead to anxieties and stressful feelings about change.

While success can be a source of satisfaction, it also can be stressful because some individuals may fear that achievement will place them in another social, academic, or social class and they will lose friendships.

Some individuals actually avoid success because they want to continue conforming to their group.

Expectations for success are stressful because they correlate with people's fear of failure. An inability to reach what people regard as success may reflect unfavorably on their self-image and SELF-ESTEEM.

Certain PERSONALITY types are driven toward success. The TYPE A PERSONALITY, for example, is associated with intense drives for success. Such individuals have competitive feelings, are extremely goal oriented, take on multiple commitments, and become preoccupied with meeting deadlines. Often, after serious illness, such individuals learn to relax more and redirect their drives, placing more value on family and friendships.

SOURCE:
Van Fleet, James K. *Lifetime Guide to Success With People.* Englewood Cliffs, N.J.: Prentice-Hall, 1995.

sudden infant death syndrome (SIDS) SIDS, or "crib death," is the sudden and unexplained death of an infant. Infants who are victims of SIDS are usually between the ages of two to four months, when they who stop breathing during a normal sleeping period. Ninety percent of all victims die within the first four months, but SIDS may strike children as old as one year.

According to Phipps Cohe, public affairs director, National SIDS Alliance, one infant every hour or one out of every 500 babies born in the United States succumbs to SIDS. Out of 36 industrialized nations, the United States ranks 20th in infant mortality; a large number of these deaths are attributed to SIDS.

Although causes of SIDS are unknown, it is not caused by childhood vaccines, suffocation, vomiting, or choking. Research projects are under way to determine predictive factors that may prevent future deaths.

Parents who have lost a child to SIDS find SUPPORT GROUPS helpful.

See also GRIEF.

FOR FURTHER INFORMATION:
American Sudden Infant Death Syndrome Institute
275 Carpenter Drive
Atlanta, GA 30328
Phone: (800) 232-SIDS; (800) 232-7437

National Sudden Infant Death Syndrome
  Foundation
10500 Little Patuxent Parkway
Columbia, MD 21044
Phone: (301) 964-8000; (800) 221-SIDS;
(800) 221-7437

Sudden Infant Death Syndrome Clearinghouse
8201 Greensboro
McLean, VA 22102
Phone: (703) 821-8955

suicide Killing oneself voluntarily and intentionally. In some cases, suicide is the consequence of DEPRESSION and stress. It is a subject that is a stressful one for many people to talk about, and a verdict of suicide certainly is not one that the family wants to hear.

Suicide is the eighth leading cause of DEATH in the United States and the second most frequent cause of death for young people in the 15–25 age group. About 12% of those who threaten or attempt suicide actually kill themselves. Current statistics may understate the actual occurrence of suicide. For example, there may be suicidal intentions behind many auto and other accidents. Additionally, because of insurance coverage issues and legal criteria for classifying cause of death, suicide may not be recorded as the cause in many cases.

Preventing suicide
Suicide is a manifestation of depression that can be successfully treated. People who show signs of depression and express hopelessness or suicidal impulses should be encouraged to get immediate professional help in order to avoid a crisis. If a suicidal crisis does occur, the

family should remove all weapons and lethal means from the home, including prescription drugs, and the individual threatening suicide should not be left alone at any time.

One of the most difficult challenges clinicians face is preventing the suicide of their patients. Such psychiatric clinicians routinely deal with patients whose diagnoses indicate a high risk for suicide. The physician, psychotherapist, or mental health worker is sometimes the only person who recognizes suicidal intent. Studies have shown that from 40% to 75% of suicidal individuals see a physician within six months to a year preceding their self-destructive acts. A number of studies have pointed out that even while receiving psychiatric treatment, psychiatric hospitalization or treatment with psychotropic drugs, patients do commit suicide.

Evidence seems to support the contention that most suicides occur in the context of psychiatric illness. However, the absence of psychiatric treatment at the time of suicide does not necessarily preclude the existence of a serious mental disturbance; severely depressed patients may appear symptom-free just prior to suicide. This may lead to an erroneous assumption that the individual is "normal" at the time of suicide.

Additionally, the presence of real or perceived physical illness may be significant in the assessment of suicidal risk. In malignant or incurable illness, two critical suicidal periods seem to be those of: a) uncertainty while diagnosis and prognosis are still at issue, and b) shock following the first realization of the upheavals and suffering, actual or fantasized, that are to follow.

Depression and suicide

Individuals who have serious depression are high suicide risks. Symptoms may include feelings of hopelessness, helplessness, and emptiness, especially with severe anxiety or panic attacks, sleep disturbance, weight loss, complete loss of interest, loss of sexual interest, impairment of function, delusional guilt, neglect of personal appearance and cleanliness, and inability to make decisions. Generally, the risk of suicide appears to be greatest in the early course of depressive illness (first three episodes).

Common instances of increased suicidal risk in depressed individuals are associated with separation or loss. The loss does not necessarily have to be a death of a loved one, but may be simply a temporary loss such as home or job or temporary separation such as from therapist, money, or love.

The "failure situation" ranks high as a precursor of suicide. This situation may occur when one is trying to regain or attain a higher level of function, such as starting a job or returning to college. Also, the failure factor ranks high when individuals try to meet higher expectations of themselves or others.

Recognizing suicide intentions

A characteristic of a chronically suicidal person is repeated communication of a wish to die or suicidal thoughts. However, this in itself is not sufficient to distinguish the high- from the low-risk individual, since the majority of the much larger group of people who attempt but do not complete suicide also convey intent in advance.

Personalities of many suicidal individuals have shown tendencies toward rigid thinking, which does not allow for alternatives in a crisis; PERFECTION in all undertakings is a personality trait that is carried to a pathological extreme.

A suicidal individual often shows intense dependency as an underlying life-style dynamic. This dependency may be notable throughout all spheres of the suicidal individual's life-style where inordinately excessive demands are made on others for constant attention, affection, and approval, and where the individual feels unable to cope for himself, thereby needing continual supervision and guidance.

Recognizing youth at risk

There are some specific clues to predict suicide among youngsters or adolescents. For example, they are more likely to communicate with those in their peer group than with their parents. They may give away a prized possession with the comment that they will not be needing it anymore. They may be more morose and isolated than usual. Although there may be signs of insomnia, worry, and anorexia, the youngster may not have all the classical signs of depression.

One study listed symptoms occurring in 25 college-age suicides in order of their frequency: despondency, futility, lack of interest in school work, tenseness around people, insomnia, suicidal communications, fatigue and malaise without apparent organic cause, feelings of inadequacy or unworthiness, and brooding over the death of a loved one.

Having a gun in the home may increase the risk that a psychologically troubled teen will commit suicide, according to David A. Brent, M.D., in the *Journal of the American Medical Association* (December 1991). Dr. Brent and colleagues noted that the odds that potentially suicidal adolescents will kill themselves are raised 75-fold when a gun is kept in the house. They commented on differences between teen suicides and that of adults. For teens, they said, a suicide attempt may be an attempt to communicate that they are in great pain, although they may be ambivalent about wanting to die. For such adolescents, ready access to a firearm may guarantee that their plea for help will not be heard.

Suicide and the aging population

A federal study published during 1991 showed that from 1980 to 1986, suicides by Americans aged 65 and older jumped 23% for men and 42% for African-American men. The rate for white women rose 17%, while there were too few suicides among African-American women

---

> ### RECOGNIZING CHARACTERISTICS OF SUICIDAL INDIVIDUALS
>
> - Depressed mood; hopeless-helpless
> - Disturbed sleep patterns and appetite disturbances
> - Anger, hostility
> - Ambivalence; impaired concentration
> - Withdrawn, isolative behavior
> - Constricted thought processes; tunnel vision
> - Psychomotor agitation or psychomotor retardation
> - Anxious; attentive to internal stimuli
> - Verbalizes suicidal thoughts or plans and references to death
> - Gives away possessions; impulsive behaviors

---

to show a meaningful trend. A study in Illinois under a grant from the American Association of Retired People Andrus Foundation showed that the great majority of the elderly who committed suicide were physically healthy. However, 79% had shown symptoms of a major treatable psychiatric illness, usually depression or ALCOHOLISM.

Assisted suicide

In 1991, *Final Exit,* a "how-to" book by Derek Humphry, executive director of the Hemlock Society (a group aimed at promoting death-with-dignity), was published. He emphasized that his controversial book for the terminally ill was not meant for unhappy or depressed people.

Many mental health professionals were concerned that this book and others may legitimize suicide for troubled people with undiagnosed depression who could be treated if their illnesses were diagnosed correctly. Many expressed fear that such books could increase suicide rates, particularly among the elderly who are not terminally ill. However, according to David Clark, past president, American Society of Suicidology (an organization dedicated to preventing suicide), many people, when they recover from an attempted suicide, are extraordinarily glad that someone did not help them die.

In March 1990, physicians writing in the *New England Journal of Medicine* about "The Physician's Responsibility toward Hopelessly Ill Patients" held that "it is not immoral for a physician to assist in the rational suicide of a terminally ill person." Two of the 12 authors of the paper dissented from this statement.

In 1990, Michigan physician Dr. Jack Kevorkian assisted in the suicide of an Oregon woman said to have ALZHEIMER'S DISEASE. He provided her with a device that she activated to administer a lethal dose of drugs. Questions were raised about Dr. Kevorkian's ability to confirm the patient's diagnosis, about the patient's ability to make an informed decision, and about the circumstances. The event took place in a van parked on a side road in Michigan, far from the patient's family and outside any institution. Many subsequent "assisted" suicides by Dr. Kevorkian and others have taken place throughout the 1990s.

See also AFFECTIVE DISORDERS.

FOR FURTHER INFORMATION:
American Academy of Child and Adolescent Psychiatry
3615 Wisconsin Avenue, NW
Washington, DC 20016
Phone: (202) 996-7300

American Association of Suicidology
2459 South Ash Street
Denver, CO 80222
Phone: (303) 692-0985

American Psychiatric Association
1400 K Street NW
Washington, D.C. 20005
Phone: (202) 682-6000

National Alliance for the Mentally Ill
2101 Wilson Blvd. (Suite 302)
Arlington, VA 22201
Phone: (703) 524-7600

National Committee on Youth Suicide Prevention
666 Fifth Avenue (13th floor)
New York, NY 10103
Phone: (212) 677-6666

National Institute of Mental Health
5600 Fishers Lane
Rockville, Maryland 20857
Phone: (301) 443-4513

National Mental Health Association
1021 Prince Street
Alexandria, VA 22314–2932
Phone: (703) 684-7722; (800) 969-NMHA

SOURCES:
Brent, David A., et al. "Teens More Likely to Commit Suicide When Gun Is in Home." *Journal of the American Medical Association,* December 3, 1991.
Fawcett, Jan, William A. Scheftner, Louis Fogg, et al. "Time-Related Predictors of Suicide in Major Affective Disorder." *American Journal of Psychiatry* 147, no. 9 (September 1990).
Garrison, Jayne. "Rushing Heaven's Door." *Health,* May-June 1997.
Humphry, Derek. *Final Exit: The Practicalities of Self-Deliverance and Assisted Suicide for the Dying.* Secaucus, N.J.: Carol Publishing, 1991.
Kahn, Ada P., and Jan Fawcett. *Encyclopedia of Mental Health.* New York: Facts On File, 1993.
Katz, Marvin. "Critics Fear Misuse of Suicide Books." *Bulletin, American Association of Retired Persons.* 32, no. 11 (December 1991).
"Should the Doctor Ever Help?" *Harvard Health Letter* 16, no. 10 (August 1991).

sunlight Light from the sun, which helps plants grow and helps elevate people's moods. Soaking up the sun's rays has been a favorite American pastime for many years. Lying in the sun was believed to be a great way to relax and escape from the stress of everyday life. The sun not only made people feel good, it also contributed to a tanned, outdoor look. That was before the dangers of ultraviolet rays were understood, said the American Academy of Dermatology (AAD) in its pamphlet, *The Sun and Your Skin,* published in 1994. Now it is known that too much sun can cause wrinkles, freckles, skin texture changes, dilated blood vessels, and skin CANCER.

Recommendations to prevent skin damage
It is important to avoid overexposure to the sun because the sun produces both visible

and invisible rays, known as ultraviolet-A (UVA) and ultraviolet-B (UVB). Both cause suntan, sunburn, and sun damage. There is no "safe" UV light. People should use protection against the sun whenever outdoors. While the harmful UV rays are more intense in the summer, at higher altitudes, and near the equator, effects of the sun are also increased by wind and reflections from water, sand, and snow. Even on cloudy days, UV radiation reaches Earth.

The AAD recommends avoiding deliberate sunbathing and wearing a wide-brimmed hat, sunglasses, and protective clothing if it is necessary to be in the sun, and to use a sunscreen at all times. A sunscreen works by absorbing, reflecting, or scattering the sun's rays on the skin. Choosing the right sunscreen can be a source of stress because so many choices are available. All sunscreens, whether they are ointments, gels, creams, lotions, or wax sticks, are labeled with SPF (sun protection factor) numbers. The higher the SPF, the greater the protection from sunburn caused by most UVB rays. Some sunscreens, called "broad spectrum," block out both UVA and UVB rays.

Protecting against effects of the sun should start by avoiding the peak hours of the sun—usually between 10 A.M. and 4 P.M. Sunscreens should be applied about 20 minutes before going outdoors and should be reapplied about every two hours after swimming or strenuous activities.

Skin cancer

While too much sun can cause painful sunburn, age the skin with wrinkles, freckles, and sunspots, set off allergic reactions such as rashes, hives, and blisters, and cause cataracts, the worst possible effect is skin cancer. There are three common types of skin cancer: basal cell carcinoma, squamous cell carcinoma, and melanoma.

Estimates indicate that approximately 700,000 Americans develop skin cancer every year. Fortunately, most skin cancers can be detected and cured if found early. Dermatologists recommend periodic self-examinations; watching the patterns of moles, freckles, and "beauty marks"; and being alert to changes in the number, size, color, and shape of pigmented areas. Contact a dermatologist if changes occur.

Effects of too little sunlight

Too little sunlight in the environment, such as in northern locations during winter months, can result in a form of depression known as SEASONAL AFFECTIVE DISORDER. Treatment involves going to a place with a brighter atmosphere, or using specially designed light treatments.

See also AFFECTIVE DISORDERS; BODY IMAGE; CHRONIC ILLNESS; CLIMATE; DEPRESSION.

FOR FURTHER INFORMATION:
American Academy of Dermatology
930 Meacham
Schaumburg, IL 60172-4965
Phone: (708) 330-0230

superiority complex An unrealistic and exaggerated belief of a person that he or she is better than others. Such a complex is a source of stress for the individual as well as others. In some people, this is a compensation mechanism for unconscious feelings of low SELF-ESTEEM or inadequacy. For example, bullies who push other children around act like that because, in reality, they have low self-esteem.

Some adults with a superiority complex seem to be snobbish, but they are really covering up for an inadequacy, such as lack of a college education.

See also INFERIORITY COMPLEX.

superstition Beliefs that have survived since ancient times regarding the mysteries of nature. Superstitions abound among cultures around the world; many people who still hold superstitious beliefs become stressed when they allow their superstitions to take over their life.

Many odd and amusing notions and customs persist; some are harmless and some are harmful. Scientific thinking supersedes the superstitious because modern science believes that everything in nature has a natural cause and that laws of nature can explain cause and effect.

Superstitious beliefs are more common among people with little education, but even well-educated people have a tendency to cling to superstitious beliefs. For example, hotels and other commercial buildings sometimes avoid numbering the 13th floor because many persons believe it is unlucky. Fridays that fall on the 13th day of the month are considered unlucky. If your ears burn, it means someone is talking about you. Bad luck follows walking under a ladder, breaking a mirror, or having a black cat cross your path. It is supposed to be good luck if one finds a penny or a four-leaf clover. Stressful interactions may arise between family members or friends when one clings to these old superstitions and another counters them with more practical explanations.

See also ACCULTURATION; TABOOS.

support groups Individuals with the same experience about a specific health or social concern who join together to help each other by sharing experiences and advice and by providing emotional support for each other.

Support groups exist for patients as well as spouses and family members in almost every medical or social category. For example, individuals with MANIC-DEPRESSIVE DISORDER began an organization that now has become nationwide, with chapters in many cities. Individuals with CHRONIC FATIGUE SYNDROME (CFS) have done the same, with the result that sufferers no longer need feel alone with their problems. There are support groups for parents of children with specific diseases, as well as groups for spouses of ALZHEIMER'S DISEASE patients and for middle-age people who care for ELDERLY PARENTS.

Many physicians recommend that patients join support groups because the sharing with others can be effective and augment any therapies provided by medical means.

An additional benefit of belonging to a support group for a particular concern is that one can stay up-to-date on progress as researchers work toward better treatments or legislators work on the issues. Many groups circulate articles from popular and scientific publications and bring in experts to discuss their latest findings.

According to Karyn Feiden, author of *Hope and Help for Chronic Fatigue Syndrome*, benefits of support groups generally fall into three major areas: informing and educating the general public, and particularly patients, their families, and the medical community; counseling and consoling those who have been diagnosed with a particular disorder; and organizing and advocating for the cause at local and national levels.

Support groups for breast cancer patients

David Spiegel, M.D., Stanford University School physician and faculty member, pioneered work with support groups for BREAST CANCER patients. In 1991, at the national meeting of Y-ME (a breast CANCER advocacy organization), he reported conclusions of a 15-year study of 86 metastatic breast cancer patients.

> While we know that psychosocial support affects outcome in terms of length of survival, the mechanism by which it does so is not clear. However, results of this study strongly suggest that psychosocial support can improve the quality of life for cancer patients, is inexpensive and easy to organize, and should be a standard part of care.
>
> Social support is an important stress buffer and is strongly related to survival. The risk of cancer and cancer mortality is higher if one is not socially integrated. The ratio may be as high as 2:1. For men, marital status is a protective factor, with married men at the lowest risk. For women, the best protective

factor is relationships with women friends and relatives. . .

When patients manage STRESS better, it may allow their bodies to devote more resources to fighting illness. This comes not by denying the illness and wishing it away, but by managing life, relationships with family and physicians, one's own feelings about having a terminal illness as fully as possible, and making their lives fuller and richer. Such techniques are not a cure for cancer, but there is some evidence that they may prolong survival.

From our support groups as well as other studies, we know that mutual support should be encouraged. There was a tremendous power among the women with the same problem. Most people don't understand DEATH, feel isolated and that they are already dead. Enhancing mutual support made these women feel more a part of humanity.

A bonding develops quickly because women in the group know what others' fears are like; this helps to normalize their reactions and relationships with each other. People feel awkward talking about cancer because they find it hard to deal with anxiety about death. "We found that it was not death itself, but the process of dying, including losing physical CONTROL, an inability to do what they did before, and PAIN, that were most difficult for the women to face. Thus there was a series of problems, not just one problem. However, there are some constructive things one can do, for example, work out a living will, improve means of pain control, and talk with one's physician about ongoing care.

"We were concerned that putting women with metastatic cancer together might demoralize some of them. Instead, direct confrontation with death led the women to discussions of positive coping strategies and no decline in mood."

The criteria for inclusion in the randomized prospective study was that women agreed to attend weekly support groups for a year. Fifty

women were randomly assigned to the support group situation; 36 were assigned to their routine cancer care. The women had comparable kinds of initial surgery, similar initial staging, comparable degrees of metastatic spread, similar courses of chemotherapy and disease-free intervals (three years for both groups).

Therapy groups included 8–10 women and two therapists who met weekly for an hour and a half. Intervention focused on direct confrontation of fears of dying and death, realistic assessment of prognosis, and development of new coping strategies for interaction with physicians, family, and friends.

Overall, patients in the treatment group showed a reduction in total mood disturbance while those in the control group worsened in terms of tension, fears, anxiety, confusion, and fatigue. The treatment group coped substantially better, and experienced less denial, significant reductions in mood disturbance, fewer phobic symptoms, and less pain.

Both the treatment and control groups had routine oncologic care. At 10-year follow-up, only three of the original 86 patients were still alive, and death records were obtained for the other 83. Survival from the time of randomization and onset of intervention was 36.6 months for the treatment group, compared with 18.9 months for the control group. Four years after randomization, all of the control patients had died and one-third of the intervention sample were still alive. There was a difference in survival from the first metastases, 43 months vs. 58 months.

In explaining the survival differences between the two groups, Dr. Spiegel said that women who are less depressed may eat better, exercise more, take better care of themselves, and may encourage physicians to be more assiduous in treatment. "We now call this supportive-expressive group therapy. The theme is how the women face their futures, not their pasts," said Dr. Spiegel.

See also BEHAVIOR THERAPY; CHRONIC ILLNESS; DEPRESSION.

SOURCES:

Feiden, Karyn. *Hope and Help for Chronic Fatigue Syndrome.* New York: Prentice-Hall, 1990.

Kahn, Ada P. "Psychosocial Support Influences Survival of Cancer Patients." *Psychiatric News,* October 1991.

Kreiner, Anna. *Everything You Need to Know About Creating Your Own Support System.* New York: Rosen Publishing Group, 1996.

Locke, Steve and Douglas Colligan. *The Healer Within.* New York: New American Library, 1986.

sympathetic nervous system (SNS)   One of two divisions of the autonomic nervous system. The system controls many involuntary activities of the glands, organs and other parts of the body and readies it for coping with suddenly occurring situations. The SNS is very involved in stress responses, as it is responsible for preparing people for fighting, fleeing, action, or sexual climax.

The SNS includes connections from the eyes to the urogenital organs. Typical sympathetic changes take place during heavy exertion or when facing extremely stressful situations. The pupils widen to facilitate vision, the arteries constrict to supply more blood to the muscles and the brain, heartbeat increases, ADRENALINE is secreted to increase metabolism, the skin perspires to eliminate waste products, and stomach and intestinal activities cease so that energy can be directed elsewhere.

See also FIGHT OR FLIGHT RESPONSE.

symptom   An indication of an illness or mental distress noticed by the sufferer. For example, symptoms of stress may be sleeplessness, fatigue, difficulty concentrating, or irritability. A symptom is different from a sign, which is an indication of a disorder noticed on an objective basis by another person, such as a physician. A group of symptoms as well as signs is sometimes referred to as a SYNDROME. An example is post-traumatic stress syndrome, which includes a wide range of symptoms, such as nightmares, feelings of claustrophobia, and an inability to concentrate; the physician may notice increased heartbeat, rapid breathing, and other signs during examination.

syndrome   A group of SYMPTOMS or signs that occur together and make up a particular disorder. For example, the syndrome that leads a physician to diagnose extreme stress in an individual, may include elevated blood pressure, difficulty sleeping, loss of weight, inability to concentrate, lack of interest in sexual activity, as well as others.

syphilis   See SEXUALLY TRANSMITTED DISEASES.

systematic desensitization   See BEHAVIOR THERAPY.

T

taboos Ideas, concepts, or practices that are not discussed or carried out openly by a given culture are referred to as taboos. Some taboos are so specific to a culture that they are difficult for outsiders to understand. The source or reason for a taboo may be unknown or forgotten; taboos may have given groups of people moral and ethical codes by which they lived.

Certain taboos that are common to many cultures are a source of stress. For example, references to the dead and DEATH are frequently avoided, made in hushed tones, or accompanied by a ritual gesture or phrase; SUICIDE is not discussed in many cultures, nor is INCEST, so much so, that reference to the behavior and to the act itself may have been suppressed. During the 1990s in the United States there were revelations that incest had a higher incidence than previously thought. As a consequence, the taboo to speak out and protest about it was, to a large extent, lifted.

Some taboos evolve from social hierarchies, such as the Hindu caste system, which rigidly regulates contact among the castes. Other taboos are related to rulers or persons in authority. For example, on a visit to the United States, Queen Elizabeth II accepted a friendly, but highly irregular, hug from a woman who was not familiar with royal protocol.

Other taboos involve sex roles and contact between the sexes such as the exclusion of women from male clubs. Cleanliness, especially of food, and bodily functions, such as excretion or MENSTRUATION, give rise to taboos in many cultures; Native American tribes confined their women to a specific lodge during their menstrual periods.

The word *taboo* is derived from the language of the Polynesian people, meaning "forbidden" or "dangerous." It is the term used for behavior related to their king. He was thought to be so full of power or *mana* that his shadow, parts of his body, and even objects that he touched were considered dangerous.

See also SUPERSTITION.

SOURCES:
Douglas, Mary. "Taboo," in Cavendish, Richard, ed., *Man, Myth and Magic,* vol. 10. New York: Marshall Cavendish, 1983; 2767–71.
Gregory, W.E. "Taboos," in Corsini, Raymond J. *The Encyclopedia of Psychology,* vol. 3. New York: Wiley, 1984; 398.

tachycardia Rapid beating of the heart, over 100 beats per minute in an adult. Most people experience 60 to 100 beats a minute, with an average of 72 to 78 beats. It is normal for tachycardia to occur under some conditions, such as vigorous EXERCISE or sexual activity. However, tachycardia is sometimes associated with AGORAPHOBIA, ANXIETY, PANIC ATTACKS AND PANIC DISORDER. People who already feel stressed, anxious, or fearful may become even more so when they become aware that their heart is beating rapidly. Under such circumstances they may fear that they are having a HEART ATTACK and, along with the rapid heartbeat, experience symptoms such as difficulty in BREATHING, PALPITATIONS, and DIZZINESS.

Other reasons for tachycardia at rest are hyperthyroidism, coronary heart disease, a high intake of CAFFEINE, and treatment with an anticholinergic and some decongestant drugs.

t'ai chi A physical, mental, and spiritual practice that uses movement to balance energy, and helps achieve and maintain harmony within oneself. Those who practice t'ai chi say that it aids them to develop more mental and spiritual energy, feel more overall vitality, and obtain relief from stress.

T'ai chi is an outgrowth of Chinese martial arts, spirituality, and Chinese medicine, and has been practiced for more than 2,000 years. As a martial art and a popular meditative practice, it is often called MEDITATION in motion. According to Chinese philosophy, to do t'ai chi is to connect the individual with nature through movement. It is considered "great shadow boxing," which draws on Taoist beliefs in the interdependence of the body and the mind. In the open spaces and parks of China today, millions of young and old people practice t'ai chi, gently swaying, gliding, and stepping.

Benefits of t'ai chi

Practitioners of t'ai chi usually experience deep and restful sleep. Their nervous system is soothed and calmed. The gentleness of t'ai chi ensures that they do not suffer strains and other muscular injuries, but instead develop greater strength, flexibility, and suppleness. Some athletes use t'ai chi as a way of warming up.

People who perform t'ai chi move all their joints and exert more energy than it appears. Through the use of slow BREATHING, individuals can pace some of the systems of their body. They can stabilize their heartbeat, the exchange of oxygen and carbon dioxide, and the secretion and absorption of endocrine fluids. The movements also improve health by assisting the flow of blood, creating tranquillity for the entire nervous system, and through deep concentration, fostering deep peace of mind.

United States researchers have been studying the physical and mental benefits of t'ai chi, particularly for older people, many of whom suffer from a lack of balance and experience falls. In an article in the *Journal of the American Geriatric Society* (May 1996), an evaluation of a 15-week course taken by 72 men and women over age 70 showed that t'ai chi not only improved their balance, but also helped these people abort falls by teaching them to cope with missteps and precarious positions. Another study, reported in the *Harvard Health Letter* (July 1997), said that older adults who practiced t'ai chi had significantly lower blood pressure readings after the exercise and a decreased fear of falling.

T'ai chi classes

Books and videos on t'ai chi are available, but the best way to learn t'ai chi is in classes held in t'ai chi studios, adult education courses at high schools and colleges, YMCAs and YWCAs, and senior adult centers. Many people combine t'ai chi with other forms of exercise.

See also ALTERNATIVE THERAPIES.

tantrums Fits of ANGER usually experienced by children, although some adults, particularly those who have mental disorders, also experience these physical outbursts. Tantrums can happen anywhere. Anyone who has ever witnessed children throwing a tantrum in public sympathizes with the stress and FRUSTRATION felt by their parents. Although physical outbursts are a normal part of childhood development, they are no less embarrassing for parents who must manage a child's loss of CONTROL, and their own loss as well.

Childhood tantrums come in many forms—usually a combination of screaming, stomping around, writhing on the floor, and breaking or wielding handy objects. Children may be angered by being unable to deal with new experiences or frustrated by a perceived obstacle. For example, objects they might want to handle can be too dangerous, too complex, or too delicate for their small fingers.

When children learn that the world does not center on them nor does it necessarily revolve around what they want, a tantrum is the way in which they may revolt. They are protesting against limitations on their behavior set by their parents and society. Fortunately for parents, most children outgrow their tantrums and eventually learn how to interact with their environment in a more mature way.

See also HOSTILITY; PARENTING.

teenage pregnancy   See PREGNANCY; UNWED MOTHERS.

teeth grinding   Known medically as bruxism, a HABIT many people practice when they feel stressed or anxious. Some people grind their teeth during the day and some do it only at night.

For about 5% of the population, teeth grinding causes serious consequences. For example, it is possible to grind the enamel off the teeth, making them more susceptible to cavities and very sensitive to heat and cold. Years of grinding can cause facial and jaw pain from fatigued muscles. Grinding also may damage the joint between the jaw and the cranium (temporomandibular joint). When a person eats, the muscles responsible for chewing exert just enough pressure to hold in place the disk of cartilage that cushions the joint. When the person grinds his or her teeth, this disk gradually becomes displaced, causing soreness, inflammation and even ARTHRITIS.

Dentists can prepare plastic retainer-like appliances called mouth guards or night guards that prevent grinding. Many people find that RELAXATION therapy, GUIDED IMAGERY, HYPNOSIS, and BIOFEEDBACK also help to relieve this unwanted habit.

See also TEMPOROMANDIBULAR JOINT SYNDROME.

telemarketers   See RANDOM NUISANCES.

television   A popular form of entertainment and education that has been available for about 40 to 50 years. In the 1990s, sitting in front of the television set occupies so many Americans for so long that they have been labeled "couch potatoes." The average American adult watches over 30 hours of television a week. While a common reason for watching TV is RELAXATION, a major study indicated that the longer viewers spent in front of the screen, the more stress they felt, because of guilt over frittering away their time or avoiding responsibilities.

An additional source of stress felt by many Americans involves both the purchase of TV sets and selection of TV programming. When buying a TV/VCR, people do not have time to deal with the brand clutter on the retail shelves and to determine the best price offered by competitive dealers. A similar competition for TV viewers exists among the various TV networks and the growing number of cable channels. An example of this is the tremendous increase in television talk shows that occurred during the 1990s, many of which seek the same TV audience market and often run concurrently during the daytime and evening hours.

Estimates indicate that early in the 21st century, there will be as many as 250 cable and network channels from which viewers will be able to choose. This dilemma, plus the production of digital TVs, which will make current sets obsolete, will have viewers stressed for years to come.

temporomandibular joint syndrome (TMJ)   TMJ occurs when the ligaments and muscles that control and support the jaw, face, and head do not work together properly. The disorder can be brought on by a spasm of the chewing muscles, teeth grinding (bruxism), or clenching the teeth as a response to STRESS and tension.

Symptoms of TMJ may include tenderness of the jaw, HEADACHES and dull, aching facial pain, jaws that lock, pain brought on by chewing or yawning, and a clicking or popping noise when opening the jaw.

Psychological counseling sometimes helps individuals overcome the underlying causes of tension and cope better with the stresses in their lives. Some people try GUIDED IMAGERY and RELAXATION exercises.

Treatment may include relieving pain by applying moist heat to the face, taking muscle-relaxant drugs, and using a bite splint at night to prevent teeth clenching and grinding. Some individuals undergo orthodontia to correct their bite while others undergo surgery on the jaw.

See also MEDITATION; TEETH GRINDING.

tendinitis An inflammation of a tendon, usually caused by injury. Because people who are under stress often do not pay attention to their bodies' signals, they increase the possibility that they are sitting, standing, and moving in ways that can lead to tendinitis. Precautions are necessary, particularly when people bend or lift. Additionally, people under stress are less likely to take the time to exercise regularly, leaving the muscles more vulnerable to strain when used for strenuous effort.

Those most at risk for tendinitis perform repetitive motions for long periods of time. The repeated motions may be at work or during sports activities. Under most conditions, their bodies may be able to handle the repetitiveness; however, if they are under the demand of deadlines and other stressors, or fail to rest, stretch or relax at regular intervals, tendinitis may occur.

Exercising—which includes conditioning, stretching, and relaxation—can help to reduce the muscular symptoms of stress, and should be continued even after aches and pain disappear. When muscles are strong and healthy, they are far better able to tolerate the tensions that occur in everyday living.

See also REPETITIVE STRESS INJURY.

tension headache See HEADACHES.

terrorism The systematic use of terror as a means of coercion is a worldwide problem.

Terrorism makes many people fearful and apprehensive about traveling and trusting strangers. It increases their levels of stress in airports and other public places; long waits often ensue because of security checks that are not fail-safe.

The bombing of the Federal Building in Oklahoma City in 1995 was an example of terrorism that killed many people and terrorized countless others, particularly those working in government buildings around the world. Hostage taking, which has made the headlines many times in the latter 1990s, is an act of terrorism.

Terrorists are individuals who are fanatical about their cause and often have no concern for their victims or for their own lives. Most terrorist groups are supported by governments who find terrorism an effective and inexpensive way to wage wars in comparison to the high cost of a conventional military force.

In 1986, then-vice president George Bush's Task Force on Combating Terrorism defined terrorism as: "The unlawful use or threat of violence against persons or property to further political or social objectives. It is usually intended to intimidate or coerce a government, individuals, or groups to modify their behavior or politics." Terrorism aimed at United States diplomats had increased dramatically in the 20 years before the Bush report.

While little can be done to protect against most types of terrorism, certain precautions, such as awareness of surroundings in public places and of unusual, out-of-place people, should be taken. Knowing that there will be long waits for baggage searches, passport checks, and other forms of questioning at airports, buildings, and other security checks to ensure safety should help to reduce an individual's levels of stress.

See also HOSTAGES; POST-TRAUMATIC STRESS DISORDER.

therapeutic touch A nontraditional therapy (alternative or complementary) developed by

Dr. Dolores Krieger, professor of nursing at New York University, in which she relieves the pain and distress of illness by passing her hands over the patient. It is also known as healing touch and is derived from the laying-on of hands. Her method is described in her book *The Therapeutic Touch, How to Use Your Hands to Help or to Heal.*

Since the mid-1970s, Dr. Krieger has conducted courses in therapeutic touch and taught thousands of people. New York University offers a fully accredited graduate course at the master's level, designed to formally teach the process of therapeutic touch and to investigate how and why it works. In addition, more than 50 universities offer formal instruction in therapeutic touch, usually as part of the curriculum for nurses' training.

How the technique works

The healer eases into an altered state of consciousness while focusing energy on the patient, then slowly passes his or her hands about four to six inches above the patient's body in an effort to sense a transfer of energy. The healer scans the body for an area of temperature change as an indication that part of the body is troubled, then lays hands on the affected area, while the patient senses a change in temperature, perhaps a feeling of deep heat, in the area being touched.

According to Dr. Krieger, at the very least, the method produces a relaxation response in the patient and works well for inflammation, musculoskeletal problems, and psychosomatic disorders. Explanation by healers whose patients have been helped say that energy passes between themselves and their patients. Skeptics believe that this healing has a PLACEBO EFFECT, but it seems to work for some individuals.

Historically, physicians touched their patients far more than they do today with the advent of so many highly technical diagnostic machines. Until the invention of the stethoscope in the mid-1800s, physicians pressed their naked ears to the bodies of patients to listen for heartbeats and other internal sounds. This intimate gesture probably had a soothing effect on the patient, much as therapeutic touch has today. As author Lewis Thomas wrote in *The Youngest Science,* "It is hard to imagine a friendlier human gesture, a more intimate signal of personal concern and affection, than the close-bowed head affixed to the skin."

Now, many nurses and other health care practitioners, including body therapists, realize the need for human touch and practice healing touch either knowledgeably or unconsciously, along with massage and other techniques.

See also ALTERNATIVE THERAPIES; BODY THERAPIES; MASSAGE THERAPY.

SOURCES:
Locke, Steven and Douglas Colligan. *The Healer Within.* New York: New American Library, 1986.
Macrae, J. *Therapeutic Touch: A Practical Guide.* New York: Alfred A. Knopf, 1988.
Thomas, Lewis. *The Youngest Science.* New York: Viking Press, 1983.

therapy   See PHARMACOLOGICAL APPROACH; PSYCHOTHERAPIES.

tic   An involuntary, repetitive movement of a muscle or muscle groups, mostly affecting the face, shoulders, or arms. Typical tics are blinking, twitching of the mouth, and shoulder shrugging. They are also a characteristic of Gilles de la Tourette Syndrome, a disorder of the nervous system that is characterized by tics and involuntary noises.

Tics are often the result of a minor psychological disturbance and may begin during childhood, affecting three times as many boys as girls. They are worsened by stress or by drawing attention to them. Tics appear to release emotional tension, so voluntary control is of questionable value. Tics usually stop within a year of onset, but some cases last to adulthood.

In some individuals, stress-induced tics can be overcome with BEHAVIOR THERAPY, GUIDED IMAGERY, HYPNOSIS, or RELAXATION training.

FOR FURTHER INFORMATION:
Tourette Syndrome Association
42–40 Bell Boulevard
Bayside, NY 11361
Phone: (800) 237-0717

time management Realistically prioritizing projects and avoiding procrastination. Time management was a "catchword" during the 1980s and 1990s as organizations strived to educate employees, particularly middle managers, to avoid the STRESS caused by a growing need to define business priorities and deal with the paper pile-up in their in-boxes. Seminars on time management were often sponsored by date book and planning calendar manufacturers who offered products as solutions to the time management problem. However, it persists and is compounded today by staff reductions that add responsibilities to existing jobs and by computerization that has raised the standards for quality and promises to reduce time and effort, when in fact the opposite is often true.

Another aspect of time management is the growing stress of balancing career and family. While this is applicable to both men and women, it is a particular problem for the working mother (both married and single) who continues to have major responsibility for running the home and caring for the chil-

---

**TIME MANAGEMENT TIPS
TO REDUCE STRESS**

- Set realistic goals; don't overestimate what you can do.
- Don't procrastinate.
- Establish priorities; make lists.
- Pace yourself; set "time-outs."

---

dren, as she shares in meeting the family's income needs.

See also PERFECTION; WORKPLACE.

tiredness See CHRONIC FATIGUE SYNDROME.

tM See MEDITATION; TRANSCENDENTAL MEDITATION.

TMJ See TEMPOROMANDIBULAR JOINT SYNDROME.

tobacco See SMOKING.

toilet training A process of teaching a child to use the toilet for urination and bowel movements. It can be an exercise in stress and anxiety for both the child and the parent because children generally will become toilet trained when they are ready. There is little to gain in speeding up the toilet-training process at a very early age or holding the child to a rigid, demanding schedule.

Some professionals connect toilet training, if it occurs when a child is too young or is too harsh in its administration, with later behavior that is obedient but resentful. On the other hand, a child whose toilet training was delayed may develop a self-centered personality.

Even when trained, accidents happen and children can revert to soiling or wetting, particularly when they are anxious or under stress. The best advice for parents is to begin toilet training at a reasonable age; view the training as an educational experience; exhibit a great deal of patience; support performance with praises and rewards; and accept occasional accidents even after training is completed.

See also BEDWETTING; PARENTING.

toxic shock syndrome See MENSTRUATION.

traffic See RANDOM NUISANCES.

transactional analysis (TA) Group or individual therapy in which the goal is to develop an individual's identity and independence and help him or her develop better COPING skills to interact with others. TA was developed by Eric Berne, a Canadian-born American psychoanalyst (1910–70), and described by Thomas A. Harris in the book *I'm OK, You're OK: A Practical Guide to Transactional Analysis* (1969).

In TA, all behavior, thinking, feeling, and experience is categorized into three ego states: parent (critical and/or loving), adult (practical and evaluative) and child (feelings, such as dependency, fun-loving, and caring). All three states are considered to serve a valuable purpose. Individuals can learn to identify which ego state is in control by identifying both nonverbal changes and verbal changes such as voice tone and use of expressions and words.

See also PSYCHOTHERAPIES.

SOURCE:
Harris, Thomas A. *I'm OK, You're OK: A Practical Guide to Transactional Analysis.* New York Harper & Row, 1969.

transcendental meditation (TM)   One of the Western world's oldest and most scientifically documented techniques known to elicit the RELAXATION response. TM is a revised and simplified form of YOGA and is the method on which most other MEDITATION techniques are based.

Developed by Maharishi Mahesh Yogi, TM is based on ancient Hindu writings. It was introduced into the United States in the early 1960s by Herbert BENSON, M.D., who studied people who practiced TM and developed his own methods for eliciting relaxation. His method is described in his book, *The Relaxation Response.*

Typically, a TM meditator spends two 20-minute periods a day sitting quietly with eyes closed and attention focused totally on the verbal repetition of a special sound or "mantra." Repetition of the mantra blocks distracting thoughts. The effect achieved is better

relaxation and relief from stress. TM has also been referred to as *mystic union.*

See also ALTERNATIVE THERAPIES.

SOURCE:
Yogi, Mahesh. *Science of Being and Art of Living: Transcendental Meditation.* New York: Meridian, 1995.

transfer   See MOVING.

travel   See AIRPLANES; RANDOM NUISANCES; VACATIONS.

trial judges   See JUDICIAL PROCEEDINGS.

trichotillomania   See HABITS; HAIR LOSS; HAIR-PULLING.

tricyclic antidepressants   See DEPRESSION; PHARMACOLOGICAL APPROACH.

Type A personality   Refers to hard-driving, fast-paced, and fast-talking individuals characterized by impatience, aggression, and ambition. They are workaholics, extremely competitive and filled with feelings of ANXIETY, WORRY, ANGER, and HOSTILITY. Type A people constantly worry about problems they cannot solve, a self-destructive type of behavior that can lead to FRUSTRATION and BURNOUT.

Many of these individuals neglect family responsibilities in favor of working and tending to business interests. They tend to feel guilty if not working and take little pleasure in other activities. They may take on multiple commitments and become preoccupied with meeting deadlines. These attitudes lead to stress upon the family and interpersonal relationships. Some researchers believe that Type A people have individualistic traits that set them apart from others, tend to be suspicious, and lack emotional support that comes from close relationships.

The Type A personality pattern was found to double the risk of developing heart disease, particularly in men under the age of 60. The power of the Type A behavior pattern to predict heart disease has been shown in many countries, with the data from Belgium, China, India, Japan, and Lithuania. Even when account is taken of other heart disease risk factors, such as cigarette smoking, HIGH BLOOD PRESSURE, and elevated serum cholesterol, the Type A pattern appears to contribute a further risk in many, but not all, people.

Researchers are studying the relationship of Type A behavior to other health outcomes. In the United States study of air traffic controllers, Type A personalities had experienced 38% more mild and moderate illnesses from all causes than their colleagues. Furthermore, Type As had a frequency of injury three-and-a-half times higher than those with other behavior patterns. The important information from this study is the knowledge that risks can be measured quantitatively and that recommendations can be made to change people's behavior patterns and thus lower risks of both heart attacks and injuries.

Many individuals make efforts to change their personality traits after a serious illness, and, as a result, relax more and take advantage of their leisure in enjoyable ways. Studies involving Type A individuals show that they can change their behavior by learning RELAXATION techniques, developing a sense of HUMOR, and making other life-style changes, thus becoming a combination of Type A and Type B personalities.

A study reported by psychologist D. Ariel Kerman, Ph.D., in her book, *The H.A.R.T. Program: Lower Your Blood Pressure Without Drugs,* indicated that researchers at Duke University found that when Type A personalities participated in a walking/jogging program (three miles per day, three days a week), their Type A characteristics became less dominant in their lives.

Type B personality   A Type B individual usually has personality traits that enable him or her to enjoy activities that are not necessarily competitive. Type Bs are not particularly goal-oriented, do not constantly worry about work, and, when they are working, do so without agitation or sense of urgency.

Relationship of Type A and B personalities to stress and employment

Successful executives are often people who can move back and forth between the Type A and Type B characteristics, depending on the situation. These combined personality types are scattered fairly evenly among top and middle management.

For optimal coping with stress, it seems that a combination of the A and B traits may be best. These individuals can enjoy a balanced life with aspects of work, family, love FRIENDS, recreation, and fun.

See also HOBBIES.

SOURCES:
Armand, M., Jr., ed. *The New Harvard Guide to Psychiatry.* Cambridge: Belknap Press of Harvard University, 1988.
Kerman, D. Ariel. *The H.A.R.T. Program: Lower Your Blood Pressure Without Drugs,* New York: HarperCollins, 1992.
Pelletier, Kenneth. *Healthy People in Unhealthy Places.* New York: Delacorte Press, 1984.

Type C personality   Individuals who have Type C personalities refuse to let any negative feeling show. They usually seem happily in CONTROL and do not express emotion,

---

TAKING THE STRESS OUT OF TYPE C PERSONALITIES

- Be aware of your emotions; get psychotherapeutic help if necessary.
- Be able to express your anger in a constructive way.
- Become more assertive; learn how to say "no" when you want to.
- Develop RELAXATION techniques that work best for you.

especially regarding ANGER, fear, sadness, or even joy.

Type Cs tend to be patient and cooperative and are highly focused on meeting other people's needs while showing little or no concern for their own. Usually, Type Cs tend to stay in stressful situations, such as bad marriages or frustrating jobs, longer than other people. They don't recognize their emotions and may not even realize when they are under STRESS. However, their bodies produce stress hormones, including cortisol, which has been known to suppress the immune system.

Because they don't express their emotions, Type C people do not produce natural opiates, the brain chemicals that have a pain-killing effect similar to artificial drugs such as morphine. This, too, reduces the overall effectiveness of their immune system.

According to psychologist Lydia Temoshok, Ph.D., author of *The Type C Connection: The Behavioral Link to Cancer and Your Health*, Type C personalities often are in the relapse group when compared with recoveries by individuals in other personality categories.

See also ASSERTIVENESS TRAINING; CODEPENDENCY; DEPRESSION; SELF-ESTEEM.

SOURCE:

Temoshok, Lydia. *The Type C Connection: The Behavioral Links to Cancer and Your Health*. New York: Random House, 1992.

ulcers See PEPTIC ULCER.

underachievement An individual who is of average or superior ability but performs poorly in school or at work is an underachiever. Underachievement may be applied to specific areas such as arithmetic or reading ability or failure to advance in a chosen field; it is a source of stress for the person involved as well as parents, teachers and employers.

Underachievement may be a result of faults in the academic environment. For example, large class sizes or school systems lacking personnel and techniques to address cases of poor performance may cause or exacerbate a child's learning problems. Teachers who have personality conflicts with certain students can contribute to their poor performance by ignoring them. Underachievement, particularly in very bright students, may result from BOREDOM when the teacher does not stimulate them or challenge their abilities. Average or bright students with short attention spans can also appear to be below normal.

Underachievement can also result from a child's relationship with his/her parents. Parents who are high achievers themselves may have unrealistic expectations for their children. This creates a vicious cycle in which the child's low SELF-ESTEEM as a reflection of parental attitudes causes his even poorer performance. Parents with average abilities who produce a child with exceptional intelligence may not understand and even discourage their child's superior performance. Family problems such as DIVORCE, conflict, death, or serious illness of a parent may cause poor performance.

Children may also become underachievers because they are perceived as different and are not socially well-adjusted to their PEER GROUP. Such factors as exceptionally high intelligence, ethnic or religious difference, a financial status that is far above or below classmates, or very mature or immature behavior patterns may set a child apart, limit friendships, and lower school performance. Achievement is also reduced when a child desires to become a member of the gang so badly that he/she associates with troublemakers or other students who perform poorly in school.

See also PERFECTION.

SOURCES:
Dejnozka, Edward. "Underachievement," in *American Educator's Encyclopedia.* Westport, Conn.: Greenwood Press, 1982.
Thiel, Ann, Richard Thiel, and Penelope B. Grenoble. *When Your Child Isn't Doing Well in School.* Chicago: Contemporary Books, 1988.

unemployment Unemployment relates to all people who want to work but have been unable to find jobs—those who have worked but are laid off, recent high school and college graduates, people with disabilities, the poor and uneducated, women returning to the workplace after child-rearing, and retirees who need additional income and/or stimulation. Because unemployment often means financial hardship, it can cause STRESS not only for the people directly involved, but also for their spouses, children, parents, and friends.

Unemployment is also a source of stress for those who have jobs but are constantly threatened with losing them. However, a 1995 poll conducted by Towers Perrin, a management consulting firm, found that most workers are "amazingly stress hardy, pragmatic and coping with the uncertainties of corporate

America." The poll also showed that one measure of a worker's adjustment to today's climate of job instability is that less than half of the workers surveyed expect to spend their entire careers with one company. Among those under age 34, only one-third counted on retiring from their present employer.

According to Leana and Feldman in their book, *Coping with Job Loss*, "Unemployment as a fact of life will continue, if not worsen. Current statistics on unemployment and layoffs underestimate the dimensions of the problem. Even with unemployment at six percent, there would still be seven million people out of work. Because government statistics do not include the discouraged job seekers (individuals who have stopped applying for new positions) and those who have joined the expanding ranks of the permanently unemployed, these figures vastly underrepresented the number of people actually out of work."

Leana and Feldman also reported that among the many situational factors influencing how a person reacts to a stressful life event, such as losing a job, perception of unemployment levels has a "substantial influence." They write, "The higher workers perceive the unemployment rates in their communities and/or professions to be, the more pessimistic they will be about the prospects for finding new jobs, especially ones at equal pay."

Fran Lowry, in *Canadian Medical Association Journal* (February 1995), says, "Now when unemployment is still an important problem in many parts of the country [Canada], idle hands are making more work for physicians. People who are out of work make more visits to their physicians for a variety of complaints. Areas of high unemployment also report a higher incidence of alcohol use, and more marital and family abuse and violence. Because unemployment causes stress, it can have bad health consequences not only for the

unemployed but for the people who are closest to them."

See also GENERAL ADAPTATION SYNDROME; LAYOFFS; LIFE CHANGE SELF-RATING SCALE.

SOURCES:

Leana, Carrie R. and Daniel C. Feldman. *Coping with Job Loss: How Individuals, Organizations and Communities Respond to Layoffs.* New York: Lexington Books, 1992.

Lowry, Fran. "Larger Private Sector Role in Health Care Needed Now, Think Tank Warns." *Canadian Medical Association Journal* 154, no. 4 (February 15, 1995): 549–5.

unwed mothers A woman who becomes pregnant and delivers a baby out of wedlock is referred to as an unwed mother. She faces many stresses in making a myriad of decisions. In most cases, she has several options to consider. She may choose to either terminate the pregnancy with a legal ABORTION or have the child, then choose between single parenthood or giving the child up for ADOPTION.

Depending on her relationship with the baby's father, the unwed mother may also choose marriage. Research on this option has shown various results. It was once believed that a "shotgun" marriage was a poor choice, both because of the failure rate of such marriages and because the wife frequently dropped out of school. However, studies of this type of marriage in the 1990s showed a fairly high success rate, often dependent on the father being older than the mother and having finished school.

Changing social standards and even the examples of celebrities have encouraged unwed mothers to keep and raise their babies, but they still must face problems of providing financial support, coping with illness and other childhood problems, while working and being responsible for child-rearing alone.

Often grandparents participate very actively in decision-making about an out-of-wedlock PREGNANCY and also in rearing the child. The results of their decision-making depend on the flexibility of their attitudes. However, if a child is reared by one's grandparents it adds several stressors to the picture. The unwed woman and her parents may have different ideas of appropriate behavior, with resultant mixed messages for the child. Also, the grandparents may be at an age and stage of life at which having a young child around interferes with their long-planned activities.

Pregnancy by choice: single women

In addition to women who unintentionally become pregnant, an increasing number of single women choose unwed motherhood. Some single women "feel the biological time clock ticking." That means they are in their late thirties, have not yet found a man to marry, and want to have a child. These single women may choose adoption; or to become impregnated by a man whom they know but will not marry, sometimes even retaining a friendly relationship with the man. Still others may choose artificial insemination, but must recognize the reluctance of some doctors to inseminate single women and the psychological difficulties of knowing very little or nothing about the father of their child. In all of these cases, even though social standards are changing, unwed mothers still must eventually cope with the possibility that their children may feel different because they lack fathers. They may face many questions growing up in a peer group of children who have two known parents, even though many of these children will be in stepfamilies or merged families.

Child Trends, an agency that conducted a study at the request of Congress as part of a debate over welfare cuts, reported that about a third of the 1.2 million births across the United States in 1993 were to unmarried mothers. About 30% of those mothers were teenagers; 60% of them were white. The percentage of unwed white women giving birth is rising faster than it is for minorities. The total number of unmarried women giving birth jumped 54%, or about 5% a year, during the 1980s.

See also BIOLOGICAL CLOCK; PARENTING.

urinary incontinence   Inability to control the evacuation of liquids from the body. It affects people of all age groups; an overwhelming number of them are women. Incontinence is a cause of extreme stress for the individual who must cope with a problem that can mean personal FRUSTRATION, emotional devastation, social isolation, and physical discomfort.

Incontinence in women

According to a study by the National Institutes of Health in 1996, 26% of women aged 30 to 59 have experienced episodes of urinary incontinence. The most common form, *stress* incontinence, occurs when the pelvic floor muscles become weak and no longer support the bladder. Without support, such everyday events as laughing, coughing, or lifting a heavy object apply stress or pressure to the bladder. In younger women, childbirth often causes the weakening of the pelvic floor muscles; estrogen deficiency brought on by MENOPAUSE is often a cause of this weakness in older women.

Urge incontinence usually occurs during involuntary bladder contractions, which may be caused by a variety of problems, including urinary infections. Help is available from urogynecologists (gynecologists who are specially trained in problems of the urinary tract). Surgical techniques for correcting the problem have advanced dramatically in the latter part of the 20th century. Exercises are also sometimes prescribed (Kegel exercises) by gynecologists to help restore muscle strength, particularly in milder cases. These exercises involve tightening the urinary muscles (as if to stop urination) repeatedly for 5–10 minutes at a time, with repetitions several times a day.

Urinary incontinence is sometimes a symptom of nervousness and tension. In many cases, anxiety can affect one's control over urinating, causing one to either feel the urge very frequently, or to be unable to void even though the urge seems present.

Understanding the mechanisms for the problem can help one cope with its attendant stressful factors. A thorough examination by a physician is essential to determine possible physical causes.

Male incontinence

In males, the cause of incontinence is frequently an enlarged prostate gland, which presses on and blocks the duct through which urine leaves the body. As more urine accumulates in the bladder and dilates it, the bladder cannot hold any more and it dribbles out. After surgical removal of the prostate, nerves controlling the urinary sphincter may be damaged, leaving a man incontinent. Radiation treatment for cancer also sometimes contributes to male incontinence.

Symptoms of a prostate problem in a man include having trouble emptying the bladder, getting up several times a night to urinate, taking longer than usual to start and, after starting, noticing a very slow stream, dribbling after finishing, and having the urge to void again just after voiding, or rectal pain. Any man experiencing these symptoms should consult a physician.

Elderly people sometimes develop urinary incontinence because of neurological reasons, such as after a stroke or a spinal-cord injury. In some cases, a diuretic prescribed for high blood pressure or heart failure may increase the output of urine and lead to incontinence.

Bladder training

The National Institute on Aging recommends steps for bladder training to help some individuals control the voiding reflex by teaching them to urinate at scheduled times. When starting the program, the scheduled times are every 30 minutes to one hour. Over a period

---

HOW TO TAKE THE STRESS OUT OF INCONTINENCE

- Keep a diary for a week or so noting how often you urinate, how often you leak, and what you are doing at the time of the incontinent episode. You may notice a pattern, either in the length of time you are able to wait between episodes or in the circumstances surrounding these episodes.
- If you find that you are wet every hour or two, empty your bladder as completely as you can every 30 to 60 minutes.
- Try to stop the urge to void at unscheduled times by relaxing or distracting yourself. For example, if you are at home, do a small household task until the urge to urinate passes; then void according to your planned schedule.
- If you become too uncomfortable to wait until the scheduled time, go and use the toilet, but void again at the next scheduled time.
- Reward yourself for staying on schedule. It takes effort, practice, and patience.
- Keep a daily log to track your progress. If you are aware of fewer incontinent episodes and have been able to void on schedule for about a week, extend the times between voiding periods by 30 minutes or so each week.
- Extend the intervals until you reach a comfortable schedule, such as two-and-a-half to three hours between voidings.
- If bladder training doesn't help, ask your physician about other forms of treatment, such as medications or surgery. A combination of several therapies may be the most helpful.

---

of six week to several months, the time between trips increases.

In the late 1990s, advertisements for "adult diapers" and products to hide the problem of incontinence attest to the fact that urinary incontinence is a common problem, and as the elderly population increases, the prevalence of the problem will also increase. According to the *Harvard Health Letter*, many people resign themselves to wearing adult diapers or pads because they mistakenly believe that urinary incontinence is a normal part of aging. Others are too embarrassed to bring it up at their doctor's attention or they fear that invasive tests and surgery might result. Those who have the condition can benefit from discussing the problem with a caring and knowledgeable physician.

See also BEDWETTING.

FOR FURTHER INFORMATION:
The SIMON Foundation
P.O. Box 815
Wilmette, IL 60091
Phone: (847) 864-3913

Help for Incontinent People (HIP)
P.O. Box 8310
Spartanburg, SC 29305
Phone: (800) BLADDER

V

vacations Breaks from the usual routine, sometimes involving travel, sightseeing, visiting friends or relatives, or remaining at home and just doing nothing. Many people who feel very stressed by work or family responsibilities look forward to vacations and anticipate relaxation and escape from stress. According to *The Complete Guide to Your Emotions and Your Health,* "getting away from it all, breaking free from routine, can bring a new perspective to old dilemmas, put a positive charge in your mental outlook, and help to fan those waning embers of enthusiasm. You'll get to know yourself a little better. When you come home, you'll be happier, healthier, and much more effective in coping with stress."

Vacations as a source of stress

However, vacations do not always result in stress reduction; they can add to an individual's stress load. First there is stress that comes from the choice of how to travel: by car, train, ship, or plane, and making those reservations can be stressful, too. Packing presents difficulties and ensuring those left behind are taken care of can give parents many anxious moments that continue all through the vacation. When grandparents take on the responsibilities of caring for the children, INTERGENERATIONAL CONFLICTS may result.

Delays of trains and planes, missed connections, and accommodations not up to expectations can be stressful. Bad weather can do more than dampen one's spirits, as it affects the enjoyment of many sights. Additionally, interpersonal relationships are really put to the test on vacations, when friends in couples or other groupings are together every day. These and many other vacation stressors can make you wish you'd stayed at home.

See also CLIMATE; HOBBIES; RANDOM NUISANCES; RECREATION.

SOURCES:
Curtis, Richard. *Taking Off.* New York: Harmony Books, 1981.
Padus, Emrika. *The Complete Guide to Your Emotions and Your Health: Hundreds of Proven Techniques to Harmonize Mind and Body for Happy, Healthy Living.* Emmaus, Pa.: Rodale Press, 1992.

HOW VACATIONS CAN HELP RELIEVE STRESS

- Afford a release from the daily routine.
- Provide opportunities for relaxation.
- See new sights, enjoy beauty, and have different experiences.
- Learn new skills; participate in an adventure.
- Anticipate pleasure and remember the joy.

Valium Trade name for an antianxiety drug chemically known as diazepam and in a class of drugs called the benzodiazepines. Valium is effective in the management of extreme stress that accompanies generalized anxiety disorder and panic disorder in appropriately selected patients. It is also sometimes used for skeletal muscle relaxation, seizure disorders, preanesthetic medication or intravenous anesthetic induction, and for alleviating symptoms during alcohol withdrawal.

Valium has been used more extensively in treating more conditions than any of the other benzodiazepines. The drug is subject to abuse and may produce physical dependence after prolonged use.

See also BENZODIAZEPINE DRUGS; DEPRESSION; PHARMACOLOGICAL APPROACH.

venereal diseases See HERPES SIMPLEX VIRUS; SEXUALLY TRANSMITTED DISEASES.

verbal slips See SLIPS OF THE TONGUE.

volunteerism Involves making the personal choice to give of time or effort to some cause. These causes include a vast range of concerns, beliefs, attitudes, and needs of the diverse American population. There is a wide variety of options open to individuals, making it possible for them to find something to volunteer for that meets a real need. At the same time, it fits what they like to do or gives them an opportunity to learn. This "right match" is what most often brings fulfillment and may bring relief from personal stress to the volunteer.

Often during life's major transitions, such as loss of a loved one, moving to a new community, loss of a job, or divorce, individuals experience great loneliness. According to Marlene Wilson, in her book, *You Can Make A Difference,* during these times, volunteering can be a very helpful and healing experience, because it is in the reaching out to others that people "get out" of themselves and remove themselves from their own personal sources of stress.

According to a 1993 Gallup survey on volunteering, 89.2 million people in the United States were volunteers; of those, 48% were adults averaging 4.2 hours a week. Two-thirds of the adult volunteers were employed. Volunteers gave two and a half times more to charities than non-volunteers.

See also HOBBIES; RETIREMENT.

FOR FURTHER INFORMATION:
Volunteer Management Associates
320 South Cedar Brook Road
Boulder, CO 80304
Phone: (303) 447-0558; (800) 944-1470

SOURCE:
Wilson, Marlene. *You Can Make a Difference!* Boulder: Volunteer Management Associates, 1990.

W

war neurosis Symptoms of anxiety caused by the extreme emotional and physical stresses of wartime experiences, including bombings, exposure to combat conditions, and internal conflicts over killing. Symptoms include ANXI-ETY, nightmares, irritability, DEPRESSION, and fears. The term has been generally replaced with POST-TRAUMATIC STRESS DISORDER. The term "war neurosis" or "shell shock" was commonly used after World War I and into the mid-20th century.

weather See CLIMATE; SEASONAL AFFECTIVE DISORDERS.

weekend depression A type of DEPRESSION that some individuals experience when away from their work. Particularly for some individuals who live alone, facing solitude creates a stressful situation.

To overcome the stresses of being alone, as well as the change in mood from the work week when one is surrounded by people, individuals can schedule pleasurable activities with FRIENDS or like-minded others so that they will not spend the entire weekend alone. Weekend depression should be distinguished from chronic depression, or SEASONAL AFFEC-TIVE DISORDER, which affects some individuals during dark months of the year.

See also AFFECTIVE DISORDERS; PHARMACO-LOGICAL APPROACH.

weight gain and loss Weight gain and loss are sometimes related to EATING DISORDERS such as anorexia nervosa or bulimia. Many individuals become worried and impose stress on themselves because of concern about their weight. Acceptance of oneself and one's body shape contributes to reduction of stress.

Concern about one's weight is often related to one's mental perception of BODY IMAGE and SELF-ESTEEM. Some individuals who fear gaining weight practice bulimia, the "bingeing and purging" syndrome, in which they gorge themselves and then induce vomiting.

See also DIETING.

Weil, Andrew American physician and author; known for his work in promoting ALTER-NATIVE THERAPIES and his books dealing with MIND-BODY CONNECTIONS. Among his best-selling books that include tips for beating stress are *8 Weeks to Optimum Health* and *Spontaneous Healing.* He advocates self-administered, commonsense cures such as eating less fat, getting more exercise, and reducing stress. He also suggests herbalism, acupuncture, naturopathy, osteopathy, chiro-practic, and hypnotism.

See also ALTERNATIVE THERAPIES.

wet dreams Nocturnal emissions from the penis during sleep. Nocturnal emissions or ejaculations are part of normal adolescent development and are caused by accumulated normal tensions that find release while the young man is asleep. For a young man who does not understand the normal processes of PUBERTY, these events can be stressful. A solid foundation of sex education is essential.

See also DREAMS.

"white coat" hypertension See HIGH BLOOD PRESSURE.

women Today, both women and men face daily stresses about family, relationships, has-sles at work and in traffic, loan repayments, and uncertainties about the future. However, traditionally, the roles of women in society were homemaking and child-rearing. It was not until the latter part of the 20th century that these roles were expanded to include increasing participation in business, the military, government, and other fields previously considered "men's fields." The change in women's roles has led in many cases to stress for women and for the men in their lives, as competition between the sexes increases, jealousies over being the provider in the family occur, and males feel an increasing loss of power and CONTROL over women in their personal and professional lives.

For different women and at different times, stressors may vary; they may be emotional, physical, or environmental. An emotional stressor may be a RELATIONSHIP concern, a physical stressor may be an illness or pain, and an environmental stressor may be noise or air pollution. The same stresses that a woman meets with equanimity at one time may be overwhelming and a threat to her wellness at another. In reacting to stressful situations, women have choices: be overwhelmed, adjust, or adapt. Without adjustment or adaptation, cumulative demands may lead to lower resistance to illness.

Statistically, women live longer than men. Paradoxically, women report more sick days and minor physical illnesses, and are more prone to ANXIETY and DEPRESSION than men; women make more visits to physicians' offices. For many women, some complaints such as stomach and digestive problems, HEADACHES and sleeping difficulties may be traced to the cumulative effect of personal stressors.

Gender-related stressors

Different stressors occur at different stages of a woman's life; responses vary between women. Some young women are concerned about physical and breast development, MENSTRUATION, and then PREGNANCY and PARENTING. Young women face DATING in this age of an epidemic of SEXUALLY TRANSMITTED DIS-

EASES and AIDS and contemplation of MARRIAGE at a time when 50% of marriages end in DIVORCE. During their twenties, thirties, and forties, some women's stressors may include the BIOLOGICAL CLOCK, INFERTILITY, child care, balancing home and work, and the GLASS CEILING in the corporate world.

BABY BOOMERS are reaching midlife. Many midlife women find MENOPAUSE stressful. Conflicting research reports on use of hormone replacement therapy make arriving at an informed decision a real dilemma. Midlife women also may face caring for their own ELDERLY PARENTS and in many cases the parents of their partners. At all ages, many women cope with being alone if they do not marry, as well as after divorce or widowhood.

Additional contemporary societal stressors also include delayed marriages, two-career relationships, later childbearing, single parenting, remarriages and reconstituted families, adult children returning home, coping with a husband or partner's loss of job, husband's early retirement, one's own unplanned retirement, chemical dependencies of self or partner, DOMESTIC VIOLENCE, crime victimization, rising costs of living, and proposed cuts in Medicare. By the year 2000 more than 19 million women will be over the age of 65 and many of them will not have planned for the financial implications of old age.

More stress: men or women?

Until women went to work in great numbers, there was a popular notion that working men experienced more stress than women. At the same time, men were viewed as deriving satisfaction and SELF-ESTEEM from their work. Now nearly half of America's workforce is female; while many may be deriving satisfaction from work, others experience gender-related work stressors. Women may be in low-pay jobs or in situations in which they have little AUTONOMY or receive SEXUAL HARASSMENT from the bosses and colleagues.

Wives or single mothers who now have the dual role of balancing commitments to family *and* work are often tired, and may feel inadequate because they can't live up to their own expectations on all fronts.

At home, women may be shouldering the greater proportion of household chores and child care responsibility, despite an increasing number of "househusbands" and cooperative partners. For many women, home is not always the place to relax. A team from Cornell Medical Center in New York City found that men's blood pressure tended to fall as soon as they went home, while women's blood pressure, particularly that of working mothers, experienced no decline and in some cases rose. Researchers at the Karolinska Institute in Stockholm, Sweden, found that men and women's blood pressures varied with their emotions. The men's tended to rise most sharply when they were angry, while the women's rose when they were anxious.

The term "Type A personality," relating to a hard-driving behavior pattern, was originally applied to men. It was thought that the effects of such behavior in men led to high blood pressure and heart disease. Some women exhibit Type A personalities, but it is more prevalent in employed women than among women who work at home. According to the American Heart Association, the incidence of heart disease in women is increasingly recognized, and heart problems are the number-one killer of postmenopausal women.

Traditionally, many women have been socialized to be the family nurturers and caregivers. They may be conciliatory rather than assertive (Type C personality). Some hide their anger rather than provoke an argument. They are haunted with guilt feelings, such as "I should." From advertising and media messages, many are dissatisfied with their BODY IMAGE, accounting for money spent on fad diets and weight-loss programs that do not work.

Coping successfully with stress
There are a variety of effective means of COP-ING for women on an everyday basis as well as during particularly stressful situations. Techniques include MEDITATION, use of audio-tapes for progressive relaxation, GUIDED IMAGERY, BIOFEEDBACK, JOURNALING, YOGA, and MASSAGE THERAPY. Jogging, walking, swimming, tennis, bicycle riding, dancing, and aerobic exercise groups also are effective. They are activities that use up the extra adrenaline stimulated by stress, help distract from stressors, leave muscles relaxed, and increase a sense of control.

Women who cope well with stress have learned to be more assertive, to say "no" when they want to, to prioritize demands on them, make choices, and leave guilt feelings behind. They develop a more positive self-image regarding their bodies, and more realistic expectations of their roles at work and within the family. Increasingly, women are realizing that PERFECTION on all fronts can't be achieved, but adequate planning and preparation will move them in that direction. They solve problems instead of worrying about them; some problems may be best handled by acceptance while others may require action. They learn to anticipate certain predictable stressors, such as upcoming holidays or starting a new job. They fight fatigue and keep their energy high with good nutrition and regular exercise. They learn to find HUMOR in the mundane. They avoid "burnout" by taking time to take care of themselves.

Women: stresses of aging and poverty
Women made up 58% of the elderly population and 74% of the poor elderly population in 1990. Although the poverty rate among older Americans declined in the last 25 years of the 20th century, a significant number of women over 65 are poor. Many women were either homemakers all their lives or moved in and out of jobs as they cared for children or parents or both and missed out on promotions

and pay raises. When they reenter the work force, they start again at the lowest echelons of their work area and this affects them at pension time.

Because many women worked in lower-wage jobs, they do not have company-sponsored pension plans. According to the Older Women's League, only 13% of women receive a private pension, compared to 33% of men. While the average pension benefit for a man is $7,415 a year, for women it is $3,683. African-American women get the smallest amount, with half receiving less than $1,908 a year, according to the Pension Rights Center based in Washington, D.C.

Women's Social Security checks are lower than men's. According to the Social Security Administration, in 1995 the average monthly benefit for retired men was $767 and for women it was only $567.

Many women have little or no savings. According to Commerce Department figures, more than one-quarter of elderly women living alone fall below the poverty line, compared to 5% of older married couples.

See also AGING; HAVING IT ALL; INTIMACY; WOMEN'S MOVEMENT; WORKING MOTHERS.

SOURCES:

Genasci, Lisa. "For Many Women, the Ending Is Not So Happy." *Chicago Tribune*, August 30, 1995.

Kahn, Ada P. "Woman and Stress." *Sacramento Medicine*, September 1995.

women's movement   Activities undertaken during the 1960s, 1970s, and early 1980s to elevate WOMEN from inferior positions in business, the professions, and social clubs, and to gain equal pay with men in the same work. Additionally, activities during the women's movement were geared to help women gain freedom from the sexual double standard, and from total responsibility for childrearing and homemaking. The women's movement imposed stresses on women entering previously dominated domains and on men who

for the first time experienced side by side working with, studying with, or socializing with women.

The movement worked toward less overall dominance by men and against the traditional stereotype of women as dependent, passive, and fragile. It has enabled a generation of women to follow career paths not open to their mothers or grandmothers, to enjoy motherhood at the same time, and to participate in previously male-dominated professional and social organizations. At the same time, WORKING MOTHERS and women professionals have experienced unique stresses in their lives.

The SEXUAL REVOLUTION, during which women began to express sexuality with an increase in pre-marital and extramarital relationships, was an outgrowth of the women's liberation movement.

Significant steps in the women's liberation movement include publication of *The Feminine Mystique* (1963) by Betty Friedan, which exploded the myth of the happy housewife, passage of the Equal Pay Act by the U.S. Congress in 1963, the founding of the National Organization for Women (1966), the first accredited women's studies course at Cornell University (1969), publication of *Sexual Politics* (1970) by Kate Millett, the founding of the National Women's Political Caucus (1971), the historic *Roe* v. *Wade* decision by the U.S. Supreme Court legalizing abortion (1973), the election of the first woman governor in her own right (Ella Grasso, Connecticut, 1974), the declaration of 1975 as the International Year of the Woman by the United Nations, the First National Women's Conference in Houston (1977), the march in 1978 of nearly 100,000 women in Washington to support extension of the Equal Rights Amendment, the appointment of Sandra Day O'Connor as the first woman to become an associate justice of the U.S. Supreme Court, and the candidacy of Democrat Geraldine Ferraro for vice president in 1984.

The International Women's Conference held in Beijing in 1995, which brought together many women from Third World countries as well as developed nations, was another development in the women's movement.

SOURCE:
Cott, Nancy F. *The Grounding of Modern Feminism.* New Haven: Yale University Press, 1989.

work flow   See workplace.

working mothers   Many working MOTHERS are stressed by role conflicts between home and employment responsibilities. Despite these conflicts, they have feelings of self-fulfillment and realize economic advantages. Many find cooperation from their husbands or other family members helpful.

Working mothers are a major issue to employers. At the end of the 1990s, 46% of the total work force was female. Almost 60% of all women 16 years and older held down jobs. On a national level, WOMEN earned 71.6% of men's wages, according to a 1994 study by Women Employed.

Because there are so many working mothers, DAY CARE facilities have become widespread. For many women, placing children in day-care facilities is a stressful and GUILT-ridden experience, which they must work through to come to terms with the reality of trying to remain in the work force as well as raise a family.

In 1995, *Working Mother* magazine released its 10th annual list of the nation's top 100 companies for working mothers. The rankings indicate "family friendly" characteristics of many employers, including provision of day care, summer camps, scholarships, flexible work hours, and care for a child's special needs. However, for many who work at less-enlightened companies, the WORKPLACE remains a difficult and stressful place when it comes to balancing family and careers. Even at companies that make a major commitment

to family issues, there is a point beyond which few businesses are willing to go.

According to Anne Ladky, executive director of Women Employed, a Chicago-based advocacy group, if a parent has to leave work on time a certain number of nights a week to pick up a child, there is still some bias against him or her. Additionally, when companies add family benefits, they do so because either the field or the geographical area is competitive when it comes to hiring and retaining employees.

A conference on "Work, Stress and Health" held in 1995, sponsored by the American Psychological Association, the National Institute of Occupational Safety and Health, the U.S. Office of Personnel Management, and the U.S. Department of Labor's Occupational Safety and Health Administration, focused on issues relating to working mothers. Research reported at that conference pointed to two competing hypotheses, according to Nancy L. Marshall, of Wellesley College's Center for Research on Women. One is the "scarcity hypothesis," which presumes that people have a limited amount of time and energy and that women with competing demands suffer from overload and inter-role conflict. The other, the "enhancement hypothesis," theorizes that the greater self-esteem and social support people gain from multiple roles outweigh the costs.

Results of other studies were cited. Theorists suggested that having children gives working women a mental and emotional boost that childless women lack. However, having children also increases work and family stress, and indirectly may increase symptoms of DEPRESSION.

According to Ulf Lundberg, University of Stockholm, the "total workload scale" leads to the conclusion that women typically spend much more time working at paid and unpaid tasks than men. Age and occupational level do not make much difference in terms of

---

**TIPS FOR WORKING MOTHERS
TO REDUCE STRESS**

- Prioritize your home and work projects.
- Develop realistic expectations for yourself
  and others.
- Delegate projects to others in the family.
- Know that you have choices.
- Identify your key stressors and ways to
  reduce them.
- Learn to say NO to excessive demands at
  home or at work.
- Ask for help when you need it.
- Realize that perfection is not a realistic goal.
- Make time for your own physical, emotional,
  and spiritual needs.
- Find humor in everyday situations; learn to
  laugh more.

---

women's total workload. What matters is whether they have children. In families without children, men and women both work about 60 hours a week. However, as soon as there is a child in the family, total workload increases rapidly for women. In a family with three or more children, women typically spend 90 hours a week in paid and unpaid work, while men typically spend only 60, according to Lundberg.

Lundberg's research indicated that women's stress is determined by the interaction of conditions at home and at work, whereas men respond more selectively to situations at work and they seem to be able to relax more easily once they get home.

See also COPING; HAVING IT ALL; PARENTING; WOMEN'S MOVEMENT.

SOURCE:
Lev, Michael, and Bonnie Rubin, "For Some Working Mothers, Some Improvement." *Chicago Tribune*, September 12, 1995.

workplace Stress at the workplace occurs for most people in varying degrees and for many varied reasons. Some people are stressed because they have too much work, while others are stressed because they are bored due to not enough work. COWORKERS and interactions with coworkers and the boss can lead to stress. Additional sources of stress include environmental situations, such as noise, poor lighting or lack of fresh air, as well as the FRUSTRATION of being underpaid and overworked.

Contemporary technological stressors at the workplace range from back strain due to sitting at a computer terminal, to REPETITIVE STRESS INJURIES (CARPAL TUNNEL SYNDROME) from use of computers, to standing on a manufacturing assembly line.

Each occupation carries with it particular stresses, many of which are hidden by the employees. For example, many secretaries may resent doing the same chores over and over. Data processors may be bored with their work. Physicians find regulations imposed on them by managed care companies and insurance companies stressful. Accountants find the tax preparation season particularly stressful, while air traffic controllers are under constant pressure every minute while at work. LAWYERS must meet the demands of their clients as well as their superiors in their law firms.

The issue of CONTROL is an important one in determining level of workplace stress. Those who feel they have more control over their situations, such as flexibility with work schedule, or decision-making about setting their own deadlines, may experience less stress than those who have no sense of control. PERSONAL SPACE is another issue. Workers who feel they have no privacy may feel more stressed than those who have offices or spaces with doors.

Jobs with fairly controllable situations include computer programmer, writer, artist, appliance repairperson, and truck driver. While these jobs can be very demanding, the minute-to-minute pace may be unhurried. Certain positions may be slow-paced but with uncontrollable factors. These include janitor, security guard, and bus driver. Fast-paced and controllable professions include some physicians in private practice, business executives, and city administrators. Fast-paced and uncontrollable professions include waiter, cashier, firefighter, and nurse.

Job mismatches can lead to stress. For some individuals, leaving the job is the solution. However, for many, that solution is not practical. Most people cannot walk away from their professions or businesses. The more realistic solution is learning to cope with the current pressures.

Coping with workplace stress

Some of the stresses of workplace relationships can be eased by taking certain actions. Listen carefully when someone is speaking to you instead of planning your response as they are speaking. Careful LISTENING can help prevent misunderstandings, which might make you angry. Additionally, ask for FEEDBACK, which is another person's perception of what you are doing or saying. Feedback is not evaluative or judgmental. Speak with your coworkers or superiors at an appropriate place and time. Do not initiate a difficult conversation without appropriate privacy. Finally, always ask for a clear statement of performance expectations. Confront a superior with questions about job role and expected outcomes.

In the late 1990s, workers have been faced with additional stresses of possible and actual DOWNSIZING of corporations during which many employees are laid off, necessitating early retirement by many and finding new jobs by others. The term "right-sizing" has arisen to mean scaling down the number of employees to an efficient and profitable level.

See also AUTONOMY; BOREDOM; COPING; JOB CHANGE; JOB SECURITY; LAYOFFS; WOMEN; WORKING MOTHERS.

SOURCES:

Adams, Scott. *The Dilbert Principle: A Cubicle's-Eye View of Bosses, Meetings, Management Fads and Other Workplace Afflictions.* New York: Harper-Business, 1997.

Field, Tiffany, Olga Quintino, et al. "Job Stress Reduction Therapies." *Alternative Therapies* 3, no. 4 (July 1997).

Murphy, Lawrence R. "Stress Management in Work Settings: A Critical Review of the Health Effects." *American Journal of Health Promotion* 11, no. 2 (November-December 1996): 112–35.

Peterson, Michael. "Work, Corporate Culture, and Stress: Implications for Worksite Health Promotion. *American Journal of Health Behavior* 21, no. 4 (1997): 243–52.

Rosch, Paul J. "Measuring Job Stress: Some Comments on Potential Pitfalls." *American Journal of Health Promotion* 11, no. 6 (July-August 1997): 400–01.

worry   A state of mental uneasiness, distress, or agitation due to concern for a past, impending, or anticipated stressful event, threat, or danger. Some degree of worrying is a common, everyday occurrence for most people. For some people, however, excessive worry adds to their stress levels. Individuals who have ANXIETY DISORDERS tend to worry more than others. For example, people who have AGORAPHOBIA may worry about what will happen if they go out of their homes, or people with a PHOBIA may worry about what will happen if they encounter a phobic object or situation.

Worrying may be called negative imagery, because the worrier focuses on negative images or worst-case scenarios (CATASTROPHIZES). Worrying to excess can be an unhealthy stressor because it causes the body to react; the heart pounds, breathing quickens, and sweating may occur. For some individuals, GUIDED IMAGERY techniques, through which they imagine themselves in a given situation with a pleasant outcome, may be useful. Additionally, RELAXATION techniques, such as MEDITATION and BIOFEEDBACK, may be helpful. In a relaxed state, individuals can think more constructively and in a more organized manner.

See also ANXIETY; COPING; GENERAL ADAPTATION SYNDROME; STRESS MANAGEMENT.

REDUCE STRESS: WORRY LESS

- When you try not to worry about something, it is likely that you will worry about it more. It may be advantageous to stay with the worry and really concentrate on it, because you may stop worrying and begin solving your problem.
- Make a distinction between matters you can do something about and those you cannot.
- Instead of asking yourself repeatedly "what if . . .," write down a number of possible solutions to a specific problem and then list the advantages and disadvantages of each idea.
- Use a diversionary technique, such as going for a walk, doing some other form of exercise, playing a musical instrument, or listening to music. Doing so will help you organize your thoughts and come up with possible solutions. The best solutions may occur when you are not thinking about the immediate problem.
- Various forms of psychotherapy and self-help can relieve the stresses of excessive worrying for many people.

SOURCES:
Diamond, David. "Bound to Worry." *Health,* July-August 1992.
Padus, Emrika, ed. *The Complete Guide to Your Emotions and Your Health,* rev. Emmaus, Pa.: Rodale Press, 1992.

writer's block   An obstacle to the free expression of ideas on paper; between the thought and the recording of it, there is an interruption in the flow. When a block occurs, the writer may feel stressed, frustrated, and stuck. Unable to go on while waiting for an inspiration, the writer may have self-doubts about his or her capabilities, hopes, and even future.

Many writers suffer from writer's block at one time or another. The block may involve an inability to get started with a writing project, or to set words down on paper; it may occur in the middle of a project and the writer will feel unable to go on. Writers may be concerned about the validity of their topic, ability to communicate on paper, and acceptance by teachers, readers, or publishers.

Too much STRESS can paralyze the writer, and too little stress can lead to apathy. The ideal state of mind, the one that unblocks, was called "eustress," or good stress, by Hans SELYE, the Canadian author of *The Stress of Life* (1956) and *Stress Without Distress* (1974). That middle point in the stress spectrum is the state of relaxed concentration accompanied by energy. Because writing can be hard work, one must be in the right mental framework to take risks and to have confidence and SELF-ESTEEM regarding one's own abilities.

Overcoming the stress of writer's block
Writing usually involves several steps: incubation, planning, research, organization, first draft, incubation, revision, and final draft. Before starting, the writer unconsciously develops ideas and insights for the written material; this is the important incubation process. To bring these ideas out of the mind and onto paper, and break writer's block, he or she must reach a state of relaxed, energized concentration in which self-criticism is set aside and there is room for creative thoughts.

There are a number of exercises one can perform to help reach the state of energized relaxation. Physical EXERCISE energizes and is conducive to a relaxed state of mind. MEDITATION and imagery exercises are also very useful in reducing stress and minimizing the self-doubt that obstructs expression. Proper nutrition and enough SLEEP are similarly important to the writer.

Another way to avoid writer's block is to avoid people who are critical of the writer's work or ideas in the early stage of the project. While their criticisms may be helpful later, early in the project criticism may be stifling.

See also CREATIVITY; FRUSTRATION.

SOURCE:
Sloane, Beverly LeBov. "Creativity." *Town Hall of California Reporter,* March-April 1987, 6–7.

X

Xanax The trade name for alprazolam, a tria-zolobenzodiazepine compound with antianxiety and sedative-hypnotic actions. It is approved by the U.S. Food and Drug Administration for use in panic disorder and generalized ANXIETY DISORDER. Studies suggest that alprazolam also has antidepressant activity in moderate depression.

See also BENZODIAZEPINE DRUGS; AGORAPHOBIA; DEPRESSION; PANIC ATTACKS AND PANIC DISORDER; PHARMACOLOGICAL APPROACH.

yoga A system of Indian philosophy and practice that is used as a stress management technique by many people. The word *youga* means "union" and teaches the means by which one can learn to commune with universal energy. Humans consist of both material and nonmaterial entities; the material entity is the physical body and the nonmaterial entities are the mind and the soul. Yoga attempts to bring together the body, mind, and soul, or the physical side, the social side (life in action), and the spiritual side.

There are several types of yoga with varying emphasis on physical, mental, and social activity. Different paths for developing the mind are based on the fact that the mind has three different aspects: knowing, feeling, and willing. A popular type of yoga practiced in the United States is *hatha yoga,* which involves regulation of the mind and body through different breathing exercises. There are over 200 balanced physical postures (*asanas*) to EXERCISE every muscle in the body. They are planned to maintain flexibility of the body, teach physical and mental control, and are useful for RELAXATION. There are exercises for tapping into *kundalini* (a large reservoir of energy thought to be situated at the base of the spinal cord).

Research studies have indicated that yoga is useful in the area of hypertension, coronary heart disease, anxiety disorders, asthma, and diabetes.

See also ALTERNATIVE THERAPIES; EXERCISE; MEDITATION.

youngest children See BIRTH ORDER; SIBLING RELATIONSHIPS.

Z

Zen   A form of Buddhism used as a basis for RELAXATION and STRESS MANAGEMENT; it is concerned with the individual meaning of a person's life rather than just removal of symptoms or improvement of his or her adjustment to life. The goal of Zen is pursued through contemplation of the nature of humankind. With this process, individuals release tensions and experience oneness with the universe.

See also ALTERNATIVE THERAPIES; MEDITATION; TRANSCENDENTAL MEDITATION.

BIBLIOGRAPHY

Acquired Immunodeficiency Syndrome (AIDS)

Andre, Pierre. *People, Sex, HIV & AIDS. Social, Political, Philosophical and Moral Implications.* Huntington, W.Va.: University Press, 1995.

Banta, William F. *AIDS in the Workplace; Legal Questions and Practical Answers.* New York: Lexington Books, 1993.

Donovan, Catherine A., and Elizabeth Stratton. "Changing Epidemiology of AIDS." *Canadian Family Physician.* 40 (August 1994).

Douglas, Paul Harding, and Laura Pinsky. *The Essential AIDS Fact Book.* New York: Pocket Books, 1996.

Epstein, Steven. *Impure Science. AIDS, Activism and the Politics of Knowledge.* Berkeley: University of California Press, 1996.

Faison, Brenda S. *The AIDS Acquired Immunodeficiency Syndrome Handbook: A Complete Guide to Education and Awareness.* Durham, N.C.: Designbase Publishing, 1991.

Gifford, Allen. *Living Well with HIV & AIDS.* Palo Alto, Calif.: Bull Publishers, 1997.

Goldfinger, Stephen E., ed. "AIDS: A Glimmer of Hope." *Harvard Health Letter* 20, no. 9 (July 1995).

McKenzie, Nancy F., ed. *The AIDS Reader: Social, Political and Ethical Issues.* New York: Meridian, 1991.

Sirimarco, Elizabeth. *AIDS.* New York: M. Cavendish, 1994.

Stewart, Gail. *People with AIDS.* San Diego: Lucent Books, 1996.

Addictions (See also ALCOHOLISM; SMOKING)

Carroll, Marilyn. *Cocaine and Crack.* Hillside, N.J.: Enslow Publishers, 1994.

Nuckols, Cardwell C. *Cocaine. From Dependency to Recovery.* Blue Ridge Summit, Pa.: Tab Books, 1989.

Agoraphobia See also ANXIETY AND ANXIETY DISORDERS; PHOBIAS

Ballenger, Janes C., ed. *Biology of Agoraphobia.* Washington, D.C.: American Psychiatric Press, 1984.

Frampton, Muriel. *Agoraphobia: Coping with the World Outside.* Wellingstorough, Northamptonshire, England: Turnstone Press, 1984.

Goldstein, Alan J. *Overcoming Agoraphobia: Conquering Fear of the Outside World.* New York: Viking, 1987.

Paolino, Adele. *Agoraphobia: Are Panic and Phobias Psychological or Physical?* Winona, Minn.: Apollo Books, 1984.

Scrignar, Chester R. *From Panic to Peace of Mind: Overcoming Panic and Agoraphobia.* New Orleans: Brunn Press, 1991.

Alcoholism

Berger, Gilda. *Alcoholism and the Family.* New York: F. Watts, 1993.

Dick, R. *New Light on Alcoholism.* Corte Madera, Calif.: Good Book Publishing, 1994.

Liehelt, Robert A. *Straight Talk About Alcoholism.* New York: Pharos Books, 1992.

O'Brien, Robert, and Morris Chafetz. *The Encyclopedia of Alcoholism.* New York: Facts On File, 1982.

O'Farrell, Timothy J., Carolyn A. Weyand, with Diane Logan. *Alcohol and Sexuality: An Annotated Bibliography on Alcohol Use, Alcoholism and Human Sexual Behavior.* Phoenix: Oryx Press, 1983.

Rosenberg, Maxine B. *Not My Family: Sharing the Truth About Alcoholism.* New York: Bradbury Press, 1988.

Seixas, Judith S., and Geraldine Youcha. *Children of Alcoholism: A Survivor's Manual.* New York: Crown Publishers, 1985.

St. Clair, Harvey R. *Recognizing Alcoholism and Its Effects: A Mini-Guide.* New York: Karger, 1991.

Varley, Chris. *Alcoholism.* New York: M. Cavendish, 1994.

Alternative therapies   See also MIND-BODY CONNECTIONS

Baker, Sarah. *The Alexander Technique: The Revolutionary Way to Use Your Body for Total Energy.* New York: Bantam Books, 1978.

Bensky, Dan, and Andres Gamble. *Chinese Herbal Medicine, Materia Medica.* Seattle: Eastland, 1986.

Bloomfield, Frena. *Chinese Beliefs.* London: Arrow Books, 1983.

Butt, Gary, and Frena Bloomfield. *Harmony Rules.* London: Arrow Books, 1985.

Christi, Hakim. *The Traditional Healer's Handbook: A Classic Guide to the Medicine of Avicenna.* Rochester, Vt.: Healing Arts Press, 1991.

Eisenberg, David. *Encounters with Qi: Exploring Chinese Medicine.* New York: Norton, 1985.

Eisenberg, D., et al. "Unconventional Medicine in the United States: Prevalence, Costs, and Patterns of Use." *New England Journal of Medicine* 328 (1993): 246–52.

Facklam, Howard. *Alternative Medicine: Cures or Myths?* New York: Twenty-First Century Books, 1996.

Feldenkrais, Moshe. *Awareness Through Movement.* New York: Harper & Row, 1977.

Fradet, Brian. *Stress, Anxiety and Depression/The Natural Medicine Collective.* New York: Dell Publishing, 1995.

Frawley, David. *Ayurvedic Healing: A Comprehensive Guide.* Salt Lake City: Passage Press, 1989.

Frawley, David, and Vasant Lad. *The Yoga of Herbs: An Ayurvedic Guide to Herbal Medicine.* Santa Fe: Lotus Press, 1986.

Gordon, James S. *Manifesto for a New Medicine: Your Guide to Healing Partnerships and Wise Use of Alternative Therapies.* Reading, Mass.: Addison-Wesley, 1996.

Heyn, Birgit. *Ayurveda The Indian Art of Natural Medicine & Life Extension.* Rochester, Vt.: Healing Arts Press, 1990.

Kaminski, Patricia, and Richard Katz: *Flower Essence Repertory. A Comprehensive Guide to North American and English Flower Essences for Emotional and Spiritual Well-Being.* Nevada City, Calif.: Flower Essence Society, 1994.

Krieger, D. *Therapeutic Touch: How to Use Your Hands to Help or to Heal.* Englewood Cliffs, N.J.: Prentice-Hall, 1979.

Lad, Dr. Vasant. *Ayurveda: The Science of Self-Healing – A Practical Guide.* Santa Fe: Lotus Press, 1984.

McGill, Leonard. *The Chiropractor's Health Book: Simple Natural Exercises for Relieving Headaches, Tension and Back Pain.* New York: Crown, 1995.

Morrison, Judith M. *The Book of Ayurveda.* New York: Fireside, 1995.

Morton, Mary, and Michael Morton. *5 Steps to Selecting the Best Alternative Medicine.* Novato, Calif.: New World Library, 1996.

Reid, Daniel. *The Complete Book of Chinese Health and Healing.* Boston: Shambhala, 1994.

Rondberg, Terry A. *Chripractic First: The Fastest Growing Healthcare First . . . Before Drugs or Surgery.* Chandler, Ariz.: Chiropractic Journal, 1996.

Ryman, Danielle. *Aromatherapy: The Complete Guide to Plant and Flower Essences for Health and Beauty.* New York: Bantam Books, 1991.

Sachs, Judith. *Nature's Prozac: Natural Therapies and Techniques to Rid Yourself of Anxiety, Depression, Panic Attacks & Stress.* Englewood Cliffs, N.J.: Prentice-Hall, 1997.

Turner, Roger Newman. *Naturopathic Medicine: Treating the Whole Person.* Northamptonshire, England: Thorsons Publishers, 1984.

Anorexia nervosa   See EATING DISORDERS.

Anxiety and anxiety disorders   See also PHOBIAS; OBSESSIVE-COMPULSIVE DISORDER; POST-TRAUMATIC STRESS DISORDER

Agras, M.W. *Panic: Facing Fears, Phobias, and Anxiety.* New York: W.H. Freeman, 1985.

Barlow, D.H. *Anxiety and Its Disorders: The Nature and Treatment of Anxiety and Panic.* New York: Guilford Press, 1988.

Barlow, D.H., and J.A. Cerny. *The Psychological Treatment of Panic.* New York: Guilford Press, 1988.

Bassett, Lucinda. *From Panic to Power.* New York: HarperCollins, 1995.

Beck, Aaron. *Anxieties and Phobias.* New York: Basic Books, 1985.

Bourne, Edmund J. *The Anxiety and Phobia Workbook.* Oakland: New Harbinger, 1990.

Gold, Mark S. *The Good News About Panic, Anxiety & Phobias.* New York: Bantam Books, 1990.

Goodwin, D.W. *Anxiety.* New York: Oxford University Press, 1986.

Gorman, J.M., M.R. Leibowitz, and D.F. Klein. *Panic Disorders and Agoraphobia.* Kalamazoo: Current Concepts in Medicine, 1984.

Marks, Isaac. *Living with Fear.* New York: McGraw-Hill, 1980.

Nardo, Don. *Anxiety and Phobias.* New York: Chelsea House, 1992.

Ornstein, Robert, and David S. Sobel. "Calming Anxiety, Phobias and Panic." *Mental Medicine Update* 3, no. 3 (1994).

Ross, Jerilyn. *Triumph Over Fear: A Book of Help and Hope for People with Anxiety, Panic Attacks, and Phobias.* New York: Bantam Books, 1994.

Sheehan, David. *The Anxiety Disease and How to Overcome It.* New York: Charles Scribner & Sons, 1984.

Taylor, C. Barr, and Bruce Arnow. *The Nature and Treatment of Anxiety Disorders.* New York: Free Press, 1988.

Warneke, Lorne. "Anxiety Disorders: Focus on Obsessive-Compulsive Disorder." *Canadian Family Physician* 39 (July 1993).

Wolman, Benjamin and George Sticker. *Anxiety and Related Disorders: A Handbook.* New York: John Wiley and Sons, 1991.

Arthritis

Cohen, Darlene. *Arthritis—Stop Suffering, Start Moving.* New York: Walker, 1995.

Lorig, Kate. *Living a Health Life with Chronic Conditions: Self-management of Heart Disease, Arthritis, Stroke, Diabetes, Asthma, Bronchitis, Emphysema & Others.* Palo Alto, Calif.: Bull Publishing, 1994.

Lorig, Kate, and James Fries. *Arthritis Helpbook,* 3rd ed. Reading, Mass.: Addison-Wesley, 1990.

McCarty, Daniel J., and William J. Koopman, eds. *Arthritis and Allied Conditions: A Textbook of Rheumatology,* Philadelphia: Lea & Febiger, 1993.

Trien, Susan F., and David Pisetsky. *The Duke University Medical Center Book of Arthritis.* New York: Fawcett, 1992.

Asthma

Adams, Francis V., *The Asthma Sourcebook: Everything You Need to Know.* Los Angeles: Lowell House/Contemporary Books, 1995.

Altman, Nathaniel. *What You Can Do About Asthma.* New York: Dell, 1991.

Hyde, Margaret O., and Elizabeth H. Forsyth. *Living with Asthma.* New York: Walker, 1995.

Shayevitz, Myra, and Berton Shayevitz. *Living Well with Chronic Asthma, Bronchitis, and Emphysema.* Yonkers, N.Y.: Consumer Reports Books, 1991.

Biofeedback

Basmajian, John V., ed. *Biofeedback: Principles and Practice for Clinician.* Baltimore: Williams & Wilkins, 1983.

Brown, Barbara. *Stress and the Art of Biofeedback.* New York: Harper & Row, 1977.

Karlins, Marvin, and Lewis M. Andrews. *Biofeedback: Turning on the Powers of Your Mind.* Philadelphia: J.B. Lippincott, 1972.

Olton, D.S., and A.R. Noonberg. *Biofeedback: Clinical Applications in Behavioral Medicine.* Englewood Cliffs, N.J.: Prentice-Hall, 1980.

Cancer

Anderson, Greg. *50 Essential Things to do When the Doctor Says It's Cancer.* New York: Plume, 1993.

Dollinger, Malin, Ernest H. Rosenbaum, and Greg Cable. *Everyone's Guide to Cancer Therapy.* Kansas City, Mo.: Andrews and McMeel, 1991.

Dreifuss-Kattan, Esther. *Cancer Stories; Creativity and Self-Repair.* Hillsdale, N.J.: Analytic Press, 1990.

Fiore, Neil A. *The Road Back to Health: Coping with the Emotional Aspects of Cancer,* rev. Berkeley, Calif.: Celestial Arts, 1991.

Marchetti, Albert. *Beating the Odds: Alternative Treatments That Have Worked Miracles Against Cancer.* Chicago: Contemporary Books, 1988.

McAllister, Robert M., S.T. Horowitz, and R.T. Gilden. *Cancer.* New York: Basic Books, 1993.

Morra, Marion, and Eve Potts. *Triumph: Getting Back to Normal When You Have Cancer.* New York: Avon Books, 1990.

Mullan, Fitzhugh, and Barbara Hoffman, eds. *Sharing the Journey: An Almanac of Practical Resources for Cancer Survivors.* Yonkers, N.Y.: Consumer Reports Books, 1990.

Sontag, Susan. *Illness as Metaphor and AIDS and Its Metaphors.* New York: Doubleday, 1990.

Temoshok, Lydia, and Henry Dreher. *The Type C Connection: The Behavioral Links to Cancer and Your Health.* New York: Random House, 1992.

Terkel, Susan Neiburg, and Marlene Lupiloff-Brass. *Understanding Cancer.* New York: F. Watts, 1993.

Complementary medicine　See ALTERNATIVE THERAPIES; MIND-BODY CONNECTIONS

Depression and manic-depressive disorder

Baskin, Valerie D. *When Words Are Not Enough: The Women's Prescription for Depression and Anxiety.* New York: Broadway Books, 1997.

Bohn, John, and James W. Jefferson. *Lithium and Manic Depression: A Guide,* rev. Madison, Wis.: Lithium Information Center, University of Wisconsin, 1990.

Burns, David D. *Feeling Good: The New Mood Therapy.* New York: Morrow, 1980.

DePaulo, J. Raymond, and Keith Ablo. *How to Cope with Depression: A Complete Guide for You and Your Family.* New York: McGraw-Hill, 1989.

Greist, John H., and James W. Jefferson. *Depression and Its Treatment: Help for the Nation's #1 Mental Problem,* rev. New York: Warner Books, 1992.

Papolos, Demitri, and Janic Palolos. *Overcoming Depression.* New York: Harper & Row, 1987.

Quinn, Brian. *The Depression Sourcebook.* Los Angeles: Lowell House, 1997.

Robbins, Paul R. *Understanding Depression.* Jefferson, N.C.: McFarland 1993.

Warneke, Lorne. "Management of Resistant Depression." *Canadian Family Physician* 42 (October 1996): 1973.

Whybrow, Peter C. *A Mood Apart: Depression, Mania and Other Afflictions of the Self.* New York: Basic Books, 1997

Divorce　See MARRIAGE AND DIVORCE

Eating Disorders

Abraham, Suzanne. *Eating Disorders: The Facts.* Oxford: Oxford University Press, 1984.

Cassell, Dana K. *Encyclopedia of Obesity and Eating Disorders.* New York: Facts On File, 1994.

Heater, Sandra Harvey. *Am I Still Visible?: A Woman's Triumph Over Anorexia Nervosa.* White Hall, Va.: White Hall Books, 1983.

Kinoy, Barbara P., ed. *Eating Disorders: New Directions in Treatment and Recovery.* New York: Columbia University Press, 1994.

Mitchell, James E., ed. *Anorexia Nervosa and Bulimia: Diagnosis and Treatment.* Minneapolis: University of Minnesota Press, 1985.

Neuman, Patricia A. *Anorexia Nervosa and Bulimia: A Handbook for Counselors and Therapists.* New York: Van Nostrand Reinhold, 1983.

Orbach, Susie. *Hunger Strike: an Anorexic's Struggle as a Metaphor for Our Age.* New York: Norton, 1986.

Romeo, Felicia F. *Understanding Anorexia Nervosa* Springfield, Ill.: C.C. Thomas, 1986.

Sacker, Ira M. *Dying to Be Thin.* New York: Warner Books, 1987.

Sonder, Ben. *Eating Disorders: When Food Turns Against You.* New York: F. Watts, 1993.

White, Marlene B. *Bulimarexia: The Binge/Purge Cycle.* New York: Norton, 1983.

Winokur, G. *Depression: The Facts.* New York: Oxford University Press, 1981.

Woodman, Marion. *The Owl Was a Baker's Daughter: Obesity, Anorexia Nervosa, and the Repressed Feminine, a Psychological Study.* Toronto: Inner City Books, 1980.

Fertility/Infertility   See also PREGNANCY

Domar, A.D., M.M. Seibel, and H. Benson. "The Mind/Body Program for Infertility: A New Behavioral Treatment Approach for Women with Infertility." *Fertility and Sterility* 53 (1990): 246–49.

Liebmann-Smith, Joan. *In Pursuit of Pregnancy: How Couples Discover, Cope With, and Resolve Their Fertility Problems.* New York: Newmarket Press, 1987.

Mahlstedt. P. "The Psychological Component of Infertility." *Fertility and Sterility* 43 (1985): 335–46.

Seibel, M.M., ed. *Infertility: A Comprehensive Test.* Norwalk, Conn.: Appleton & Lange, 1990.

Guided imagery   See also ALTERNATIVE THERAPIES; MIND-BODY CONNECTIONS

Achterberg, Jeanne. *Imagery in Healing: Shamanism and Modern Medicine.* San Francisco: Shambhala Publications, 1985.

Burns, David. *Feeling Good: The New Mood Therapy.* New York: Avon Books, 1992.

Epstein, Gerald. *Healing Visualizations, Creating Healing Through Imagery.* New York: Bantam Books, 1989.

Rossman, Martin L. *Healing Yourself: A Step-by-Step Program for Better Health Through Imagery.* New York: Walker, 1987.

Samuels, Michael. *Healing with the Mind's Eye.* New York: Random House, 1992.

Siegel, Bernie. *Love, Medicine and Miracles.* New York: Harper & Row, 1986.

———. *Peace, Love and Healing.* New York: Harper & Row, 1986.

Simonton, O. Carl, Stephanie Matthew-Simonton, and James L. Creighton. *Getting Well Again.* New York: Bantam Books, 1981.

Headaches

Attansio V., F. Andrasik, and E.G. Blanchard. "Cognitive Therapy and Relaxation Training in Muscle Contraction Headache: Efficacy and Cost-effectiveness." *Headache* 27 (1987): 254–60.

Blanchard, E.B., K.A. Appelbaum, et al. "Placebo-controlled Evaluation of Abbreviated Progressive Muscle Relaxation and of Relaxation Combined with Cognitive Therapy in the Treatment of Tension Headache." *Journal of Consulting and Clinical Psychology* 58 (1990): 210–15.

Blanchard, E.B., N.L. Nicholson, et al. "The Role of Regular Home Practice in the Relaxation Treatment of Tension Headache." *Journal of Consulting and Clinical Psychology* 59 (1991): 467–70.

Diamond, Seymour. *The Hormone Headache: New Ways to Prevent, Manage, and Treat Migraines and Other Headaches.* New York: MacMillan, 1995.

Inlander, Charles B., and Porter Shimer. *Headaches: 47 Ways to Stop the Pain.* New York: Walker, 1995.

Maas, Paula, and Deborah Mitchell. *The Natural Health Guide to Headache Relief: The Definitive Handbook of Natural Remedies for Treating Every Kind of Headache Pain.* New York: Pocket Books, 1997.

Minirth, Frank B., with Sandy Dengler. *The Headache Book.* Nashville: Nelson Publishers, 1994.

Solomon, Seymour, and Steven Fraccaro. *The Headache Book.* Yonkers, N.Y.: Consumer Reports Books, 1991.

Health, wellness, and stress

Barsky, Arthur J. *Worried Sick: Our Troubled Quest for Wellness.* Boston: Little, Brown, 1988.

Benson, Herbert. *The Wellness Book: The Complete Guide to Maintaining Health and Treating Stress-Related Illness.* Secaucus, N.J.: Carol Publishing, 1992.

Bohm, David *Wholeness and the Implicate Order.* London: Ark, 1980.

Campbell, Joseph. *The Inner Reaches of Outer Space.* New York: Alfred Van Der Marck, 1985.

Capra, Fritjof. *The Turning Point.* New York: Bantam, 1982.

Castenada, Carlos. *The Art of Dreaming.* New York: Harper Collins, 1993.

Dubos, Rene. *Mirage of Health.* New York: Anchor Books, 1959.

Hoffer, Eric. *The True Believer.* New York: Harper and Row, 1951.

Illich, Ivan. *Medical Nemesis: The Expropriation of Health.* New York: Pantheon, 1982.

Ornstein, Robert, and David Sobel. *The Healing Brain: Breakthrough Discoveries About How the Brain Keeps Us Healthy.* New York: Simon & Schuster, 1987.

Pelletier, Kenneth R. *Sound Mind, Sound Body: A Model for Lifelong Health.* New York: Simon and Schuster, 1994.

Peterson, Christopher, and Lisa M. Bossio. *Health and Optimism.* New York: Macmillan, 1991.

Simonton, Carl. *Getting Well Again.* New York: Bantam Books, 1978

Starr, Paul. *The Social Transformation of American Medicine.* New York: Basic Books, 1982.

Strasburg, Kate, et al. *The Quest for Wholeness: An Annotated Bibliography in Patient-Centered Medicine.* Bolinas, Calif.: Commonweal, 1991.

Stutz, David, and Bernard Feder. *The Savvy Patient: How to Be an Active Participant in Your Medical Care.* Yonkers, N.Y.: Consumer Reports Books, 1990.

Weil, Andrew. *Eight Weeks to Optimum Health: Proven Program for Taking Full Advantage of Your Body's Healing Power.* New York: Alfred A. Knopf, 1997.

Wolinsky, Stephen. *Quantum Consciousness: The Guide to Experiencing Quantum Psychology.* Norfolk, Conn.: Bramble Books, 1993.

Heart Attack

Dembroski, T.M., et al. "Components of Hostility as Predictors of Sudden Death and Myocardial Infarction in the Multiple Risk Factor Intervention Trial." *Psychosomatic Medicine* 51 (1989): 514–22.

Friedman, Meyer, and Diane Ulmer. *Treating Type A Behavior and Your Heart.* New York: Fawcett, 1985.

Kerman, D. Ariel. *The H.A.R.T. Program: Lower Your Blood Pressure Without Drugs.* New York: HarperCollins Publishers, 1992.

Ornish, Dean. *Dr. Dean Ornish's Program for Reversing Heart Disease.* New York: Ballantine, 1992.

Williams, Redford. *The Trusting Heart: Great News About Type A Behavior.* New York: Times Books/Random House, 1989.

Holistic medicine See ALTERNATIVE THERAPIES; MIND-BODY CONNECTIONS

Hypnosis

Callan, Jean. "Hypnosis: Trick or Treatment?" *Health,* May/June 1997.

Erickson, M.H., and E.L. Rossi. *Hypnotherapy: An Exploratory Casebook.* New York: Irvington, 1979.

Hadley, Josie, and Carol Staudacher. *Hypnosis for Change.* Oakland, Calif.: New Harbinger Publications, 1996.

Haley, J. *Advanced Techniques of Hypnosis and Therapy: Selected Papers of Milton H. Erickson, M.D.* New York: Grune & Stratton, 1967.

Lankton, S.R., ed. *Ericksonian Hypnosis: Application, Preparation, and Research.* New York: Brunner/Mazel, 1988.

Rhue J.W., S.J. Lynn, and I. Kirsch, eds. *Handbook of Clinical Hypnosis.* Washington, D.C.: American Psychological Association, 1993.

Rossi, E.L. *The Psychology of Mind-Body Healing: New Concepts of Therapeutic Hypnosis.* New York: Norton, 1993.

Imagery See GUIDED IMAGERY

Immune system See also PSYCHONEUROIMMUNOLOGY

Borysenko, M. "The Immune System: An Overview." *Annals of Behavioral Medicine* 9 (1987): 3–10.

Cohen, S., D.A.J. Tyrrell, and A.P. Smith. "Psychological Stress and Susceptibility to the Common Cold." *New England Journal of Medicine* 325 (1991): 606–12.

Herbert, Tracy B. "Stress and the Immune System." *World Health,* March-April 1994.

Locke, Steven, and Douglas Colligan. *The Healer Within,* New York: New American Library, 1986.

Job loss See WORKPLACE

Marriage and divorce

Briscoe, D. Stuart. *Marriage Matters! Growing Through the Differences and Surprises of Life Together.* Wheaton, Ill.: H. Shaw, 1994.

Gottman, John Mordechai. *Why Marriages Succeed or Fail: What You Can Learn From the Breakthrough Research to Make Your Marriage Last.* New York: Simon & Schuster, 1994.

O'Neill, Nena, and George O'Neill. *Open Marriage: A New Life Style for Couples.* New York: M. Evans, 1972.

Roleff, Tamara L., and Mary E. Williams, ed. *Marriage and Divorce.* San Diego: Greenhaven Press, 1997.

Simpson, Eileen B. *Late Love: A Celebration of Marriage After Fifty.* Boston: Houghton Mifflin, 1994.

Meditation See also MINDFULNESS MEDITATION

Benson, Herbert. *Beyond the Relaxation Response.* New York: Berkeley Press, 1985.

———. *The Relaxation Response.* New York: Avon Books, 1975.

Borysenko, Joan, and J. Duscher. *On Wings of Light: Meditations for Awakening to the Source.* New York: Warner Books, 1992.

Chopra, Deepak. *Ageless Body, Timeless Mind.* New York: Crown, 1993.

———. *Creating Affluence: Wealth Consciousness in the Field of All Possibilities.* San Rafael, Calif.: New World Library, 1993.

———. *Creating Health: How to Wake Up the Body's Intelligence.* Boston: Houghton Mifflin, 1991.

———. *Quantum Healing.* New York: Bantam, 1989.

———. *Unconditional Life.* New York: Bantam, 1992.

Connor, Danny, with Michael Tse. *Qigong, Chinese Movement & Meditation for Health.* York Beach, Me.: Samuel Weiser, 1992.

Cousins, Norman. *The Healing Heart.* New York: Norton, 1983.

Denniston, Denise, and Peter McWilliams. *The TM Book: Transcendental Meditation, How to Enjoy the Rest of Your Life.* Allen Park, Mich.: Versemonger Press, 1975.

Dossey, L. *Meaning and Medicine: A Doctor's Tales of Breakthrough and Healing* New York: Bantam, 1991.

———. *Recovering the Soul.* New York: Bantam, 1989.

———. *Space, Time and Medicine.* Boston: Shambhala, 1982.

Dychtwald, K. *Bodymind.* Los Angeles: Tarcher, 1986.

Goleman, Daniel. *The Meditative Mind.* Los Angeles: Tarcher, 1988.

Levey, Daniel. *The Fine Arts of Relaxation, Concentration and Meditation.* London: Wisdom Publications, 1987.

Mahesh Yogi, Maharishi. *Science of Being and Art of Living: Transcendental Meditation.* New York: Meridian, 1995.

Nuernberger, Phil. *Freedom From Stress.* Honesdale, Pa.: Himalayan International Institute of Yoga Science and Philosophy, 1985.

Trungpa, Chogyam. *Shambhala: The Sacred Path of the Warrior.* Boston: Shambhala, 1984.

Mindfulness meditation (insight meditation)

Goldstein, Joseph, and Jack Kornfield. *Seeking the Heart of Wisdom: The Path of Insight Meditation.* Boston: Shambhala, 1987.

Hanh, Thich Nhat. *Being Peace.* Berkeley: Parallax Press, 1987.

———. *The Miracle of Mindfulness: A Manual of Meditation.* Boston: Beacon Press, 1976.

———. *The Sun My Heart.* Berkeley: Parallax Press, 1988.

Kabat-Zinn, Jon. *Full Catastrophe Living: Using the Wisdom of Your Body and Mind to Face Stress, Pain and Illness.* New York: Delacorte Press, 1991.

———. *Wherever You Go, There You Are.* New York: Hyperion, 1994.

Levine, Stephen. *A Gradual Awakening.* Garden City, N.Y.: Anchor/Doubleday, 1979.

Suzuki, Shunryu. *Zen Mind, Beginner's Mind.* New York: Weatherhill, 1986.

Mind-body connections See also ALTERNATIVE THERAPIES; PSYCHONEUROIMMUNOLOGY

Benson, Herbert. *Beyond the Relaxation Response.* New York: Berkeley Press, 1985.

———. *The Relaxation Response.* New York: Avon Books, 1975.

Borysenko, Joan. *Guilt Is the Teacher, Love Is the Lesson.* New York: Warner Books, 1991.

———. *Minding the Body, Mending the Mind.* New York: Bantam, 1988.

Cannon, Walter. *The Wisdom of the Body.* New York: Norton, 1939.

Chopra, Deepak. *Perfect Health.* New York: Harmony Books, 1990.

———. *Quantum Healing: Exploring the Frontiers of Mind/Body Medicine.* New York: Bantam Books, 1989.

Cousins, Norman. *Anatomy of an Illness as Perceived by the Patient.* New York: Norton, 1979.

———. *Head First: The Biology of Hope and the Healing Power of the Human Spirit.* New York: Viking Penguin, 1990.

———. *The Healing Heart.* New York: Norton, 1983.

Dienstfrey, Harris. *Where the Mind Meets the Body.* New York: HarperCollins, 1991.

Dossey, Larry. *Space, Time and Medicine.* Boston: Shambhala, 1982.

Goleman, Daniel, and Joel Gurin, eds. *Mind Body Medicine: How to Use Your Mind For Better Health.* Yonkers, N.Y.: Consumer Reports Books, 1993.

Gordon, James S., et al. *Mind, Body and Health: Toward an Integral Medicine.* New York: Human Sciences Press, 1984.

Locke, Steven E., and Douglas Colligan. *The Healer Within: The New Medicine of Mind and Body.* New York: Dutton, 1986.

Moyers, B. *Healing and the Mind.* New York: Doubleday, 1993.

Ornstein, Robert, and David Sobel. THE HEALING BRAIN. New York: Simon & Schuster, 1988.

Pelletier, Kenneth R. *Holistic Medicine: From Stress to Optimum Health.* Magnolia, Mass.: Peter Smith, 1984.

———. *Mind as Healer, Mind as Slayer,* rev. New York: Delacorte, 1992.

———. *Sound Mind, Sound Body: A New Model for Lifelong Health.* New York: Simon & Schuster, 1994.

Siegel, Bernie. *Love, Medicine and Miracles.* New York: Harper and Row, 1986.

———. *Peace, Love and Healing.* New York: Harper and Row, 1989.

Williams, Redford. *The Trusting Heart: Great News About Type A Behavior.* New York: Times Books, 1989.

Nutrition

Brody, Jane. *Jane Brody's Nutrition Book.* New York: W.W. Norton, 1981.

Brown, Judith E. *Everywoman's Guide to Nutrition.* Minneapolis: University of Minnesota Press, 1991.

Finn, Susan Calvert, and Linda Stern. *The Real Life Nutrition Book: Making the Right Food Choices Without Changing Your Life-Style.* New York: Penguin Books, 1992.

Haas, Robert. *Eat Smart, Think Smart: How to Use Nutrients and Supplements to Achieve Maximum Mental and Physical Performance.* New York: HarperCollins, 1994.

Kotsanis, Frank N., and Maureen A. Mackey, eds. *Nutrition in the '90s: Current Controversies and Analysis,* vol. 2. New York: M. Dekker, 1994.

Manahan, William O. *Eat For Health: A Do-It-Yourself Nutrition Guide for Solving Common Medical Problems.* Tiburon, Calif.: H.J. Kramer, 1988.

Quilllan, Patrick. *Beating Cancer with Nutrition.* Tulsa: Nutrition Times Press, 1994.

Tessler, Gordon S. *Lazy Person's Guide to Better Nutrition.* La Jolla, Calif.: Better Health Publishers, 1984.

Werbach, Melvyn. *Healing Through Nutrition: A Natural Approach to Treating 50 Common Illnesses with Diet and Nutrients.* New York: HarperCollins, 1993.

Obsessive-compulsive disorder   See also ANXIETY AND ANXIETY DISORDERS

Alper, Gerald. *The Puppeteers: Studies of Obsessive Control.* New York: Fromm, 1994.

Reyes, Karen. "Obsessive-Compulsive Disorder: There Is Help," *Modern Maturity,* November-December 1995.

Occupational stress   See WORKPLACE

Pain

Bogin, Meg. *The Path of Pain Control.* Boston: Houghton Mifflin, 1982.

Corey, David, with Stan Solomon. *Pain: Free Yourself for Life.* New York: NAL-Dutton, 1989.

Melzack, Ronald, and Patrick Wall. *The Challenge of Pain.* New York: Penguin Books, 1988.

Stacy, Charles B., et al. *The Fight Against Pain.* Yonkers, N.Y.: Consumer Reports Books, 1992.

Sternbach, Richard A. *Mastering Pain: A Twelve-Step Program for Coping with Chronic Pain.* New York: Putnam, 1987.

Panic attacks and panic disorder   See ANXIETY AND ANXIETY DISORDERS

Pharmacological approach

Appleton, William S. *Prozac and the New Antidepressants: What You Need to Know About Prozac, Zoloft, Paxil, Luvox, Wellbutrin, Effexor, Serzone, and More.* New York: Plume, 1997.

Bloomfield, Harold H., and Peter McWilliams. *How to Heal Depression.* Los Angeles: Prelude Press, 1994.

Fieve, Ronald R. *Prozac.* New York: Avon, 1994.

Turkington, Carol. *Making the Prozac Decision: A Guide to Antidepressants.* Los Angeles: Lowell House, 1994.

Wilkinson, Beth. *Drugs and Depression.* New York: Rosen, 1994.

Phobias   See also ANXIETY AND ANXIETY DISORDERS

Bourne, Edmund J. *The Anxiety & Phobia Workbook.* Oakland, Calif.: New Harbinger Publications, 1995.

Doctor, Ronald M., and Ada P. Kahn *Encyclopedia of Phobias, Fears and Anxieties.* New York: Facts On File, 1989.

DuPont, Robert L. *Phobia: A Comprehensive Summary of Modern Treatments.* New York: Brunner/Mazel, 1982.

Jampolsky, Gerald. *Love Is Letting Go of Fear.* New York: Bantam Books, 1979.

Marks, Isaac M. *Fears, Phobias, and Rituals.* Oxford: Oxford University Press, 1987.

———. *Living with Fear.* New York: McGraw-Hill, 1980.

Marshall, John R. *Social Phobia: From Shyness to Stage Fright.* New York: Basic Books, 1994.

Monroe, Judy. *Phobias: Everything You Wanted to Know, But Were Afraid to Ask.* Springfield, N.J.: Enslow Publishers, 1996.

Nardo, Don. *Anxiety and Phobias.* New York: Chelsea House, 1992.

Zane, Manuel D., and Harry Milt. *Your Phobia.* Washington, D.C.: American Psychiatric Press, 1984.

Post-traumatic Stress Disorder (PTSD)   See also ANXIETY AND ANXIETY DISORDERS

Catherall, Donald Roy. *Back from the Brink: A Family Guide to Overcoming Traumatic Stress.* New York: Bantam Books, 1992.

Egendorf, A. *Healing from the War: Trauma and Transformation After Vietnam.* Boston: Houghton Mifflin, 1985.

Eitinger, Leo, and Robert Krell, with Miriam Rieck. *The Psychological and Medical Effects of Concentration Camps and Related Persecutions on Survivors of the Holocaust.* Vancouver: University of British Columbia Press, 1985.

Eth, S., and R.S. Pynoos. *Post-Traumatic Stress Disorder in Children.* Washington, D.C.: American Psychiatric Press, 1985.

Lindy, Jacob D. *Vietnam: A Casebook.* New York: Brunner/Mazel, 1987.

Peterson, Kirtland C., Maurice F. Prout, and Robert A. Schwarz. *Post-traumatic Stress Disorder: A Clinician's Guide.* New York: Plenum Press, 1991.

Porterfield, Kay Marie. *Straight, Talk About Post-Traumatic Stress Disorder: Coping with the Aftermath of Trauma.* New York: Facts On File, 1996.

Sonnenberg, S.M., A.S. Blank, and J.A. Talbott, eds. *The Trauma of War: Stress and Recovery in Vietnam Veterans.* Washington, D.C.: American Psychiatric Press, 1985.

Van der Kolk, B.A., ed. *Post-Traumatic Stress Disorder: Psychological and Biological Sequelae.* Washington, D.C.: American Psychiatric Press, 1984.

Pregnancy

Kitzinger, Sheila. *The Complete Book of Pregnancy and Childbirth. Mississauga,* Ontario: Random House of Canada, 1996.

Psychology, contemporary   See also ALTERNATIVE THERAPIES; MIND-BODY CONNECTIONS; PSYCHONEUROIMMUNOLOGY

Berne, Eric. *Games People Play.* New York: Grove Press, 1964.

Borysenko, Joan. *Guilt Is the Teacher, Love Is the Lesson.* New York: Warner Books, 1990.

Bradshaw, John. *Bradshaw On: The Family.* Deerfield Beach, Fla.: Health Communications, 1988.

———. *Healing the Shame That Binds You.* Deerfield Beach, Fla.: Health Communications, 1988.

Cousins, Norman. *The Healing Heart.* New York: Avon Books, 1984.

Csikzentmihalyi, Mihaly. *Flow: The Psychology of Optimal Experience.* New York: Harper Collins Perennial, 1991.

Peck, M. Scott. *The Road Less Traveled.* New York: Simon and Schuster, 1978.

Wolinsky, Stephen H. *Quantum Consciousness: The Guide to Experiencing Quantum Psychology.* Norfolk, Conn.: Bramble Books, 1993.

Psychoneuroimmunology

Ader, Robert, D. Felton and N. Cohen, eds. *Psychoneuroimmunology.* 2nd ed. San Diego: Academic Press, 1990.

Bohm, David. *Wholeness and the Implicate Order.* London: Routledge and Kegan Paul, 1980.

Cousins, Norman. *Anatomy of an Illness.* New York: Bantam Books, 1981.

Kiecolt-Glaser, J.K., and R. Glaser. "Psychoneuroimmunology: Can Psychological Interventions Modulate Immunity?" *Journal of Consulting and Clinical Psychology* 60 (1992): 569–75.

Relaxation

Agras, W.S., et al. "Relaxation Training for Essential Hypertension at the Worksite: II: The Poorly Controlled Hypertensive." *Psychosomatic Medicine* 49 (1987): 264–73.

Benson, Herbert. *Beyond the Relaxation Response.* New York: Berkeley Press, 1985.

———. *The Relaxation Response.* New York: Avon Books, 1975.

———. *Your Maximum Mind.* New York: Times Books, 1987.

Benson, Herbert, Eileen M. Stuart, and staff of the Mind/Body Medical Institute. *The Wellness Book: The Comprehensive Guide to Maintaining Health and Treating Stress-Related Illness.* New York: Carol, 1992.

Blumenfeld, Larry, ed. *The Big Book of Relaxation: Simple Techniques to Control the Excess Stress in Your Life.* Roslyn, N.Y.: Relaxation Company, 1994.

Davis, Martha, Elizabeth Robbins Eshelman, and Matthew McKay. *The Relaxation and Stress Reduction Workbook.* Oakland, Calif.: New Harbinger Publications, 1995.

Self-esteem

Hazelton, Deborah M. *Solving the Self-Esteem Puzzle.* Deerfield Beach, Fla.: Health Communications 1991.

Hillman, Carolynn. *Recovery of Your Self-Esteem.* New York: Simon & Schuster, 1992.

Johnson, Carol. *Self-Esteem Comes in All Sizes.* New York: Doubleday, 1995.

Kahn, Ada P., and Sheila Kimmel. *Empower Yourself: Every Woman's Guide to Self-Esteem.* New York: Avon Books, 1997.

Lindenfield, Gael. *Self-Esteem.* New York: HarperPaperbacks, 1997.

Minchinton, Jerry. *Maximum Self-Esteem: The Handbook for Reclaiming Your Sense of Self-Worth.* Yanzant, Miss.: Arnford House Publishers, 1993.

Porat, Frieda. *Self-Esteem: The Key to Success in Work and Love.* Saratoga, Calif.: R & E Publishers, 1988.

Prato, Louis. *Be Your Own Best Friend. How to Achieve Greater Self-Esteem, Health, and Happiness.* New York: Berkeley Books, 1994.

Steinem, Gloria. *Revolution From Within: A Book of Self-Esteem.* Boston: Little, Brown, 1992.

Smoking

Buckley, Christopher. *Thank You for Not Smoking.* New York: Random House, 1994.

Hammond, S. Katharine. "Environmental Tobacco Smoke Presents Substantial Risk in Workplaces." *The Journal of the American Medical Association,* September 26, 1995.

Liesges, Robert C., and Margaret DeBon. *How Women Can Finally Stop Smoking.* Alameda, Calif.: Hunter House, 1994.

Mowat, David L., Darlene Mecredy, Frank Lee, et al. "Family Physicians and Smoking Cessation." *Canadian Family Physician* 42 (October 1996): 1946.

Pietrusza, David. *Smoking.* San Diego: Lucent Books, 1997.

Rogers, Jacquelyn. *You Can Stop Smoking.* New York: Pocket Books, 1995.

Sanders, Pete, and Steve Myers. *Smoking.* Brookfield, Conn.: Copper Beech Books, 1996.

Social support and self-help

Feiden, Karyn. *Hope and Help for Chronic Fatigue Syndrome.* New York: Prentice-Hall, 1990.

Kahn, Ada P. "Psychosocial Support Influences Survival of Cancer Patients." *Psychiatric News,* October 1991.

Kreiner, Anna. *Everything You Need to Know About Creating Your Own Support System.* New York: Rosen, 1996.

Locke, Steve, and Douglas Colligan. *The Healer Within.* New York: New American Library, 1986.

Pilisuk, Marc, and Susan H. Parks. *The Healing Web: Social Networks and Human Survival.* Hanover, N.H.: University Press of New England, 1986.

Spiegel, David. *Living Beyond Limits.* New York: Times Books, 1993

White, Barbara J., and Edward J. Madara. *The Self-Help Sourcebook: Finding & Forming Mutual Aid Self-Help Groups.* Denville, N.J.: American Self-Help Clearinghouse, St. Clares-Riverside Medical Center, 1992.

Stress and stress management

Antonovsky, A. *Unraveling the Mystery of Health: How People Manage Stress and Stay Well.* San Francisco: Jossey-Bass, 1987.

Brammer, L.M. *How to Cope with Life Transitions: The Challenge of Personal Change.* New York: Hemisphere Publishing, 1991.

Bridges, William. *Managing Transitions: Making the Most of Change.* Reading, Mass.: Addison-Wesley, 1991.

———. *Transitions: Making Sense of Life's Changes.* Reading, Mass.: Addison-Wesley, 1980.

Colin, Stacey. "How to Find Your Stress Hot Spots." *McCall's,* September 1994.

Cuban, Barbara. "Getting the Best of Stress." *Diabetes Forecast,* June 1989, 43.

Eliot, Robert S. *From Stress to Strength: How to Lighten Your Load and Save Your Life.* New York: Bantam Books, 1994.

Eliot, Robert, and Dennis Breo. *Is It Worth Dying For?* New York: Bantam Books, 1987.

Faelten, Sharon, and David Diamond. *Take Control of Your Life: A Complete Guide to Stress Relief.* Emmaus, Pa.: Rodale Press, 1988.

Feder, Barnaby J. "A Spreading Pain, and Cries for Justice." *The New York Times,* June 5, 1994.

Flint, Robert S. *From Stress to Strength: How to Lighten Your Load and Save Your Life.* New York: Bantam Books, 1994.

Gordon, James S. *Stress Management.* New York: Chelsea House Publishers, 1990.

Hafen, B.Q., et al. *The Health Effects of Attitudes, Emotions and Relationships.* Provo, Utah: EMS Associates, 1992.

Lark, Susan M. *Anxiety and Stress. A Self-Help Program.* Los Altos, Calif.: Westchester, 1993.

Lehrer, Paul M., and Robert L. Woolfolk, eds. *Principles and Practice of Stress Management,* 2nd ed. New York: Guilford Press, 1993.

Maddi, Salvatore, and Suzanne Kobasa. *The Hardy Executive: Health Under Stress.* Homewood, Ill.: Dow Jones-Irwin, 1984.

Miller, Lyle H., and Alma Dell Smith. *The Stress Solution: An Action Plan to Manage the Stress in Your Life.* New York: Pocket Books, 1993.

Ornish, Dean. *Stress, Diet, and Your Heart.* New York: Holt, Rinehart and Winston, 1983.

Padus, Emrika, ed. *The Complete Guide to Your Emotions and Your Health.* Emmaus, Pa.: Rodale Press, 1992.

Patel, Chandra. *The Complete Guide to Stress Management.* New York: Plenum Press, 1991.

Roggenbuck Gillespie, Peggy. *Less Stress in 30 Days: An Integrated Program for Relaxation.* New York: New American Library, 1986.

Sapolsky, Robert M. *Why Zebras Don't Get Ulcers.* New York: W.H. Freeman & Company, 1994.

Seaward, Brian Luke. *Managing Stress: Principles and Strategies for Health and Wellbeing; Managing Stress: A Creative Journal.* Boston: Jones and Bartless Publishers, 1994.

Selye, Hans. *The Stress of Life,* rev. New York: McGraw-Hill, 1978.

———. *Stress Without Distress.* New York: Lipincott, 1974.

Snyder, Solomon H., ed. *Stress Management.* New York: Chelsea House Publishers, 1990.

Visualization   See GUIDED IMAGERY

Women

Berg, Barbara J. *The Crisis of the Working Mother.* New York: Summit Books, 1986.

Freudenberger, Herbert, and Gail North. *Women's Burnout: How to Spot It, How to Reverse It, and How to Prevent It.* Garden City, N.Y.: Doubleday, 1985.

Kahn, Ada P. "Women and Stress." *Sacramento Medicine,* September 1995.

Lerner, Harriet Goldhor. *The Dance of Anger.* New York: Harper & Row, 1985.

———. *The Dance of Intimacy.* New York: Harper & Row, 1989.

Long, B.C., and C.J. Haney. "Coping Strategies for Working Women: Aerobic Exercise and Relaxation Interventions." *Behavior Therapy* 19 (1988): 75–83.

Powell, J. Robin. *The Working Woman's Guide to Managing Stress.* Englewood Cliffs, N.J.: Prentice-Hall, 1994.

Siress, Ruth Hermann. *Working Women's Communications Survival Guide: How to Present Your Ideas With Impact, Clarity, and Power and Get the Recognition You Deserve.* Englewood Cliffs, N.J.: Prentice-Hall, 1994.

Witkin-Lanoil, Georgia. *The Female Stress Syndrome: How to Become Stress-Wise in the '90s.* New York: Berkley Books, 1991.

Workplace

Adams, Scott. *The Dilbert Principle: A Cubicle's-Eye View of Bosses, Meetings, Management Fads and Other Workplace Afflictions.* New York: HarperBusiness, 1997.

Arrobe, Tanya. "Reducing the Cost of Stress: an Organizational Model" *Personnel Review* 19 (Winter 1990).

Brown, Stephanie. *Preventing Computer Injury: The Hand Book with KeyMoves Software.* New York: Ergonome, 1993.

Buono, Anthony F., and James L. Bowditch. *The Human Side of Mergers and Acquisitions: Managing Collisions Between People, Cultures and Organizations.* San Francisco: Jossey Bass Publishers, 1989.

Donkin, Scott W. *Sitting on the Job: How to Survive the Stresses of Sitting Down to Work—A Practical Handbook.* Boston: Houghton Mifflin, 1986.

Frankenhaeuser, Marianne. "The Psychophysiology of Workload, Stress, and Health: Comparison Between the Sexes." *Annals of Behavioral Medicine* 13 (4): 197–204.

Karasek, Robert, and Tores Theorell. *Health Work: Stress, Productivity: and the Reconstruction of Working Life.* New York: Basic Books, 1990.

Leana, Carrie R., and Daniel C. Feldman. *Coping with Job Loss: How Individuals, Organizations and Communities Respond to Layoffs.* New York: Lexington Books, 1992.

Meyer, G.J. *Executive Blues: Down and Out in Corporate America.* New York: Franklin Square Press, 1997.

Murphy, Lawrence R. "Stress Management in Work Settings: A Critical Review of the Health Effects." *American Journal of Health Promotion,* 11, no. 2 (November/December 1996).

Paulsen, Barbara. "Work and Play: A Nation Out of Balance." *Health,* October 1994.

Peterson, Michael. "Work, Corporate Culture, and Stress: Implications for Worksite Health Promotion." *American Journal of Health Behavior* 21, no. 4 (1997): 243–52.

Riley, Anne W., and Stephen J. Zaccaro, ed. *Occupational Stress and Organizational Effectiveness.* New York: Praeger, 1987.

Rosch, Paul J. "Measuring Job Stress: Some Comments on Potential Pitfalls." *American Journal of Health Promotion* 11, no. 6 (July/August 1997).

Rosen, Robert. *The Healthy Company.* Los Angeles: Jeremy P. Tarcher, 1991.

Schnall, Peter L., Carl Pieper, and Joseph E. Schwartz. "The Relationship Between Job Strain, Workplace Disastolic Blood Pressure, and Left Ventricular Mass Index: Results of a Case-control Study." *Journal of the American Medical Association* 263, no. 7 (April 11, 1990).

Schor, Juliet. *The Overworked American: The Unexpected Decline of Leisure.* New York: Basic Books, 1991.

Shalowitz, Deborah. "Another Health Care Headache: Job Stress Could Strain Corporate Budgets." *Business Insurance* 25 (May 20, 1991).

Snyder, Don J. *The Cliff Walk: A Memoir of a Lost Job and a Found Life.* Boston: Little, Brown, 1997.

Veninga, Robert L., and James P. Spradley. *The Work Stress Connection.* New York: Ballantine Books, 1981.

Walker, Cathy. "Workplace stress." *Canadian Dimension* 27 (August 1993).

Wolf, Stewart G. Jr., and Albert J. Finestone. *Occupational Stress.* Littleton, Mass.: PSG Publishing, 1986.

Yoga

Devananda, Swami Vishnu. *The Swivananda Companion to Yoga.* New York: Fireside/Simon & Schuster, 1983.

Groves, Dawn. *Yoga for Busy People: Increase Energy and Reduce Stress in Minutes a Day.* Emeryville, Calif.: New World Library, 1995.

Iyengar, Geeta S. *Yoga: A Gem for Women.* Palo Alto, Calif.: Timeless Books, 1990.

Lad, Vasant, and David Frawley. *The Yoga of Herbs,* Santa Fe.: Lotus Press, 1986.

Taylor, Louise. *A Woman's Book of Yoga: A Journal for Health and Self-Discovery.* Boston: Charles F. Tuttle, 1993.

Terkel, Susan Neiburg. *Yoga Is For Me.* Minneapolis: Lerner Publications, 1987.

Vishnudevananda, Swami. *The Complete Illustrated Book of Yoga.* New York: Crown/Julian Press, 1960.

INDEX

Numbers in **boldface** indicate major treatment of a topic

A

AA *See* Alcoholics Anonymous
AAD *See* American Academy of Dermatology
AAHA *See* American Animal Hospital Association
AAMI *See* age-associated memory impairment
AARP *See* American Association of Retired Persons
ABA *See* American Bar Association
abortion **1–2,** 231, 273, 274, 348
absenteeism **2**
    alcohol and 25
    back pain and 53–55
    burnout and 71–72
    employee assistance programs and 136
    school avoidance 296
    in shift work 310
abuse **123–25,** 299, 352
    addiction 11–12, 352
    of alcohol 24–27
    ambivalence and 35–36
    effect on self-esteem 299
ACA *See* American Chiropractic Association
Academy for Guided Imagery, The 155
access to care **2–3**
acculturation **3–4,** 229, 236
Accutane 5
acne **4–5**
Acne (AAD publication) 6
acquired immunodeficiency syndrome (AIDS) **6–9,** 305, 307
    adultery and 13
    dating and 122, 304, 310
    marijuana as treatment 215
    prevention of 92, 296
    rape and 285
    See also human immunodeficiency virus (HIV)
acrophobia 9
ACSM *See* American College of Sports Medicine
ACTH *See* adrenocorticotrophic hormone
acupressure **9,** 65, 164, 219, 310
acupuncture **9–11,** 65, 77, 138, 164, 184, 310
Adaptation to Life (Valliant) 95
addiction 10, **11–13,** 87, 150, 180
    See also alcohol and alcoholism; anxiety; behavior therapy
ADEAR Center Alzheimer's Disease Education and Referral 35

adenosine 73
Ader, Robert 279
ADHD *See* attention-deficit/hyperactivity disorder
Administration on Aging 17
adolescents **282–83**
    acne 4–5
    with AIDS 7–8
    autonomy of 50
    with depression 15, 115–16
    peer pressure of 253–54
    pregnant **272–73,** 348–49
    puberty 354
    shyness 312
    smoking 318
    suicide of 330, 332
Adopting Your Child (Reynolds) 12, 13
adoption **12,** 211, 348, 349
ADRDA *See* Alzheimer's Disease and Related Disorders Association
adrenaline (epinephrine) **13,** 36, 73, **139–41,** 145, 174, 262, 337
adrenergic nervous system 21
adrenocorticotrophic hormone **9**
adultery **13**
advance directives **108–9,** 138
Advances: The Journal of Mind-Body Health 328
advertising **13–14,** 139, 254
Aerobics and Fitness Association of America 141
affective disorders **14–16,** 111
    See also specific affective disorders
affirmation 74
age-associated memory impairment (AAMI) 33, 147, 223
age discrimination **17–18**
Age Discrimination in Employment Act of 1967 17
Ageless Body, Timeless Mind (Chopra) 80, 81
aggression 18, **43–44,** 49, 124
aging **18–19,** 80–81
    Alzheimer's disease and 33–35
    arthritis and 42–43
    deafness and 106
    sex drive and 302
    women and 356–57
    See also elderly parents
Aging Myths (Kra) 223
agoraphobia **19–23,** 87, 265, 321
Agoraphobia (Frampton) 23
AIDS *See* acquired immunodeficiency syndrome
AIDS-Hotlines National AZT Hotline 8, 186
airplanes and airports **23–24**

crowds and 20, 21, 85, 352
flight cancellations and delays 324, 352
motion sickness and 234–35
terrorism and 341
See also jet lag
Al-Anon 27
alcohol and alcoholism **24–28,** 223, 259
    acculturation and 3
    addiction 11–12
    agoraphobia and 23
    among elderly 332
    among homeless 176
    codependancy and 87
    depression and 298
    in dysfunctional families 128
    genetic factors and 25
    nutrition affected by 242
    treatment for 10, 50, 56–59
    See also support groups
Alcoholics Anonymous (AA) 27, 87, 135, 136, 151, 312
Alexander, Matthias 28
Alexander technique **28,** 53–55
allergies 28–30, 44–46, 69–71, 116, 190
alopecia 157
Alpern, Lynne 187
alprazolam (Xanax) 22, 24, **30,** 60, 251, 262, 362
Alternative Medicine: Cures or Myths? (Facklam) 33
Alternative Medicine: The Definitive Guide (Burton Goldberg Group) 33, 247
alternative therapies **30–33,** 246–47
    for addiction 11
    for cancer 279
    for diabetes 117
    for headaches 164
    homeopathy and 178
    mind-body connections and 229, 354
    See also specific therapies
Alternative Therapies 204, 243, 259, 280, 328, 360
Alzheimer, Alois 33
Alzheimer's Association 35
Alzheimer's disease **33–35,** 142, 191, 222, 333
Alzheimer's Disease and Related Disorders Association (ADRDA) 34, 35
Alzheimer's Disease International 35
AMA *See* American Management Association; American Medical Association

AMA Book of Womancare (Holt & Weber) 2
AMA Handbook on Mental Retardation (Grossman) 227
ambivalence **35–36**
amenorrhoea 226
American Academy of Allergy and Immunology 29, 30
American Academy of Child and Adolescent Psychiatry 333
American Academy of Dermatology (AAD) 5, 117, 157, 170, 174, 268, 333, 334
American Academy of Facial Plastic and Reconstructive Surgery 96
American Academy of Pain Medicine 249
American Animal Hospital Association (AAHA) 258
American Association for the Study of the Headache 164
American Association of Naturopathic Physicians 239
American Association of Retired People Andrus Foundation 332
American Association of Retired Persons 19, 75–76, 138
American Association of Suicidology 333
American Association on Mental Deficiency 227
American Bar Association (ABA) 25, 138
American Cancer Society 75, 319
American Chiropractic Association (ACA) 79
American College of Allergy and Immunology 30
American College of Nurse-Midwives 274
American College of Obstetricians and Gynecologists 61, 78, 274
American College of Sports Medicine (ACSM) 171
American Demographics 105, 292
American Dental Association 110, 111
American Diabetes Association 118
American Dietetic Association 119
American Educator's Encyclopedia (Dejnozka) 347
American Fertility Society 196
American Foundation for Homeopathy 178
American Gastroenterological Association 119
American Hair Loss Council 157